Difficult Cases in Endourology

Ahmed M. Al-Kandari • Mahesh Desai
Ahmed A. Shokeir • Ahmed M. Shoma
Arthur D. Smith
Editors

Difficult Cases in Endourology

Springer

Editors
Ahmed M. Al-Kandari, M.D., FRCS(C)
Department of Surgery
Kuwait University
Jabriyah
Kuwait City
Kuwait

Mahesh Desai, M.S., FRCS
Department of Urology
Muljibhai Patel Urological Hospital
Nadiad
Gujarat
India

Ahmed A. Shokeir, M.D., Ph.D., FEBU
Department of Urology
Urology and Nephrology Center
Mansoura University
Mansoura
Egypt

Ahmed M. Shoma, M.D.
Department of Urology
Urology and Nephrology Center
Mansoura University
Mansoura
Egypt

Arthur D. Smith, M.D.
Department of Urology
Smith Institute for Urology
Hofstra North Shore – Long Island
Jewish Health System
New Hyde Park
NY
USA

ISBN 978-1-4471-6882-9 ISBN 978-1-84882-083-8 (eBook)
DOI 10.1007/978-1-84882-083-8
Springer London Heidelberg New York Dordrecht

Printed on acid-free paper

Springer is part of Springer Science+Business Media (www.springer.com)

I would like to dedicate this book to the very important people in my life. These people are:

- *First of all, my mother, whose support and prayers I am still enjoying. I can never repay my mother no matter what I do for her in the future.*
- *I also am very grateful to my father, who died several years ago but was so supportive of my becoming a physician.*
- *Finally, I wish to express my appreciation to my life companion, my wife Somayah, mother of my children, who continues over the years to be my support and encouragement in my self-development and who has stood with me during all the difficult periods of my life.*

Ahmed M. Al-Kandari, M.D., FRCS(C)

Preface

The idea of this book, *Difficult Cases in Endourology*, came about from my feeling that a concise book with a practical approach toward the common endourologic procedures and their difficulties was needed. It is of utmost importance that the urologists who are interested in doing endourologic procedures have a good knowledge of the difficulties and complications associated with these procedures and be prepared to deal with them.

It is a great honor for me to collaborate with world experts in endourology, such as the founder of the Endourologic Society, Dr. Arthur Smith. I am honored to be one of his previous fellows in his distinguished Smith Institute for Urology at the Hofstra North Shore-Long Island Jewish Health System. Dr. Smith continues to encourage endourologic training, research, and educational activities all over the world.

Endourology cannot be discussed without a tribute to outstanding urologists and scientists such as our coeditor Dr. Mahesh Desai, who contributed tremendously to this important subspecialty. His endourologic contribution was and continues to be a major reference for this important specialty.

I am also honored to work at and collaborate with the distinguished Mansoura Urology Center in Egypt. There, I have the privilege to work with our two other distinguished coeditors, Dr. Ahmed Shokeir, who is the editor of the *Arab Journal of Urology*, and Dr. Ahmed Shoma, who is a well-known world-class endourologist.

We are pleased to have with us as contributors a group of world experts in endourology who have definitely enriched the book.

I am confident that this book will be an excellent, handy, and practical resource for residents, fellows, and urologists interested in pursuing and performing endourologic procedures.

Finally, we do hope that this book will be an important, practical, and helpful reference in the important and technically demanding subspecialty of endourology.

Ahmed M. Al-Kandari, M.D., FRCS(C)

Contents

Contributors

Ahmed Abed, M.D. Department of Urology, Urology and Nephrology Center, Mansoura University, Mansoura, Egypt

Ahmed M. Al-Kandari, M.D., FRCS(C) Department of Surgery, Kuwait University, Jabriyah, Kuwait City, Kuwait

Khalid Matar Al-Otaibi, MBBS, FRCSC Department of Urology, University of Dammam, Khobar, Saudi Arabia

Abdelghaffar S. Arafa, MCS, MRCS Department of Urology, Alsalam International Hospital, Bned Elgar, Dasma, Kuwait

Demetrius H. Bagley, M.D., FACS Department of Urology, Thomas Jefferson University Hospital, Philadelphia, PA, USA

Tamer S. Barakat, M.D. Department of Urology, Urology and Nephrology Center, Mansoura University, Mansoura, Egypt

Ahmad Samy Bedair, M.D. Department of Urology, Faculty of Medicine, Cairo University, Giza, Egypt

Amit Satish Bhattu, M.S. Department of Urology, Muljibhai Patel Urological Hospital, Nadiad, Gujarat, India

Michael Blute, M.D. Department of Urology, Smith Institute for Urology, Hofstra North Shore –Long Island Jewish Health System, New Hyde Park, NY, USA

Hakan Çakir, M.D. Department of Urology, Acibadem Fulya Hospital, Istanbul, Turkey

Jacob Howard Cohen, M.D., MPH Department of Urology, Lenox Hill Hospital, New York, NY, USA

Francisco Pedro Juan Daels, M.D. Department of Urology, Instituto Universitario del Hospital Italiano de Buenos Aires, Buenos Aires, Argentina

Mahesh Desai, M.S., FRCS Department of Urology, Muljibhai Patel Urological Hospital, Nadiad, Gujarat, India

Amit Doshi, MBBS, M.S. Department of Urology, Muljibhai Patel Urological Hospital, Nadiad, Gujarat, India

Brian Duty, M.D. Department of Urology, Smith Institute for Urology, Hofstra North Shore – Long Island Jewish Health System, New Hyde Park, NY, USA

Ahmed S. El-Hefnawy, M.D. Department of Urology, Urology and Nephrology Center, Mansoura University, Mansoura, Egypt

Ahmed R. El-Nahas, M.D. Department of Urology, Urology and Nephrology Center, Mansoura University, Mansoura, Egypt

Mohamed M. Elsaadany, M.D., M.Sc. Department of Urology, Urology and Nephrology Center, Mansoura University, Mansoura, Egypt

Ahmed Mohamed Elshal, M.D. Department of Urology, Urology and Nephrology Center, Mansoura University, Mansoura, Egypt

Raguram Ganesamoni, M.S., MRCS, MCh Department of Urology, Muljibhai Patel Urological Hospital, Nadiad, Gujarat, India

Arvind P. Ganpule, M.S., DNB, MNAMS Department of Urology, Muljibhai Patel Urological Hospital, Nadiad, Gujarat, India

Ehud Gnessin, M.D. Department of Urology, Hebrew University of Jerusalem and Shaare Zedek Medical Center, Jerusalem, Israel

Michael Grasso III M.D. Department of Urology, Lenox Hill Hospital, New York, NY, USA

Department of Urology, Medical College of New York, New York, NY, USA

Joseph A. Graversen, M.D. Department of Urology, University of California, Irvine, Orange, CA, USA

Mantu Gupta, M.D. Department of Urology, Columbia University, New York, NY, USA

Ahmed M. Harraz, M.D. Department of Urology, Urology and Nephrology Center, Mansoura University, Mansoura, Egypt

Zhaohui He, M.D., Ph.D. Department of Urology, Minimally Invasive Surgical Center, The First Affiliated Hospital of Guangzhou Medical College, Haizhou District, Guangzhou, China

Kelly A. Healy, M.D. Department of Urology, Thomas Jefferson University Hospital, Philadelphia, PA, USA

Hamdy Mohamed Ibrahim, M.D. Department of Urology, Faculty of Medicine, Fayoum University, Giza, Egypt

Brandon K. Isariyawongse, M.D. Department of Urology, Glickman Urological and Kidney Institute, Cleveland Clinic Foundation, Cleveland, OH, USA

Panagiotis Kallidonis, M.D. Department of Urology, University Hospital of Patras, Rion, Patras, Greece

Ahmed M. Labib, MBBCh, M.Sc. Department of Anesthesia, Ain-shams University, Cairo, Egypt

Xun Li, M.D. Department of Urology, Minimally Invasive Surgical Center, The First Affiliated Hospital of Guangzhou Medical College, Haizhou District, Guangzhou, China

Evangelos Liatsikos, M.D., Ph.D. Department of Urology, University Hospital of Patras, Rion, Patras, Greece

James E. Lingeman, M.D. Department of Urology, Methodist Hospital, Indianapolis, IN, USA

Jessica A. Mandeville, M.D. Department of Urology (4SE), Lahey Clinic Medical Center, Burlington, MA, USA

Shashikant Mishra, M.S., DNB Department of Urology, Muljibhai Patel Urological Hospital, Nadiad, Gujarat, India

Manoj Monga, M.D., FACS Department of Urology, Glickman Urological and Kidney Institute, Cleveland Clinic Foundation, Cleveland, OH, USA

Stevan B. Streem Center for Endourology and Stone Disease, Cleveland, OH, USA

Adam C. Mues, M.D. Department of Urology, New York University School of Medicine, New York, NY, USA

Zeph Okeke, M.D. Department of Urology, Smith Institute for Urology, Hofstra North Shore – Long Island Jewish Health System, New Hyde Park, NY, USA

Zhamshid Okhunov, M.D. Department of Urology, Smith Institute for Urology, Hofstra North Shore – Long Island Jewish Health System, New Hyde Park, NY, USA

Yasser Osman, M.D. Department of Urology, Urology and Nephrology Center, Mansoura University, Mansoura, Egypt

Soroush Rais-Bahrami, M.D. The Arthur Smith Institute for Urology, Hofstra North Shore - Long Island Jewish School of Medicine, New Hyde Park, NY, USA

Donnaline Richman, MN, JD Department of Urology, Fager & Amsler, LLP, Syracuse, NY, USA

James H. Robb, M.B.A. Department of Urology, Donald J Fager & Associates, Inc., Medical Liability Mutual Insurance Company, New York, NY, USA

Ravindra B. Sabnis, M.S., MCH Department of Urology, Muljibhai Patel Urological Hospital, Nadiad, Gujarat, India

Ahmed A. Shokeir, M.D., Ph.D., FEBU Department of Urology, Urology and Nephrology Center, Mansoura University, Mansoura, Egypt

Ahmed M. Shoma, M.D. Department of Urology, Urology and Nephrology Center, Mansoura University, Mansoura, Egypt

Arthur D. Smith, M.D. Department of Urology, Smith Institute for Urology, Hofstra North Shore – Long Island Jewish Health System, New Hyde Park, NY, USA

Shady A. Soliman, M.D. Department of Urology, Urology and Nephrology Center, Mansoura University, Mansoura, Egypt

Guohua Zeng, M.D., Ph.D. Department of Urology, Minimally Invasive Surgical Center, The First Affiliated Hospital of Guangzhou Medical College, Haizhou District, Guangzhou, China

Sinan Zeren, M.D. Department of Urology, Acibadem Fulya Hospital, Istanbul, Turkey

Introduction

1

Ahmed M. Al-Kandari

Endourology is the branch of urologic surgery concerned with closed procedures for visualizing or manipulating the urinary tract [1]. This field has evolved tremendously over the past few years. The term was popularized by Dr. Arthur Smith, one of the editors of this book. Dr. Smith as well as other pioneers in this field throughout the world have contributed significantly to innovations in this subspecialty, especially after the founding of the Endourological Society [2].

With this book, the editors have created a handy reference for urologists, residents, and fellows interested in expanding their experience in endourology. In this introductory chapter, I will walk you through the contents to focus on the most important aspects and provide commentary about them.

Issues related to percutaneous renal surgery including stone removal, treatment of ureteropelvic junction obstruction, and treatment of renal pelvic urothelial tumors are the main subjects of this book. Also covered are the different difficult conditions encountered in these procedures. Ureteroscopy will be discussed as well, along with its various aspects and difficulties.

It is well known that anesthesia during surgical procedures is the key for successful patient outcome without major or minor complications, and thus, a chapter covers the selection of anesthesia, especially general anesthesia during percutaneous renal surgery. It is also important to know all the anesthetic options available for cases, including epidural, spinal or hemispinal, or local anesthesia during percutaneous renal surgery.

An adequate time frame for optimal preoperative preparation, for example, for PCNL for large kidneys stones, is essential. This should include proper control for all comorbid conditions if present, such as diabetes, hypertension, pulmonary diseases, as well as cardiac problems. Patients who are on anticoagulants or antiplatelets should discontinue these medications for the proper time interval before percutaneous renal surgery in order to avoid significant bleeding [3].

The issue of prone versus supine percutaneous renal surgery will be addressed since this is an important aspect, especially when prolonged prone position may compromise the respiratory condition of certain cases. Obviously, if one is used to the prone approach as most endourologists in the world are, then preparing for the supine approach with careful understanding of the anatomy and technique and with the assistance of an experienced surgeon in the supine approach is essential and will allow for a safer choice in selected cases. The issue of maximizing access to the ureteropelvic system, especially in complex stone cases or in cases with combined ureteral and renal pathology, is important, as stones with ureteropelvic junction obstruction warrant consideration of efficient patient positioning. Some surgeons prefer prone with open legs and access to urethra and

A.M. Al-Kandari, M.D., FRCS(C)
Department of Surgery, Kuwait University,
Jabriyah, Kuwait City 13110, Kuwait
e-mail: drakandari@hotmail.com

A.M. Al-Kandari et al. (eds.), *Difficult Cases in Endourology*,
DOI 10.1007/978-1-84882-083-8_1, © Springer-Verlag London 2013

kidney. Others prefer supine to mild lateral position with lithotomy to access the urethra and kidney. In all these circumstances, the avoidance of all position-related complications is vital. The use of antiembolic stockings or a pneumatic compression device to avoid deep venous thrombosis especially in lengthy procedures is recommended. Additionally, padding, avoidance of pressure on the extremities, and proper positioning are essential in order to avoid neuropraxias [4].

For percutaneous renal surgery (since there is a potential blood loss), preoperative blood cross matching is essential. Occasionally, when patients have comorbid conditions and after a lengthy procedure, it may be safer to observe the patient overnight in the intensive care unit.

With regard to percutaneous renal surgery and the procedure of choice for most large (over 2 cm) renal and upper ureteric stones [5], several important aspects warrant emphasis:

1. Prone versus supine position
2. General versus epidural anesthesia
3. Fluoroscopic versus ultrasound-guided renal puncture
4. Balloon versus telescopic tract dilatation
5. Ultrasound versus pneumatic versus laser lithotripsy
6. Type of drainage tube for the kidney or keeping it tubeless
7. Size of working puncture size (small or mini versus standard)
8. Options for tract access
9. Postoperative imaging follow-up plan
10. Duration for postoperative hospital stay
11. Management of postpercutaneous renal surgery complications including septic and nonseptic complications

These issues will be discussed in detail from a practical perspective in order to maximize usefulness.

To reach a successful percutaneous renal surgery outcome, the following points deserve close attention and will be covered in detail in subsequent chapters:

1. Complete preoperative imaging assessment and prior accurate selection of the site of access according to the individual patient body and anatomy as well as the stone location, burden, and shape
2. A thorough and honest explanation regarding the stone-free rate after percutaneous renal surgery and the possibility of the need for a second-look operation or shock wave lithotripsy or the need for blood transfusion
3. Well-oriented and experienced anesthesia team
4. Well-trained assistants and nurses
5. Well-oriented X-ray technician to facilitate the movement of the C-arm with different desired angles during the case
6. Blood product preparation
7. Complete availability of equipment and instruments as well as disposables, plus a fully capable operating and circulating nursing staff
8. Careful manipulations in the kidney with security of the guidewire and sheath, gentle movement of the rigid instruments, and careful and vigilant manipulation to avoid mucosal tears or perforations that may complicate the case
9. Use of warm saline irrigation with moderate height and avoidance of any pressure with irrigation
10. Careful observation of blood loss, close monitoring of vital signs, and invasive monitoring if needed, with immediate correction of any abnormality; consideration of expediting and terminating the procedure without delay with nephrostomy tube insertion if major complications occur in order to minimize patient morbidity

Obviously, since most urologists use X-ray for renal access and tract dilation (although sometimes this is done by an interventional radiologist), the importance of following the radiation safety precautions for the urologist and his or her team cannot be overemphasized [6].

In this book, we will also discuss the issue of percutaneous renal surgery for treating ureteropelvic junction obstruction. This technique is very effective for this condition, but proper case selection is important, and patients should be excluded from having this technique when the following are present:

1. Large very dilated renal pelvis
2. Poor renal function as per nuclear scan studies
3. Very high insertion or obvious crossing vessel (although some authors argue against that) [7]

After gaining access in ureteropelvic junction obstruction cases, the choice of endopyelotomy is that of the surgeon's, although we recommend, based on personal experience, the holmium laser due to the fine accurate cut it provides with bloodless field, making this tool very helpful for achieving the goal. It is worth mentioning that one indication for endopyelotomy is after failed previous pyeloplasty [8].

Percutaneous renal surgery for transitional cell carcinoma is reserved for a very select group of patients who have a solitary kidney or impaired renal function with low-grade bulky malignancy. The small low-grade upper tract urothelial tumor burden can be managed with flexible ureteroscopy and laser with excellent results, but obviously the need for rigorous follow-up is essential [9].

Percutaneous renal surgery is also a successful procedure for treatment of bulky renal stones in children, although shock wave lithotripsy was found to be successful in children as well and should be considered. With regard to instruments for percutaneous renal surgery in children, some urologists use small-caliber sheaths and instruments, while others use standard adult instruments with equally safe and effective outcomes [10].

Ureteroscopy has undergone tremendous improvements since it started decades ago, and these improvements benefitted from the technology that led to better optics, miniaturization, use of camera, and flexible ureteroscopy. Along with the development of the scopes, there were significant improvements in the disposables used to achieve a successful minimally invasive ureteroscopy. This included the use of hydrophilic guidewires, the use of nitinol small-caliber baskets, and the use of a grasper which allowed successful access to any location in the pelvicaliceal system, obviously with the easy and excellent assistance of the flexible scopes. The use of small-caliber laser fibers has allowed successful disintegration of most renal stones. The use of ureteral access sheaths has facilitated easy and frequent approach to the upper urinary tract, especially in retrograde management of bulky renal stones.

Ureteroscopy has been shown in multiple reports to be safe and effective in treating ureteral stone problems that can arise in pregnancy. Detailed description of possible approaches in this challenging patient group will be illustrated.

Issues related to endourology training will be discussed. The following methods to expand one's learning of and experience with endourological procedures will be covered:

1. Joining a residency program with a well-established endourological reputation
2. Doing a clinical endourology fellowship
3. Attending different endourological conferences
4. Visiting experts and observing them in action
5. Inviting experts to operate at your facility

The medicolegal issues related to endourological procedures are essential to allow the urologist to practice in a safe environment. Being an expert endourologist may also provide an opportunity to be a scientific expert in legal cases.

Since we are members of the Endourological Society, we are obliged to do further research to improve our outcomes in endourological practice, and we are encouraged to join the scientific efforts of the Clinical Research Office of the Endourological Society (CROES) [11]. Such participation will ultimately improve of our practice and will be reflected positively in the outcomes in our patients.

References

1. Dorland's Medical Dictionary for Health Consumers. Philadelphia: WB Saunders; 2007.
2. WWW.Endourology.org.
3. Gross AJ, Bach T. Preoperative percutaneous stone surgery in patients receiving anticoagulant therapy. J Endourol. 2009;23(10):1563–5.

4. Patel A, Fuchs GJ. Air travel and thromboembolic complications after percutaneous nephrolithotomy for staghorn stone. J Endourol. 1998;12(1):51–3.
5. Bandi G, Best SL, Nakada SY. Current practice patterns in the management of upper urinary tract calculi in the north central United States. J Endourol. 2008;22(4):631–6.
6. Majidpour HS. Risk of radiation exposure during PCNL. Urol J. 2010;7(2):87–9.
7. Stein RJ, Gill IS, Desai MM. Comparison of surgical approaches to ureteropelvic junction obstruction: endopyeloplasty versus endopyelotomy versus laparoscopic pyeloplasty. Curr Urol Rep. 2007;8(2):140–9.
8. Patel T, Kellner CP, Katsumi H, Gupta M. Efficacy of endopyelotomy in patients with secondary ureteropelvic junction obstruction. J Endourol. 2011;25(4):587–9.
9. Keeley Jr FX, Bibbo M, Bagley DH. Ureteroscopic treatment and surveillance of upper urinary tract transitional cell carcinoma. J Urol. 1997;157(5):1560–5.
10. Dogan HS, Kilicarslan H, Kordan Y, Celen S, Oktay B. Percutaneous nephrolithotomy in children: does age matter? World J Urol. 2011;29(6):725–9.
11. de la Rosette J. A platform for global endourological research. J Endourol. 2009;23(10):1551–3.

Anesthetic Considerations During Endourologic Surgery

2

Ahmed M. Labib and Ahmed M. Al-Kandari

Introduction

Urologic surgeries include procedures ranging from "minor" day-case-based procedures to major procedures, causing marked hemodynamic changes. These surgeries have undergone many improvements in the last two decades. A good example of minimally invasive surgical procedures is percutaneous nephrolithotomy (PCNL) and ureteroscopic (URS) lithotripsy. PCNL facilitates a direct approach to calculi with few traumas to the kidneys and surrounding structures than open surgery, and it is the treatment of choice for kidney stones >2 cm, staghorn calculi, and multiple kidney calculi. The techniques used in PCNL have improved, and efforts have been made to decrease morbidity, analgesic needs, and hospitalization time. In a study of hemodynamic changes during general anesthesia during a series of PCNL for staghorn stones, the operation was found to be a challenge because of the possibility of fluid absorption, dilutional anemia, hypothermia, or significant blood loss [1].

A.M. Labib, MBBCh, M.Sc.
Department of Anesthesia, Ain-shams University, Cairo, 11371, Egypt
e-mail: libboo@hotmail.com

A.M. Al-Kandari, M.D., FRCS(C) (✉)
Department of Surgery, Kuwait University, Jabriyah, Kuwait City 13110, Kuwait
e-mail: drakandari@hotmail.com

Preoperative Anesthetic Considerations

Preoperative optimization of patients, evaluation of comorbid conditions, and preparing the patient to be in optimal condition at the time of surgery are essential. Endourologic procedures are mostly elective, and a thorough evaluation with proper time scheduling is important.

Occasionally, elderly patients require anesthesia for endourologic surgeries. In that group, cardiovascular and respiratory diseases are common. Subsequently, patients must be assessed and optimized as much as possible [2].

The urologist at times must consider operating on high-risk patients. These are patients who typically have a high score according to the American Society of Anesthesia (ASA score). A study looked into the outcome between low ASA score (2 or less) versus a score that was higher than 2. This included the patients who needed PCNL. The overall complication rate was similar when comparing the high-risk (12.1 %) and low-risk (12.3 %) groups ($P=0.41$). The stone-free rate for the high-risk group was 61 % compared with 92 % for the low-risk group ($P=0.028$). It was concluded that PCNL can be safely performed in the high-risk preoperative patient population [3].

Next, we enumerate the important preoperative measures that must precede PCNL:

1. The anesthetist who will provide anesthesia for PCNL cases as well as the urologist should be familiar with the case and understand the

A.M. Al-Kandari et al. (eds.), *Difficult Cases in Endourology*,
DOI 10.1007/978-1-84882-083-8_2,

potential complications and be prepared to deal with them.

2. Knowledge of the detailed history of the patient and knowledge of the past history of other medical problems, especially diabetes mellitus, hypertension, ischemic heart disease, renal impairment, and pulmonary problems, are essential. Also, it is very important to know if the patient developed any general complications, for example, bleeding and hypothermia, during similar procedures in the past, since patients are prone to recurrent urinary stone disease.
3. Detailed knowledge of medication history, especially antiplatelets and anticoagulants, is essential. It is contraindicated to do PCNL on patients who are still on anticoagulants.
4. A thorough physical examination including vital signs and body habitus, especially in obese patients, is essential before PCNL.
5. Any patient with other chronic medical problems requiring PCNL should be referred to the physician and specialist for further evaluation.
6. The common important investigations needed before PCNL include the following:
   - Complete blood count (CBC).
   - Full biochemical profile.
   - Coagulation profile including PT, PTT, and, occasionally, bleeding time.
   - Electrocardiogram (ECG), chest X-ray, and possibly echocardiogram in patients with history of heart problem.
   - Urine analysis and culture.
   - Absence of infection is essential before operation.
7. Patients are instructed to take their antihypertensive or heart medications the morning of surgery with sips of water. They should not take their insulin and oral hypoglycemic medications in the morning of surgery. At that time, blood sugar is checked, and, if it is elevated, then short-acting insulin is given or a sliding scale is started with IV fluids.
8. The use of anti-embolic leg stockings or compression bandages is encouraged, especially when a lengthy procedure is anticipated. Subsequently, pneumatic leg compression devices if available are a good alternative to decrease the risk of deep vein thrombosis. It is better to strap the legs so they do not fall (Fig. 2.1).
9. The use of prophylactic IV antibiotics is a standard practice, and this may include second- or third-generation cephalosporin. This is typically given at time of induction of anesthesia.

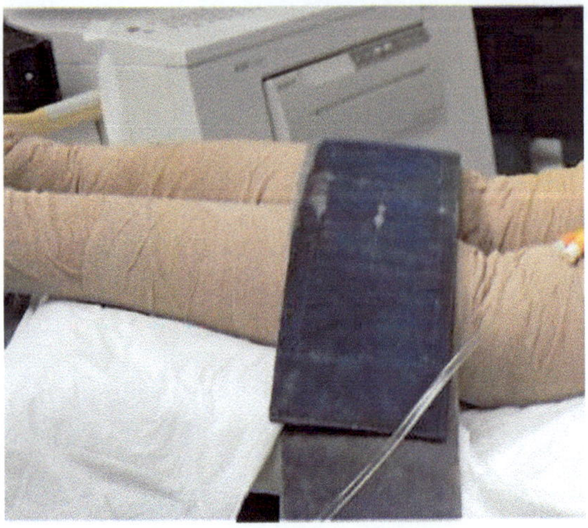

Fig. 2.1 Compression bandage on lower limbs with strap during PCNL in prone position

Important Anesthetic Considerations Regarding the Urogenital System

It is absolutely essential for the anesthetist and important for the urologist to have knowledge about the innervations of the urogenital system, especially when planning for spinal, epidural, or less common local anesthesia during PCNL. Knowledge about the effects of commonly used anesthesia drugs as well as the hemodynamic effects and urine output changes is also very helpful for patient care.

Pain Conduction Pathways of the Urogenital System

The parts of the urogenital system that are in the abdomen receive nerve supply from the autonomic nervous system through sympathetic and parasympathetic pathways. Pelvic urinary organs

Table 2.1 Pain conduction pathways of the urogenital system

Organ	Sympathetics, spinal segments	Parasympathetics	Spinal levels of pain conduction
Kidney	T8–L1	CN X (vagus)	T10–L1
Ureter	T10–L2	S2–4	T10–L2
Bladder	T11–L2	S2–4	T11–L2 (dome), S2–4 (neck)
Prostate	T11–L2	S2–4	T11–L2, S2–4
Penis	L1 and L2	S2–4	S2–4
Scrotum	NS	NS	S2–4
Testes	T10–L2	NS	T10–L1

Reproduced with permission from Malhotra et al. [4]
NS not significant for nociceptive function

and genitalia are supplied by the autonomic and somatic nerves (Table 2.1).

Innervation of the Urogenital System

Sympathetic fibers to the kidney originate as preganglionic fibers from the eighth thoracic through the first lumbar segments and converge at the celiac plexus and aorticorenal ganglia. Postganglionic fibers to the kidney are mainly from the aorticorenal and celiac ganglia (Fig. 2.2). Parasympathetic input is from the vagus nerve [6]. Some anesthetics can cause a reversible transient depression in renal function. Renal blood flow, GFR, urine output, and urinary sodium excretion are decreased (Table 2.2).

Positioning

Anesthesiologists have a serious responsibility for the proper positioning of patients under anesthesia. A patient's positioning requires cooperation of many – anesthesiologists, surgeons, and nurses – to ensure patient safety and well-being while providing surgical exposure. Whenever possible during anesthesia, patients should be placed in a position that they can tolerate while awake.

Prone Position During PCNL

Most urologists use prone positioning during PCNL. In the prone position, the legs have to be in plane with the torso, so hemodynamic reserve is maintained; however, if there is any marked lowering of the legs or tilt of the entire table, venous return may be augmented or decreased, accordingly [7].

We commonly use soft pillows under the chest and pelvis to allow for a better space for the abdomen to move during respiration. Attention must be paid to the ability of the abdomen to hang free and to move with respiration.

When mobilizing the patient to a prone position, care must be taken to avoid pulling on IV cannulae. The legs should be flexed slightly at the knees and hips and padded. The head can be supported facedown and rested on a soft pillow or special head piece that would accommodate the face with the tube or the face turned to the side (Figs. 2.3 and 2.4). The anesthesiologist is responsible for coordinating the move and for repositioning the head. Both arms can be positioned at the patient's sides and tucked in the neutral position. More padding is needed under the elbow to prevent ulnar nerve compression. The arms are not to be abducted more than 90° to prevent excessive brachial plexus stretching. We prefer to use gel pads under any pressure point as much as possible.

The dependent's eyes must be checked frequently for external compression. The head is kept in a neutral position using a horseshoe headrest or a surgical pillow. Careful attention to the eyes must be given during the prone position. Eye care is especially essential in the prone position since there has been documented increase in intraocular pressure in one study; this is a risk in

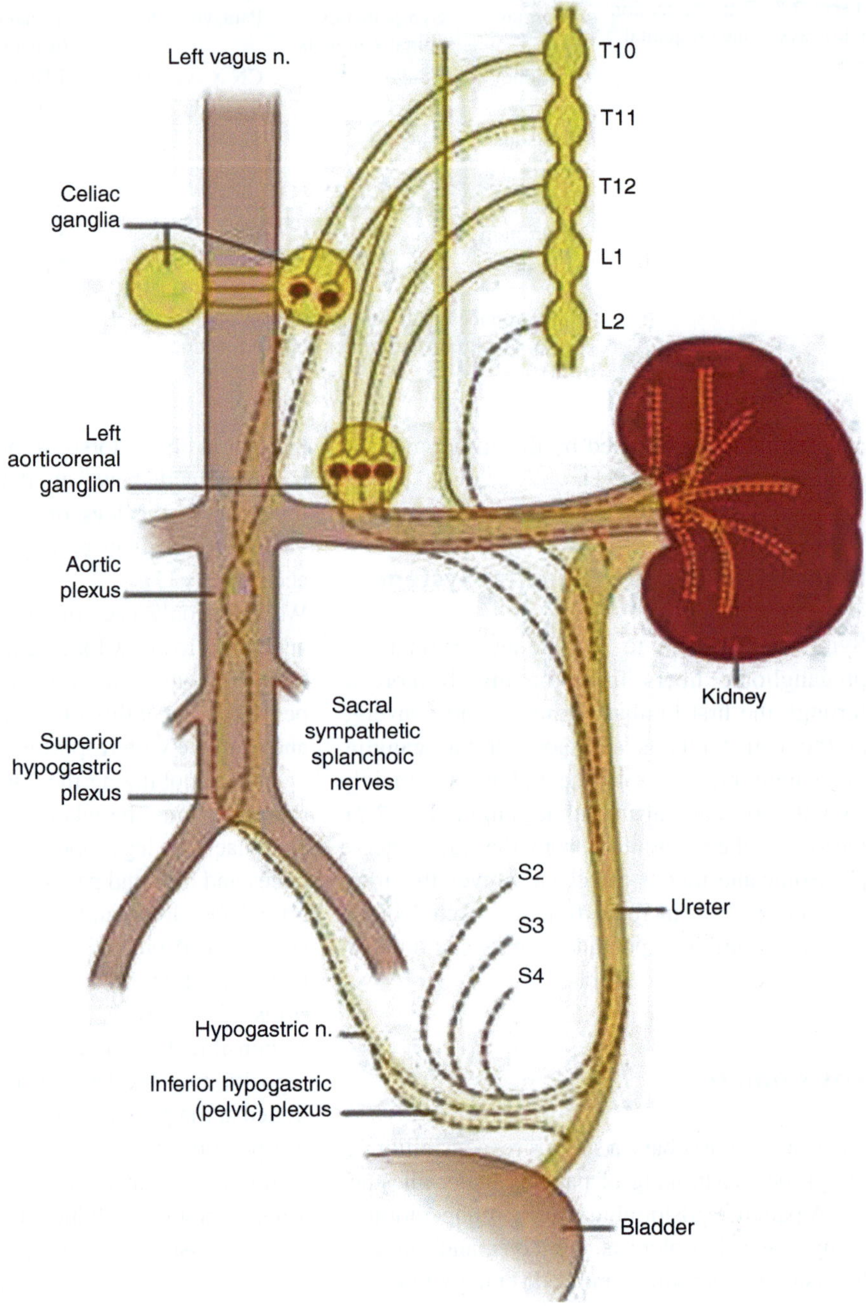

Fig. 2.2 Autonomic and sensory innervation of the kidney and ureters. *Solid line* indicates preganglionic fibers; *dashed line* indicates postganglionic fibers; *dotted line* indicates sensory fibers (Reproduced with permission from Gee and Ansell [5])

glaucoma patients and may cause visual impairment. Intraocular pressure has a linear relationship with time of the procedure [9].

The urologist must ensure that he or she has allowed for table space for the C-arm X-ray machine so that it can move and reach the entire target field easily.

The prone position is especially risky for morbidly obese patients; their respiration is already compromised, and they are difficult to reposition

Table 2.2 Various anesthetics' effects on renal function

	RBF	GFR	Urine output	Urine solutes
General anesthesia	↓	↓	↓	↓
Intravenous anesthetics				
Thiopental	↔	↓	↓	↓
Midazolam	↔	↔	↓	↔
Fentanyl/droperidol	↔	↔	↓	↓
Fentanyl (high dose)	↔	↔	↔	↔
Inhaled anesthetics				
Halothane	↔	↓	↓	↓
Enflurane	↓	↓	↓	↓
Ioflurane	↔	↓	↓	↓
PEEP	↓	↓	↓	0
Regional anesthesia				
Epidural (with epinephrine)	↓	↓	↓	0
Epidural (without epinephrine	↔	↔	↔	0
Spinal	↔	↔	↔	0

Reproduced with permission from Malhotra et al. [4]
Key: no significant change, *o* significant data, decrease, *GFR* glomerular filtration rate, *PEEP* positive end-expiratory pressure, *RBF* renal blood flow

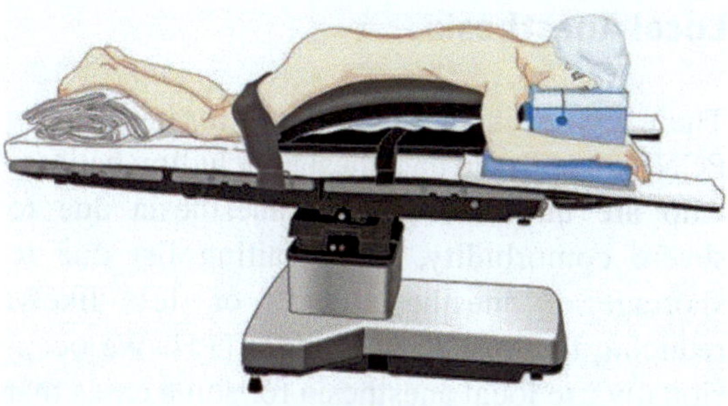

Fig. 2.3 Prone position with Wilson frame. Arms are abducted less than 90° whenever possible. Pressure points are padded, and chest and abdomen are supported away from the bed to minimize abdominal pressure and preserve pulmonary compliance. Soft head pillow has cutouts for eyes and nose and a slot to permit endotracheal tube exit. Eyes must be checked frequently (Reproduced with permission from Cassola and Woo Lee [8])

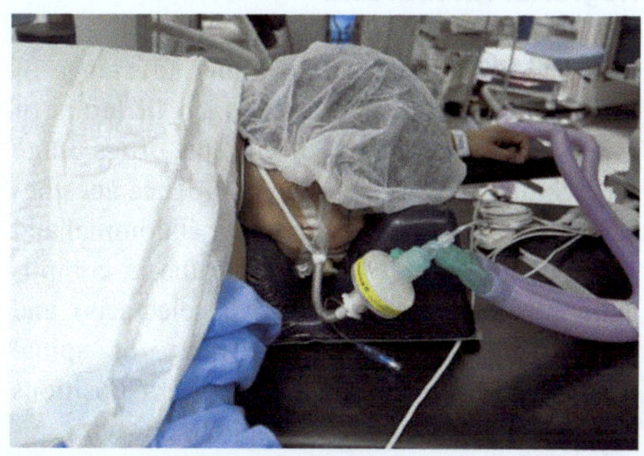

Fig. 2.4 A patient in prone position after being intubated with a special head support with gel pad and empty in the inside to avoid any eye or tube compression

quickly. These patients will benefit from supine or modified supine position.

Types of Anesthesia for PCNL

PCNL is mostly performed under general anesthesia, but recently, a trend toward regional anesthesia is increasing. There are studies proving that local anesthesia with patient sedation can be used for selected cases.

Commonly, the urologist puts the patient in the lithotomy position for cystoscopy and ureteral catheterization with fixation of a urethral catheter. Then the patient is commonly put in the prone position, although some urologists prefer supine or modified supine position; this will be discussed in another chapter.

General Anesthesia

General anesthesia with positive pressure ventilation and muscle relaxation is usually used for PCNL since the patient has to lie in an uncomfortable position during the relatively long procedure. Due to the prone position and the possibility of increased intra-abdominal pressure, endotracheal tube (ETT) is recommended.

Anesthesia induction may be intravenous or inhalational, and rapid sequence induction is preferred in patients known to have autonomic neuropathy. Large bore intravenous access is preferred because of the risk of unexpected hemorrhage. In high-risk patients, especially in complex cases such as PCNL for staghorn stones, we as well as our anesthetist prefer invasive monitoring, for example, central venous line as well as arterial line.

Regional Anesthesia

Regional anesthesia has the same advantage of general anesthesia in the abdomen in terms of avoiding the anaphylaxis of multiple drugs usage [10]. Spinal anesthesia proved to reduce anesthesia charges on patients with lower abdominal and limb surgeries [11]. General anesthesia complications – such as pulmonary (atelectasis) and neurologic (brachial plexus injury or spinal injury), especially during changing of positions – are more common than complications with spinal anesthesia [12]. General anesthesia may be challenging in situations such as PCNL with staghorn calculi because of fluid absorption and electrolyte imbalance possibility, so regional anesthesia is a good alternative [9].

Achieving a good postoperative outcome can be accomplished in most patients, regardless of the anesthetic technique used; however, early postoperative recovery of patients can be influenced by anesthesia, and, because the aim is to discharge patients from hospitals safely as early as possible, the anesthesia choice matters [13].

Spinal anesthesia in adults is typically given with bupivacaine 15 mg, fentanyl 25 μg, which are injected intrathecally at L3–L4 interspace. After this, the head of the patient is kept down for 5–10 min. Subsequently, the anesthesia level is checked. The patient is then put in lithotomy position, and cystoscopy and ureteral catheterization are done. The patient is then put in prone position while awake. Sedation with protection of the airways is done to reduce anxiety. This is given either as midazolam 1 mg or diazepam 2.5 mg IV. In a study comparing general versus regional anesthesia during PCNL, the authors concluded that combined spinal-regional anesthesia is a feasible technique in PCNL operations because the efficacy and safety were not affected [6]. Furthermore, in a prospective trial comparing general versus combined spinal-epidural anesthesia (CSEA) during PCNL, CSEA was shown to be as effective and as safe as PCNL under GA. Patients who undergo PCNL under CESA require lesser analgesic dose and have a shorter hospital stay [14].

Local Anesthesia

There are occasional indications for performing PCNL under local anesthesia, including patients who are unfit for general anesthesia due to severe comorbidity, long waiting list due to shortage of anesthesia staff, or, less likely, reducing the cost of anesthesia [15]. We occasionally use local anesthesia for some cases that are second-look PCNLs in which less manipulation is anticipated.

Pain during PCNL is believed to be caused by dilatation of the renal capsule and parenchyma and is not believed to be due to stone disintegration. Therefore, the renal capsule is the target of local anesthesia. Lignocaine is infiltrated at the renal entry site to block the renal capsule [16].

Local anesthesia with IV sedation including the sedative effect of diazepam and the analgesic effect of pethidine seems to be sufficient in order to perform PCNL in cooperative patients with optimal renal stone size and a dilated upper urinary tract [15].

We have used local anesthesia successfully in second-look PCNLs. These patients have an established tract, and the use of local anesthesia with IV sedation could be a very useful method in these cases.

Monitoring

Monitoring of respiratory and cardiovascular systems is important because of the risks occurring due to patient positioning and the risk of bleeding or complications during PCNL. The decision for invasive blood pressure monitoring using an arterial line or central venous pressure depends on the patient's preoperative condition, as we mentioned earlier. Attention must be given to maintaining the patient's temperature as normal as possible by using warm blankets, warm intravenous fluids, and mattresses. This is essential in order to avoid hypothermia, which is a risk associated with PCNL especially when cold irrigation fluids are used. It is important to use warm irrigation during PCNL.

Since irrigation fluid is part of routine PCNL cases, it is important to be aware of the amount of the fluids used, the level of irrigation height, and the duration of surgery and to recognize the consequences of fluid absorption. A study on fluid absorption during PCNL showed that fluid absorption occurred in 78 % of patients and 28 % absorbed volumes in excess of 1 l. This was found during a study using ethanol 1 % with saline irrigation [17].

It is also important for the urologist as well as the anesthetist to assess patient breathing during the recovery period after PCNL cases. In addition, assessment of the abdomen for any distention is important to rule out intraperitoneal fluid extravasation which may affect breathing. One should be careful after lengthy procedures, especially when perforation of the renal collecting system occurred. It is our preferred practice to keep the post-PCNL cases that are older (above 60 years of age), high-risk patients, and complex cases, that is, those with multiple punctures or who had significant bleeding, in the intensive care unit overnight for proper monitoring and observation.

Indications for Blood Transfusion During or After PCNL

Here we now list the indications for blood transfusion during or after PCNL:

1. If the patient has a borderline hemoglobin (Hb) and if the patient is elderly and excessive bleeding is noticed, one may consider blood transfusion earlier.
2. If, during the case or in recovery, it was found that the patient bled significantly and tachycardia and hypotension developed, then the surgeon must conclude the case, commence a tamponade catheter or nephrostomy, and then give a blood transfusion.
3. If, during the recovery observation period, the patient is found hypotensive and this is not drug related and immediate Hb has dropped, then we prefer to perform a transfusion earlier.

Renal Precautions During PCNL

Care must be taken to avoid factors compromising renal function, especially in patients whose functions are already impaired. Surgery is a major risk factor, as well as hypotension, sepsis, dehydration, and nephrotoxic drugs. Care of renal function is also essential when performing PCNL in a solitary kidney. Monitoring the urine output during the case as well as early in the postoperative period could be difficult; therefore, follow-up of serum creatinine levels is essential.

Pulmonary Complications Post-PCNL

Damage to the pleura causing pneumothorax or hydrothorax can occur during PCNL. This is a risk when supracostal renal access is chosen. Due to the proximity of the pleural cavity to the kidneys, there is a risk of pleurotomy, especially with upper pole kidney access. In order to prevent pneumothorax, percutaneous access above the 12th rib must be performed near the end of the rib. The collecting system, if entered in supracostal puncture, is to be accessed over the lateral portion of ribs at the time of complete expiration.

The anesthesiologist has to be aware of an increase in airway pressure and ETCO2 and/or the possibility of a decrease in SPO2. A chest X-ray is recommended after PCNL. Fluoroscopic monitoring of the chest is a sensitive way for timely diagnosis of pneumothorax intraoperatively [18]. A chest X-ray is typically done in the recovery period, and when there is a significant peumothorax, pleural effusion, or hemothorax, a chest tube is introduced.

Anesthetic Considerations During Ureteroscopy

Ureteroscopy is commonly done under general as well as regional anesthesia. Doing it under local anesthesia with IV sedation is possible. Recently, URS under local anesthesia, with or without sedation, has become a viable option for a high percentage of correctly selected patients. For those patients who then require deeper sedation or general anesthesia, anesthesia can be induced quickly with new agents such as remifentanil, propofol, and desflurane without a prolonged postoperative recovery period [19]. Since the effectiveness and morbidity of ureteroscopic lithotripsy under local anesthesia are comparable to those of many other previous reports and since most of the patients could tolerate the pain of the procedure, we suggest that ureteroscopic lithotripsy can be performed effectively and safely under local anesthesia [20].

Anesthesia for Cystoscopy

Cystoscopy is the most common procedure in urologic day-case practice. A meta-analysis of nine studies which compared patients treated with intraurethral plain gel and patients treated with intraurethral 2 % lignocaine showed no statistically significant treatment effect [21]. Sedation combined with Entonox (50 % O_2 + 50 % N_2O) improved young patients' tolerance to flexible cystoscope. Rigid cystoscope may require general anesthesia due to scope diameter and bladder distension. Spinal anesthesia is better in patients with COPD if they can lie supine without coughing. In our experience, flexible cystoscopy is well tolerated in both male and female adult patients under local anesthesia only.

Lithotomy Position

The lithotomy position is used during rectal, gynecologic, and urologic surgeries. Hips are flexed 80–100° from the trunk, and the legs are abducted 30–45° from the midline. Knees are flexed until the lower legs are parallel to the torso, and the legs are held by supports or stirrups, usually calf support style or using a "candy cane" knee crutch (Figs. 2.5 and 2.6). Lithotomy position requires coordinated positioning of the lower limbs by two assistants to avoid lumbar spine torsion. Both legs have to be raised together, and the knees and hips must be flexed simultaneously. After the surgery, the patient has to be returned to the supine position in a similar coordinated manner.

The lithotomy position may cause serious physiologic changes. When the legs are raised, preload increases, causing a transient increase in cardiac output and intracranial pressure to a lesser degree in otherwise healthy patients. Also, lithotomy position causes the abdominal

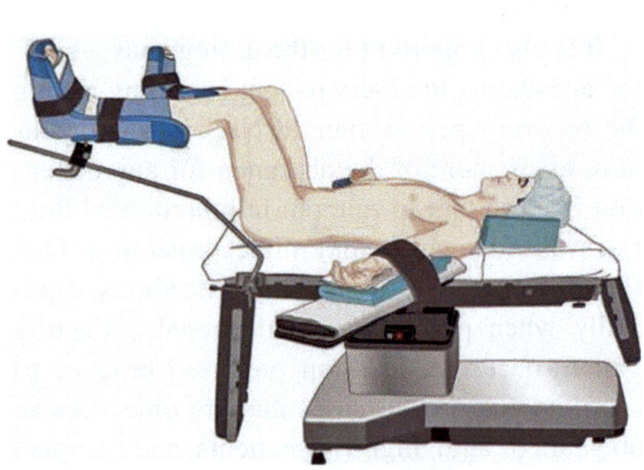

Fig. 2.5 Lithotomy position. Hips are flexed 80–100° with lower leg parallel to body. Arms are on armrests away from hinge point of foot section (Reproduced with permission from Cassola and Woo Lee [8])

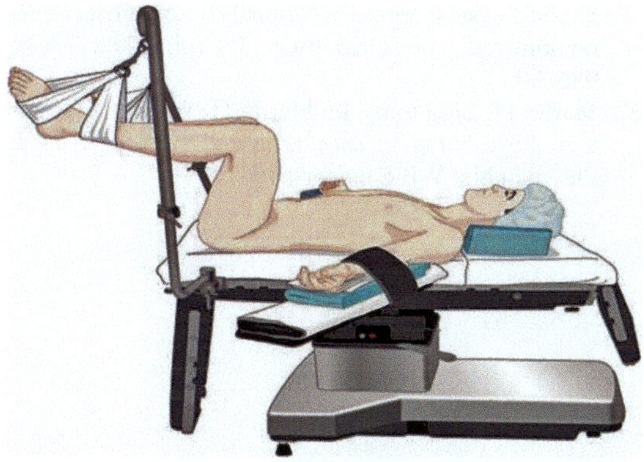

Fig. 2.6 Lithotomy position with "candy cane" supports (Reproduced with permission from Cassola and Woo Lee [8])

viscera to displace the diaphragm upward, reducing lung compliance and potentially resulting in a decreased tidal volume. If obesity is present, abdominal pressure may significantly increase enough to obstruct venous return to the heart [22].

Summary

The urologist who is interested in doing endourologic procedures such PCNL and URS is required to understand the important anesthetic-related issues. These include proper preoperative evaluation and optimization of patients. Knowledge of important aspects of positioning and repositioning from supine to lithotomy to prone position is essential. Intraoperative and postoperative monitoring of patients is vital to ensure safe and successful outcome.

References

1. Rozentsveig V, Neulander EZ, Roussabrov E, Schwartz A, Lismer L, Gurevich B, Klein Y, Weksler N. Anesthetic considerations during percutaneous nephrolithotomy. J Clin Anesth. 2007;19(5):351–5.
2. Cherian VT, Tomlinson AA. Preoperative optimization. In: Cashman JN, editor. Preoperative assessment. London: BMJ Books; 2001. p. 93–132.
3. Patel SR, Haleblian GE, Pareek G. Percutaneous nephrolithotomy can be safely performed in the high-risk patient. Urology. 2010;1(75):51–5.
4. Malhotra V, Sudheendra V, Diwan S. Anesthesia for renal and genitourinary systems. In: Miller RD, editor. Miller's anesthesia. 6th ed. Philadelphia: Elsevier/Churchill Livingstone; 2005.
5. Gee WF, Ansell JF. Pelvic and perineal pain of urologic origin. In: Bonica JJ, editor. The management of pain. 2nd ed. Philadelphia: Lea & Febiger; 1990. p. 1368–78.
6. Anderson KJ, Kabalin JN, Cadeddu JA. Surgical anatomy of the retroperitoneum, kidneys, and ureters. In: Wein AJ, Kavoussi LR, Novick AC, Partin AW, Peters CA, editors. Campbell-Walsh urology. 9th ed. Philadelphia: WB Saunders; 2007. p. 3–37.
7. Lumb AB, Nunn JF. Respiratory function and ribcage contribution to ventilation in body positions commonly used during anesthesia. Anesth Analg. 1991;73:422–6.
8. Cassola L, Woo Lee J. Patient positioning and anesthesia. In: Miller RD, editor. Miller's anesthesia. 6th ed. Philadelphia: Elsevier/Churchill Livingstone; 2005.
9. Agah M, Ghasemi M, Roodneshin F, Radpay B, Moradian S. Prone position in percutaneous nephrolithotomy and postoperative visual loss. Urol J. 2011;8(3):191–6.
10. Singh I, Kumar A, Kumar P. "Ambulatory PCNL" (tubeless PCNL under regional anesthesia) – a preliminary report of 10 cases. Int Urol Nephrol. 2005; 37:35–7.
11. Montamat SC, Cusack BJ, Vestal RE. Management of drug therapy in the elderly. N Engl J Med. 1989; 321:303–9.
12. Basiri A, Mehrabi S, Kianian H, Javaherforooshzadeh A. Blind puncture in comparison with fluoroscopic guidance in percutaneous nephrolithotomy: a randomized controlled trial. Urol J. 2007;4:79–83.
13. Rozentsveig V, Neulander EZ, Roussabrov E, et al. Anesthetic considerations during percutaneous nephrolithotomy. J Clin Anesth. 2007;51:24–7.
14. Singh V, Sinha RJ, Sankhwar SN, Malik A. A prospective randomized study comparing percutaneous nephrolithotomy under combined spinal-epidural anesthesia with percutaneous nephrolithotomy under general anesthesia. Urol Int. 2011;87(3):293–8.
15. Evangelos A, Anastasios K, Stavros G, Vassilios T, Michael M. Feasibility of percutaneous nephrolithotomy under assisted local anaesthesia: a prospective study on selected patients with upper urinary tract obstruction. Eur Urol. 2007;51:224–8.
16. Dalela D, Goel A, Singh P, Shankhwar SN. Renal capsular block: a novel method for performing percutaneous nephrolithotomy under local anesthesia. J Endourol. 2004;18:544–6.
17. Malhotra SK, Khaitan A, Goswami AK, Gill KD, Dutta A. Monitoring of irrigation fluid absorption during percutaneous nephrolithotripsy: the use of 1 % ethanol as a marker. Anaesthesia. 2001;56(11): 1103–6.
18. Vsevolod R, Endre Z, Efim R, et al. Anesthetic considerations during percutaneous nephrolithotomy. J Clin Anesth. 2007;19:351–5.

19. Cybulski PA, Joo H, Honey RJ. Ureteroscopy: anesthetic considerations. Urol Clin North Am. 2004; 31(1):43–7.
20. Park HK, Paick SH, Oh SJ, Kim HH. Ureteroscopic lithotripsy under local anesthesia: analysis of the effectiveness and patient tolerability. Eur Urol. 2004;45(5):670–3.
21. Patel AR, Jones JS, Babineau D. Lidocaine 2 % gel versus plain lubricating gel for pain reduction during flexible cystoscopy: a meta-analysis of prospective, randomized, controlled trials. J Urol. 2008;179(3): 986–90.
22. Martin JT. Lithotomy. In: Martin JT, Warner MA, editors. Positioning in anesthesia and surgery. 3rd ed. Philadelphia: WB Saunders; 1997.

Difficulties in Instrumentation of Endourologic Procedures

3

Ahmed M. Al-Kandari

Introduction

Endourologic surgery has become successful in achieving its goals through the significant development of instruments and disposables. Obviously, one of the major improvements occurred in the optics and their miniaturization. Subsequently, a thorough understanding of the important details of the instruments and disposables is essential in efficient endourologic surgery. In this chapter, the emphasis will be mostly related to ureteroscopy (URS) and percutaneous nephrolithotomy (PCNL), with discussion of common instruments and important disposables. A few practical points regarding associated problems and solutions will be discussed.

Guidewires

Guidewires are the key instruments for successful endourologic procedures. These are used either through a retrograde approach in ureteroscopy or an antegrade approach through the percutaneous renal route.

While it has been proposed by some groups that routine use of a safety wire is not required [1, 2], we believe that the presence of a safety wire does not add to any significant morbidity, while also maintaining emergency access to the urinary tract throughout the procedure.

Numerous guidewires are commercially available. In general, they differ in size, tip design, surface coating, and shaft rigidity. An ideal guidewire requires little force to flex in response to resistance and requires a large force to perforate tissue. A slippery hydrophilic guidewire is used to obtain access to the ureter or to bypass an impacted calculus or a tight stricture area, whereas a stiffer guidewire that is less likely to slip out is used to straighten a tortuous ureter or to pass instruments and access sheaths into the upper collecting system [3]. The stiff wires are also typically less likely to be bent during repeated maneuvers, especially in percutaneous renal surgery.

In a study comparing different guidewires, nine available guidewires were compared: the Roadrunner® PC and polytetrafluoroethylene (PTFE) wire (Cook Urological, Spencer, IN), the Glidewire®, the Bentson-type 15-cm flexible tip PTFE-coated wire and the Amplatz Super Stiff™ (Boston Scientific Microvasive, Miami, FL), Urowire XF™, the Bentson guidewire and the Amplatz guidewire (Applied Medical, Rancho Santa Margarita, CA), and the PTFE-coated Bard® guidewire (Bard Urological Division, Covington, GA) [4]. The study found that the Glidewire (Fig. 3.1) required the greatest force to puncture in an in vitro model, whereas the Amplatz Super Stiff wire (Fig. 3.2) was the most resistant to bending. This indicated that in this

A.M. Al-Kandari, M.D., FRCS(C)
Department of Surgery, Kuwait University, Jabriyah, Kuwait City 13110, Kuwait
e-mail: drakandari@hotmail.com

A.M. Al-Kandari et al. (eds.), *Difficult Cases in Endourology*,
DOI 10.1007/978-1-84882-083-8_3, © Springer-Verlag London 2013

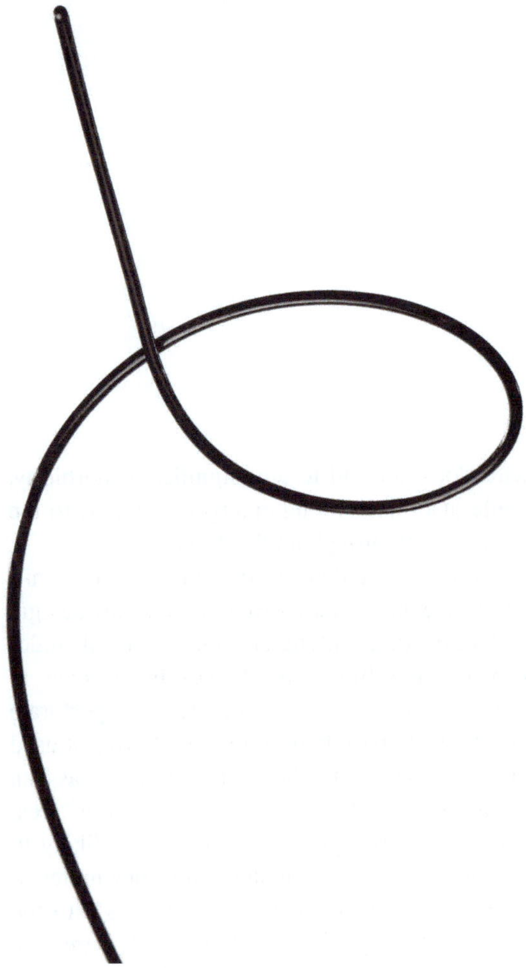

Fig. 3.1 Guidewire: hydrophilic (Image courtesy of Boston Scientific Corporation. Opinions expressed herein are those of the author alone and not necessarily Boston Scientific Corporation)

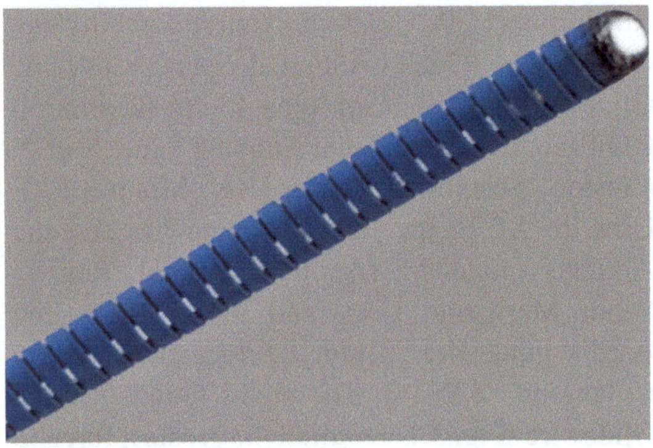

Fig. 3.2 Guidewire: Amplatz Fixed Core Super Stiff™ wire (Permission for use granted by Cook Medical Incorporated, Bloomington, IN)

in vitro model, the Glidewire would be the safest wire for initial access and the Amplatz Super Stiff would be the best wire for passing instruments and repeated maneuvers. In general, floppy tip and nitinol-based guidewires appear to be best used for access with an emphasis on tip flexibility and a low friction coating, while the stiffer shaft guidewires are selected for coaxial passage of catheters, stents, and sheaths [4].

Hybrid wires incorporating features of different glidewires (a hydrophilic distal tip for bypassing an obstructing stone, a kink-resistant body, and a flexible proximal tip for backloading of instruments) have been developed [5]. In one study which evaluated two hybrid wires, the Bard NiCore™ and Boston Scientific Sensor™, it was reported that neither hybrid wire was as stiff as the Boston Scientific Amplatz Super Stiff, suggesting the importance of continued reliance on this wire for passage of ureteral access sheaths and large stents [5].

Difficulties and problems with guidewires are as follows:

1. *Wrong site of insertion*: It is essential when training nurses and assistants that attention is paid to the site of the floppy tip of the guidewire so that the stiff wire tip is not advanced first, as this may lead to perforation. It is always a good habit to push the end gently on the palm to see if it is stiff or floppy.
2. *Wire slippage*: It is of utmost importance to secure the guidewires during endourologic procedures since this secures safe entrance to the urinary system especially when visibility is decreased. Thus, the following points are important to secure the guidewires:
   (a) Exchange hydrophilic wires with standard wires as soon as the aim of their usage is achieved since they tend to be very slippery.
   (b) When using standard wires, make sure that enough coil of the proximal end is made under fluoroscopy, especially when exchanging instruments or removing balloons.
   (c) Keep the distal end of the wire in a secure spot covered or clipped under the drape.

(d) Using double wires during ureteroscopy or percutaneous renal surgery is of great help to avoid inadvertent slippage.
(e) Using through and through guidewire (the extra stiff one) especially during percutaneous renal surgery is our preferred approach since it guarantees security.

3. *Difficulty with wire insertion*:
(a) J-tip wires are not commonly easy to pass through the ureteric orifice, but when hydrophilic, they may be best to advance in tortuous ureter. In order to overcome the difficulty of using them in orifice introduction, use them over a ureteric catheter, typically 5F, as this can be helpful.
(b) When a ureteric stone is impacted, then blind wire passage may be difficult. In such a case, ureteroscopy and pushing the stone gently or even fragmenting it with laser until access is developed can be helpful to passing the guidewire.

4. *Maintaining sterile field with guidewires*: It is very essential to maintain a sterile field during endourologic procedures, but, because of the nature of guidewires to slip partially and because of continuous manipulation and the changing of instruments and disposables, care must be taken to avoid obvious wire contamination. The following points are worth remembering:
(a) Always drape the C-arm of the X-ray machine with a sterile sheath.
(b) Cover and secure the safety wires.
(c) If the safety wire partially slips and touches an unsterile field, we do not advise exchanging the wire. Instead, hold the end with gauze, clean it with antiseptic (Betadine solution) and then cover the wire.
(d) We typically use prophylactic antibiotics during all our endourologic procedures.

5. *Managing bent wires*: Bent guide wires are a challenge for endourologic procedures especially during percutaneous renal dilatation of the tract and occasionally during D-J stent insertion. Subsequently, we advise the following:
(a) Use extra stiff guidewires during percutaneous renal surgery to avoid wire bending.
(b) If the guidewire during ureteroscopy is noted and D-J stent insertion is noted, it is better to change it over a ureteric catheter.
(c) Guidewire manipulations must be monitored by fluoroscopy especially during D-J stent insertion in order to avoid curling in the bladder.

6. *Curling wire in the bladder*: This is a simple but time-wasting problem if not identified readily. This typically can happen when the wire which is inserted from the ureteric orifice and is advanced to the kidney, when it is readvanced with fluoroscopic control, or when a double-J stent is also advanced without being at the orifice. The solution is to use fluoroscopy, pull back the wire, and then redirect it in proper position.

Ureteral Access Sheath

Ureteral access sheath is one of the important disposables used for ease of introduction of different ureteroscopes as well of multiple entries and manipulations during ureteroscopy (Fig. 3.3). Alternatively, a flexible ureteroscope can be passed over the guidewire. Use of a ureteral access sheath has been shown to lower irrigation pressure, reduce operative time, facilitate

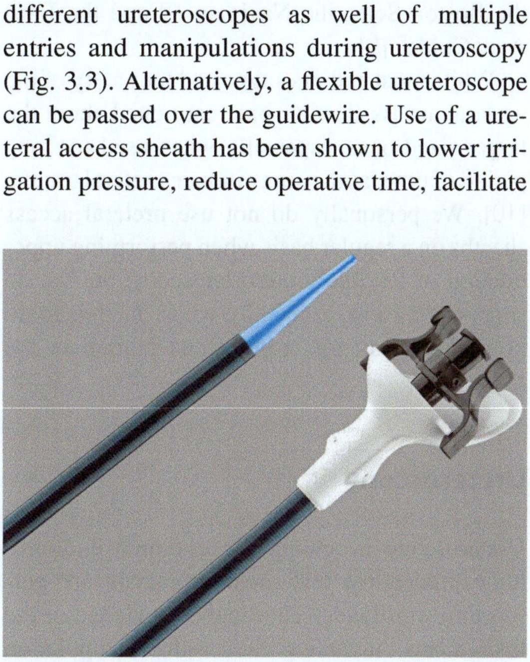

Fig. 3.3 Flexor® reteral access sheath (Permission for use granted by Cook Medical Incorporated, Bloomington, IN)

ureteral re-entry, and improve ureteroscope longevity [6].

Factors that are important to clinical application include a lubricated outer coating to facilitate entry, a low friction inner coating for easy ureteroscope insertion, and a reinforced wall to decrease sheath kinking and buckling.

In one study, no significant difference in the overall successful placement of the applied reinforced and the nonreinforced access sheaths was shown; in that study, most patients were previously stented, which assists in easier stent placement [7].

Another study presented a comparison between two common access sheaths, the 12/15 Fr Applied Access Forte® XE (Applied Medical) and the 12/14 Fr Cook Flexor®, in a clinical setting [8]. The study noted that the device failure rate was 44 % for the applied sheath and 0 % for the Cook sheath. In each case of device failure, the Cook sheath allowed successful completion of the procedure. In a subsequent analysis, the Cook Flexor remained the most resistant to buckling while the Gyrus ACMI Uropass® (Southborough, MA) was most resistant to kinking when compared with the Boston Scientific Navigator™ and the Bard AquaGuide® [9].

While most authors suggested the safety of the ureteral access sheath, some cautioned about the larger-sized ones, especially when used for long period of time, as they may induce ureteral trauma [10]. We personally do not use ureteral access sheaths on a regular basis when performing upper ureteral or flexible ureterorenoscopy, but we do support their use, especially when one has to do laser lithotripsy for larger stone burden in the kidney.

Ureteroscopy

Ureteroscopy is among the common endourologic procedures that most urologists are performing worldwide. Thorough knowledge of the instruments, including their safe manipulation during surgery and the process of sterilization, is essential to increase instrument durability, especially when dealing with the flexible ureteroscope.

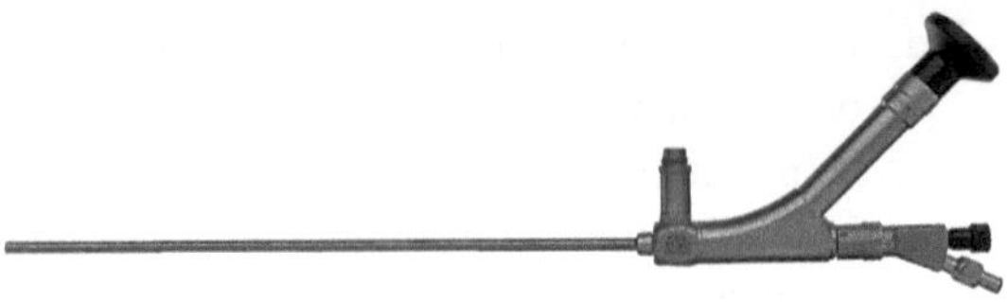

Fig. 3.4 Semirigid ureteroscope (© 2012 Photo Courtesy of KARL STORZ Endoscopy-America, Inc)

Semirigid ureteroscopy (Fig. 3.4) is commonly used for the lower ureter and sometimes in the middle and upper ureters, especially in dilated ureters and commonly in developing countries due to cost and maintenance issues of flexible ureteroscopes.

Advances in ureteroscope design have resulted in smaller scopes with increasing deflection capabilities and easier access to lower pole calices. The effectiveness of ureteroscopes is highly dependent on the size and type of accessory instruments in the working channel [11]. The flexible ureteroscope (Fig. 3.5) remains one of the most fragile instruments in urology and should be handled carefully by experienced personnel. A study suggested that flexible ureteroscope durability can be increased by sterilization by the urology staff and not by a central sterilization department [12].

Flexible Fiberoptic Ureteroscopes

Flexible fiberoptic ureteroscopes are essential instruments that allow minimally invasive intervention for the upper urinary tract. This includes ureteroscopic stone treatment for the upper ureter and kidney, retrograde endopyelotomy, and ureterorenoscopic management of upper tract tumors. Different manufacturers have produced different flexible ureteroscopes with emphasis on miniaturization and durability.

A study compared four new generation ureteroscopes: the Gyrus ACMI DUR®-8 Elite, the Storz Flex-X2 9 (Tuttlingen, Germany), the Olympus URF-P5 (Center Valley, PA), and the Wolf 7325.076 (Knittlingen, Germany). The Wolf scope had the smallest tip size at 6.0 Fr, while the ACMI had the largest shaft size at 10 Fr. The Storz and Wolf scopes had superior

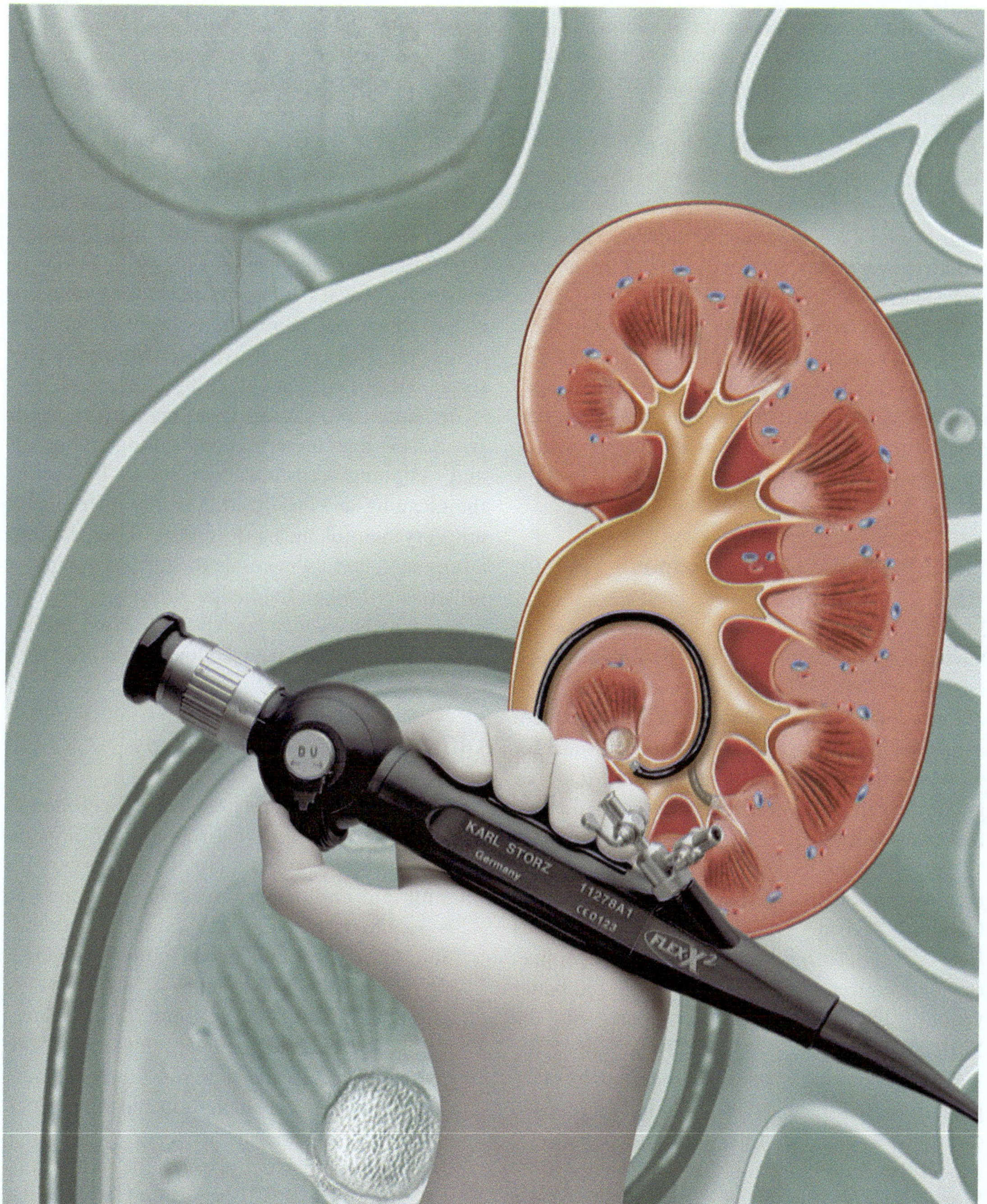

Fig. 3.5 Flexible ureteroscope (© 2012 Photo Courtesy of KARL STORZ Endoscopy-America, Inc)

deflection and torsion stiffness, whereas irrigation was superior with the shorter ACMI scope and inferior with the longer Olympus scope. The double lever deflection of the ACMI increased the difficulty of stone manipulation. The Wolf and the Olympus scopes had the superior optical quality, while the Olympus scope had the least illumination [13].

Another study evaluated the durability of different flexible ureteroscopes – the Stryker Flexvision™ U-500 (Kalamazoo, MI), the Wolf Viper, the Olympus URF-P5, and the Gyrus ACMI DUR®-8 Elite – in a randomized trial [14]. The ACMI required major repair after the fewest mean number of cases (5.3). While the Stryker and the Wolf scopes each experienced early catastrophic failure (fewer than ten cases) in one of three sites, this occurred at all sites for the ACMI [3].

In a study comparing the Wolf flexible ureteroscopes (the Wolf Cobra dual-channel (3.3 Fr) to the Wolf Viper single channel (3.6 Fr) scope) [15], it was found that the dual-channel scope had better flow and deflection when larger instruments were used [16].

Flexible Digital Ureteroscopes

Flexible fiberoptic ureteroscopes continue to have problems with vision, illumination and durability. With advancements in technology, digital ureteroscopes were invented with camera at the tip [17]. These were associated with a larger working channel for instrument passage and irrigation, which is a common problem with flexible fiberoptic scopes.

Some studies looked into the digital flexible ureteroscopes. This included the Gyrus ACMI/ Olympus Invisio® DUR®-D and the Olympus URF-V digital ureteroscopes in a prospective, randomized trial [18]. The URF-V offered better visibility and maneuverability compared with the DUR-D. In 9 % of cases of the digital scopes, the URF-P5 fiberoptic scope was required to complete the cases since stones could not be reached due to the larger size of the digital scope.

Another study compared the performance of the Storz 11274AA flexible fiberoptic ureteroscope to the Olympus URF-V digital flexible ureteroscope. After 22 procedures in each group, a deflection loss was present for the fiberoptic ureteroscopes while no change was noted with the digital ureteroscope [19].

A study evaluated the efficacy of a laser fiber protection system in preventing damage to the DUR-D ureteroscope. The system functions by recognizing the blue covering of the laser fiber and disabling the laser generator if the fiber is drawn into the scope, thereby preventing inadvertent firing. The system was 100 % effective in shutting down the laser prior to entry into the ureteroscope. The system was less effective if bleeding was present or if blue dyes, such as indigo carmine, were used. Damage at the tip of the scope if the laser fiber is pulled into the working channel may still occur if the laser fiber breaks within the scope, which may happen at the point of maximal deflection. That system was developed specifically for the DUR-D and not other digital scopes [20].

In summary, careful handling of the more fragile flexible ureteroscopes during operation and assigning well-trained nurses to look after the cleaning and sterilization of the instruments are very helpful means to ensure more durable equipment. It is always essential to have a standby ureteroscope when the budget allows in order to overcome the sudden unexpected scope failure that can happen in a busy endourologic practice.

Difficulties with Ureteroscopy

The difficulties with ureteroscopy are as follows:

1. *Difficulty in insertion*: In nondilated ureters, the use of a small diameter ureteroscope, semirigid or flexible, especially less than 8, is required to avoid ureteral orifice dilatation. Otherwise, balloon dilatation is needed. Obviously, the presence of a guidewire is essential to facilitate a safe entry into the ureter. If a prominent enlarged middle lobe of the prostate is noted and found to be an obstacle to rigid ureteroscope insertion and if one does not have a flexible ureteroscope, then resection of that prostatic lobe may be required to solve this difficulty. If one cannot advance the available rigid ureteroscope, then stenting the ureter and coming back after a few weeks is always helpful in passive dilatation.
2. *Difficulty in visibility*: Difficulty in visibility during ureteroscopy can happen especially during the following situations:
   (a) Traumatic manipulations with wire of other disposables.

(b) Lithotripsy with most modalities. Managing such a problem is commonly done by increasing the irrigation which can be done by various methods including syringes, manual or automatic irrigation. Avoiding traumatic manipulation is important for avoidance of poor visualization. Occasional bladder fullness can affect visualization, and this can be overcome with different methods including use of access sheath, use of small catheter in the bladder, or use of a sheath of cystoscope in the bladder.

(c) Difficulties due to irrigation leakage from the scope. This can be overcome by using a fresh tight nipple or special adapters, especially with nitinol basket or laser fiber (Fig. 3.6).

(d) Defective lens. The operating room nurses should check the lenses of all operative endoscopes and send any defective lens out for repair. The availability of extra scopes is essential in order to overcome the urgent need for replacement.

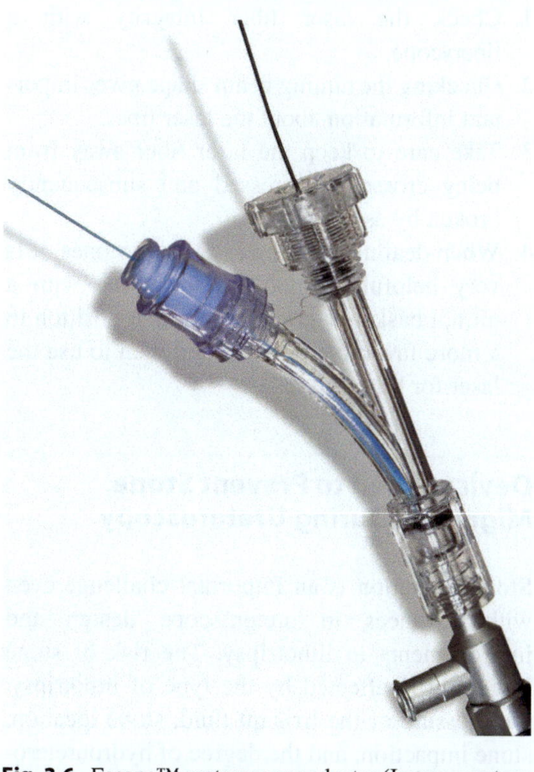

Fig. 3.6 Escape™ ureteroscope adapter (Image courtesy of Boston Scientific Corporation. Opinions expressed herein are those of the author alone and not necessarily Boston Scientific Corporation)

Intracorporeal Lithotripsy During Ureteroscopy

During ureteroscopy, either semirigid or flexible, it is essential to have an intracorporeal lithotripsy device. Pulling a big stone intact is a dangerous movement that should be discouraged. Whenever the stone is found to be bigger than the tip of ureteroscope on fluoroscopy, it is essential to disintegrate the stone.

The important features of a good intracorporeal machine during URS lithotripsy are the small caliber that fits the small scopes, less retropulsion, and less tissue trauma. The two commonly used intracorporeal lithotripters during URS nowadays are pneumatic and laser. The least used are the electrohydraulic and ultrasonic because of tissue trauma and a bigger probe, respectively. Presently the Holmium:YAG is the standard lithotripsy machine during URS (Fig. 3.7). The Holmium:YAG is effective against all types of stones with a depth of penetration of less than 0.5 mm and provides higher stone-free rates and smaller size fragments. The Holmium:YAG causes less stone retropulsion compared with pneumatic machine [21].

When using laser lithotripsy, one must be familiar with laser fibers. This includes knowledge of sizes, single versus reusable (Fig. 3.8), and familiarity with irrigation control and proper positioning of the fiber on stones. Knowledge of the best power setting for lithotripsy is essential. In general for flexible ureteroscopy, it is better to use the smallest fiber in order to maximize deflection and irrigant flow, which will result in better visibility and efficient ureteroscopy.

When studying 24 Holmium:YAG laser fibers of different sizes from various manufacturers [22], Mues et al. compared small (150–300 μm) and medium (300–400 μm) fibers separately. They noted that of the small core fibers – the SureFlex™ LLF-150 (AMS, Minnetonka, MN) and LLF-273, the OptiLite™ SMH1020F (Cook Medical), and the Dornier LG

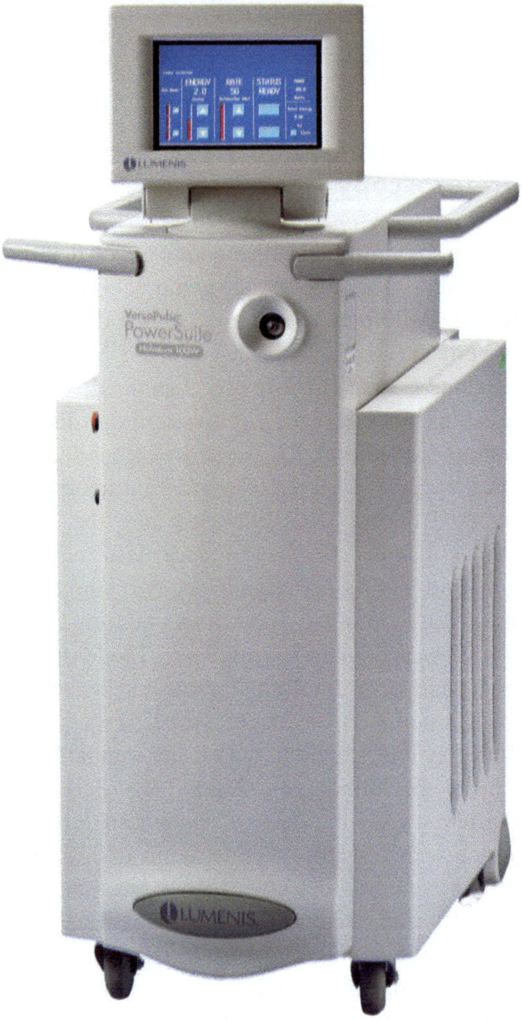

Fig. 3.7 Lumenis® high power laser machine (Courtesy of Lumenis® Surgical, Germany, GmbH)

Super 270 (Wessling, Germany) – had the highest rate for failure. In the medium fiber group, the SureFlex LLF-365 and the Accuflex™ 365 (Boston Scientific) had the highest failure rate. Interestingly, the reusable Lumenis® 365 fiber (Yokneam, Israel) had a higher failure rate compared with the single-use fiber.

Another study further evaluated multiple reusable fibers including the Laser Peripherals 270, the Laser Peripherals 365, the Lumenis Slimline™ 270, and the Lumenis Slimline 365. Thirty-seven laser fibers were required for 541 endoscopic procedures. The 365 μm fibers had significantly more uses than the 270 μm fibers.

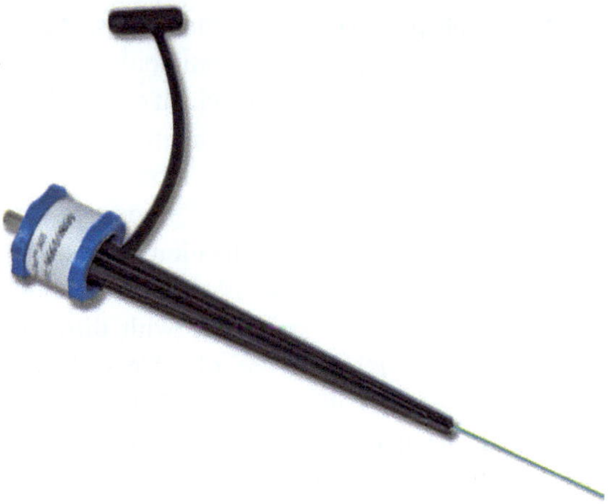

Fig. 3.8 Laser fibers 365, 200 Mic (Courtesy of Lumenis® Surgical, Germany, GmbH)

The reusable Lumenis Slimline 270 was found not to be cost effective [14].

The following are important areas of attention when using laser during ureteroscopy:

1. Check the laser fiber integrity with a fiberscope.
2. Checking the aiming beam shape gives important information about the laser fiber.
3. Take care to keep the laser fiber away from being crossed or pressed and subsequently broken by assistants.
4. When dealing with lower caliceal stones, it is very helpful to mobilize the stone with a nitinol basket or grasper from that position to a more favorable position and then to use the laser for lithotripsy.

Devices Used to Prevent Stone Migration During Ureteroscopy

Stone migration is an important challenge even with advances in ureteroscope design and improvements in lithotripsy. The risk of stone migration is affected by the type of lithotripsy, the pressure of the irrigant fluid, stone location, stone impaction, and the degree of hydroureteronephrosis. Different devices have been designed to decrease stone retropulsion and increase ureteroscopic efficiency.

The Escape® nitinol stone retrieval basket (Boston Scientific) (Fig. 3.9) is helpful to capture stones and allows for simultaneous laser lithotripsy. In a study of patients who underwent ureteroscopic laser lithotripsy using the Escape basket [23], laser lithotripsy of stone held in a basket decreased stone migration; however, it also decreased manipulation of the tip of the ureteroscope. In general, this approach is recommended if a stone becomes entrapped in the basket at the time of extraction [24].

Another interesting device is the Stone Cone® (Boston Scientific) (Fig. 3.10), which is a ureteral occlusion device used to prevent retropulsion of stones larger than 2–3 mm during lithotripsy. It consists of a 0.43-mm nitinol wire with a 3 Fr PTFE cover with the distal sheath shaped in a concentric coil fashion. The stone cone is resistant to pneumatic or electrohydraulic lithotripsy but can also be disrupted by the holmium laser.

In a study that evaluated the Stone Cone over a 3-year period [25], 133 patients were identified, and only two cases of residual retropulsed fragments greater than 2 mm were found. Of 105 cases of semirigid ureteroscopy, no case required conversion to flexible ureteroscopy secondary to stone migration. However, it was emphasized that patients with ureteropelvic junction stones or proximal hydroureteronephrosis greater than 10 mm were not included. This could be a limitation for stone cone usage.

The Cook NTrap® (Cook Urological) (Fig. 3.11) is a 2.6 Fr device with a deployable backstop. Clinical experience has not been reported in the literature, while some effect has been demonstrated in laboratory studies. That study evaluated the Stone Cone and Cook NTrap in the laboratory [26]. It was noted that stone retropulsion was decreased and fragmentation efficiency increased compared with a control group.

In another important study, comparison of four ureteral occlusion devices was done. This included the PercSys® Accordion® (Fig. 3.12) (Percutaneous System, Palo Alto, CA), the Stone Cone (7 and 10 mm) and the Cook NTrap in a ureteral model [27]. The PercSys Accordion is a

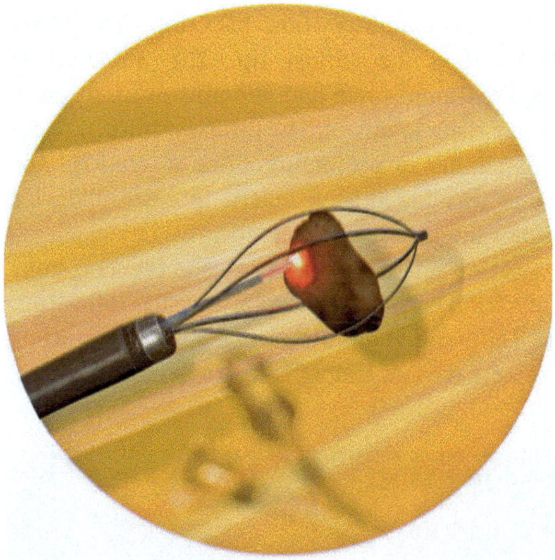

Fig. 3.9 Escape® nitinol basket (Image courtesy of Boston Scientific Corporation. Opinions expressed herein are those of the author alone and not necessarily Boston Scientific Corporation)

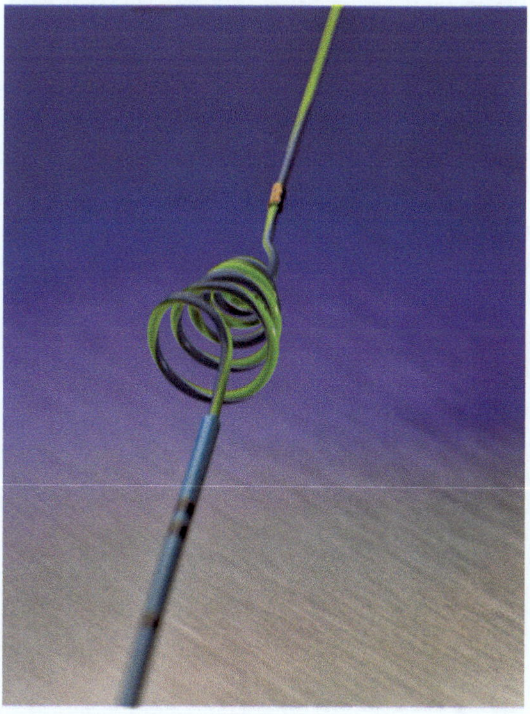

Fig. 3.10 Stone Cone™ (Image courtesy of Boston Scientific Corporation. Opinions expressed herein are those of the author alone and not necessarily Boston Scientific Corporation)

2.9 Fr polyurethane film backstop. The Cook NTrap had the stiffest tip. The Stone Cone required more force and attempts at insertion in comparison to others. The efficacy of the devices was similar in preventing stone migration. The same was found with regard to ease of device removal with stone fragments.

Issues related to devices that prevent stone migration during ureteroscopy are the following:

1. The issue of extra cost that is added to using these devices should be taken in consideration.
2. Proper selection of these devices is important to utilize them optimally.
3. Use of a holmium laser instead of a pneumatic device could minimize the retropulsion and decrease the need for these devices.
4. If retropulsion and stone migration happens during stone lithotripsy, then the urologist should be prepared to deal with it, for example, by using a flexible ureteroscopy and nitinol retrieval devices.

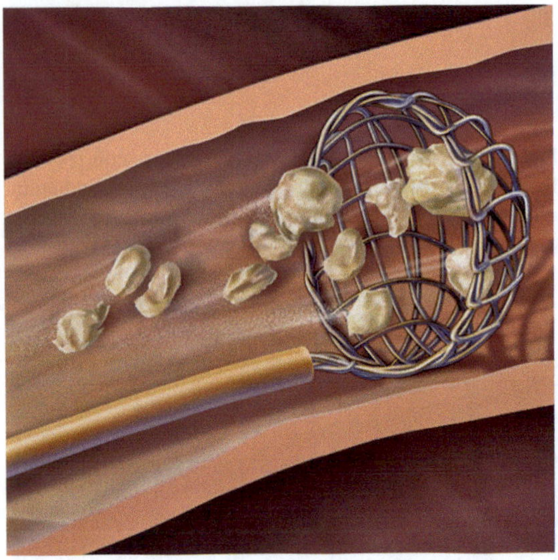

Fig. 3.11 The Cook NTrap® (Permission for use granted by Cook Medical Incorporated, Bloomington, IN)

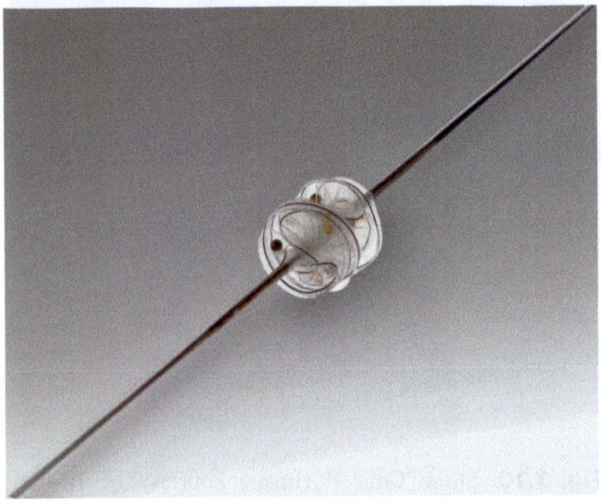

Fig. 3.12 PercSys® Accordion® (Courtesy of PercSys®, Palo Alto, CA)

Retrieval Devices Used During Ureteroscopy

Currently, different stone baskets are available. Important differences between baskets include wire material and stiffness, size, radial dilation force to open in the ureter, configuration, and ability to capture or disengage a stone. Although old baskets were tipped, the development of tippless baskets is superior for stone extraction from renal calices. Nitinol baskets are the most common baskets used in flexible ureteroscopy. They are unique in being less rigid when compared with stainless steel and allow for greater deflection and ease of stone disengagement. Also, special forceps such as Graspit® (Boston Scientific) (Fig. 3.13) are of great help during flexible ureterorenoscopy and help in mobilizing lower caliceal stones in a better position for laser lithotripsy.

In a study that evaluated several baskets, it was found that the Cook NCircle® had a more linear opening and closing dynamic, making for a more controlled opening and closing [28]. The Sacred Heart Halo baskets were strongest for radial dilation force, while the Cook NCircle 3.2 Fr had the strongest force for application through a

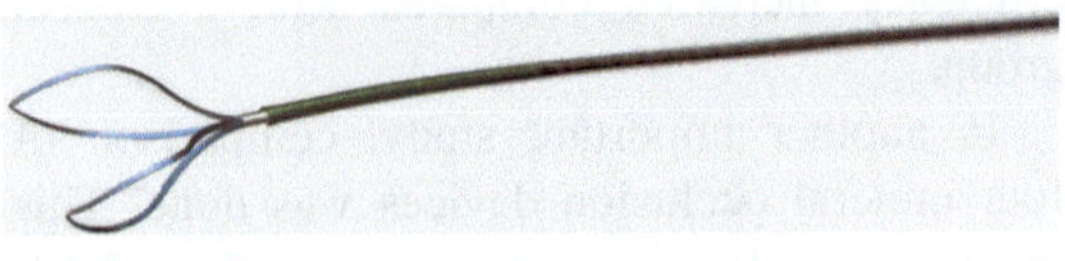

Fig. 3.13 The Graspit® forceps (Image courtesy of Boston Scientific Corporation. Opinions expressed herein are those of the author alone and not necessarily Boston Scientific Corporation)

semirigid ureteroscope [29]. Furthermore, the Sacred Heart Halo was more efficient in calyceal models while the Cook NCircle 3.0 Fr helped efficient stone engagement in ureteral models [30, 31]. On the other hand, the Cook NCompass™ helped to capture stones less than 1 mm due to the webbing feature [3].

Efficient flexible scope deflection, especially in the lower pole of the kidney, with clear visibility due to efficient irrigation, has necessitated some companies to develop smaller baskets. A good example is the 1.5 Fr Sacred Heart Halo, which allowed for significantly higher irrigant flow rate [6].

A study evaluated the radial dilation capabilities of three small stone baskets including the Boston Scientific Optiflex® (1.3 Fr), the Cook NCircle Nitinol Tipless Stone Extractor (1.5 Fr), and the Sacred Heart Halo (1.5 Fr) [32]. As mentioned previously, the Sacred Heart Halo had the highest radial dilation force compared with the other baskets [33]. This is important to remember when using these smaller baskets, especially when there is ureteral stricture or edema.

Percutaneous Nephrolithotomy

Percutaneous nephrolithotomy (PCNL) is the operation of choice for the management of large or multiple renal stones. Different instruments and disposables have undergone important improvements and innovations that have led to more safe and successful outcomes especially during PCNL.

Rigid Nephroscope

The standard nephroscope is the main instrument used in PCNL (Fig. 3.14). Various lengths and sizes are available as well as right and oblique angle working channels. Important aspects related to use of a rigid nephroscope are as follows:

1. Some nephroscopes differ in the site of working channel angle and the amount the forceps opening, for example, Storz versus Wolf.

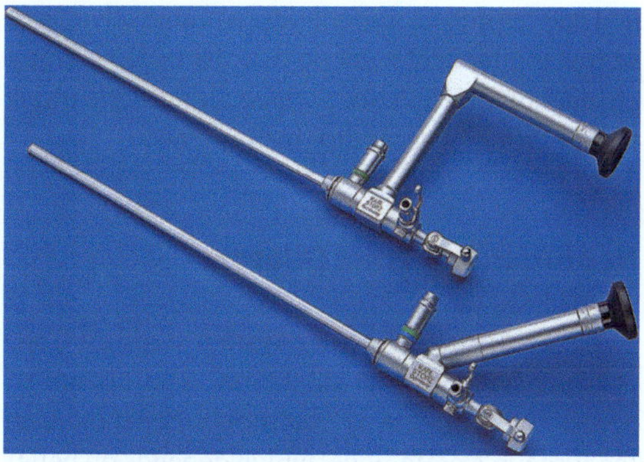

Fig. 3.14 Rigid nephroscope (© 2012 Photo Courtesy of KARL STORZ Endoscopy-America, Inc)

2. It is good practice to prepare and connect the nephroscope with all attachments (light cable, irrigation tubing, camera) before starting the renal puncture. This is important in order to avoid delay, especially if bleeding is encountered.
3. A long nephroscope is useful in obese patients to overcome the long distance from the skin to the renal collecting system.
4. In pediatric cases, especially in those who have small body weight, it is very helpful to use small nephroscopes, which are available.
5. Typically, when the time comes for nephroscope usage during PCNL, the surgeon moves the C-arm away to make it more convenient to move around, except when residual stones are being followed, when the C-arm can be brought in.
6. The rigid nephroscope is a rigid instrument, and the surgeon must be careful not to use excessive torque on the kidney since this may cause excessive renal trauma and bleeding. And if a greater angle is required to search for residual stones, then the use of a flexible nephroscope should be considered.

Improvements in rigid nephroscopes involved the provision of different sizes as stated before. Interest in development resulted in a new digital nephroscope, the Invisio Smith nephroscope from Gyrus ACMI. This was used clinically during PCNL for the removal of caliceal stones [34–36]. This scope had an integrated light source and camera. It was perceived by the operators to be lighter and had improved ergonomics. Another advantage of that digital nephroscope was the large working channel of the 15 Fr size, which allowed the insertion of different accessory instruments.

Nephrostomy Tract Dilators

Entrance of the collecting system during PCNL is dependent on tract dilatation. The choice of access tract dilation is commonly dependant on the surgeon's preference, which depends on belief and experience, and the availability of necessary equipment, which is cost dependant. The common dilators used during PCNL are balloon, Amplatz Teflon, or metal Alken dilators.

In a study comparing balloon dilatation (Fig. 3.15) with Amplatz dilation (Fig. 3.16) of the nephrostomy tract in a group of patients [34], there was no difference in blood loss or operative time. There was no significant difference in failure rates between these two common techniques. It is always helpful to be familiar with all dilation techniques, and one can alternate techniques in case one fails. Obviously, cost consideration is important. One should note that the failed cases could be related to balloons with less pressure being used in this study.

An interesting study compared the expansion of balloon dilators under extrinsic compression simulating retroperitoneal scar tissue [35]. The Bard X-Force®, the Boston Scientific Microvasive Amplatz Tractmaster™, and the Cook Ultraxx™ were tested. While all balloons performed well under low constrictive forces, the Bard X-Force (30 atm) and the Cook Ultraxx performed best under the higher constrictive loads.

Difficulties and problems with dilators are listed below:

1. The development of a short, straight access in the collecting system is key in successful tract dilatation.
2. The absolute confirmation that the guidewire is in the collecting system cannot be overemphasized before tract dilatation.
3. The use of either a very secure access wire, for example, in the ureter or two wires, is essential for security of the access.

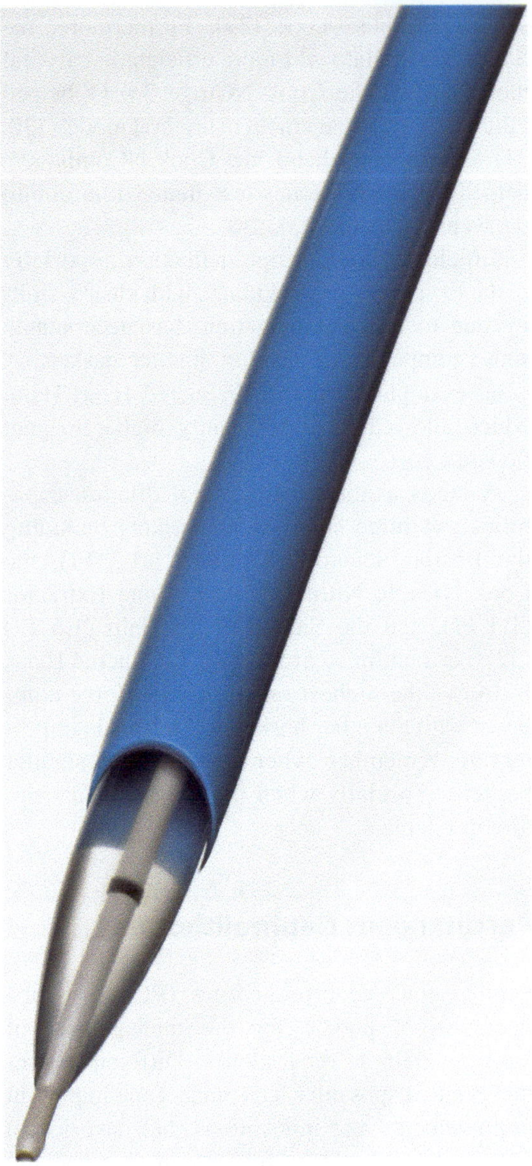

Fig. 3.15 Balloon dilator (Image courtesy of Boston Scientific Corporation. Opinions expressed herein are those of the author alone and not necessarily Boston Scientific Corporation)

4. The use of extrastiff guidewire is essential in tract dilatation especially in redo cases.
5. Amplatz dilators: Commonly in developing countries these dilators are reused after being sterilized, although this is not recommended by the manufacturers. This practice has been found to be safe in terms of infection and quality of the instrument. A common problem

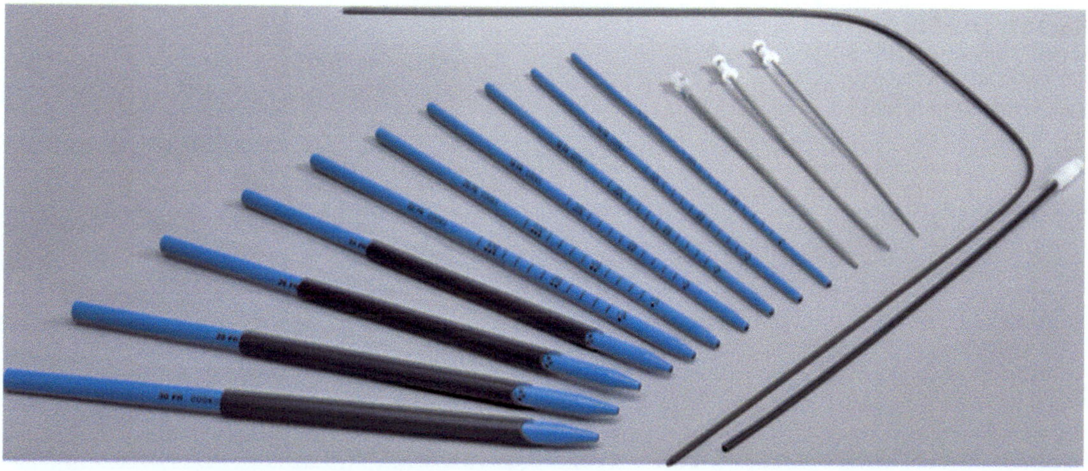

Fig. 3.16 Amplatz dilators (Permission for use granted by Cook Medical Incorporated, Bloomington, IN)

noted in these situations is the tear of the dilator tip, which renders them difficult to be passed and subsequently may bend the guidewire and cause the dilatation to be difficult. Therefore, a thorough inspection of these reused disposables is essential to avoid problems. Obviously, single use of these disposables is a better practice that will confirm the better quality of instrument.

6. Balloon dilators:
   (a) Difficulty to fully inflate: Although uncommon, this is quite important to observe, is that there is disappearance of the waist on the balloon, which will allow easy sheath insertion. If this happens, then one can use the Kelly or artery forceps to open the fascia which is commonly the site of such a problem, especially in previously operated cases. Also, it is important to open the skin well and preferably to open the fascia sharply before balloon insertion. Sometimes the cause of difficulty to inflate is simple, which is poor connection and leakage at syringe connections.
   (b) Inflating the balloon without the sheath on: this simple mistake can cause problems with balloon usage, since it has to be reinserted and refilled. It is essential to supervise the preparation of the balloon to avoid such mistakes.
   (c) Underdilatation: Since the balloons commonly have the radio-opaque mark more proximal from the tip, and since the tip is conical, there is a possibility of under dilatation. This can be overcome by redilating with Amplatz or metal dilators or gently spreading with forceps and inserting the sheath over the wire, especially when the tip of the sheath is close to the renal collecting system.

Intracorporeal Lithotripsy During PCNL

Intracorporeal lithotriptors are essential equipment for any PCNL. In our view and especially in a busy endourology center, it is very helpful to have all the tools of lithotripsy that will help render the patient stone-free. The most common equipment used for intracorporeal lithotripsy during PCNL are ultrasonic and pneumatic lithotripters. The ultrasonic device has the advantage of lithotripsy with continuous suction to aspirate stone fragments. This is especially helpful in soft stones like struvite. It also has the advantage of being on top of the stone so the stone can be disintegrated and sucked, thus preventing stone migration. On the other hand, the pneumatic device has the advantage of being the most powerful and can fragment all kinds to stones efficiently and safely. But its disadvantages are

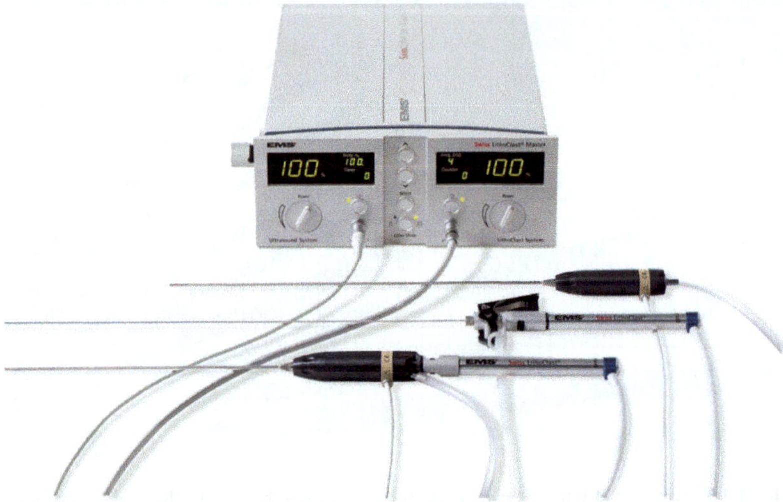

Fig. 3.17 LithoClast® Master (Courtesy of E.M.S., Electro-Medical Systems S.A., Nyon, Switzerland)

stone migration and the need for individual fragment removal.

Currently, there are devices that include features of both modalities. The LithoClast® Master (EMS, Nyon, Switzerland) (Fig. 3.17), also known as the LithoClast Ultra (Boston Scientific) in North America, is a combination ultrasonic and pneumatic lithotripter. The addition of the LithoPump® suction (EMS) and Vario handpiece (EMS) to the LithoClast Select Series is thought to improve vision and allow higher power output, respectively. There is an improved suction channel which is straight in pure ultrasound mode and at a 45° angle in combination mode. This modification is helpful to reduce probe clogging, which can be cumbersome.

With regard to other models of lithotriptors, the Gyrus ACMI CyberWand™ is an ultrasonic lithotripter that contains two separate probes which vibrate at two different frequencies to fragment stones. The probes are of different length, which cause a ballistic effect. The CyberWand is almost twice as fast compared with the LithoClast Master in an in vitro model with regards to stone penetration [35].

Other lithotriptors include the Cook LMA Stonebreaker™, which is a pneumatic lithotripter. It is a portable lightweight device. In one study, it was successful in fragmenting all stone types. KUB stone-free rates were reported to be 100 % [36].

An interesting study that compared different lithotripters used during percutaneous treatment of upper ureteric stones included the holmium laser, the pneumatic lithotripter and the Swiss LithoClast Master [37, 38]. While the study noted that the operative time was shorter and the stone-free rates were higher with the LithoClast Master and the holmium laser, there was a 16 % incidence of ureteral strictures in the patients treated with the high energy holmium laser at 1-year follow-up. This is more than what we typically notice with laser lithotripsy during proximal ureteroscopy. It could be related to the types of upper ureteric stones, which could be impacted, or to the technique chosen.

Retrieval Devices Used During PCNL

Commonly, most urologists use standard two prong rigid forceps during PCNL (Fig. 3.18). Three prong forceps are also available. Important points to review when using rigid standard stone forceps during PCNL are as follows:

1. If the stone fragment is bigger than the forceps jaw, stop and fragment it further.
2. Removing small fragments helps to visualize and work better during stone lithotripsy.
3. Care must be taken with grasping large fragments to avoid breaking the forceps jaws.

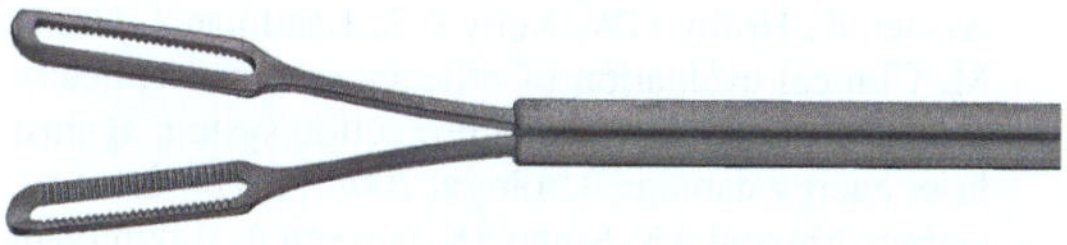

Fig. 3.18 Two prong rigid nephroscope forceps (© 2012 Photo Courtesy of KARL STORZ Endoscopy-America, Inc)

4. It is always important to have standby forceps since forceps may break during the case.
5. When grasped, the stone should be in sight at all times.
6. Care must be taken not to grasp mucosa or perforate since this may complicate the case by causing bleeding or extravasation, respectively.
7. Avoid the temptation to use grasper forceps for stone removal under fluoroscopy only, which some urologists do, as this may cause more injury to the kidney.
8. It is always essential to have your assistant hold the sheath and wire during stone fragment retrieval to avoid inadvertent removal.
9. If the stone and forceps are stuck in the sheath: This also may happen when attempting to remove a large stone fragment. One may attempt steady pulling or one may leave the stone in the sheath to fragment further. Less commonly, when a secure guidewire is in the collecting system, one may attempt to remove the stone, forceps, and sheath as one block after securing the guidewire.
10. Broken forceps during stone retrieval: This can happen, and one must always be careful to observe the integrity of the forceps, especially the two prongs. If a broken instrument is noticed, then you must confirm that the piece is removed out of the renal collecting system.

Other disposable devices have been developed to help stone retrieval during PCNL, but they are less commonly used, probably due to cost issues, and since most endourologists are more used to standard forceps. An example is the Cook Perc NCircle, which is a tipple, nitinol stone basket designed for PCNL (Fig. 3.19). In an in vitro study comparing the Storz 3-prong grasper with the Cook Perc NCircle, it was proven that the Perc NCircle was faster in stone extraction with less chance of inadvertent sheath removal [39]. Further clinical trials are required to verify these findings before making a clinical recommendation. Obviously, any technological advancement is welcome to increase the efficiency and safety of PCNL.

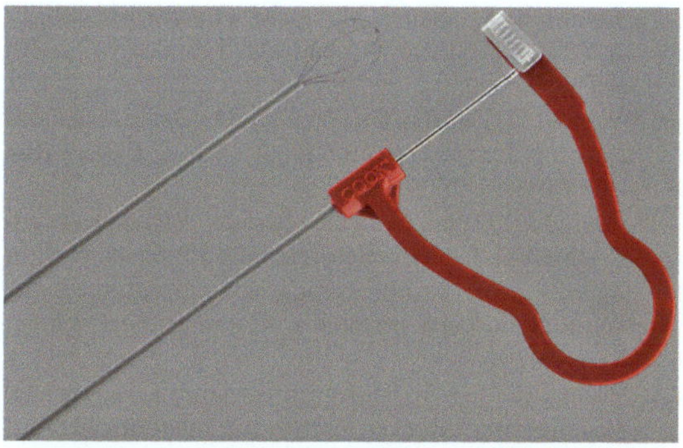

Fig. 3.19 Perc NCircle® (Permission for use granted by Cook Medical Incorporated, Blomington, IN)

Summary

Knowledge of the important instruments and disposables used during endourologic procedures is essential for safe and successful outcome. If one decides to perform endourologic surgery, then the availability of essential tools is a must. Understanding the potential problems of these instruments and disposables is important in order to face these difficulties when they occur.

References

1. Dickstein RJ, Kreshover JE, Babayan RK, Wang DS. Is a safety wire necessary during routine flexible ureteroscopy? J Endourol. 2010;24:1589–92.
2. Eandi JA, Hu B, Low RK. Evaluation of the impact and need for use of a safety guidewire during ureteroscopy. J Endourol. 2008;22:1653–8.
3. Holden T, Pedro RN, Hendlin K, Durfee W, Monga M. Evidence-based instrumentation for flexible ureteroscopy: a review. J Endourol. 2008;22:1423–6.
4. Clayman M, Uribe CA, Eichel L, Gordon Z, Mcdougall EM, Clayman R. Comparison of guide wires in urology. Which, when and why? J Urol. 2004;171: 2146–50.

5. Hendlin K, Korman E, Monga M. Guidewires: lubricity and shaft stiffness (abstract). J Endourol. 2010; 24:PS4–14.
6. Weiland D, Canales BK, Monga M. Medical devices used for ureteroscopy for renal calculi. Expert Rev Med Devices. 2006;3:73–80.
7. Shields JM, Tunuguntla HS, Bhalani VK, Ayyathurai R, Bird VG. Construction-related differences seen in ureteral access sheaths: comparison of reinforced versus nonreinforced ureteral access sheaths. Urology. 2009;73:241–4.
8. Monga M, Best S, Venkatesh R, Ames C, Lieber D, Vanlangendock R, et al. Prospective randomized comparison of 2 ureteral access sheaths during flexible retrograde ureteroscopy. J Urol. 2004;172:572–3.
9. Pedro RN, Hendlin K, Durfee WK, Monga M. Physical characteristics of next-generation ureteral access sheaths: buckling and kinking. Urology. 2007;70: 440–2.
10. Delvecchio FC, Auge BK, Brizuela RM, Weizer AZ, Silverstein AD, Lallas CD, Pietrow PK, Albala DM, Preminger GM. Assessment of stricture formation with the ureteral access sheath. Urology. 2003; 61(3):518–22; discussion 522.
11. Bach T, Geavlete B, Herrmann TR, Gross AJ. Working tools in flexible ureterorenoscopy – influence on flow and deflection: what does matter? J Endourol. 2008; 22:1639–43.
12. Semins MJ, George S, Allaf ME, Matlaga BR. Ureteroscope cleaning and sterilization by the urology operating room team: the effect on repair costs. J Endourol. 2009;23:903–5.
13. Paffen ML, Keizer JG, De Winter GV, Arends AJ, Hendrikx AJ. A comparison of the physical properties of four new generation flexible ureteroscopes: (De)flection, flow properties, torsion stiffness, and optical characteristics. J Endourol. 2008;22:2227–34.
14. Knudsen BE, Pedro R, Hinck B, Monga M. Durability of reusable Holmium: Yag laser fibers: a multicenter study. J Urol. 2011;185:160–3.
15. Haberman K, Ortiz O, Chotikawanich E, Monga M. A dual channel flexible ureteroscope: in vitro evaluations of deflection flow, luminescence and resolution (abstract). J Endourol. 2010;24:PS1–13.
16. Ortiz-Alvarado O, Haberrman K, Chotikawanich E, Monga M. The Cobra dual-channel flexible ureteroscope: novel function, novel applications. J Endourol. 2011;25(9):1411–4.
17. Andonian S, Okeke Z, Smith AD. Digital ureteroscopy: the next step. J Endourol. 2008;22:603–6.
18. Shah K, Monga M, Knudsen BE. Prospective randomized trial comparing two flexible digital ureteroscopes: Gyrus ACMI/Olympus Invisio DUR-D and Olympus URF-V (abstract). J Endourol. 2010;24: PS28–28.
19. Multescu R, Geavlete B, Georgescu D, Geavlete P. Conventional fiberoptic flexible ureteroscope versus fourth generation digital flexible ureteroscope: a critical comparison. J Endourol. 2010;24:17–21.
20. Xavier K, Hruby GW, Kelly CR, Landman J, Gupta M. Clinical evaluation of efficacy of novel optically activated digital endoscope protection system against laser energy damage. Urology. 2009;73:37–40.
21. Garg S, Mandal AK, Singh SK, Naveen A, Ravimohan M, Aggarwal M, et al. Ureteroscopic laser lithotripsy versus ballistic lithotripsy for treatment of ureteric stones: a prospective comparative study. Urol Int. 2009;82:341–5.
22. Mues AC, Teichman JM, Knudsen BE. Evaluation of 24 Holmium:Yag laser optical fibers for flexible ureteroscopy. J Urol. 2009;182:348–54.
23. Kesler SS, Pierre SA, Brison DI, Preminger GM, Munver R. Use of the escape nitinol stone retrieval basket facilitates fragmentation and extraction of ureteral and renal calculi: a pilot study. J Endourol. 2008;22:1213–7.
24. Teichman JM, Kamerer AD. Use of the Holmium:Yag laser for the impacted stone basket. J Urol. 2000;164: 1602–3.
25. Eisner BH, Dretler SP. Use of the stone cone for prevention of calculus retropulsion during Holmium:Yag laser lithotripsy: case series and review of the literature. Urol Int. 2009;82:356–60.
26. Lee HJ, Box GN, Abraham JB, Deane LA, Elchico ER, Eisner BH, et al. In vitro evaluation of nitinol urological retrieval coil and ureteral occlusion device: retropulsion and Holmium laser fragmentation efficiency. J Urol. 2008;180:969–73.
27. Ahmed M, Pedro RN, Kieley S, Akornor JW, Durfee WK, Monga M. Systematic evaluation of ureteral occlusion devices: Insertion, deployment, stone migration, and extraction. Urology. 2009;73: 976–80.
28. Monga M, Hendlin K, Lee C, Anderson JK. Systematic evaluation of stone basket dimensions. Urology. 2004;63:1042–4.
29. Hendlin K, Lee C, Anderson JK, Monga M. Radial dilation force of tipless and helical stone baskets. J Endourol. 2004;18:946–7.
30. Lukasewycz S, Hoffman N, Botnaru A, Deka PM, Monga M. Comparison of tipless and helical baskets in an in vitro ureteral model. Urology. 2004;64: 435–8.
31. Lukasewycz S, Skenazy J, Hoffman N, Kuskowski M, Hendlin K, Monga M. Comparison of nitinol tipless stone baskets in an in vitro caliceal model. J Urol. 2004;172:562–4.
32. Korman E, Hendlin K, Monga M. Next-generation nitinol stone baskets: radial dilation force and dynamics of opening (abstract). J Endourol. 2010;24: PS28–31.
33. Andonian S, Okeke Z, Anidjar M, Smith AD. Digital nephroscopy: the next step. J Endourol. 2008;22: 601–2.
34. Gonen M, Istanbulluoglu OM, Cicek T, Ozturk B, Ozkardes H. Balloon dilatation versus Amplatz dilatation for nephrostomy tract dilatation. J Endourol. 2008;22:901–4.

35. Hendlin K, Monga M. Radial dilation of nephrostomy balloons: a comparative analysis. Int Braz J Urol. 2008;34:544–6.
36. Pugh JW, Canales BK. New instrumentation in percutaneous nephrolithotomy. Indian J Urol. 2010;26: 389–94.
37. Rane A, Kommu SS, Kandaswamy SV, Rao P, Aron M, Kumar R, et al. Initial clinical evaluation of a new pneumatic intracorporeal lithotripter. BJU Int. 2007; 100:629–32.
38. Zhu Z, Xi Q, Wang S, Liu J, Ye Z, Yu X, et al. Percutaneous nephrolithotomy for proximal ureteral calculi with severe hydronephrosis: assessment of different lithotriptors. J Endourol. 2010;24:201–5.
39. Hoffman N, Lukasewycz SJ, Canales B, Botnaru A, Slaton JW, Monga M. Percutaneous renal stone extraction: in vitro study of retrieval devices. J Urol. 2004;172:559–61.

Percutaneous Management of Calyceal Diverticula: An American Experience

4

Jessica A. Mandeville, Ehud Gnessin, and James E. Lingeman

Introduction

Calyceal diverticula are smooth-walled, nonsecretory, urothelium-lined cavities within the parenchyma of the kidney. These cavities communicate with the collecting system via an infundibulum ("neck") off of a calyceal fornix, through which urine can flow in a retrograde fashion. Calyceal diverticula are congenital in nature and thought to be the result of failed degeneration of small ureteric buds. They occur with equal frequency in men and women and do not appear to have a predilection for side (right versus left). They can be identified on 0.21–0.45 % of intravenous pyelogram (IVP) studies. The great majority of these diverticula are unilateral and located in the upper pole (70 %) of the involved renal unit. Diverticula are more frequently develop in the posterior aspect of the kidney but can also be found in anterior locations [1–5].

While many patients with calyceal diverticula are asymptomatic, these diverticula can become problematic over time. Calyceal diverticula are known to be associated with flank pain, hematuria, recurrent urinary tract infections, and calculus formation. Recurrent urinary tract infections will be identified in 25 % of patients with known diverticula, and poor drainage via a narrow infundibulum can result in sepsis, abscess formation, and eventual parenchymal damage [2]. Calculi can be expected to develop in 9.5–50 % of diverticula [1, 2]. These calculi are highly unlikely to pass spontaneously, generally owing to the small caliber nature of the diverticular necks. While asymptomatic diverticula can be managed expectantly, general indications for treatment include pain, recurrent urinary tract infections, hematuria, stones, or compression and damage of surrounding renal parenchyma (generally seen with large diverticula) [1, 2, 5].

J.A. Mandeville, M.D.
Department of Urology (4SE), Lahey Clinic Medical Center,
41 Mall Road, Burlington, MA, 01805, USA
e-mail: jessica_mandeville@hotmail.com

E. Gnessin, M.D.
Department of Urology, Hebrew University of Jerusalem and Shaare Zedek Medical Center,
Jerusalem, 91031, Israel
e-mail: ehud.gnessin@gmail.com

J.E. Lingeman, M.D. (✉)
Department of Urology, Methodist Hospital,
1801 North Senate Blvd, Suite 220, Indianapolis, IN, 46202, USA
e-mail: jlingeman@iuhealth.org

Treatment of Calyceal Diverticula

Previously, treatments for calyceal diverticula were performed using invasive, open surgical techniques such as unroofing and marsupialization procedures, diverticulectomy or partial nephrectomy. Today, less invasive modalities are available for the treatment of calyceal diverticula including extracorporeal shock wave lithotripsy

A.M. Al-Kandari et al. (eds.), *Difficult Cases in Endourology*,
DOI 10.1007/978-1-84882-083-8_4, © Springer-Verlag London 2013

(ESWL), ureteroscopy, laparoscopy, and percutaneous nephrolithotomy (PNL).

ESWL may provide symptomatic pain relief in some patients, but stone clearance rates of only 4–58 % are reported in the literature [1–5]. Due to its inferior success rates when compared to other minimally invasive treatment modalities, ESWL is generally not recommended for the treatment of stones in diverticula but could be considered in rare instances of small, stone-containing diverticula with wide infundibula. An additional drawback of ESWL in the management calyceal diverticula is the inability to treat the underlying anatomic abnormality, which allows for continued risk of stone formation and recurrent urinary tract infections [1, 3].

Ureteroscopic management of calyceal diverticula was first described in 1989 [6]. This approach first requires retrograde ureteroscopic identification of the diverticular ostium followed by balloon dilation or incision of the neck. Subsequently, treatment of any contained stones can be carried out with some form of lithotripsy (i.e., electrohydraulic, laser, or simultaneous extracorporeal shock wave lithotripsy). Stone clearance rates reported in the literature vary widely (30–83 %) as do symptom resolution rates (35–100 %) [5–8]. Pitfalls to this procedure include inability to identify small diverticular ostia and difficulty in treating lower pole diverticula due to limitations in the flexion capabilities of ureteroscopes that are currently available on the market.

Laparoscopy has limited indications for the management of calyceal diverticula and has traditionally been employed for the management of large, anteriorly located diverticula with minimal surrounding normal renal parenchyma. Associated operative times are significantly longer when compared to other minimally invasive techniques, even in expert hands.

Percutaneous management of symptomatic calyceal diverticula is consistently associated with higher stone-free (85–100 %) and symptom resolution rates (~85 %) [1, 3, 8]. At the time of PNL, electro-cautery fulguration of the diverticulum can also be carried out, allowing for complete or near-complete collapse of the cavity. Additionally, identification of the diverticulum via retrograde contrast instillation is not necessarily required, as needle access to the diverticulum can often be achieved by direct puncture onto a stone within the cavity. Despite the excellent results achieved with percutaneous management of calyceal diverticula, many urologists are not comfortable with the procedure for various reasons. These include the possibility of thoracic complications (hemo- or hydrothorax) associated with supracostal access for upper pole diverticula, increased risk of bleeding associated with anteriorly located lesions (increased amount of parenchyma traversed), and perceived difficulty with safely maintaining wire access within the confined space of the diverticulum. Here we describe our technique for the percutaneous management of calyceal diverticular stones and diverticular ablation via a sub-costal access. This technique is also suitable for stones located in dilated calyces (hydrocalyces) with stenotic infundibula. In this scenario, access to the calyx of interest is obtained using our diverticular access technique and wire access to the ureter can subsequently be achieved with the use of flexible or rigid nephroscopy.

Sample Cases

Case 1
A 41-year-old female with a history of bilateral vesico-ureteral reflux, reflux nephropathy, and right renal atrophy underwent bilateral ureteral reimplantation at the age of 22 months. She presented with a 2-year history of intermittent left-sided flank pain. She additionally reported two episodes of gross hematuria possibly associated with the passage of fine, gravel-like material. She had recurrent urinary tract infections as a child, but denied any infections over the past 10–15 years. She denied a personal or family history of nephrolithiasis. An abdominal plain X-ray (KUB – Fig. 4.1a) revealed a 1.4 × 1.0 cm calcification in the region of the upper pole of the left kidney. A follow-up IVP study (Fig. 4.1b) revealed that the calcification was located within an upper pole calyceal diverticulum. Scarring of

the upper pole of the left kidney and right renal atrophy were also noted.

Case 2

An otherwise healthy 64-year-old male presented with several months of intermittent right-sided flank pain. He denied a personal history of nephrolithiasis but did report a history of stone disease (type unknown) in his son. A non-contrast computed tomography scan (NCCT) of the abdomen and pelvis revealed the presence of an approximately 2-cm calculus in a dilated upper pole calyx of the right kidney. Bilateral incomplete collecting system duplication was also noted. A follow-up IVP study (Fig. 4.2a, b) confirmed the presence of the large stone within an upper pole calyx of the right kidney. This study also demonstrated bilateral collecting system duplication with joining of the ureters at the L2–L3 vertebral level.

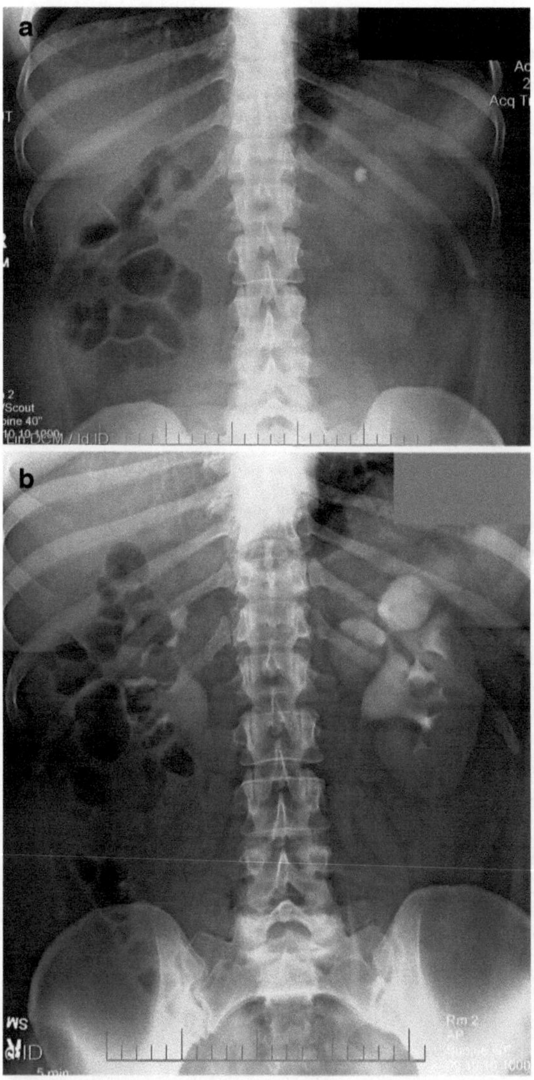

Fig. 4.1 (**a**) KUB of patient described in Case 1 demonstrating a calcification in the region of the upper pole of the left kidney. (**b**) IVP of the patient described in Case 1 demonstrating that the calcification is located within an upper pole calyceal diverticulum

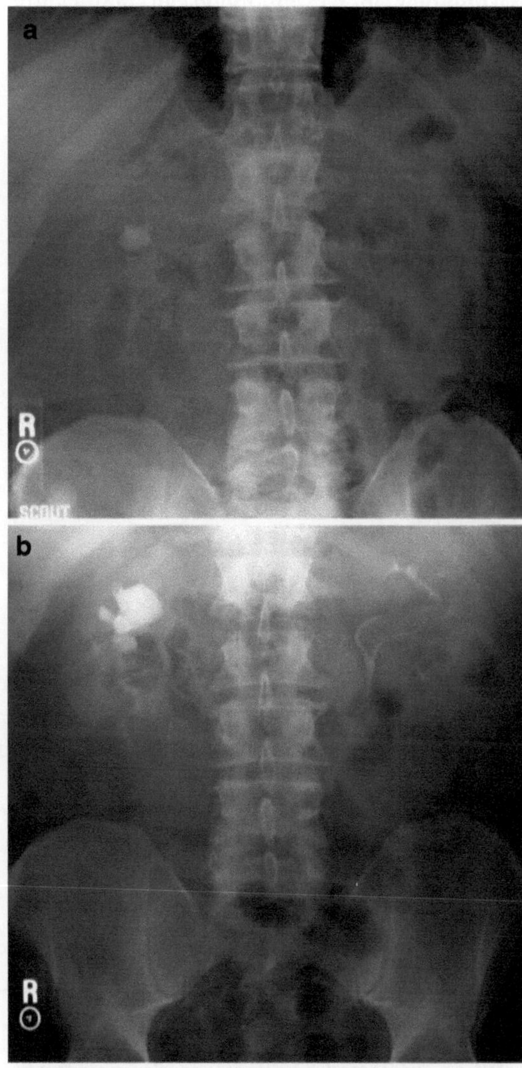

Fig. 4.2 (**a**) KUB of the patient described in Case 2 demonstrating a calcification in the region of the upper pole of the right kidney. (**b**) IVP of the patient described in Case 2 demonstrating that the calcification is located in a dilated upper pole calyx. This image also demonstrates the presence of bilateral incomplete collecting system duplication

Both collecting systems were extremely delicate and the stone-containing calyx was also noted to have a very narrow caliber infundibulum.

Decision Making

The patient described in Case 1 has several characteristics that make PNL the most reasonable option for management. The history of prior ureteral reimplantation in childhood can significantly increase the challenge of obtaining retrograde access to the kidney. Additionally, due to the size and location of the stone within a diverticulum, ESWL would not allow for adequate stone clearance. Similarly, the patient described in Case 2 also has complex and delicate collecting system anatomy, which would also make retrograde access much more difficult. Again, the large size and location of the stone within a dilated calyx with a stenotic infundibulum would make ESWL a poor choice for management. Therefore, it was recommended that both patients undergo PNL for treatment of their stone burden.

Preoperative Evaluation

All patients being prepared for percutaneous renal surgery should have a urine sample sent for culture and antibiotic susceptibility. All patients, including those with negative preoperative urine cultures, should receive 1 week of broad-spectrum oral antibiotic treatment prior to undergoing PNL. This is done with the intent of covering bacteria which may be harbored within a poorly draining diverticulum or within a stone. Additionally, all patients should receive parenteral broad-spectrum antibiotic coverage perioperatively, and the antibiotic should be tailored according to sensitivity reports for patients in whom preoperative urine cultures were positive.

When indicated, patients with significant comorbidities should be evaluated by the necessary medical services (i.e., cardiology or pulmonary medicine) to determine if they are appropriate candidates for general anesthesia and the stress of a surgical procedure. Additionally, recommendations for postoperative management of preexisting medical conditions can be obtained. Finally, a thorough review of all of the patient's medications should be performed and any antiplatelet or anticoagulant therapy should be discontinued for at least 1 week when possible.

Patient Positioning

After the administration of general endotracheal anesthesia, a 16 French Foley catheter is placed under sterile conditions. The patient is then transitioned onto the operating table in the prone position. The arm contralateral to the kidney being treated ("down arm") is carefully padded and positioned by the patient's side. The ipsilateral arm ("up arm") is padded and abducted with the elbow positioned at 90° (Fig. 4.3). The patient is then securely taped to the operating table, prepped, and draped in a sterile fashion. A C-arm fluoroscopic unit is covered sterilely and maneuvered over the patient from the side opposite of the kidney being treated.

Obtaining Access to the Diverticulum (or Hydrocalyx)

The C-arm fluoroscopic unit is used to initially identify the stone-containing diverticulum. The stone is then used as the target for obtaining

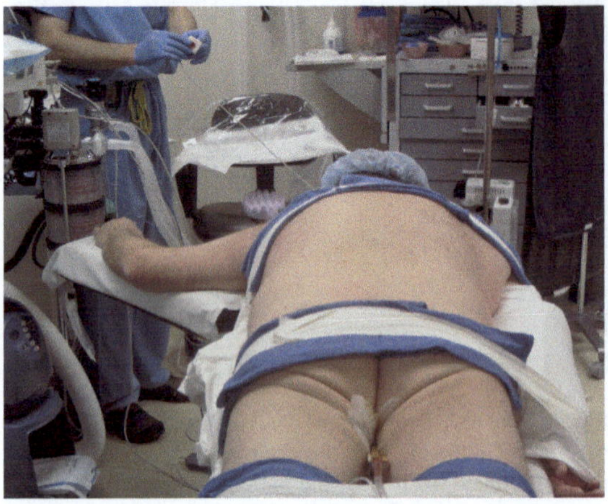

Fig. 4.3 Patient positioned to undergo left-sided PNL

direct percutaneous access with an 18 gauge diamond-tipped needle. A biplanar, fluoroscopic triangulation technique is employed to direct needle placement into the diverticulum [9]. Mediolateral adjustments of the needle, which elucidate the point of entry into the stone-containing diverticulum, are made with the C-arm directed parallel to the needle (anterior-posterior view). Cephalad and caudal needle adjustments, which demonstrate the depth of penetration, are made with the C-arm rotated as obliquely as possible in relation to the axis of the needle. It is important to maintain the needle orientation in one plane while adjustments are made in the second plane. This can be facilitated by the surgeon resting his or her arm on the patient's torso to stabilize the line of puncture. Once the direction of puncture is appropriately aligned in both planes, the needle is advanced with the C-arm rotated obliquely in order to monitor the depth of penetration. The anesthesiologist is asked to hold the patient's respirations prior to and during advancement of the needle in order to minimize respiratory motion of the kidney. Before the renal capsule is entered (the point at which the kidney begins to move with further advancement of the needle), final adjustments to the direction of puncture are made in both planes. The needle is then advanced into the stone-containing diverticulum with the C-arm again rotated obliquely [9].

It is preferable to obtain needle access to the diverticulum from an infracostal approach whenever possible in order to avoid the potential pleural complications associated with supracostal access. Infracostal access to upper pole diverticula (or solitary stone-containing hydrocalyces) can be achieved in nearly all cases, keeping in mind that a more medial puncture site and steep cephalad angulation for the direction of puncture will be required.

Non-Stone-Containing Diverticula/ Diverticula with Radiolucent Stones

In the case of symptomatic diverticula that do not contain stones (or contain stones which are not visible on fluoroscopy), instillation of contrast into the cavity is necessary in order to obtain needle access. Cystoscopic placement of a ureteral catheter and instillation of contrast material will often allow for retrograde opacification of the targeted diverticulum. However, if the diverticulum has a very small caliber infundibulum, this may not be possible. In this instance, ultrasound or CT guided preprocedure opacification of the diverticulum by the interventional radiology service can provide the visual target necessary for obtaining percutaneous access in the operating room. Opacification of the diverticulum should be performed with the patient in the prone position, using a 20 gauge spinal needle. It is important not to overdistend the diverticulum, as this can cause extravasation of contrast material and lead to difficulty with fluoroscopically targeting the cavity [4, 10].

Working Wire and Safety Wire Placement

Once needle access is achieved, a 0.035-in., J-tipped, removable core guide wire (Boston Scientific, Natick, MA) is advanced through the needle and coiled in the diverticulum under fluoroscopic guidance (Fig. 4.4a). A J-tipped removable core wire is ideal for initial access because the flexible distal end of the wire can be adapted to the size of the diverticulum. Additionally, the wire proximal to the removed core is stiff enough to allow for subsequent dilation of the percutaneous tract. It is imperative that the wire be carefully advanced into the diverticulum under fluoroscopic guidance for several reasons. First, it allows the surgeon to confirm that a portion of stiff wire is within the diverticulum so that subsequent tract dilation can be safely performed. Second, it is useful in preventing backwall perforation of the diverticular cavity with the stiff portion of the wire, which can lead to bleeding and obscured visualization. After the J-tipped wire is appropriately positioned in the diverticulum, an 8/10 French coaxial dilator (Boston Scientific, Natick, MA) is sequentially passed over the wire and into the cavity under fluoroscopic guidance, again taking great care not to advance the stiff end of the wire or the dilator through the back of the diverticulum. Once the 10 French component of the coaxial dilator is appropriately advanced within the diverticulum, the 8 French dilator is removed. Finally, a second J-tipped removable core wire is advanced through the 10 French dilator and coiled into the diverticulum to serve as a safety wire. The 10 French dilator is removed, and tract dilation can be safely performed (Fig. 4.4b) [1].

Tract Dilation

A balloon dilator (NephroMax™ Balloon, Boston Scientific, Natick, MA) is advanced over the working wire, again under fluoroscopic guidance, to ensure that neither the wire or balloon tip perforates the back wall of the diverticulum. When the balloon is appropriately positioned, it is inflated to capacity with contrast material. The balloon is then evaluated fluoroscopically to be sure there are no waists at the skin or fascial level, which would prevent passage of the access sheath over the balloon. If a waist is identified, the balloon should be deflated, and the skin incision should be dilated down to the fascial level using a hemostat. The balloon can then be repositioned and inflated. Next, a 30 French Amplatz sheath (Boston Scientific, Natick, MA) is advanced over the balloon under fluoroscopic guidance (Fig. 4.4c). For very small diverticula, it may not be possible to advance the sheath directly into the cavity due to the taper at the distal end of the balloon dilator. In these cases, endoscopic dilation of the tract and advancement of the sheath is necessary (see discussion in next section) [1].

Endoscopic Evaluation of the Diverticula (or Hydrocalyx) and Stone Treatment

A 24.5 French, rigid offset nephroscope without the external sheath (Richard Wolf, Vernon Hills, IL) is passed into the access sheath using normal saline as the irrigation fluid. For small diverticula, it is often necessary to dilate the portion of the

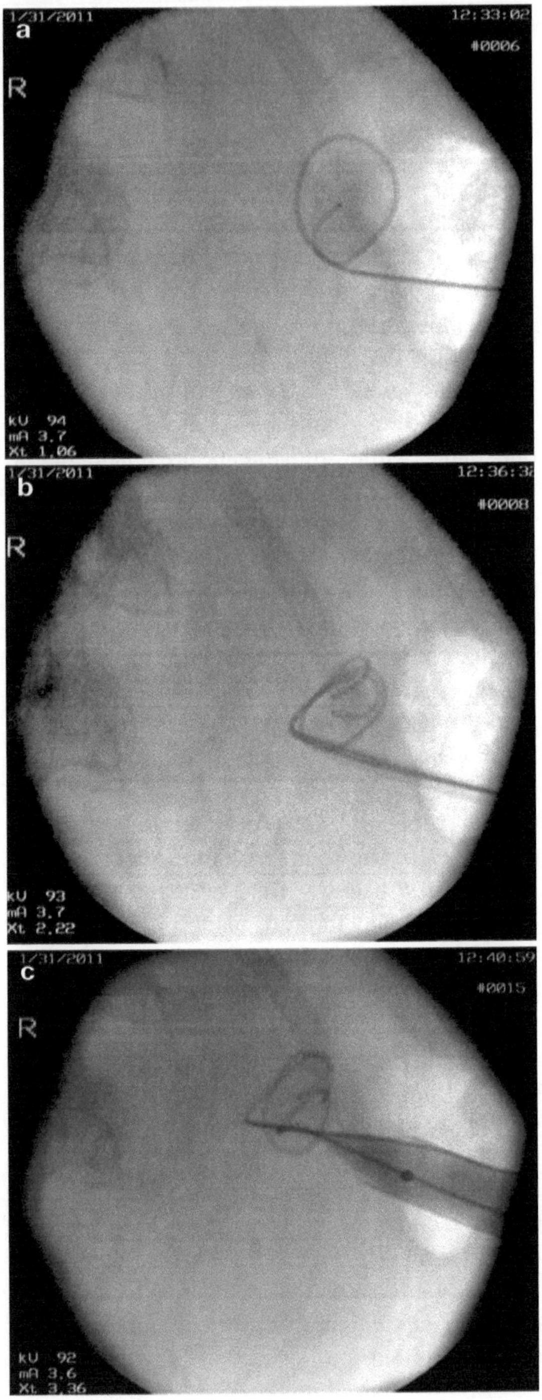

Fig. 4.4 (**a**) J-tipped removable core working wire coiled within a moderate-sized calyceal diverticulum. Note that a portion of stiff wire is within the cavity. (**b**) Working wire and safety wire coiled within the diverticulum. Stiff portions of both wires are within the cavity. (**c**) 30 French Amplatz sheath advanced over the dilating balloon up to the point of the diverticular cavity. Both J-tipped wires remain within the diverticular cavity and no back-wall perforation has occurred

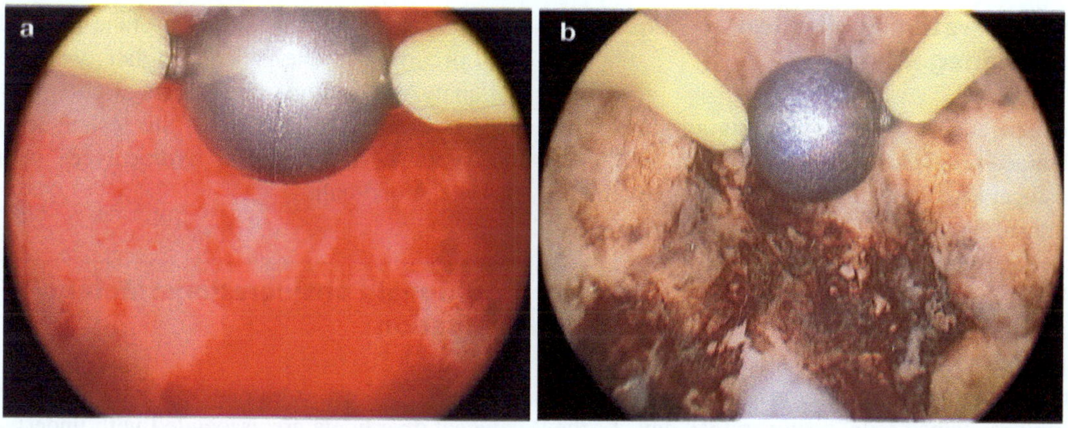

Fig. 4.5 (a) Prefulguration view of the diverticular cavity with the rollerball electrode in position. No papilla was identified to suggest that the cavity was a dilated calyx. (b) Postfulguration view of the diverticular cavity

percutaneous tract immediately preceding the cavity. This can be done by manually spreading the tract with an 11 French rigid alligator forceps. The rigid nephroscope can then be gently passed into the cavity, and the access sheath can subsequently be advanced over the nephroscope and into the lumen of the diverticulum. Once the stone material is identified a variety of techniques can be used for removal. For solitary, smaller stones, simple forceps, or basket extraction is often possible. In the case of large or numerous stones, ultrasonic lithotripsy is our preferred method for stone removal [1]. In all cases, a fragment of stone should be sent for bacterial culture and sensitivity and the remaining fragments should be sent for analysis of the crystalline composition.

Obliteration of the Diverticulum

Once the diverticulum has been entirely cleared of stone burden, the cavity should be carefully evaluated to ensure that a flattened renal papilla is not present, which would indicate that the cavity represents an obstructed calyx rather than a diverticulum. In this case, fulguration of the cavity would not be indicated. Once it is confirmed that the cavity represents a diverticulum, attention should then be turned to obliteration of the diverticular cavity. Irrigation fluid should be switched to 1.5 % glycine or 3 % sorbitol, and a 24 French resectoscope with a rollerball electrode (Karl Storz, El Segundo, CA) is assembled. The diverticular lining is then fulgurated in its entirety using a pure coagulation setting at 30 W (Fig. 4.5a, b). It is important to avoid contact of the rollerball electrode with the J-tipped wires. In our practice, we do not attempt to identify the infundibular communication to the collecting system, nor dilate it [1]. While some groups advocate dilation of the infundibulum or creation of a neoinfundibulum to the collecting system, this can cause significant bleeding and requires prolonged nephrostomy tube stenting of the infundibulum to ensure it remains patent. Additionally, the likelihood of complete obliteration of the diverticular cavity is much higher when fulguration is performed [10].

Postprocedure Drainage

After the diverticular cavity has been ablated, an 18 French red rubber catheter or a 10 French Cope loop (Cook Incorporated, Bloomington, IN) catheter is placed into the cavity. A Cope loop drainage catheter is generally reserved for diverticula that are large enough to house the loop in its entirety. Proper placement of the red rubber catheter or Cope loop within the diverticular cavity is confirmed with contrast injection under fluoroscopy prior to suturing it in place at the skin level. In the case of small diverticula, the red rubber catheter more often serves as a perinephric drain, as it frequently becomes dislodged from the cavity.

Postoperative Evaluation and Management

Postoperatively, abdominal imaging should be obtained to assess for stone-free status. NCCT on postoperative day 1 (prior to drainage catheter removal) is preferred as this allows for the detection of retained small fragments, which could ultimately cause persistent pain, leave a nidus for infection or prevent complete collapse of the diverticular cavity. In patients with no residual stone fragments and minimal output from the drainage catheter on postoperative day 1, the catheter can be removed, and the patient can be discharged home. For patients with residual fragments, a secondary procedure to remove the remaining stone burden can be performed on postoperative day 2 and the patient can then be discharged home. All patients should undergo follow-up imaging at 3 months time with renal ultrasound, IVP, or CT urography to assess for resolution of the diverticulum.

Results

At our institution the above-described technique for the percutaneous treatment of symptomatic calyceal diverticula has proven quite successful. This technique has allowed for a stone-free rate of 94.2 % after the primary percutaneous procedure. When a secondary percutaneous procedure is performed on patients with residual stone fragments identified on NCCT, a stone-free rate of 98 % has been achieved. Because our institution is a tertiary referral center, many of our patients are from out of state and obtain follow-up care with their local urologists. To our knowledge, during the course of postoperative follow-up, no patients have experienced a recurrent stone event. For the patients in whom a postoperative IVP has been available for our review, a complete diverticular resolution rate of 73.1 % has been observed. Our average operative time using this technique is 67.3 min (range 30–150 min) and the average hospital stay is 1.12 days (range 0.75–2.0 days) [10]. We have noted few complications, with a pleural effusion, perirenal hematoma, and significant pain after nephrostomy tube removal each occurring in one patient. To date, we have not analyzed the stone-free rates and complications associated with the use of this technique in the treatment of stones in hydrocalyces with stenotic infundibula.

Additional Considerations: Metabolic Evaluation

A review of the literature supports the fact that calyceal diverticula are associated with underlying metabolic abnormalities. In a 2006 report by Auge and colleagues, all patients with calyceal diverticula who underwent evaluation were noted to have a metabolic abnormality including hypercalciuria, hyperoxaluria, hypocitraturia, or hyperuricosuria. The most common abnormality noted on 24-h urine evaluation was low urine volume (<2.0 l/day) [11]. Additionally, a 2007 study by Matlaga and colleagues demonstrated similar urinary risk parameters (hypercalciuria and elevated calcium-oxalate supersaturation) in calcium-oxalate stone formers and in stone forming patients with calyceal diverticula [12]. Therefore, it is our practice to perform a metabolic evaluation prior to or 4–6 weeks after surgical intervention in all patients being treated for stone-containing calyceal diverticula. We routinely obtain a serum basic metabolic panel, calcium, and phosphorus level as well as two 24-h urine samples (collected on consecutive days). If any metabolic abnormalities are identified, they are treated appropriately (i.e., increased oral fluid intake for low urine volume or thiazide treatment for significant hypercalciuria) and repeat 24-h urine studies are then performed to assess for treatment success and stone-risk reduction.

Additional Considerations: Infection Treatment and Prevention of Recurrence

For all patients undergoing PNL for the treatment of calyceal diverticula, we generally recommend a 7-day course of culture-specific oral antibiotic in the immediate postoperative period given the fact that the poorly draining diverticula can harbor chronically infected urine. For patients in whom stone culture is positive, a prolonged antibiotic course (1–3 months) is recommended, in hopes of completely eradicating the urinary tract of the offending bacteria and preventing infection recurrence or stone regrowth.

Conclusion

Calyceal diverticula are congenital, nonsecretory cavities within the renal parenchyma, which can remain silent over a patient's lifetime or cause significant problems such as pain, hematuria, recurrent infection, or stone formation. When diverticula become symptomatic, treatment is indicated. The advent of minimally invasive technologies such as ESWL, ureteroscopy, and PNL has made the treatment of diverticula much more tolerable for the patient. To date, PNL remains the most reliable means for complete stone clearance, symptom resolution, and cavity ablation. Percutaneous treatment of calyceal diverticula presents a unique set of challenges to the urologist, as there is limited working space within the diverticular cavity and safe maintenance of wire access to the cavity can be difficult. Here we present a unique method for percutaneous treatment of calyceal diverticula, which has allowed for excellent stone-free and diverticular resolution rates with few complications.

In addition to the surgical management of diverticula, the urologist must keep in mind that there is a significant association with underlying metabolic abnormalities. Therefore, all patients treated for calyceal diverticula should undergo metabolic evaluation with serum testing and 24-h urine analysis. Any significant underlying abnormalities should be appropriately treated, and follow-up studies should be performed to assure the prescribed treatment is successful.

References

1. Kim SC, Kuo RL, Tinmouth WW, et al. Percutaneous nephrolithotomy for calyceal diverticular calculi: a novel single stage approach. J Urol. 2005;173:1194–8.
2. Gross AJ, Herman TRW. Management of stones in calyceal diverticulum. Curr Opin Urol. 2007;17:136–40.
3. Canales B, Monga M. Surgical management of the caliceal diverticulum. Curr Opin Urol. 2003;13:255–60.
4. Matlaga BR, Kim SC, Watkins SL, et al. Pre-percutaneous nephrolithotomy opacification for calyceal diverticular calculi. J Endourol. 2006;20:175–8.
5. Chong TW, Bui MHT, Fuchs GJ. Calyceal diverticula: ureteroscopic management. Urol Clin North Am. 2000;27:647–54.
6. David RD, Fuchs GJ. Flexible ureterorenoscopy, dilation of narrow caliceal neck, and ESWL: a new minimally invasive approach to stones in caliceal diverticula. J Endourol. 1989;3:3.
7. Batter SJ, Dretler SP. Ureterorenoscopic approach to the symptomatic caliceal diverticulum. J Urol. 1997;158:709–13.
8. Auge BK, Munver R, Kourambas J, et al. Endoscopic management of symptomatic caliceal diverticula: a retrospective comparison of percutaneous nephrolithotomy and ureteroscopy. J Endourol. 2002;16:557–63.
9. Lingeman JE, Matlaga BR, Evan AP. Surgical management of upper urinary tract calculi. In: Kavoussi LR, Novick AC, Partin AW, et al., editors. Campbell-Walsh urology. 9th ed. Philadelphia: Saunders/Elsevier; 2007. p. 1431–507.
10. Krambeck AE, Lingeman JE. Percutaneous management of caliceal diverticuli. J Endourol. 2009;23:1723–9.
11. Auge BK, Maloney ME, Mathias BJ, et al. Metabolic abnormalities associated with calyceal diverticular stones. BJU Int. 2006;97:1053–6.
12. Matlaga BR, Miller NL, Terry C, et al. The pathogenesis of calyceal diverticular calculi. Urol Res. 2007;35:35–40.

Managing Bleeding During Percutaneous Renal Surgery

5

Ahmed R. El-Nahas, Ahmed M. Shoma, and Ahmed A. Shokeir

Introduction

Percutaneous nephrolithotomy (PCNL) was introduced to urology practice in 1976 when Fernstrom and Johansson published their first report of percutaneous treatment of renal stones in three patients [1]. Then, the techniques of percutaneous renal access, dilatation of the tract, and stone manipulation were standardized by Alken et al. in 1981 [2]. During the following years, PCNL was reported by many authors all over the world as a minimally invasive treatment of renal stones, and percutaneous renal surgery (PRS) had become a daily urological practice [3, 4]. After the introduction and widespread availability of extracorporeal shock waves lithotripsy (SWL), it became the treatment of choice for small and noncomplex renal stones [5]. Therefore, the indications of PCNL were changed to include larger stone burden, and there were marked improvements in the techniques and instruments as well as in gaining much experience in doing PRS [6]. Currently, it is the treatment of choice for large, complex renal stones and staghorn stones because it offers better stone-free rate than SWL and lower morbidity than open surgery [7, 8].

A.R. El-Nahas, M.D. • A.M. Shoma, M.D. (✉)
A.A. Shokeir, M.D., Ph.D., FEBU
Department of Urology, Urology and Nephrology Center, Mansoura University, El Gomhoria Street, Mansoura 35516, Egypt
e-mail: ar_el_nahas@yahoo.com; ahmedshoma@hotmail.com; ahmed.shokeir@hotmail.com

The complications of PRS are specific for the procedure, and they include bleeding, injury to adjacent organs, and sepsis [9]. Bleeding complications during or after PRS are the most dangerous and life-threatening of them [10, 11]. In this chapter, we will present management of bleeding complications of PRS with special focus on identifications of risk factors and technical steps to avoid this frustrating complication.

Incidence of PRS Bleeding Complications

Blood loss is expected in PRS because some bleeding can occur during renal puncture, tract dilatation, nephroscopy, and stone disintegration. This bleeding is usually insignificant and does not interfere with visibility during stone manipulation or affect the patient's hemodynamic. Access to the pelvicalyceal system and intrarenal manipulations may traumatize interlobar or segmental renal vessels resulting in significant bleeding. It is considered a complication when blood transfusion is required. The reported incidence of transfusion after PCNL ranged between 0 and 23 % [12–16]. Osman et al. had reported on 315 patients who underwent PCNL with ultrasonography-guided renal access; the incidence bleeding was 10.8 %, but blood transfusion was not required in any patient [12]. A transfusion rate of 12 % was reported by Srivastava et al. for 1,854 patients and Lee et al. for 582 patients [13, 14], while higher rates of transfusion were observed by Martin et al.

A.M. Al-Kandari et al. (eds.), *Difficult Cases in Endourology*,
DOI 10.1007/978-1-84882-083-8_5, © Springer-Verlag London 2013

and Stoller et al. who reported 22 and 23 %, respectively [15, 16]. However, a transfusion rate of 36 % was reported by Martin et al. when they used multiple nephrostomy tracts for treatment of staghorn stones [16].

In spite of the wide variation in the reported incidence of post-PCNL transfusion rates, most of bleeding complications could be controlled with conservative measures such as clamping the nephrostomy, hydration and diuretics, hemostatic medications, and Kaye balloon tamponade [17, 18], and the need of selective renal artery angiography and embolization ranged between 0.3 and 1.4 % [3, 4, 11, 13, 14, 19, 20].

Renal Vascular Injuries During PRS

Types of Renal Vascular Injuries

Venous injury is the most common cause of intraoperative bleeding. However, it is usually mild and can be controlled with advancement of the Amplatz sheath to compress the renal parenchyma and stop bleeding or by conservative measures [11]. In contrary, arterial injuries cause severe bleeding. The most commonly detected arterial lesions were arteriovenous fistula (AVF) or arterial pseudoaneurysm. Blood passage from the high pressure of the injured artery to the injured adjacent vein results in AVF, and blood passage to the parenchyma leads to pseudoaneurysm [13]. A rare type of arterial injuries is laceration of a large branch of the main renal artery. It is the result of improper too medial puncture or overdilatation, and it leads to rapid loss of blood and may be fatal [11].

Management of Renal Vascular Injuries

Management of Intraoperative Bleeding

Venous bleeding from the renal parenchymal puncture along the tract can be stopped with the compression effect of the Amplatz sheaths over the parenchyma. The distal segment of the sheath should be within the area of the pelvicalyceal system, enabling tamponade of parenchymal bleeding. If proper placement of the sheath and removal of blood clots from the collecting system do not restore vision, then the procedure should be stopped and a wide nephrostomy tube is placed and clamped to facilitate clotting of blood inside the pelvicalyceal system with tamponade bleeding [21]. The other indication for termination of the procedure is the development of hemodynamic instability (hypotension and tachycardia) as a result of either rapid severe blood loss or continuous bleeding for a long time.

If bleeding does not stop, a Kaye tamponade balloon catheter (Cook Medical Inc., Bloomington, IN) can be used [18, 22]. The Kaye catheter is 25 cm in length with an internal lumen 14 F that allows drainage of the renal pelvis. Its balloon is 15 cm in length and 36 F in diameter when inflated. It is introduced over the guide wire through the percutaneous tract so that 2–3 cm is within the renal pelvis and then inflated with 10–12 ml of diluted contrast medium to tamponade the nephrostomy tract. It is left inflated for 2–4 days. The inflated balloon will tamponade the tract, and lumen will drain the collecting system. Alternatively, a percutaneous tract dilating balloon can be placed and inflated to tamponade the tract.

Heavy venous bleeding should be suspected when a high volume of dark colored blood drains from the tract after fluid irrigation is stopped. Injection of contrast into the collecting system in this setting will sometimes demonstrate opacification of the renal venous system. Gupta et al. described placement of a Council-tip balloon catheter that is inflated to compress renal parenchyma to tamponade venous bleeding [23].

A novel technique was described for patients with refractory tract hemorrhage by Millard et al. and named "hemostatic sandwich." In this technique, a 5-F angiographic catheter was placed through the kidney into the bladder, and a 22-F Council-tip catheter balloon was passed over this catheter and positioned so that the inflated balloon would occlude the inner surface of the nephrostomy tract. Then, a 16-F Council-tip catheter was placed over a second wire so that the balloon was just underneath the skin surface. Gelatin matrix hemostatic sealant was then injected to fill the tract. Inflation of the outer balloon completely sealed the tract, completing the hemostatic sandwich [24].

Arterial bleeding should be suspected if blood through the tract is bright red or has a pulsatile flow. Management of severe arterial bleeding that does not respond to any previous measures includes replacement of blood loss and urgent superselective renal angiograph and embolization proximal to the injured artery. In rare cases, urgent open renal exploration is warranted where the main renal artery is temporary clamped and then deep hemostatic sutures are applied to the bleeding area. Should this fail to control bleeding, partial or total nephrectomy is the last resort [10, 11].

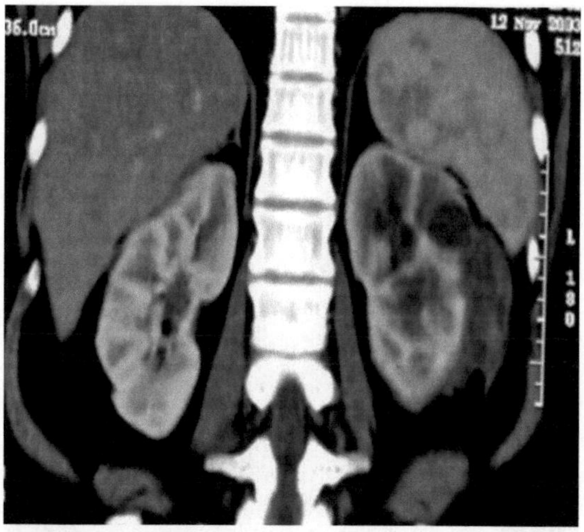

Fig. 5.1 Post-PCNL contrast-enhanced CT (coronal reformatted image) showing left perirenal hematoma

Management of Postoperative Bleeding

Postoperative bleeding may present with gross hematuria through the nephrostomy tract or through the urethra. It may be complicated with hypovolemic shock. Bleeding can occur in the immediate postoperative period, at the time of nephrostomy tube removal, or several days to weeks later [10, 11, 14, 20]. It may result from strenuous activity or restarting anticoagulation therapy. Delayed bleeding may result from rupture of arterial pseudoaneurysm [25].

Management of postoperative hematuria starts with immediate clamping of the nephrostomy if present or manual compression on the nephrostomy site with restoration if circulation collapses using crystalloids, colloids, blood, and blood product transfusion. The patients should undergo renal angiography and superselective embolization during the acute attack of bleeding.

Sometimes, there is no obvious external bleeding, and the urine looks clear in spite of internal bleeding to the retroperitoneal space. This is suspected when significant decrease of the hematocrit level is noticed after PCNL. A computed tomography (CT) scan should be performed if this diagnosis is suspected for detection of perirenal hematoma (Fig. 5.1). Conservative treatment in the form of bed rest and hemostatic drugs is successful treatment in most of cases, while blood transfusion and angiographic embolization are indicated if the hematoma is expanding or causing hemodynamic instability.

Technique of Superselective Renal Embolization

The procedure is performed under intravenous sedation with the patient in the supine position. A 21-gauge micropuncture needle is used to access the right common femoral artery. Then, a 0.035-in. J-tip guide wire is introduced, and the needle is then exchanged for a 6-F sheath over the guide wire. A Cobra catheter (Angiodynamics, Queensbury, NY) is then placed within the origin of the renal artery. A small amount of contrast is injected. Digital subtraction angiography (DSA) is performed to minimize the amount of contrast and radiation to the patient. Renal arterial anatomy is delineated, and any sources of hemorrhage are identified.

Arteriovenous fistulae are characterized by early filling of the venous system during arteriography (Fig. 5.2). Pseudoaneurysms, on the other hand, are saccular dilatations of the arterial branches (Fig. 5.3). Finally, lacerated segmental arteries are identified by contrast extravasation from a bluntly ended arterial branch (vessel cutoff).

A microcatheter (Terumo Progreat™ Microcatheter, Tokyo, Japan) is then used. Depending on the angiographic findings, the diag-

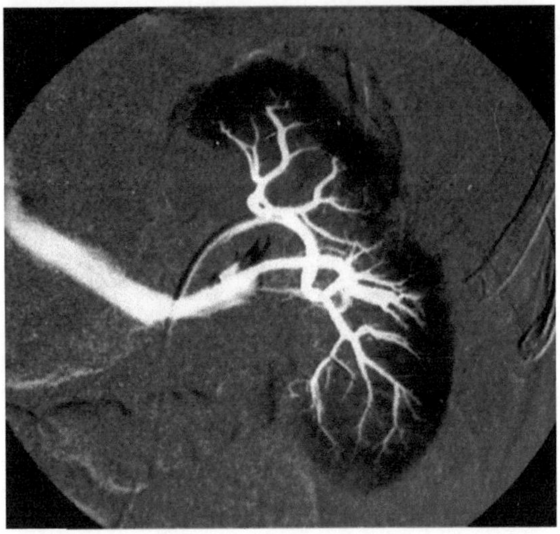

Fig. 5.2 Left superselective renal angiography showing passage of the contrast through the left renal vein due to arteriovenous fistula

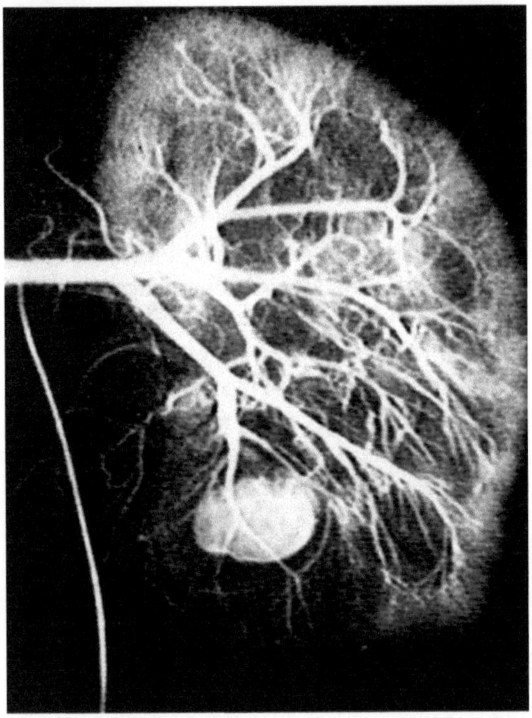

Fig. 5.3 Left superselective renal angiography showing extravasation of the contrast to form saccular dilatation from a lower arterial branch (pseudoaneurysms)

nostic microcatheter is advanced more as distally as possible through the arterial branches so that when the point of vascular disruption is embolized, as little renal parenchyma as possible is sacrificed. Platinum microcoils are the most commonly used embolization material. They are introduced through the microcatheter for embolization of the arterial branch just proximal to the site of injury [11, 21]. Gelfoam can be used for embolization alone or in combination with microcoils [13, 15]. Glue was also used as adjuvant to microcoils [26].

After placement of the microcoils, angiography is repeated through the Cobra diagnostic catheter to verify occlusion of the bleeding point and to assess the amount of parenchymal loss secondary to infraction. The catheters are removed, and pressure is applied at the site of the groin puncture [21]. After embolization, the patient will remain in bed with vital signs monitoring every 4–6 h. Ultrasonography and complete blood count are performed daily until stabilization of the condition. If bleeding recurs, another embolization session is performed [11].

Results of Superselective Renal Embolization

The success of superselective embolization to control bleeding after PCNL is very high. Martin et al. reported 87.5 % for 8 patients [19], Kessariset et al. published 90 % in 17 patients [20], and El-Nahas et al. reported 92 % in 39 patients [11], while Srivastava et al. observed 100 % success [13]. All these authors reported the need for a second embolization session in some patients either due to failure to identify the bleeding vessel in the first session or due to recurrence of bleeding.

Complication of Superselective Renal Embolization

Transfemoral arterial access complications include hemorrhage, arterial obstruction, pseudoaneurysms, and arteriovenous fistula with an incidence for each less than 0.3 % [27]. During superselective embolization, there is a risk of arterial dissection and "nontarget" embolization that can occur with migration of the embolization material [21]. Postinfarction syndrome which includes flank pain, fever, nausea, and vomiting is expected if a large arterial branch is occluded.

These symptoms are transient and can be managed symptomatically [28]. Urinary leakage from the nephrostomy site due to ischemia of the parenchyma supplied by the embolized artery was encountered and could be treated with double-J ureteral stent [11]. Postembolization rise in serum creatinine was reported in three out of nine patients with solitary kidney [29]. The long-term functional and morphological effects of embolization were evaluated by IVU and DMSA renal scans. Long-term follow-up showed functional and morphological improvements in comparison to early postembolization results [29].

Risk Factors of PRS Bleeding Complications

Identification of risk factors that affect bleeding complications of PRS is of paramount importance because avoiding them is the key to minimize bleeding. They can be divided into patient, renal, stone, and procedure-related factors.

Patients' Risk Factors

Kukreja et al. had investigated factors affecting blood loss during PCNL. The most important patients' risk factor associated with blood transfusion requirement in their study was preexisting anemia [30]. Turna et al. found that diabetic patients were prone to increased blood loss. Associated arteriosclerosis with thickened basement membranes may make such patients more prone to bleeding after the initial trauma of tract formation [31]. Other patients' factors such as age, gender, and hypertension were not risk factors [11, 30].

Renal Risk Factors

Solitary renal unit was identified by El-Nahas et al. to be an independent risk factor for severe bleeding after PCNL. Compensatory hypertrophy is a normal physiological response in a solitary kidney as the thickness of renal parenchyma increases with the increase in kidney size. Puncture and dilatation through thick renal parenchyma may increase the possibility of bleeding due to damage to more renal tissue and its vascular supply [11].

The role of previous surgical intervention (open or PCNL) for increased blood loss during PCNL has been a controversial issue. Stoller et al. and Kurtulus et al. found no significant difference in blood loss or transfusion rates in patients with and without a history of open surgery [16, 32]. On the contrary, Kukreja et al. found a significant decrease in blood loss in patients with a history of PCNL or open surgery. Cortical thinning with reduced blood flow may be responsible for this observation [30]. Other renal factors such as urinary tract infection, renal insufficiency function of the ipsilateral renal unit, and degree of hydronephrosis did not correlate with bleeding complications [30].

Stone Risk Factors

Increased stone burden was an important risk factor for bleeding complications of PCNL. Therefore, staghorn stones and stones with large surface area represent independent significant risk factors for increased blood loss [30], transfusion rate [31], and the need for embolization [11, 13, 20].

Procedure-Related Risk Factors

The technique of performing PRS is the most important influence of blood loss, transfusion rate, and bleeding complications.

Percutaneous Renal Access

Factors affecting proper percutaneous access include initial puncture, entry calyx, and number of punctures. The initial puncture can be done with a radiologist or a urologist and under ultrasonography or fluoroscopy guidance. Lam et al. showed a significant lower transfusion rate when the puncture was performed by a urologist (0 %) when compared with punctures performed by a radiologist (11 %) [33]. Watterson et al. reported higher clinically significant bleeding when the initial puncture was placed by a radiologist [34].

Kukreja et al. had found that ultrasound-guided access was associated with significantly less blood loss than fluoroscopy-guided access. They explained the reason for this by the fact that fluoroscopy-guided access requires imaging in two planes with the X-ray beam perpendicular and parallel to the puncture needle. On contrary, ultrasonography offers real-time three-dimensional monitoring of the puncture, including the needle and the collecting system, in the same plane, thereby minimizing the chance of vessel injuries [30]. However, fluoroscopic-guided punctures using multidirectional C-arm was reported to be a safe technique even in complex staghorn stones [11].

Other percutaneous-related risk factors include too medial punctures that may lead to direct injury to the posterior segmental arterial branch or puncture through an infundibulum which increases the risk of injury to segmental and interlobar vessels. Dilatation of these tracts can cause catastrophic bleeding [35].

El-Nahas et al. reported that upper calyceal puncture was a significant risk factor for severe bleeding requiring embolization. The reason for the increased incidence of vascular injury with upper calyceal puncture may be related to the oblique and longer length of the tract. In many cases, the upper calyx was superior to the site of skin puncture even if a supracostal approach was used. Therefore, an oblique and longer tract was needed (Fig. 5.4). Moreover, changing the direction of the tract to reach the renal pelvis may result in injury to the adjacent parenchyma with its vascular supply [11].

Multiple tracts were proved to be associated with more risk of bleeding complications [11, 15, 16, 30, 31]. It seems logical that the chances of damage to renal vasculature would be greater as the number of punctures increases.

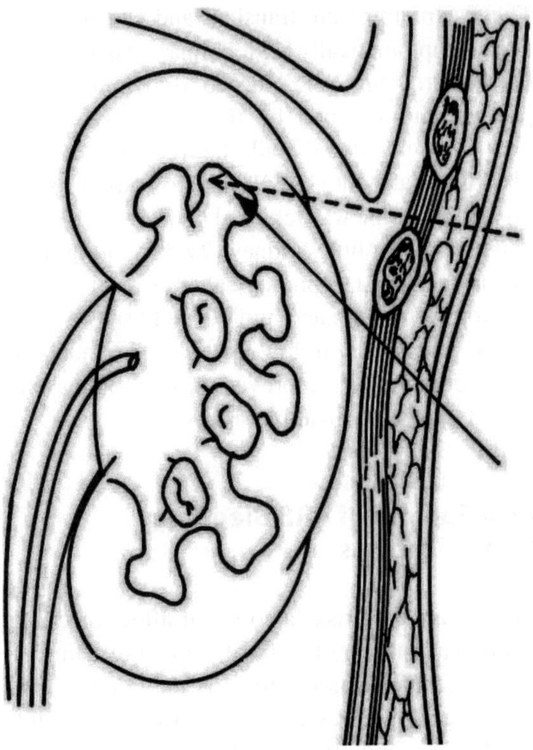

Fig. 5.4 A diagram showing short and direct percutaneous access to the upper pole through a supracostal puncture (*dashed arrow*) and an oblique and long percutaneous access to the upper pole through a subcostal puncture (*black arrow*)

Tract Dilatation

Method and extent of tract dilatation affect the degree of blood loss during PCNL. Methods of tract dilatation are the single-step balloon dilator (NephroMax™; Microvasive, Natick, Massachusetts), the Amplatz dilators, or the Alken metal telescopic sequential dilator. Stoller et al. compared telescopic metal and single-step balloon dilatation and found no significant difference in transfusion rates. Kukreja et al. compared the three methods of tract dilatation, and they observed more blood loss with statistically significant difference with Alken dilators [30], while Turna et al. [31] and Bellman and Davidoff [36] found that Amplatz dilatation system was associated with significantly more blood loss than balloon dilatation. They believe that during sequential dilator exchanges (in Amplatz dilators), the tamponade effect on the renal parenchymal tract is lost, leading to increased blood loss [31, 36].

The extent of tract dilatation was reported, by some investigator, to affect the degree of blood loss. Kukreja et al. have reported significantly less blood loss with the smaller tract (1.1 g/dl for tract size of 22 F (mini-PCNL) compared with 1.7 g/dl for tract size larger than 26 F) [30]. Feng et al. have found no difference in transfusion rates between standard PCNL (dilatation to 30 F) and mini-PCNL [37]. The advantage of small tract was overcome by longer operative times. Therefore, mini-PCNL is more useful in children with small kidneys [38], and its role in adults is restricted to kidneys with nondilated calyces and narrow infundibula or when a second tract is needed to remove residual small stones or in multiple tract procedures [30].

Intraoperative Technical Complications

Development of intraoperative complication is an important risk factor for PRS-related bleeding [30]. Perforation of the renal pelvis or the calyces was reported to be associated with increased blood loss. This may occur during dilatation of the tract or during stone disintegration [16]. Laceration of the calyceal neck (infundibulum) may damage adjacent blood vessels leading to severe bleeding. It can result from forceful manipulation of the rigid nephroscope to access stones in different calyces or pushing the large Amplatz sheath through the narrow neck of the calyx. Loss of the access tract during stone retrieval is another cause of intraoperative bleeding because of loss of the tamponade effect of the sheath over the renal parenchyma [30].

Operator Experience

The urological surgeon is responsible for optimizing renal access, tract dilatation, intrarenal manipulation, and minimizing technical errors. Operator experience was a significant predictor of the need for embolization [11]. Lam et al. reported that improved skills and flexible nephroscopy decreased transfusion rates [33].

Operative Time

Prolonged operative time was reported to be associated with increased blood loss during PCNL. The cutoff for safe operative time of PCNL is not defined, and it is decided by the endourologist judged by intraoperative events. Development of complications such as significant perforation of the pelvicalyceal system or intraoperative bleeding associated with hypotension is an indication to stage the procedure where nephrostomy tubes are placed through all unused tracts. This will allow subsequent manipulations to be performed through a mature tract. Sequential dilatation of this tract after 48 h may cause less trauma, leading to reduced bleeding and better vision during nephroscopy [30].

Staging the procedure for removal of large calculi is a controversial issue. The presence of a large stone burden was an indication of staging PCNL by Kukreja et al. [30], while two-stages may offset the correlation with blood loss. As such, the total blood loss from all the stages may be higher and be reflected in a higher transfusion rate.

Prevention of PRS Bleeding Complications

Bleeding complications of PRS cannot be completely avoided, and direct control of bleeding through the nephrostomy tracts is generally difficult. The following advices can minimize the incidence and magnitude of bleeding during and after PRS.

Proper Patient Selection and Preoperative Preparation

Bleeding complications in patients with uncontrolled hypertension, coagulopathy, and bleeding diathesis may be life-threatening. Therefore, complete blood counts and coagulation profiles must be assessed preoperatively. It is advised to avoid doing PRS for these patients and replace it with retrograde intrarenal surgery (RIRS) using ureterorenoscopy [39]. When PRS is the only option of treatment, international normalization ratio (INR) value more than 1.5 should be corrected which can be done through transfusion of fresh-frozen plasma (FFP) immediately prior to PCNL or by replacement of missing coagulation factors or platelets before intervention [35]. Preoperative transfusion of platelets is required immediately prior to PCNL when platelet concentration is below 50,000–80,000/dl [40].

In patients who are receiving anticoagulant or antiplatelet drugs, PRS can be performed with special precautions. Van Cangh et al. had divided these patients into three risk categories (high, intermediate, and low) and recommended the protocol for discontinuation of the anticoagulant drugs before intervention with replacement of low molecular weight heparin [41]. There are two major concerns about disconnection and reinitiating anticoagulation therapy: increasing risk for thromboembolic complications during the discontinuation period and the lack of knowledge about when to restart anticoagulation therapy after PRS. Keffer et al. reported that stoppage of warfarin (anticoagulant) for 5 days before PCNL with enoxaparin bridging and resuming it 5 days postoperatively and stoppage of clopidogrel and cilostazol (platelet inhibitors) for 10 days preoperatively and resuming it 5 days postoperatively was safe (7 % bleeding complications and 4 % thromboembolic complications) [42] .

Sound Techniques for PRS

The mainstay of reducing bleeding during PRS is meticulous operative technique and identification and modification of factors that may increase bleeding. The urologist is responsible for optimizing percutaneous renal access, tract dilatation, intrarenal manipulation, and minimizing technical errors.

Percutaneous Renal Access

Establishing an optimal percutaneous renal access is the most important factor in successful stone removal and minimization of blood loss during PRS. The ideal access must be straight and enter a posterior calyx at the most peripheral portion of the fornix to minimize the length of the tract through the renal parenchyma, thus limiting injury to large vessels which are condensed around the infundibulum of the calyx. This can be achieved with ultrasonographic guidance of fluoroscopic guidance using multidirectional C-arm to obtain two plains of fluoroscopy (anteroposterior and lateral). It is also advised that a urologist performs the renal access because he has a complete understanding of the intrarenal anatomy, especially the relation between the vasculature and the collecting system [30]. For urologists who do not place their own access, it is wise to perform a nephrostogram with oblique views prior to tract dilatation to ensure appropriate placement of the percutaneous nephrostomy tube.

The working J-tipped guide wire should pass easily through the infundibulum of the posterior calyx and into the renal pelvis. In contrast, direct puncture to the anterior calyx limits renal pelvic and posterior calyceal access. The working wire will often curl in the anterior calyx and not pass into the renal pelvis. The ideal tract should give access to the stone with no or minimal angulation. Therefore, we advise entering the upper calyx through a straight and direct tract when possible and avoiding excessive changes in the direction of the upper calyceal tract by using another lower calyceal puncture or flexible nephroscope to remove migrating stone fragments [11].

Tract Dilatation

Placement of two guide wires is important because a rigid one will be used for advancement of the dilators (working guide wire) and the second will be a safety guide wire in case of tract loss due to slippage or kinking of the working wire. To minimize renal pelvic perforation and excessive bleeding, the surgeon must avoid over advancement of the dilators because this may injure major vessels that are medial [16, 35]. When using the Alken dilator, each sequential dilator must be used in turn; skipping a size will tear the tissue and cause bleeding. The extent of tract dilatation must be suitable for the renal size and degree of hydronephrosis (i.e., reducing the caliber of the percutaneous tract in children and patients with nondilated collecting systems, with a narrow infundibulum and for secondary tracts in multiple-tract procedures) [35].

Intrarenal Manipulations

Meticulous and delicate manipulation during nephroscopy and stone disintegration and retrieval is of utmost importance in minimizing bleeding complications during PRS. Experience in PRS is usually needed to perform the procedure safely and effectively as well. El-Nahas et al. recommended that

PCNL should be performed by an experienced endourologist in patients at risk for severe bleeding, such as those with a solitary kidney or staghorn stones, because an experienced endourologist has the skills needed to perform proper renal access, judicious tract dilatation, and gentle manipulations using rigid and flexible nephroscopes [11].

The location of the working sheath should be noted because pushing a large sheath through a narrow calyceal neck may lead to disruption of the infundibulum and severe bleeding. Therefore, when the neck of the calyx is narrow, it is advised to dilate it before passage of the nephroscope or the sheath. The sheath can also slip out of the renal parenchyma during stone manipulation leading to loss of the renal tamponade and bleeding. This may occur during extraction of large stone fragments. So, it is safer to disintegrate a large stone into fragments smaller than the inner diameter of the sheath before extraction.

Stone disintegration must be done under direct vision, and adequate vision is only possible with sufficient irrigation. Also, the surgeon had to avoid pushing the stone during disintegration because this may lead to perforation and bleeding. Placing a second puncture when the initial tract is in a suboptimal location is important because compromise in access can lead to excessive torque forces on the kidney during stone manipulation and excessive bleeding [35].

In the postoperative period when the nephrostomy tube is ready to be removed, the surgeon needs to closely observe the patient and tube site for several minutes to ensure hemostasis. In cases where a Malecot or Cope tube is utilized, it is best to remove these under fluoroscopic guidance to minimize tissue injury and bleeding. Venous bleeding from the nephrostomy site can be managed with a pressure dressing and close observation. Brisk and bright bleeding from the tube site must alert the surgeon to a possible arterial bleeding. The patient should be stabilized and taken to the interventional radiology suite for angiographic embolization. The source of bleeding in this setting may be due to disrupted vessels or tissue bridges sheared off by the eye or lumen of the nephrostomy tube [16].

Summary

Management of bleeding complications induced by PRS includes the following: stopping the procedure; placement and clamping of a wide nephrostomy tube; administration of intravenous fluids, diuretics, and hemostatic drugs; and transfusion of blood or blood products whenever indicated. In some cases, special catheters such as Council-tip and Kaye catheters can be used. If bleeding continues in spite of previous measures, superselective renal angiography and embolization of the injured vessel are useful to control bleeding. In rare cases with severe uncontrollable bleeding, emergency exploration and suturing the bleeding renal parenchyma or doing nephrectomy can be life-saving procedure.

Bleeding complications of PRS cannot be completely avoided, but identification of risk factors is of paramount importance because avoiding them is the key to minimize PRS-induced bleeding. The following can minimize the incidence and magnitude of bleeding during and after PRS:

1. Proper patient selection and preoperative preparation.
2. The urologist is responsible for optimizing percutaneous renal access, tract dilatation, intrarenal manipulation, and minimizing technical errors.
3. The ideal percutaneous renal access must be straight and enter a posterior calyx at the most peripheral portion of the fornix.
4. The extent of tract dilatation must be suitable for the renal size and degree of hydronephrosis.
5. Meticulous and delicate manipulation during nephroscopy, stone disintegration, and retrieval.

References

1. Fernstrom I, Johansson B. Percutaneous pyelolithotomy: a new extraction technique. Scand J Urol Nephrol. 1976;10:257–9.
2. Alken P, Hutschenreiter G, Günther R, Marberger M. Percutaneous stone manipulation. J Urol. 1981;125:463–6.

3. Segura JW, Patterson DE, Le Roy AJ, Williams Jr HJ, Barrett DM, Benson Jr RC, et al. Percutaneous removal of kidney stones: review of 1,000 cases. J Urol. 1985;134:1077–81.
4. El-Kenawy MR, El-Kappany HA, El-Diasty TA, Ghoneim MA. Percutaneous nephrolithotomy for renal stones in over 1000 patients. Br J Urol. 1992; 69:470.
5. Chaussy CG, Fuchs GJ. Current state and future developments of noninvasive treatment of human urinary stones with extracorporeal shock wave lithotripsy. J Urol. 1989;141:782–9.
6. Desai M, Jain P, Ganpule A, Sabnis R, Patel S, Shervastav P. Developments in technique and technology: the effect on the results of percutaneous nephrolithotomy for staghorn calculi. BJU Int. 2009;104: 542–8.
7. Preminger GM, Assimos DG, Lingeman JE, Nakada SY, Pearle MS, Wolf Jr JS. AUA nephrolithiasis guideline panel chapter 1: AUA guideline on management of staghorn calculi: diagnosis and treatment recommendations. J Urol. 2005;17:1991–2000.
8. Al-Kohlany KM, Shokeir AA, Mosbah A, et al. Treatment of complete staghorn stones: a prospective randomized comparison of open surgery versus percutaneous nephrolithotomy. J Urol. 2005;173:469–73.
9. Michel MS, Trojan L, Rassweiler JJ. Complications in percutaneous nephrolithotomy. Eur Urol. 2007;51: 899–906.
10. Lang EK. Percutaneous nephrostolithotomy and lithotripsy: a multi-institutional survey of complications. Radiology. 1987;162:25–30.
11. El-Nahas AR, Shokeir AA, El-Assmy AM, et al. Post-percutaneous nephrolithotomy extensive hemorrhage: a study of risk factors. J Urol. 2007;177:576–9.
12. Osman M, Wendt-Nordahl G, Heger K, Michel MS, Alken P, Knoll T. Percutaneous nephrolithotomy with ultrasonography-guided renal access: experience from over 300 cases. BJU Int. 2005;96:875–8.
13. Srivastava A, Singh KJ, Suri A, Dubey D, Kumar A, Kapoor R, et al. Vascular complications after percutaneous nephrolithotomy: are there any predictive factors? Urology. 2005;66:38–40.
14. Lee WJ, Smith AD, Cubelli V, Badlani GH, Lewin B, Vernace F, et al. Complications of percutaneous nephrolithotomy. AJR Am J Roentgenol. 1987;148: 177–80.
15. Martin X, Tajra LC, Gelet A, Dawahra M, Konan PG, Dubernard JM. Complete staghorn stones: percutaneous approach using one or multiple percutaneous accesses. J Endourol. 1999;13:367–8.
16. Stoller ML, Wolf Jr JS, St Lezin MA. Estimated blood loss and transfusion rates associated with percutaneous nephrolithotomy. J Urol. 1994;152:1977–81.
17. Galek L, Darewicz B, Werel T, Darewicz J. Hemorrhagic complications of percutaneous lithotripsy: original methods of treatment. Int Urol Nephrol. 2000; 32:231–3.
18. Kaye KW, Clayman RV. Tamponade nephrostomy catheter for percutaneous nephrolithotomy. Urology. 1986;27:441–5.
19. Martin X, Murat FJ, Feitosa LC, Rouviere O, Lyonnet D, Gelet A, et al. Severe bleeding after nephrolithotomy: results of hyperselective embolization. Eur Urol. 2000;37:136–9.
20. Kessaris DN, Bellman GC, Pardalidis NP, Smith AG. Management of hemorrhage after percutaneous renal surgery. J Urol. 1995;153:604–8.
21. Rastinehad AR, Andonian S, Smith AD, Siegel DN. Management of hemorrhagic complications associated with percutaneous nephrolithotomy. J Endourol. 2009;23:1763–7.
22. Kerbl K, Picus DD, Clayman RV. Clinical experience with the Kaye nephrostomy tamponade catheter. Eur Urol. 1994;25:94–8.
23. Gupta M, Bellman GC, Smith AD. Massive hemorrhage from renal vein injury during percutaneous renal surgery: endourological management. J Urol. 1997;157:795–7.
24. Millard 2nd WW, Jellison FC, Tenggardjaja C, Ebrahimi KY, Baldwin DD. Hemostatic sandwich to control percutaneous nephrolithotomy tract bleeding. J Endourol. 2010;24:1415–9.
25. Gavant ML, Gold RE, Church JC. Delayed rupture of renal pseudoaneurysms: complication of percutaneous nephrostomy. AJR Am J Roentgenol. 1982;138: 948–9.
26. Beaujeux R, Saussine C, AL-Fakir A, et al. Superselective endovascular treatment of renal vascular lesions. J Urol. 1995;153:14–7.
27. Hessel SJ, Adams DF, Abrams HL. Complications of angiography. Radiology. 1981;138:273–81.
28. Schwartz MJ, Smith EB, Trost DW, Vaughan Jr ED. Renal artery embolization: clinical indications and experience from over 100 cases. BJU Int. 2007;99: 881–6.
29. El-Nahas AR, Shokeir AA, Mohsen T, Gad HM, El-Assmy AM, El-Diasty TA, El-Kappany HA. Functional and morphological effects of postpercutaneous nephrolithotomy superselective renal angiographic embolization. Urology. 2008;71:408–12.
30. Kukreja R, Desai M, Patel S, Bapat S, Desai M. Factors affecting blood loss during percutaneous nephrolithotomy: prospective study. J Endourol. 2004; 18:715–22.
31. Turna B, Nazli O, Demiryoguran S, Mammadov R, Cal C. Percutaneous nephrolithotomy: variables that influence hemorrhage. Urology. 2007;69:603–7.
32. Kurtulus FO, Fazlioglu A, Tandogdu Z, Aydin M, Karaca S, Cek M. Percutaneous nephrolithotomy: primary patients versus patients with history of open renal surgery. J Endourol. 2008;22:2671–5.
33. Lam HS, Lingeman JE, Newman DM, et al. Evolution of the technique of combination therapy for staghorn calculi: a decreasing role for extracorporeal shock wave lithotripsy. J Urol. 1992;148:1058–62.

34. Watterson JD, Soon S, Jana K. Access related complications during percutaneous nephrolithotomy: urology versus radiology at a single academic institution. J Urol. 2006;176:142–5.
35. Lee KL, Stoller ML. Minimizing and managing bleeding after percutaneous nephrolithotomy. Curr Opin Urol. 2007;17:120–4.
36. Bellman GC, Davidoff R. Influence of technique of percutaneous tract creation on incidence of renal hemorrhage. J Urol. 1997;157:1229–31.
37. Feng MI, Tamaddon K, Mikhail A, Kaptein JS, Bellman GC. Prospective randomized study of various techniques of percutaneous nephrolithotomy. Urology. 2001;58:345–50.
38. Desai MR, Kukreja RA, Patel SH, Bapat SD. Percutaneous nephrolithotomy for complex pediatric renal calculus disease. J Endourol. 2004;18:23–7.
39. Gross AG, Bach T. Preoperative percutaneous stone surgery in patients receiving anticoagulant therapy. J Endourol. 2009;23:1563–5.
40. Lewis S, Patel U. Major complications after percutaneous nephrostomy-lessons from a department audit. Clin Radiol. 2004;59:171–9.
41. Van Cangh P, Smith AD, Ng CS, et al. Management of difficult kidney stones. J Endourol. 2007;21:478–89.
42. Kefer JC, Turna B, Stein RJ, Desai MM. Safety and efficacy of percutaneous nephrostolithotomy in patients on anticoagulant therapy. J Urol. 2009;181:144–8.

6 Septic Complications During Percutaneous Nephrolithotomy (PCNL)

Evangelos Liatsikos and Panagiotis Kallidonis

Introduction

Percutaneous nephrolithotomy (PCNL) is a milestone for the removal of renal stones for three decades already [1]. Since the first introduction of the technique in 1976, various improvements have been proposed [2, 3]. The indications of the procedure were limited due to the introduction of extracorporeal shock wave lithotripsy (ESWL) in the 1980s [4]. Clinical experience with ESWL revealed the limitations of the technique, and the role of PCNL in the management of renal stones was redefined [5–7]. The current indications for PCNL include large, hard infected stones, obstruction-related stones, ESWL failures, and stones related with anatomical variations [8, 9]. In addition, improvements in instruments such as flexible nephroscopes, ureteroscopes, and lithotriptors (holmium/yttrium-aluminum-garnet laser, combination of ultrasound and pneumatic technology) contributed to the current high stone-free rates of PCNL which are higher than 90 % [10–12]. Flexible nephroscopes allowed the disintegration and removal of stones in calyces not accessible by the rigid nephroscopes, while advanced lithotriptors enabled the management of very hard stones [13].

In general, PCNL is considered as a safe procedure accompanied by low complication rate [8,14]. Nevertheless, the review of current literature revealed complication rate up to 83 %. The majority of complications were bleeding or fever of no clinical significance [13]. Fever following PCNL procedure has been observed in 21–32.1 % of the cases [15–18]. Septicemia represented a major complication of PCNL and was encountered in 0.9–4.7 % of the cases [13]. Recently, categorization of PCNL complications in 811 patients according to Clavien classification system was performed. Fever requiring antipyretics was the most common grade I complication and was observed in 3 % of the cases. Urinary tract infection requiring additional to prophylactic antibiotic therapy was encountered in 0.8 % of the cases (grade II complication). Urosepsis was observed in 0.3 % of the cases and was classified as a grade 4b compilation [19]. Duration of procedure, bacterial load in the urine, severity of obstruction, and presence of infected stone directly affect the incidence of urosepsis and septic shock. Sepsis is difficult to predict even if careful preoperative preparation has taken place. The source of the infection is almost always the stone itself, regardless of its nature (infection or noninfection stone). Despite the high index of suspicion, it is impossible to predict preoperatively with certainty the source of infection [20].

The pathogenesis of urosepsis associated with PCNL has been attributed to high concentrations of endotoxins released in the systemic circulation during stone manipulation resulting

E. Liatsikos, M.D., Ph.D. • P. Kallidonis, M.D. (✉)
Department of Urology, University Hospital of Patras, Rion, Patras, 26504, Greece
e-mail: liatsikos@yahoo.com; pkallidonis@yahoo.com

A.M. Al-Kandari et al. (eds.), *Difficult Cases in Endourology*,
DOI 10.1007/978-1-84882-083-8_6, © Springer-Verlag London 2013

in initiation of systemic inflammatory response. High concentrations of lipopolysaccharides have been detected in both infection and noninfection stones. Several cytokines such as interleukins, tumor necrosis factor (TNF), interferons, kinins, complement factors, and nitric oxide play role in urosepsis. The above process could be enhanced by an obstruction of the upper urinary tract due to the open pyelolymphatic and pyelovenous channels [20].

We herein discuss our experience with septic complications related to PCNL procedure while presenting current literature on the subject as well as prevention and management methods.

Difficulties

Septicemia (or bacteremia) is defined as systemic disease associated with the presence and persistence of pathogenic microorganisms or their toxins in the blood. Septicemia is usually transient, self-limited, and of little clinical significance. Instrumentation of the urinary tract is not uncommon to cause bacteremia [21]. Sepsis syndrome could follow unresolved septicemia and includes tachypnea (respirations>20/min), tachycardia (Pulse>90 min), hyperthermia (>38.3 °C) or hypothermia (<35.6 °C), white blood cell count >12,000 or <4,000/mm^3, clinical evidence of infection and evidence of inadequate organ perfusion with hypoxemia ($PaCO_2$<32mmHg), elevated plasma lactated concentration, and oliguria (<0.5 ml/kg for at least 1 h). Sepsis syndrome could result into septic shock which is presented with all of the above signs and symptoms of sepsis syndrome and additionally hypotension (systolic pressure < 90mmHg or drop of pressure by >40mmHg for at least 1 h). Sepsis syndrome and septic shock are medical emergencies. Septic syndrome without shock has been reported to have a mortality rate of 13 %. Septic shock has mortality rate of 28 %, while shock developing after sepsis syndrome has a rate of 43 % [21].

Gram-negative and gram-positive bacteria were isolated in 30–80% and 5–24 % of the cases of sepsis syndrome and septic shock, respectively. An etiologic agent was not identified in almost half of the cases. *E. coli* was the most common organism associated with bacteremia. *P. aeruginosa*, *Proteus*, *Providencia*, *Serratia*, *Acinetobacter*, and *Enterobacter* have been related to nosocomial infections. The type of organism responsible is not related to the severity of septic shock [22–24].

Fever secondary to urinary tract infection following PCNL is common presented in up to 32 % of the cases. Septicemia could be caused by an infection introduced by the access to the kidney or if the stones are infected. Fever following PCNL is significantly more frequent (and higher) in cases of infected stones (struvite or staghorn stones) in comparison to those with sterile stones [25]. Renal insufficiency is a risk factor for postoperative fever and sepsis [8, 13]. Long-lasting operation and high volume or pressure of irrigation fluid used during the procedure predispose to fever [8, 17, 25].

Intestinal and colonic injuries could result in septic complications such as peritonitis or severe urinary tract infection. Previous bowel surgery predisposes to duodenum or colonic injury, and the urologist should proceed with special care [8]. Colonic perforation has been observed in less than 1 % of PCNLs [13]. The rare case of a retrorenal colon or cases of punctures laterally to the posterior axillary line are related to colonic injury. Colonic perforation had an incidence of 0.3 % in a large series of 5,039 cases [26]. All injuries were retroperitoneal. Left side was involved in 66.6 % of the complicated cases while right was involved only in cases of horseshoe kidney or recurrent disease. Colonic injuries took place in 12 lower caliceal punctures (80 %) and lower caliceal punctures in the remaining. The latter punctures resulted in bowel lesion only in cases of horseshoe kidney or chronic colonic distension [26]. Risk factors for colonic injury are advanced patient age, presence of horseshoe kidney and left-side procedure, and risk of perforation can increase up to 1 %. [13]. Further risk factors are an inflated colon and a very thin patient. Intestinal injuries are rare during PCNL. The majority of colon laceration cases are detected postoperatively [26]. The colonic injury could be diagnosed by the presence of contrast within the colon during antegrade or retrograde pyelography as well as with abdominal computerized tomography [8]. The second and third segments of duodenum could be lacerated in the case of renal pelvis perforation during dilation, sheath placement, or stone extraction [8, 13, 27]. The presence of intestinal mucosa or contents visualized during PCNL as well as the presence of contrast within the bowel in nephrostogram should alert the surgeon.

Case Description

Several cases of septic complications have been observed during our experience with PCNL. The following special cases are discussed in an attempt to propose methods to overcome septic complications.

Case 1

A 37-year-old female was presented in the emergency department in septic condition. Fever was 39.4 °C; rigor, chills, cough, and right flank pain were present. Tachycardia and tachypnea were observed. Laboratory examination revealed 22,000 white blood cell count (92 % neutrophils), with increased SGOT/SGPT, LDH, and CRP. Slight increase in serum creatinine was also present. Blood gas examination revealed metabolic acidosis with concomitant respiratory alkalosis. Chest X-ray showed atelectasis in the lower lobe of the right lung. Abdominal ultrasound revealed pelvicaliceal dilatation of the right kidney with the presence of a stone occupying the majority of the collecting system. KUB X-ray showed the presence of a staghorn stone in the right kidney. Urinalysis demonstrated high counts of white and red blood cell count. Blood and urine cultures were obtained. Antibiotic therapy was initiated immediately and symptomatic supportive measures were taken (oxygen administration, antipyretics, etc.).

In order to elucidate the source of sepsis, chest and abdominal CT scan was performed. A fistula between the collecting system of the right kidney and the lower lobe of the ipsilateral lung was revealed. Placement of chest tube for drainage of the right thoracic cavity and of two nephrostomy tubes for decompression and drainage of the right collecting system took place. The nephrostogram performed during nephrostomy insertions confirmed the presence of fistula (Figs. 6.1 and 6.2). Purulent fluid was released during the puncture of the collecting system.

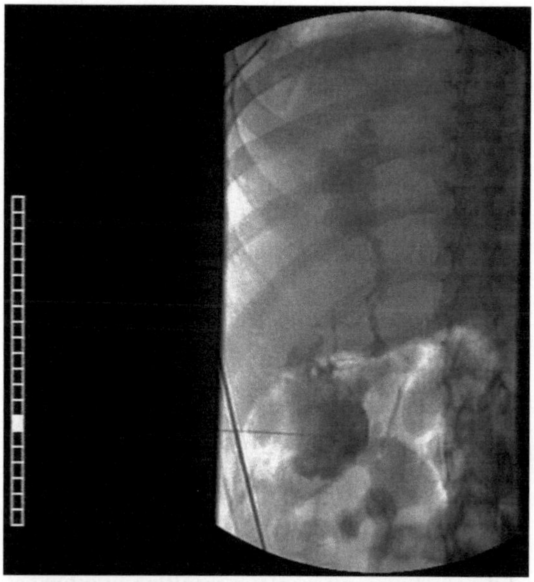

Fig. 6.1 Fistula formed between the right lung and ipsilateral pelvicaliceal system as presented in nephrostogram

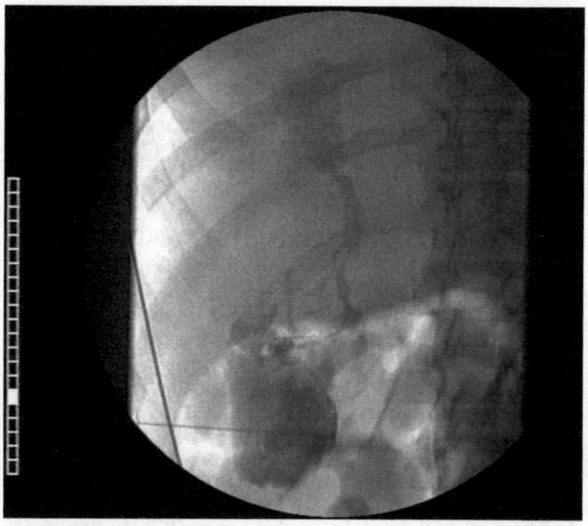

Fig. 6.2 Fistula formed between the right lung and ipsilateral pelvicaliceal system as presented in nephrostogram (magnified image)

In the following 2 days after admission, the patient significantly improved with reduction of fever, absence of rigor and chills, and limitation of flank pain. Blood gas examination was normalized. Biochemical profile improved in comparison to the initial examination. Antibiotic therapy continued and the patient was allowed to return home after 15 days. The nephrostomy tube remained in place. Three weeks after the initial incident, a nephrostogram was repeated and the fistula was not observed. PCNL followed for the clearance of the staghorn stone.

Case 2
A 55-year male patient underwent PCNL for the management of a right renal pelvic stone. During puncture and sheath placement, the dilatation of the tract was overzealous resulting in injury of the duodenum. The injury was observed during the nephrostogram as the contrast was present in the duodenum (Figs. 6.3, 6.4, and 6.5). We did not proceed further with the procedure since any additional manipulation could result in expanding the lesion. The patient was managed by nasogastric suction and nephrostomy placement in order to decompress both the collecting system of the kidney and the stomach. Antibiotics and parenteral hyperalimentation were administered. Nephrostogram was repeated 7 days after the injury and there was no leakage of contrast in the duodenum (Fig. 6.6). Two weeks after the incident, the patient underwent PCNL for stone clearance.

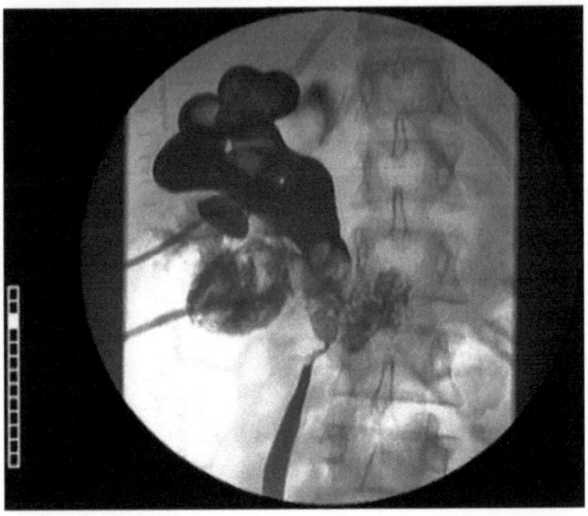

Fig. 6.3 Perforation of renal pelvis and duodenum. Note the contrast in the duodenum

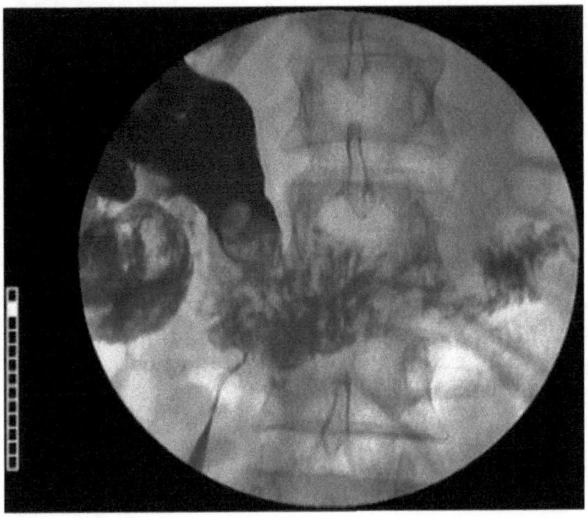

Fig. 6.4 Contrast in perforated duodenum. Clear depiction of the duodenal intraluminal morphology

Case 3
A 50-year-old female underwent PCNL for multiple stones in the right renal pelvis. No complication was observed during the procedure. On the first postoperative day, the patient complained of intense abdominal pain. Fever was present (38.2 °C). Auscultation of the abdomen revealed absence of bowel sounds, while there was increased tenderness on the right side of the abdomen. White blood cell count was high. An abdominal CT scan was performed and the presence of fluid in the peritoneal cavity was detected. The suspicion of a colonic perforation led us to perform laparotomy. A very small lesion in the ascending colon was revealed. The lesion was responsible for leakage of the colonic content in the peritoneal cavity and causing peritonitis. Colostomy was eventually performed. The postoperative course after the laparotomy was uneventful. The patient underwent reanastomosis of the colon 3 months after the colostomy procedure.

Case 4
A 42-year-old female patient underwent PCNL for multiple stones in the left pelvicaliceal system. No untoward event was observed during the procedure. On the 8th postoperative day and as the

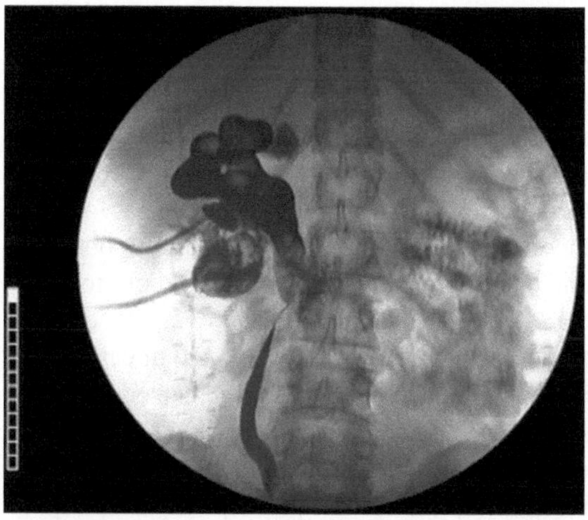

Fig. 6.5 Contrast in perforated duodenum. Clear depiction of the communication between the collecting system and the duodenum

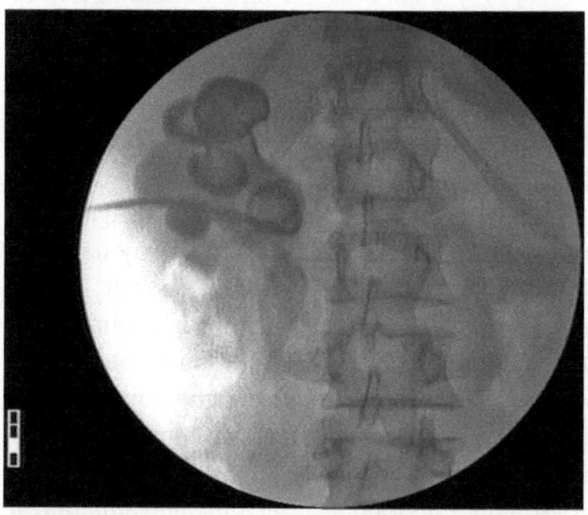

Fig. 6.6 The duodenal injury a week after the perforation

patient was already discharged, fever of 39 °C and intense left flank pain initiated. The patient presented to us with the above symptoms as well as tachycardia and tachypnea. White blood cell count was elevated with 90 % neutrophilia. CRP, SGOT/SGPT, and LDH were increased. Metabolic acidosis was present. Abdominal ultrasound showed fluid collection around the left kidney. Nephrostomy was also placed for the drainage and decompression of the collecting system. A nephrostogram was performed and perirenal collection was confirmed along with leakage from a calyx (Figs. 6.7, 6.8, and 6.9). Percutaneous drainage of

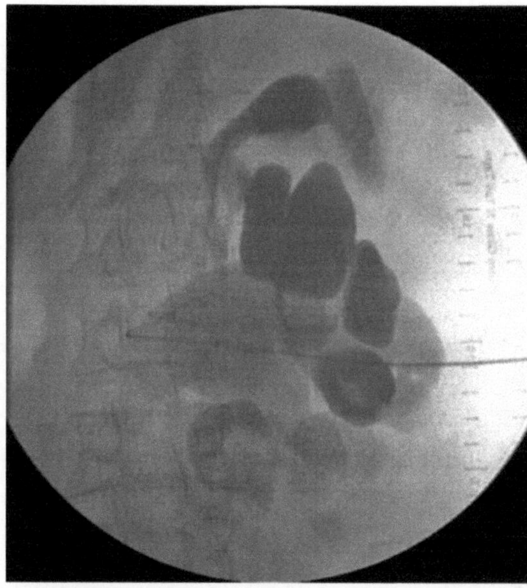

Fig. 6.7 Perforated renal calyx results in extravasation of contrast into renal abscess cavity

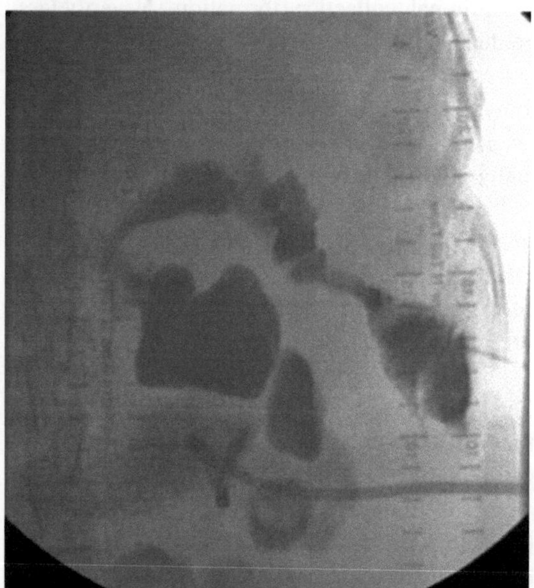

Fig. 6.8 Clear depiction of the fistula between the collecting system and the abscess cavity

purulent fluid followed which confirmed the diagnosis of perirenal abscess. Antibiotic therapy was administered. Since we routinely perform a nephrostogram before the removal of nephrostomy tube after PCNL, the current case was unusual. The postoperative nephrostogram should have

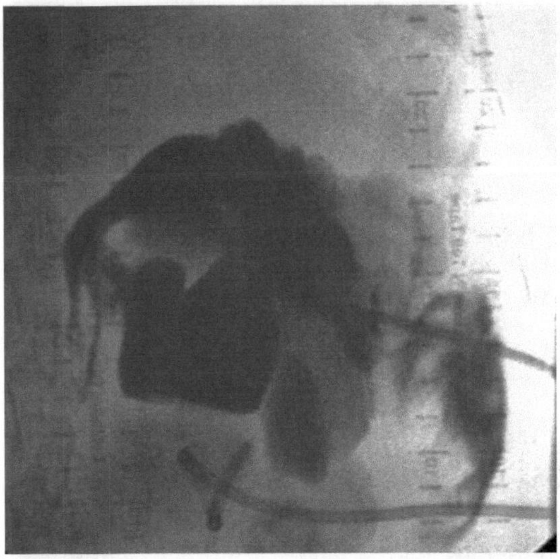

Fig. 6.9 Drainage and nephrostomy tubes inserted

detected any lesion of the pelvis which could lead to perirenal collection formation. Nevertheless, gradual leakage of fluid in the perirenal tissue took place and the following removal of the nephrostomy increased the intrapelvic pressure and resulted in a perirenal collection which was eventually infected resulting in renal abscess.

Discussion: Authors' Solution Suggested to Best Deal with These Difficulties

The majority of fever cases are managed successfully with antipyretics. Sepsis is a medical emergency with an overall mortality rate of 13 %. Forty percent of the patients decease within the first 24 h [24]. Incidence of septicemia and septic shock was higher in patients with fever, high leukocyte count, high creatinine level, diabetes mellitus, and low serum albumin level [28]. Administration of appropriate antimicrobial medication reduces mortality rate and the incidence of septic shock. The use of antibiotics, in which the responsible bacteria are not susceptible, results in poor prognosis. Thus, the proper selection of antimicrobial medication is imperative in the cases of septicemia. Etiologic agents associated with instrumentation of the genitourinary tract and indwelling catheters are *E. coli*, *Klebsiella*, *Enterobacter*, *Serratia*, *Proteus* species, and *P. aeruginosa*. Thus, the physician should consider the following antibiotics for treatment of sepsis: amikacin, tobramycin, gentamicin or alternatively ampicillin/sulbactam, piperacillin/tazobactam [29]. Multiple blood cultures for aerobic and anaerobic organisms should be obtained, and every effort should be made in order to elucidate the potential source (urine, wounds, etc.). In the case of responsible agent identification, the antimicrobial therapy should be changed (if necessary). Antimicrobial therapy should be continued until the patient is afebrile for 3–4 days and in stable clinical condition. Additional supportive measures should be taken in cases of hypotension, renal failure, and respiratory symptoms, and the patient should be admitted in intensive care unit [13].

Cases of small intestine injury could be treated conservatively with antibiotics, parenteral hyperalimentation, ureteral stenting, nasogastric suction, and formation of a controlled fistula. A large fistula should be managed with open surgery [8, 13]. Extraperitoneal colonic perforations should be managed with isolation of the gastrointestinal tract from the urinary tract. Any nephrostomy tube involving the large bowel should retracted in the colon. A separate nephrostomy tube or retrograde ureteral stent should be inserted and antibiotic medication should administered. [13, 30]. The gastrointestinal tract contains organisms such as *Bacteroides* species, *E. coli*, *Klebsiella*, *Enterobacter*, *Serratia*, and *Salmonella* which could cause sepsis. Aminoglycosides with additional clindamycin could be administered. Cefoxitin or third generation cephalosporins could be used as alternative antibiotics [29]. Conservative and minimally invasive management of colonic injuries is successful in most cases [25, 26, 31, 32]. Intraperitoneal perforation requires prompt open surgical management [13].

Advice for Better Preparation for These Difficulties

Specific recommendations for the prevention of septic complications taking place or started during PCNL:

- Prophylactic antibiotic therapy reduces septic complication events even in patients with sterile urine and noninfectious stones [8].
- Treatment of preexisting urinary tract infection is imperative since fever is significantly higher and frequent in patients with infected urinary stones (struvite, staghorn stones) [8, 25]. Antimicrobial therapy should be started at least a week prior to PCNL performance. Broad-spectrum antibiotics should be given. Urine cultures and stone bacteriology (especially in struvite stones) are expected in some cases to be different [8, 33]. Additional antibiotics for urease-producing organisms should be considered for administration.
- Staghorn stones may be associated with purulent puncture fluid (3–10 %) regardless of sterile urine culture. PCNL should be postponed. Drainage of the collecting system (ureteral stent, nephrostomy), urine culture, and appropriate antibiotic treatment should be performed for at least a week [13]. Administration of oral ciprofloxacin for 1 week before the operation reduces the risk for urosepsis in patients with stones larger than 20 mm or with dilated pelvicaliceal systems [34].
- Preoperative urinalysis and urine culture are essential.
- High pressure of the collecting system should be avoided during stone disintegration [8]. The use of working sheath that is significantly wider than the endoscope is helpful for maintaining low pressure in the collecting system since there is backflow of administrated fluids through the sheath.
- The duration of the operation should be limited under 90 min [8, 13].
- Sonographic or fluoroscopic control during puncture would limit the risk for bowel injury due to the visualization of bowel and appropriate patient selection [8, 13].
- Intestinal and colonic perforations could also be prevented by minimizing overzealous manipulations during puncture, tract dilation, and stone management. Moreover, abdominal CT scan is helpful in identifying bowel (especially the colon) anatomical relations and to avoid injury. CT scan should be performed in all patients with malformation of the kidney (horseshoe kidney).

Summary

Prevention of septic complications associated with PCNL is possible by following certain rules and by performing the technique with care. Nevertheless, these untoward events are always present in the experience of an endourologist, and the knowledge how to deal them is of critical importance. Septic complications would not result in high mortality if prompt and appropriate measures are taken.

References

1. Fernstrom I, Johansson B. Percutaneous pyelolithotomy: a new extraction technique. Scand J Urol Nephrol. 1976;10:257–9.
2. Shah HN, Kausik VB, Hegde SS, Shah JN, Bansal MB. Tubeless percutaneous nephrolithotomy: a prospective feasibility study and review of previous reports. BJU Int. 2005;96:879–83.
3. Lahme S, Zimmermanns V, Hochmuth A, Janitzki V. Minimal-invasive PCNL (mini-perc). Alternative oder Ersatz für konventionelle PCNL. Urologe A. 2008; 47:563–8.
4. Chaussy C, Schmiedt E, Jocham D, Brendel W, Forssmann B, Walther V. First clinical experience with extracorporeally induced destruction of kidney stones by shock waves. J Urol. 1982;127:417–20.
5. Segura JW. The role of percutaneous surgery in renal and ureteral stone removal. J Urol. 1989;141:780–1.
6. Rassweiler J, Alken P. ESWL 90 – state of the art: limitations and future trends of shock wave lithotripsy. Urol Res. 1990;18:13–24.
7. Rassweiler JJ, Renner C, Chaussy C, Thüroff S. Treatment of renal stones by extracorporeal shock wave lithotripsy. Eur Urol. 2001;40:54–64.
8. Skolarikos A, de la Rosette J. Prevention and treatment of complications following percutaneous nephrolithotomy. Curr Opin Urol. 2008;18:229–34.
9. Skolarikos A, Alivizatos G, De La Rosette JJMCH. Percutaneous nephrolithotomy and its legacy. Eur Urol. 2005;47:22–8.
10. Hafron J, Fogarty JD, Boczko D, Hoenig DM. Combined ureterorenoscopy and shockwave lithotripsy for large renal stone burden: an alternative to percutaneous nephrolithotomy? J Endourol. 2005;19:464–8.

11. Marguet CG, Springhart WP, Tan YH, et al. Simultaneous combined use of flexible ureteroscopy and percutaneous nephrolithotomy to reduce the number of access tracts in the management of complex renal calculi. BJU Int. 2005;96:1097–100.
12. Duvdevani M, Razvi H, Sofer M, Beiko DT, Nott L, Chew BH, Denstedt JD. Third prize: contemporary percutaneous nephrolithotripsy: 1585 procedures in 1338 consecutive patients. J Endourol. 2007;21(8): 824–9.
13. Michel MS, Trojan L, Rassweiler JJ. Complications in percutaneous nephrolithotomy. Eur Urol. 2007;51: 899–906.
14. Rudnick DM, Stoller ML. Complications of percutaneous nephrostolithotomy. Can J Urol. 1999;6:872–5.
15. Osman M, Wendt-Nordahl G, Heger K, Michel MS, Alken P, Knoll T. Percutaneous nephrolithotomy with ultrasonography- guided renal access: experience from over 300 cases. BJU Int. 2005;96:875–8.
16. Lee WJ, Smith AD, Cubelli V, et al. Complications of percutaneous nephrolithotomy. AJR Am J Roentgenol. 1987;148:177–80.
17. Dogan HS, Sahin A, Cetinkaya Y, Akdogan B, Ozden E, Kendi S. Antibiotic prophylaxis in percutaneous nephrolithotomy: prospective study in 81 patients. J Endourol. 2002;16:649–53.
18. Aron M, Yadav R, Goel R, et al. Multi-tract percutaneous nephrolithotomy for large complete staghorn calculi. Urol Int. 2005;75:327–32.
19. Tefekli A, Karadag MA, Tepeler K, et al. Classification of percutaneous nephrolithotomy complications using the modified clavien grading system: looking for a standard. Eur Urol. 2008;53:184–90.
20. Mariappan P, Tolley DA. Endoscopic stone surgery: minimizing the risk of post-operative sepsis. Curr Opin Urol. 2005;15:101–5.
21. Walsh PC, Retik AB, Vaughan Jr ED, Wein AJ, et al. Campbell's urology. 8th ed. Philadelphia: Saunders; 2002. p. 567–8.
22. Bone RC. Sepsis, the sepsis syndrome, multi-organ failure: a plea for comparable definitions. (Editorial). Ann Intern Med. 1991;114:332.
23. Calandra T, Glauser MP, Schellekens J, Verhoef J, the Swiss-Dutch J5 Immunoglobulin Study Group. Treatment of gram-negative septic shock with human IgG antibody to Escherichia coli J5: a prospective, double-blind, randomized trial. J Infect Dis. 1988;158:312.
24. Kreger BE, Craven DE, Carling PC, McCabe WR. Gram-negative bacteremia. III: reassessment of etiology, epidemiology, and ecology in 612 patients. Am J Med. 1980;68:332.
25. Takeuchi H, Ueda M, Nonomura M, et al. Fever attack in percutaneous nephrolithotomy and transurethral ureterolithotripsy. Hinyokika Kiyo. 1987;33:1357–63.
26. El-Nahas AR, Shokeir AA, El-Assmy AM, et al. Colonic perforation during percutaneous nephrolithotomy: study of risk factors. Urology. 2006;67:937–41.
27. Culkin DJ, Wheeler Jr JS, Canning JR. Nephroduodenal fistula: a complication of percutaneous nephrolithotomy. J Urol. 1985;134:528–30.
28. Leibovici L, Greenshtain S, Cohen O, et al. Toward improved empiric management of moderate to severe urinary tract infections. Arch Intern Med. 1992;152: 2481.
29. Walsh PC, Retik AB, Vaughan Jr ED, Wein AJ, et al. Campbell's urology. 8th ed. Philadelphia: Saunders; 2002. p. 571.
30. Denstedt J, Khoury S. Stone disease. In: 2nd international consultation on stone disease. Paris: Health Publications; 2008. p. 230.
31. Gerspach JM, Bellman GC, Stoller ML, Fugelso P. Conservative management of colon injury following percutaneous renal surgery. Urology. 1997;49:831–6.
32. Vallancien G, Capdeville R, Veillon B, Charton M, Brisset JM. Colonic perforation during percutaneous nephrolithotomy. J Urol. 1985;134:1185–7.
33. Ohkawa M, Tokunaga S, Nakashima T, et al. Composition of urinary calculi related to urinary tract infection. J Urol. 1992;148:995–7.
34. Mariappan P, Smith G, Moussa SA, Tolley DA. One week of ciprofloxacin before percutaneous nephrolithotomy significantly reduces upper tract infection and urosepsis: a prospective controlled study. BJU Int. 2006;98:1075–9.

Visceral Complications of Percutaneous Nephrolithotomy (PCNL)

7

Abdelghaffar S. Arafa and Ahmed M. Al-Kandari

Introduction

Percutaneous nephrolithotomy (PCNL) was introduced in the 1970s as a minimally invasive procedure in the treatment of renal stones, with further development in its technique in the ensuing years. Indications for PCNL have diminished with the appearance of extracorporeal shock wave lithotripsy (ESWL) in the early years of 1980s, but then they gradually increased [1–4]. Currently, the role of PCNL is mainly in the treatment of large, multiple, complex, and lower calyceal stones [5]. The efficacy of PCNL has increased with the improvement and introduction of new instruments such as the flexible nephroscope, the ureteroscope, and intracorporeal lithotripsy technology (ultrasound, pneumatic, and laser devices) [6, 7].

PCNL is generally considered a safe procedure with a low rate of complications [8]. Careful selection of patients and proper preparation significantly reduced the complication rates. It is very essential to evaluate the patient thoroughly with all required tests to achieve the best results with the least complications. A complete diagnostic work-up is needed that includes the basic tests of complete blood count, renal profile, coagulation profile, and urine culture. Patients typically require a blood cross match. Other imaging tests which are commonly done are:

- Plain X-ray of the abdomen or what is called kidney-ureter-bladder (KUB).
- Abdominal ultrasound.
- Intravenous urography (IVU).
- Computed tomography urography (CTU). Commonly, most centers currently do a CT scan, plain and then with IV contrast, in order to properly plan the renal access. This is by far more superior and is especially required in complex stone cases.
- Renal isotope scanning can be helpful especially when a ureteropelvic junction obstruction is present as well as when accurate renal function assessment is required to make a proper decision regarding how to manage the kidney with stones.

It is well known that the absolute contraindications of PCNL include uncorrected coagulopathy or active urinary tract infection. A patient with other medical comorbidities such as diabetes mellitus, pulmonary disease, cardiovascular disease, and morbid obesity should be evaluated carefully preoperatively. Special care needs to be considered intraoperatively and postoperatively in order to avoid complications.

A.S. Arafa, MCS, MRCS
Department of Urology, Alsalam International Hospital, Bned Elgar, Dasma, 35151, Kuwait
e-mail: dr.ghaffar@yahoo.com

A.M. Al-Kandari, M.D., FRCS(C)(✉)
Department of Surgery, Kuwait University, Jabriyah, Kuwait City 13110, Kuwait
e-mail: drakandari@hotmail.com

A.M. Al-Kandari et al. (eds.), *Difficult Cases in Endourology*,
DOI 10.1007/978-1-84882-083-8_7, © Springer-Verlag London 2013

Technique of PCNL

A brief review of PCNL technique will be included in this chapter to help review the topic. Commonly, the procedure is done under general anesthesia. After positioning in the lithotomy position, cystoscopy is done and ureteric catheterization is done. Then the patient is commonly positioned prone. Some urologists may use supine or modified supine position [5, 9, 10].

Puncture of the pelvicalyceal system is done either under ultrasound or fluoroscopy guidance and directed to the desired calyx. Effort should be made to lessen manipulations through the cortical tissue during puncture to decrease the incidence of intrarenal vascular injuries and the possibility of arteriovenous fistula formation. It is also important to decrease radiation exposure and to shorten the working tract between the calyx and skin [9]. See Fig. 7.1.

Then passage of a floppy-tipped guidewire through the puncture needle to the collecting system is done. This is followed by creation of a working tract using different dilators such as the Alken telescopic metal dilators or balloon dilator or the Amplatz sequential dilators. Subsequently, after placing a 30 F working sheath in adults, a 26 F rigid nephroscope is introduced into the kidney through this tract [12].

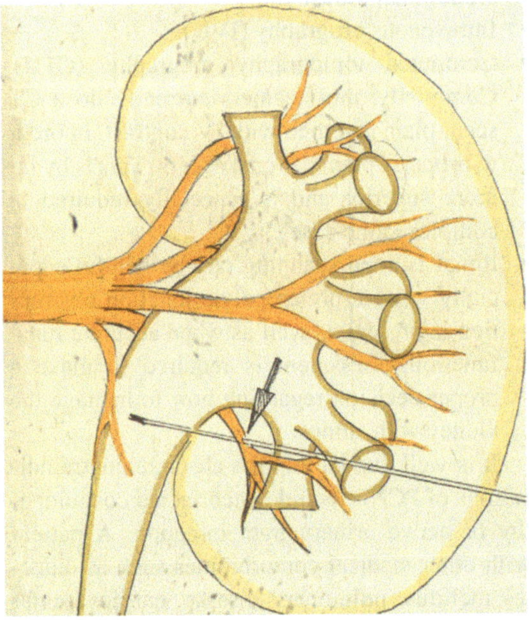

Fig. 7.1 Renal vascular anatomy. Puncture of renal pelvis or calyceal infundibulum increases risk of vascular injury. Interlobar artery (*arrow*) (Reproduced with permission from Michel et al. [11])

The number of punctures during PCNL depends on the size, number, and location of stones. Treatment strategies have changed after the appearance of ESWL (combination of PCNL with ESWL vs. multiple punctures) [3, 13]. It is well known that the complications of PCNL increase with increasing number of punctures.

Although access through the lower calyx was considered by many urologists to be the classic access, many others prefer to use multiple tracts for stone clearance, and fewer prefer upper polar access for more optimal stone manipulation in cases containing upper and lower calyceal stones. This was associated with relatively higher rates of pleural complications, given that the supracostal approach was done [14–17].

Once the stone is identified during PCNL, lithotripsy is done with ultrasound, pneumatic probe, or laser device, followed by removal of stone fragments. In case of stone migration to another calyx which is not accessible by the rigid nephroscope, flexible nephroscope can be used.

A nephrostomy tube is classically placed in the renal pelvis, and antegrade nephrostogram is performed after 24–48 h before its removal to confirm the absence of extravasation or residual obstructing stones.

Complications of PCNL

The majority of complications after PCNL are minor. Longer operative time and higher ASA scores are associated with the risk of more severe postoperative complications in PCNL [18].

Of 5,724 patients with Clavien scores, 1,175 (20.5 %) of the patients experienced one or more complications. The most frequent complications were fever and bleeding. Urinary leakage, hydrothorax, hematuria, urinary tract infection, pelvic perforation, and urinary fistula also occurred in ≥20 patients in each group. The majority of complications ($n=634$, 54.0 %) were classified as Clavien grade I. Two patients died in the postoperative period. The largest absolute increases in mean Clavien score were associated with American Society of Anesthesiologists (ASA) physical status classification IV (0.75) or III (0.34), anticoagulant medication use (0.29), positive microbiologic culture from urine (0.24), and the presence of concurrent cardiovascular disease (0.15). Multivariate regression analysis revealed that operative time and ASA score were significant predictors of higher mean Clavien scores [18].

An approach is the validated Dindo-modified Clavien system, which was originally reported by seven studies. No deviation from the normal postoperative course (Clavien 0) was observed in 76.7 % of PNL procedures. Including deviations from the normal postoperative course without the need for pharmacologic treatment or interventions (Clavien 1) would add up to 88.1 %. Clavien 2 complications including blood transfusion and parenteral nutrition occurred in 7 %. Clavien 3 complications requiring intervention occurred in 4.1 %. Clavien 4, life-threatening complications, occurred in 0.6 %. Clavien 5, mortality, occurred in 0.04 %. High-quality data on complication management of rare but potentially debilitating complications are scarce and consist mainly of case reports [19].

Complications of PCNL are either those related to the access or those related to stone removal. Causes of intraoperative complications are mainly improper selection of the patient, technical errors, or inadequate equipment. Proper selection of the patients is necessary to reduce the morbidity rates related to PCNL.

PCNL is contraindicated in patients with uncorrected coagulopathy, pyonephrosis, and urinary tract infection. Presence of medical comorbidities such as pulmonary or cardiovascular diseases, diabetes, and obesity significantly increases the risk of complications. Also, spinal deformity, malrotated kidney, horseshoe kidney, and anatomical malformations increase the difficulty of the procedure and increase the risk of suboptimal results, but these can be managed with experience.

Careful positioning on the operating table is important to reduce intraoperative complications. Putting a special cushion under the patient with some deflection increases the area between the last rib and iliac crest which enhances more easily the puncture of the kidney, but at the same time, this higher position may lead to more difficulty in using the nephroscope and the lithotripsy probe. Many urologists believe that the oblique position provides easier access to the kidney [9, 10].

Supracostal access may be required for upper calyceal stones, staghorn stones, and upper ureteric stones, but it carries an increased risk of chest complications [17]. This is lately less in frequency when only the supra 12th rib is used.

Using a J-guidewire with inner core and soft tip decreases the risk of renal pelvis perforation; however, more rigid guidewires may be required, especially if the patient had previous renal surgery [15]. This is helpful to avoid kinking of the wire and to facilitate entry into and work in the kidney.

Complications related to access include parenchymal bleeding (either major bleeding requiring intervention, bleeding requiring transfusion, or minor bleeding) and organ injuries. Complications related to stone extraction include septicemia, extravasation, and fluid absorption. Bleeding and infection are covered in two other chapters. In this chapter, we will focus on visceral complications of PCNL.

Organ Injuries

The organs commonly injured during PCNL are the pleura and the lungs, with possibility of pneumothorax and hydropneumothorax (especially with puncture above the 12th rib), the duodenum, the colon, and other abdominal organs.

Pleural and Chest Injuries

The risk of pleural and other chest injuries during PCNL rises with punctures above the level of the 12th rib. In a study by Mousavi et al. and in series of 671 cases, the pulmonary complications were estimated to be 3 (0.4 %) in pneumothorax and 2 (0.3 %) in hemothorax [20]. If the puncture comes through the pleura, the irrigation fluid and/or air and/or blood will find access to the pleura, leading to hydrothorax, pneumothorax, hydropneumothorax, or hematothorax [13, 14, 16, 17, 21].

Injury of the pleura occurs mainly during puncture and dilation of the nephrostomy tract. The fluid accumulation occurs gradually, so it could go unnoticed until the end of the procedure. Suggestive signs of pleural injury that may be observed are fluid extravasation around the nephroscope (with less return of fluid) and increase in the peak inspiratory pressure, which would be typically noted by an anesthetist. This event may be unnoticed until the patient returns to the supine position and begins to breathe spontaneously because controlled ventilation opposes the hydrothorax effects. Also, chest and abdomen are not apparent in the prone position.

The problem of course increases with the difficulty and the duration of the procedure as that means use of a large volume of irrigation fluid. It is important to measure the irrigation fluid input and output with close observation of the ventilatory pressure. Large differences between input and output and significant increase in the inspiratory pressure should alert the anesthetist about the possibility of chest problem. This will eventually lead to considering the possibility of procedure termination.

Precautions to be taken to minimize the risk of chest problems with PCNL are:

- Puncture under ultrasound guidance or after exhalation.
- Close observation of input and output of the irrigation fluid with monitoring of the ventilator pressure.
- Use of a watertight seal between the sheath of the nephroscope and the drapes to prevent escape of irrigation fluid. This fluid can be collected for accurate measurement of the balance between input and output.
- Time factor is of great importance. The procedure duration should be shortened as much as possible to decrease fluid absorption.
- The lower calyceal access is highly preferred, and use of a flexible nephroscope and/or ESWL in combination is highly helpful to reduce such complications.

The majority of cases are managed conservatively. A chest tube is inserted in cases of hydrothorax and hematothorax. Extensive surgical intervention is rarely required in these cases, and it is in the form of thoracoscopy and thoracotomy [13, 14, 16, 17, 21].

Some authors described the use of thoracoscopic-guided high PCNL puncture (ninth to tenth interspace) with routine chest tube. This resulted in excellent stone treatment outcomes and minimal thoracic side effects [22].

Abdominal Organ Injuries

Injuries of the abdominal organs are rare complications of PCNL. Adequate evaluation of the patient preoperatively and identification of high-risk patients are important for prevention of such complications. Mousavi et al. estimated that colonic perforation occurred in 2/671 cases (0.3 %) [20]. Typically, these are managed conservatively.

The risk factors for colonic perforation are:

- Left-sided procedures.
- Advanced age and female gender.
- Anatomical abnormalities such as horseshoe kidney and vertebral column anomalies such as severe scoliosis and meningomyelocele.
- Abnormal rare retrorenal colonic position (Fig. 7.2).
- Extremely thin patients.
- Colonic distension.

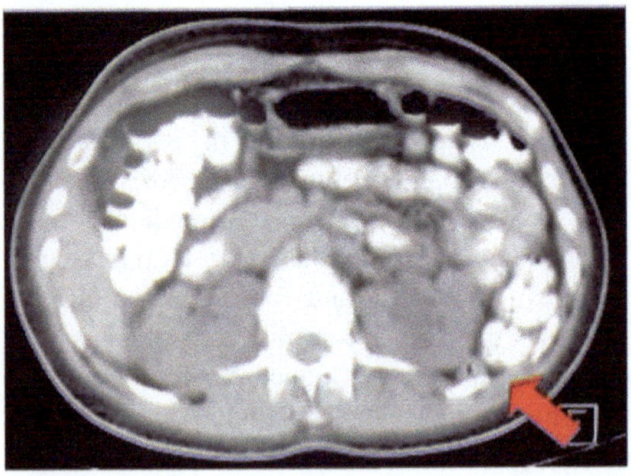

Fig. 7.2 Sagittal CAT image showing the retrorenal position of the descending colon (*arrow*) which causes risk of perforation during PCNL (Reproduced with permission from Negrete-Pulido et al. [23])

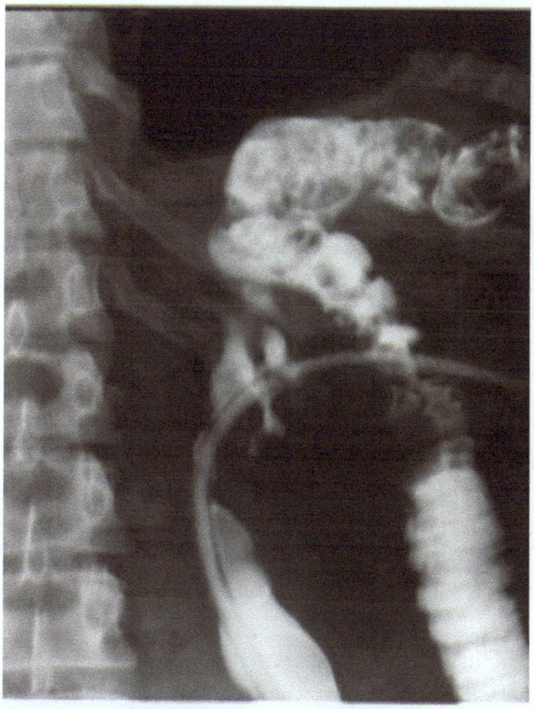

Fig. 7.3 Colonic injury after failed puncture for PCNL. Filling of the intestine by contrast agent is clear after filling nephrostomy (Reproduced with permission from Michel et al. [11])

- Previous bowel surgeries carry more risk for colonic and duodenal injuries.
- Transplanted kidney.
- Extreme lateral puncture.

These factors contribute to posterior displacement of the colon making it more liable for injuries during puncture and nephrostomy tract dilation. See Fig. 7.3. The presence of multiple risk factors in the same patient carries more risk of incidence of colonic perforation.

Although incidence of colonic perforation is rare (0.2–0.8 %), it is one of the most dangerous complications because it carries many risks such as abscess, fistula formation (either nephrocolonic or colocutaneous), peritonitis from intraperitoneal fecal soiling, and septicemia [11, 24].

Early diagnosis and early management are of extreme importance, as the majority of cases can be managed conservatively. This complication is rarely discovered intraoperatively. The patient is usually presented with postoperative pain at the puncture site, fever and gas or fecal matter leakage through the nephrostomy tract, and/or signs of peritonitis.

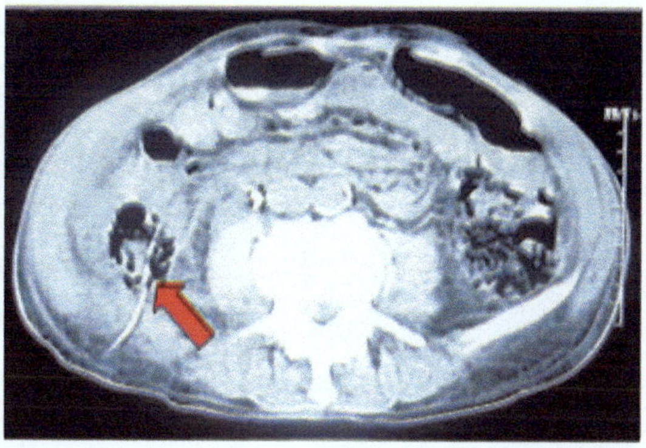

Fig. 7.4 Passage of nephrostomy tube through the ascending Colon is shown (Reproduced with permission from Negrete-Pulido et al. [23])

Antegrade nephrostogram at the end of the procedure is helpful to identify possible perforation of the colon. The best diagnostic tool for diagnosis is abdominal CT showing passage of the nephrostomy tube through the colon. If a nephrocolonic fistula is suspected after removal of nephrostomy tube, retrograde ureteropyelography is recommended to confirm diagnosis. See Fig. 7.4.

Management

In the case of extraperitoneal perforation of the colon, the urinary tract should be separated from the gastrointestinal tract (GIT) by traction of the nephrostomy tube under fluoroscopic control outside the pelvicalyceal system; the tube should be placed inside the colon, converting the nephrostomy tube into a colostomy tube [25–28]. See Fig. 7.5. Broad spectrum intravenous antibiotics should be started, and a low-fiber diet should be given.

A double J stent may be inserted for better diversion of the urinary system away from GIT. The nephrostomy tube (colostomy tube) is left until closure of the colocutaneous tract. After 7–10 days, a contrast study should be done through the colostomy tube to ensure closure of the nephrocolonic fistula before removal of the colostomy tube [29, 30].

Conservative management is successful in the majority of cases. Open surgery is required in

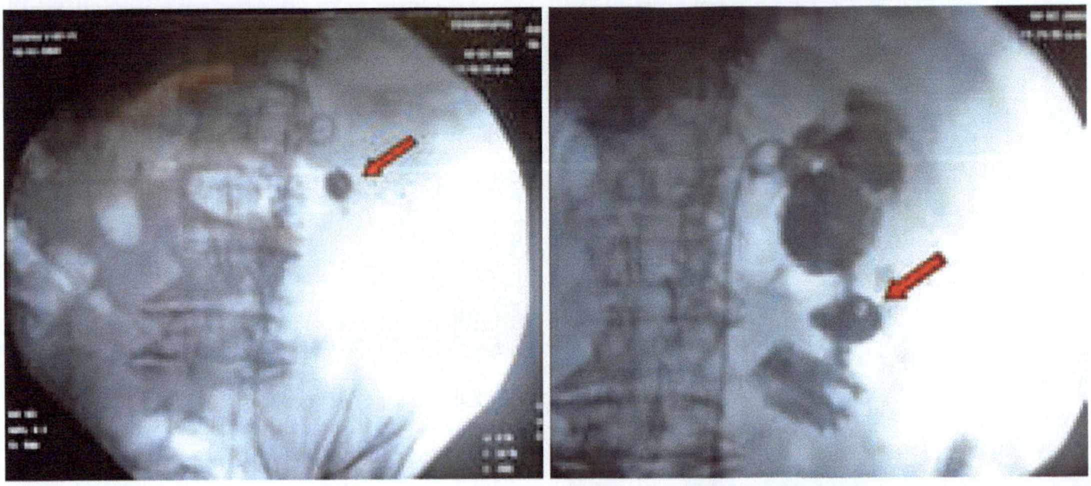

Fig. 7.5 Under fluoroscopic guidance, traction of nephrostomy catheter (*arrows*) toward the opening of the colon and conversion into a colostomy catheter after ureteral catheter insertion (Reproduced with permission from Negrete-Pulido et al. [23])

cases of intraperitoneal perforation with manifestations of peritonitis or sepsis and failure of conservative management. Primary closure of the fistula or resection anastomosis may be required for these patients. Colostomy may be an option of treatment to enhance closure of fistula especially in late diagnosis of nephrocolonic or colocutaneous fistula [31, 32].

Precautions to reduce the risk of colonic perforation in PCNL are as follows:

- Adequate preoperative assessment and high-risk patient identification.
- Preoperative abdominal CT scan as a part of the evaluation to identify the position of the colon and the safest site for access [33, 34].
- Sonographically guided puncture is helpful to ensure that the puncture is far enough away from the bowel.
- Change the puncture site if there is doubt in colonic puncture.
- Immediate postoperative nephrostogram to identify inadvertent perforation of the colon.

Splenic Injury

Splenic injury during PCNL is a very rare complication. The risk factors for this include:

- Splenomegaly
- Puncture below the last rib

Ultrasonographic-guided puncture reduces the risk of splenic injury during PCNL.

Splenic injury is a surgical emergency; in most cases, it is associated with significant bleeding. Emergency exploration and splenectomy are performed with blood transfusion to compensate the blood volume loss. Although it is rare, in rare cases conservative management was successful [35]. See Fig. 7.6 a, b.

Liver Injury

Liver injury is a very rare complication of PCNL and can occur when puncture and dilatation are done in the right side. Report of conservative management showed successful outcome in this rare condition [36].

Gall Bladder Injury

Gall bladder injury during PCNL is a very rare situation, and typically, this can happen during right-sided PCNL cases. It can happen when the access needle punctures the distended gallbladder. The surgeon will aspirate and see bile. He or she should not panic and redirect his needle mostly in a more lateral and less deep position. It is very essential to recognize the bile so that no further tract dilation is done. This incident of

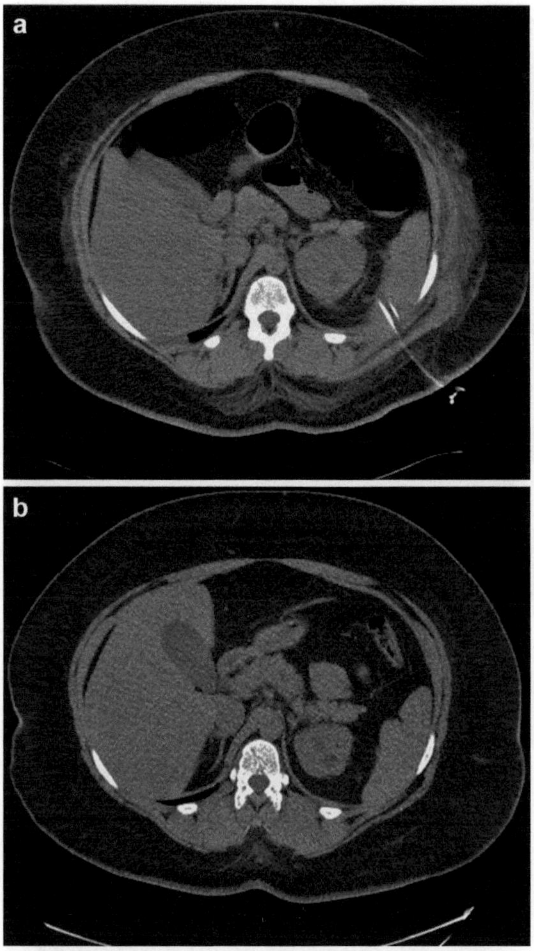

Fig. 7.6 (**a**, **b**) CT scan of abdomen. (**a**) A nephrostomy tube through spleen. (**b**) The spleen, which healed after conservative measures (Reproduced with permission from Thomas et al. [35])

gall bladder puncture will not cause any further injury.

Complications Related to Stone Removal

Complications related to stone removal include septicemia, extravasation, and fluid absorption. Septicemia and infection related to PCNL will be discussed in another chapter.

Extravasation and Fluid Absorption

Perforation of the collecting system is the leading cause of extravasation and fluid absorption.

Management of Urine Extravasation

Urine extravasation occurs in severe perforations of the pelvicalyceal system or through the nephrostomy tract leading to extraperitoneal urine collection (urinoma). Manifestations are mainly flank pain and/or swelling with or without signs of infection.

Measures for management of urine extravasation are:

- Percutaneous urinoma drainage.
- Broad-spectrum antibiotics.
- Double J stent may be required (if persistent urine leakage occurs).

Prevention can be achieved by performing the steps of the procedure under fluoroscopic control and under endoscopic clear visualization, especially during tract establishment and stone lithotripsy. Use of continuous flow irrigation system and measuring the balance between input and output of irrigation fluid can be of help. Normal saline is preferred as irrigation fluid to avoid hyponatremia if water is used. If fluid discrepancy of more than 500 ml between inflow and outflow is reached, the procedure should be terminated, and a nephrostomy tube should be placed.

Management of Intravasation of Irrigation Fluid

Intravasation of irrigation fluid during PCNL is another complication that can happen when the pelvicaliceal system is perforated. This commonly can happen in thin patients, and it may happen in children. The best time for identification is at the end of a case or during the recovery observation period. Typically, the patient has generalized abdominal distention, with pain, nausea, and vomiting when he is awake. It is of great help to do an urgent ultrasound of the abdomen, which will show free fluid in the peritoneal cavity.

The management usually depends on the condition of the patient. If it is mild distension, then just keeping the patient nil per mouth and giving him diuretics will help. Otherwise, a peritoneal drainage tube is essential and can be put under local anesthesia just under the umbilicus. The typical fluid color is watery with a bloody tinge. The patient may also require a nasogastric tube. He also needs to be put on IV antibiotics.

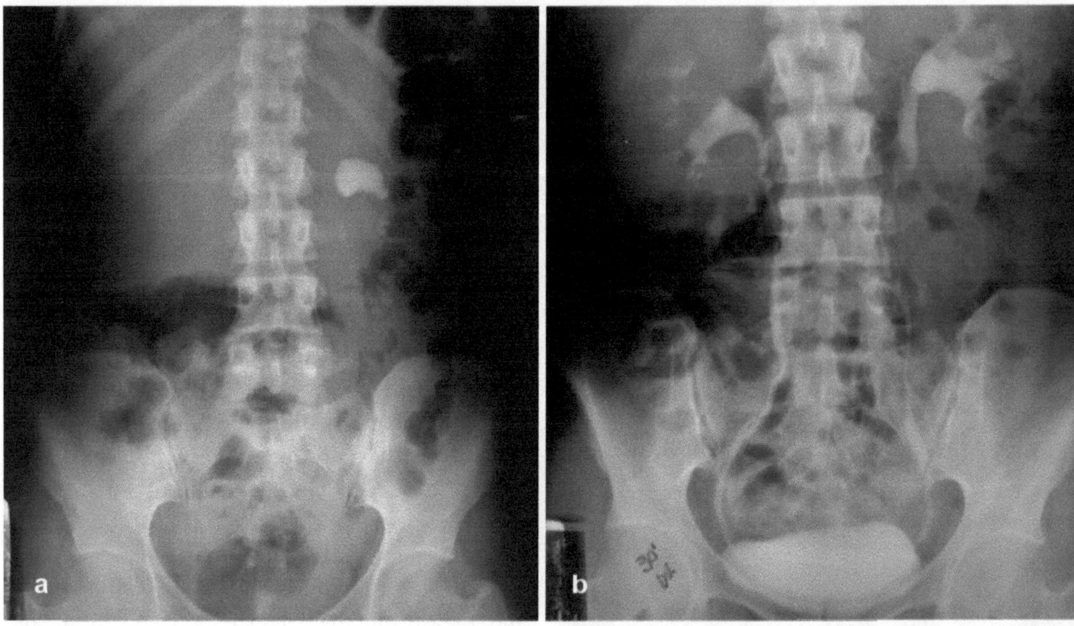

Fig. 7.7 (**a, b**) Excretory urography showing a large pelvic stone with moderate calyceal dilation, with dilated upper ureter up to stricture. (Reproduced with permission from Neto et al. [38])

Monitoring of serum electrolytes is essential especially if suspecting fluid absorption.

Proximal Ureteric Stricture

Proximal ureteric stricture is a rare complication of PCNL that can occur in cases of proximal ureteric stones or pelvic stones [37]. See Figs. 7.7 a, b and 7.8. Strictures of the pelvicalyceal system usually involve the pelviureteric junction and/or calyceal infundibulum and are estimated to be less than 1 % [39, 40].

Causes are mainly endoscopic stone manipulations, mucosal injury, and extravasation of contaminated urine [39, 40]. Pelvic perforation and urinary extravasation lead to retroperitoneal and periureteral inflammation. Ureteral scarring and ureteral stricture occur as a late complication of PCNL.

This complication can be prevented by reducing injuries of the collecting system by performing all steps under fluoroscopic guidance and clear endoscopic control, particularly during stone manipulations. Ensuring sterile urine before PCNL reduces the postoperative inflammatory response and possibility of stricture formation.

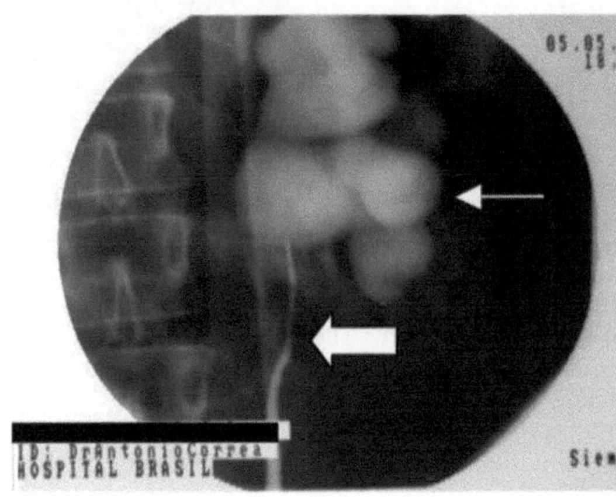

Fig. 7.8 Extensive proximal ureteral stricture (*large arrow*) with massive collecting system dilation (*narrow arrow*) (Reproduced with permission from Neto et al. [38])

Summary

Percutaneous nephrolithotomy is considered a safe procedure. Although it is a minimally invasive procedure, it has potential complications. Most of these complications are not clinically significant, such as postoperative fever, minor bleeding, or blood transfusion. Major complications are rare, such as renal hemorrhage; septicemia; adjacent organ injuries in the liver, spleen, and colon; extravasation; fluid absorption; and residual stone fragments [11, 24].

Measures taken into consideration to minimize complications of PCNL are adequate preoperative evaluation of the patient, careful puncture of the suitable calyx under ultrasound and fluoroscopic guidance, atraumatic dilation of the nephrostomy tract, minimal stone manipulations, use of flexible nephroscope for upper calyx stones or fragments, knowing when to stop and terminate the procedure, proper urologist training and experience, proper patient selection, accurate patient positioning, and adequate instruments.

References

1. Alken P, Hutschenreiter G, Guenther R. Percutaneous kidney stone removal. Eur Urol. 1982;8:304–11.
2. Segura JW, Patterson DE, LeRoy AJ, et al. Percutaneous removal of kidney stones: review of 1,000 cases. J Urol. 1985;134:1077–81.
3. Rassweiler J, Gumpinger R, Miller K, Hölzermann F, Eisenberger F. Multimodal treatment (extracorporeal shockwave lithotripsy and endourology) of complicated renal stone disease. Eur Urol. 1986;12:294–304.
4. Chaussy C, Schmiedt E, Jocham D, Brendel W, Forssmann B, Walther V. First clinical experience with extracorporeally induced destruction of kidney stones by shock waves. J Urol. 1982;127:417–20.
5. Lingeman JE, Newmark JR, Wong MYC. Classification and management of staghorn calculi. In: Smith AD, editor. Controversies in endourology. Philadelphia: Saunders; 1995. p. 136–44.
6. Hafron J, Fogarty JD, Boczko D, Hoenig DM. Combined ureteroscopy and shockwave lithotripsy for large stone burden: an alternative to percutaneous nephrolithotomy? J Endourol. 2005;19:464–8.
7. Marguet CG, Springhart WP, Tan YH, et al. Simultaneous combined use of flexible ureteroscopy and percutaneous nephrolithotomy to reduce the number of access tracts in the management of complex renal calculi. BJU Int. 2005;96:1097–100.
8. Rudnick DM, Stoller ML. Complications of percutaneous nephrolithotomy. Can J Urol. 1999;6:872–5.
9. Desai M, Ridhorkar V, Patel S, Bapat S, Desai M. Pediatric percutaneous nephrolithotomy: assessing impact of technical innovations on safety and efficacy. J Endourol. 1999;13:359–64.
10. Ng MT, Sun WH, Cheng CW, Chan ES. Supine position is safe and effective for percutaneous nephrolithotomy. J Endourol. 2004;18:469–74.
11. Michel MS, Trojan L, Rassweiler JJ. Complications in percutaneous nephrolithotomy. Eur Urol. 2007; 51(4):899–906.
12. Alken P. The telescope dilator. World J Urol. 1985;3: 7–10.
13. Rassweiler JJ, Renner C, Eisenberger F. Management of complex renal stones. BJU Int. 2000;86:919–28.
14. Netto Jr NR, Ikonomodis J, Ikari O, Claro JA. Comparative study of percutaneous access for staghorn calculi. Urology. 2005;65:659–63.
15. Kim SC, Kuo RL, Lingeman JE. Percutaneous nephrolithotomy: an update. Curr Opin Urol. 2003;13: 235–41.
16. Liatsikos EN, Kapoor R, Lee B, Jabbour M, Barbalias G, Smith AD. "Angular percutaneous renal access." multiple tracts through a single incision for staghorn calculous treatment in a single session. Eur Urol. 2005;48:832–7.
17. Gupta R, Kumar A, Kapoor R, Srivastava A, Mandhani A. Prospective evaluation of safety and efficacy of the supracostal approach for percutaneous nephrolithotomy. BJU Int. 2002;90:809–13.
18. Labate G, Modi P, Timoney A, Cormio L, Zhang X, Louie M, Grabe M, Rosette on Behalf of the Croes PCNL Study Group. The percutaneous nephrolithotomy global study: classification of complications. J Endourol. 2011;25(8):1275–80.
19. Seitz C, Desai M, Häcker A, Hakenberg OW, Liatsikos E, Nagele U, Tolley D. Incidence, prevention, and management of complications following percutaneous nephrolitholapaxy. Eur Urol. 2012;61(1):146–58.
20. Mousavi-Bahar SH, Mehrabi S, Moslemi MK. Percutaneous nephrolithotomy complications in 671 consecutive patients: a single-center experience. Urol J. 2011;8(4):271–6.
21. Eisenberger F, Miller K, Rassweiler J, editors. Stone therapy in urology. New York: Thieme Medical Publisher; 1991.
22. Finelli A, Honey RJ. Thoracoscopy-assisted high intercostal percutaneous renal access. J Endourol. 2001;15(6):581–4, discussion 584–5.
23. Negrete-Pulido OR, Molina-Torres M, Gutierrez-Aceves J. Colonic perforation during percutaneous nephrolithotomy: prevention, diagnosis and treatment. Rev Mex Urol. 2010;70(1):44–7.
24. Skolarikos A, De la Rosette J. Prevention and treatment of complications following percutaneous nephrolithotomy. Curr Opin Urol. 2008;18(2):229–34.
25. El-Nahas AR, Shokier AA, El-Assmy AM, et al. Colonic perforation during percutaneous nephrolithotomy: study of risk factors. Urology. 2006;67:937–41.
26. Gerspach JM, Bellman GC, Stoller ML, Fugelso P. Conservative management of colon injury following percutaneous renal surgery. Urology. 1997;49:831–6.
27. Vallancien G, Capdeville R, Veillon B, Charton M, Brisset JM. Colonic perforation during percutaneous nephrolithotomy. J Urol. 1985;134:1185–7.
28. Takeuchi H, Ueda M, Nonomura M, et al. Fever attack in percutaneous nephrolithotomy and transurethral ureterolithotripsy. Hinyokika Kiyo. 1987;33:1357–63.

29. Shah O, Assimos DG. Complications of percutaneous renal surgery. In: Smiths textbook of endourology. 2nd ed. Hamilton/London: BC Decker Inc; 2006. p. 159–64.
30. Goswami A, Shrivastava P, Mukherejee A, et al. Management of colonic perforation during percutaneous nephrolithotomy in horseshoe kidney. J Endourol. 2001;15(10):989–91.
31. Noor Buchholz NP. Colon perforation after percutaneous nephrolithotomy revisited. Urol Int. 2004;72(1): 88–90.
32. Nouira Y, Nouira K, Kallel Y, Feki W, Horchani A. Colonic perforation complicating percutaneous nephrolithotomy. Surg Laparosc Endosc Percutan Tech. 2006;16(1):47–8.
33. Segura JW, Patterson DE, Le Roy AJ, et al. Percutaneous removal of kidney stones: review of 1000 cases. J Urol. 1985;134(6):1077–80.
34. Neustein P, Barbaric ZL, Kaufman JJ. Nephrocolic fistula: a complication of nephrostolithotomy. J Urol. 1986;135(3):571–3.
35. Thomas AA, Pierce G, Walsh RM, Sands M, Noble M. Splenic injury during percutaneous nephrolithotomy. JSLS. 2009;13(2):233–6.
36. El-Nahas AR, Mansour AM, Ellaithy R, Abol-Enein H. Case report: conservative treatment of liver injury during percutaneous nephrolithotomy. J Endourol. 2008;22(8):1649–52.
37. Lee WJ, Smith AD, Cubelli V, et al. Complications of percutaneous nephrolithotomy. AJR Am J Roentgenol. 1987;148.
38. Neto ACL, de Mattos MHE, da Silva MNK, Wroclawski ER. Extensive ureteral stricture after percutaneous nephrolithotomy. Arch Esp Urol. 2008; 61(4):559–61.
39. Weir JM, Honey DA. Complete infundibular obliteration following percutaneous nephrolithotomy. J Urol. 1999;161:1274.
40. Wong MY. Evolving technique of percutaneous nephrolithotomy in a developing country: Singapore General Hospital Experience. J Endourol. 1998; 12:397.

8

Percutaneous Nephrolithotomy (PCNL) for Staghorn Calculi: The Rigid Approach – Overcoming the Difficulties

Arvind P. Ganpule and Mahesh Desai

Introduction

The cornerstone of management of staghorn calculi includes complete clearance of the stone with minimal morbidity. The AUA Nephrolithiasis Guidelines mentions percutaneous nephrolithotomy (PCNL) as the treatment of choice for staghorn calculi [1]. The management of staghorn calculi is one of the most challenging among endourologic procedures because the operating surgeon has to do the balancing act of complete stone clearance with minimal morbidity. In this chapter, we discuss the possible difficulties one may encounter during the procedure.

Preoperative Work-Up

Preoperative Imaging

The preoperative imaging prior to PCNL includes application and use of preoperative ultrasound, intravenous urography (IVU), and computerized tomography (CT) imaging. Each of these imaging modalities has its advantages and disadvantages.

A.P. Ganpule, M.S., DNB, MNAMS (✉)
M. Desai, M.S., FRCS
Department of Urology, Muljibhai Patel Urological Hospital, Dr. Virendra Desai Road, Nadiad 387001, Gujarat, India
e-mail: doctorarvind1@gmail.com; mrdesai@mpuh.org

Ultrasound

A preoperative ultrasound a day prior to surgery is helpful for selecting the calyx of puncture. In addition, it gives information regarding the cortex, distribution of stone burden, and the possibility of any intervening bowel and other visceral structures. This preoperative imaging modality is of particular help if one plans an ultrasound-guided puncture. A preoperative ultrasound also helps in assessing the skin to calyx distance; this assumes importance in individuals having a higher body mass index.

However, ultrasound requires special training and is a subjective examination. Moreover, in a few countries, ultrasound examination requires a radiologist to perform the examination.

Intravenous Pyelography

The IVU helps to identify the calyx of puncture preoperatively. A posterior calyx typically appears round (because of its end on appearance) and is laterally placed; the anterior calyx is medially placed and maintains the cup shape in posterior anterior plain X-ray films. IVU carries the advantage of offering information regarding the relationship of the rib cage and the kidney. This may help the surgeon to plan a supracostal or subcostal puncture preoperatively.

IVU carries the disadvantage of radiation hazards and the attendant problems with contrast injection.

3D CT Imaging and Reconstruction

With advances in CT techniques such as rapid spiral acquisition and reconstruction software, it is

A.M. Al-Kandari et al. (eds.), *Difficult Cases in Endourology*,
DOI 10.1007/978-1-84882-083-8_8, © Springer-Verlag London 2013

now possible to reproduce exactly the reconstructed images of pelvicalyceal system and the stone. In a study by Thiruchelvam et al., the 3D CT protocol helped to predict and reproduce the site, number and size of stones, optimal site for puncture, and potential hazards for placing the tracts [2]. CT carries the disadvantage of radiation and cost.

Difficulties in Rigid Approach for Staghorn Calculi

The difficulties one encounters may be in the various steps of the procedure or because of the variation in the anatomy of the patient such as skeletal anomalies, obesity, etc.

Difficulties in Gaining Access

A perfect puncture is a one that has a shortest straight tract through the cup of the calyx to the desired calyx (Fig. 8.1).

Inability to Puncture

This typically happens in cases having minimal dilation or no dilatation of the pelvicalyceal system. A lack of experience of the operating surgeon will also contribute to this difficulty.

This problem can be overcome by administration of injectable furosemide which helps in dilatation of the system. During an ultrasound-guided puncture, the calyx in question, papilla and the skin should be in one line. A gentle jiggling of the puncture needle helps in ascertaining the location of the needle in the subcutaneous tissue. When an ultrasound-guided puncture is employed, non-visualization of the needle along the tract may hamper eventual successful access.

The type of needle used also helps in overcoming the difficulties related to access. A new needle tends to deflect less, the EchoTip® needle (Cook Medical, Bloomington, IN), which has an echo reflective surface; this helps in visualizing the needle during puncture. The puncture attachment is an effective ancillary tool in avoiding deviation of the needle during puncture. During a fluoroscopic puncture, the parallax (difference in position of the needle in anteroposterior and lateral views) should be eliminated. A recent addition to the armamentarium for gaining access is the "all see through needle." This needle has a fiber-optic cable housed in the lumen; hence, real-time endoscopic visualization of the access tract is possible. Initial studies have shown the utility of this system in gaining access; however recently, this has been used for completing the procedure in a single step [3–5].

Blood at Tip of Needle (Fig. 8.2)

Often after the initial puncture, the efflux might be red. The surgeon has to distinguish between frank blood (suggesting that the needle might be

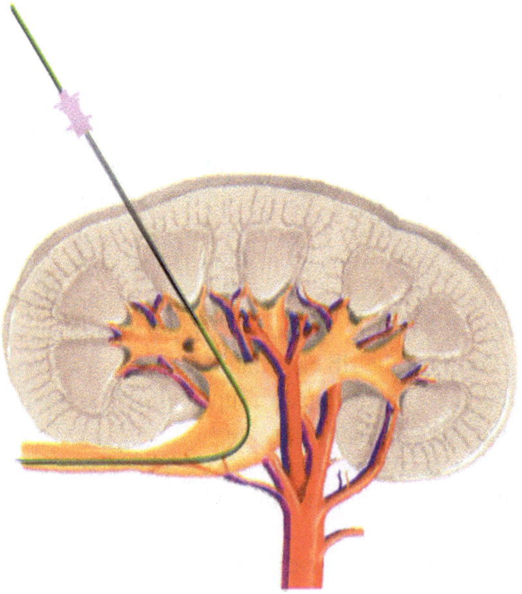

Fig. 8.1 Perfect puncture

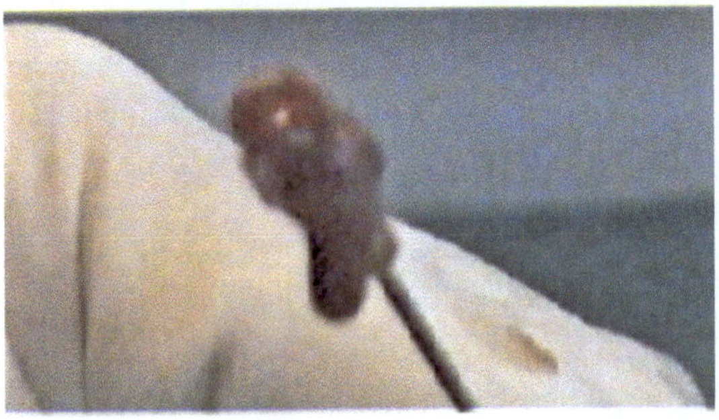

Fig. 8.2 Blood at tip of needle

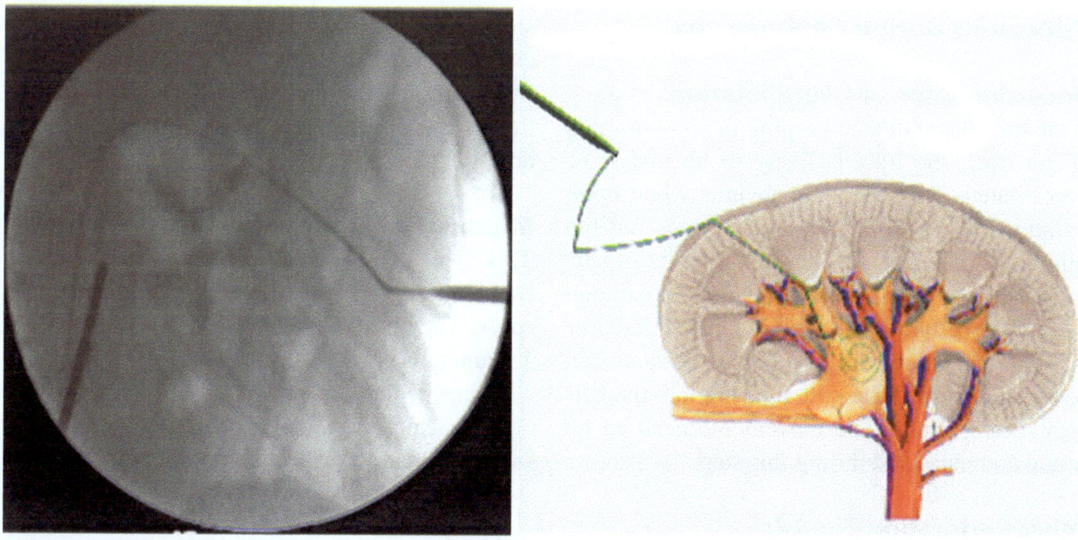

Fig. 8.3 Kinking of guidewire

in the cortex or might have hit a blood vessel) and blood mixed with urine; in the former, the puncture should not be accepted. If the efflux is blood tinged, this often happens after multiple attempts at gaining access; such an efflux (blood tinged) gets cleared after instillation of irrigation fluid from the ureteric catheter. In the latter situation after confirming the position of the needle with a contrast study, the puncture can be accepted.

Inability to Park the Guidewire

Ideally the guidewire should be parked in the ureter or a distant calyx. Often this is difficult if the access is in a stone-bearing calyx and/or the calyces are completely occupied by the stone as seen in a complete staghorn calculus. The space can be created by instillation of saline pushed through a ureteric catheter. A hydrophilic guidewire often finds its way into the desired place; however at times, it also runs the risk of slippage due to its hydrophilic coating. If the guidewire does not coil into a distant calyx, it can be passed excessively into the access calyx. If inspite of all the manipulations the guidewire does not park safely, the wire should be coiled in the calyx of entry and additional care should be exercised during dilating the tract.

Difficulties in Dilatation

Wire Kinks (Fig. 8.3)

This occurs often if a stiff guidewire is in use and/or the operator is a novice. The dilatation should always occur along the direction of the wire. Kinks are uncommon if a hydrophilic/glide wire is used. The wire often kinks at the thoracolumbar fascia. The thoracolumbar fascia should be generously incised in all cases to avoid this problem. A custom-made knife serves the purpose, and at times the same can be done with a no. 15 surgical knife.

If a wire kinks, the problem can be tackled as follows:

- The site of the kink will help determine further course of action. If it is possible to retrieve the kinked part of the wire into the fascial dilator lumen, this is done so that the guidewire can be exchanged with a new wire. Alternatively if a safety wire is in place, this is used for completing the procedure.
- If the kinks occur at multiple places, it is preferable to perform a fresh access.
- If the guidewire slips after tract dilatation, a fresh guidewire may be inserted through the tract. However if the wire slips prior to dilation and establishment of the tract, a fresh puncture should be contemplated.

Difficulties During Nephroscopy

Underdilatation or Overdilatation

If the tract is not dilated keeping in mind the axis of the tract, the tract is likely to be under- or over-dilated. This becomes obvious when upon introduction of a nephroscope, fat is visible (Fig. 8.4); one needs to decrease the rate of irrigation flow to avoid extravasation. The surgeon needs to ascertain if the tract is under-dilated or over-dilated; if the wire is in place, the same can be ascertained by following the wire into the pelvicalyceal system. The movements need to be gentle and measured during this step.

Pelvic Perforation (Fig. 8.4)

The decision regarding dealing with this situation depends on the size of the perforation and the visibility due to the presence of oozing. If the perforation is small enough to offer an unhindered completion of the procedure, the stone is cleared as swiftly as possible. However, if the perforation is large, a nephrostomy tube is placed and the procedure is staged.

Stone Clearance

The stone should be broken into large pieces so that the stone can be cleared in a minimal number of stages. The size of the pieces should be assessed depending on the size of the Amplatz sheath. A quick way to achieve complete stone clearance is use of Lithoclast® (EMS, Dallas, TX) with suction. This energy source prevents migration of the stone fragments as well as fast clearance of stones.

Migration of Stone into a Distant Calyx

This typically becomes challenging if a stone fragment migrates into upper calyx or an anterior calyx. The options available are

1. Puncture wash: This can be done in small stones which have migrated into a calyx having a short infundibulum; the success with this modality is typically better if the calyx is a nondependant calyx. A stone-bearing calyx puncture is done, and a saline wash is done which displaces the stone in a favorable position (either the initial calyx of puncture or the pelvis). This avoids excess torque on the infundibulum and the resultant bleeding.
2. Multiperc or additional tract: When the infundibulum is long and narrow puncture wash is likely to fail. In such situations, the tract can be dilated; preferably, the tract should be dilated minimally. This may be challenging if the stone is in a compact calyx.
3. Flexible instrumentation: The application of flexible instrumentation is useful if expertise and instrumentation is available. A flexible ureteroscope is useful if the pelvis is dilated;

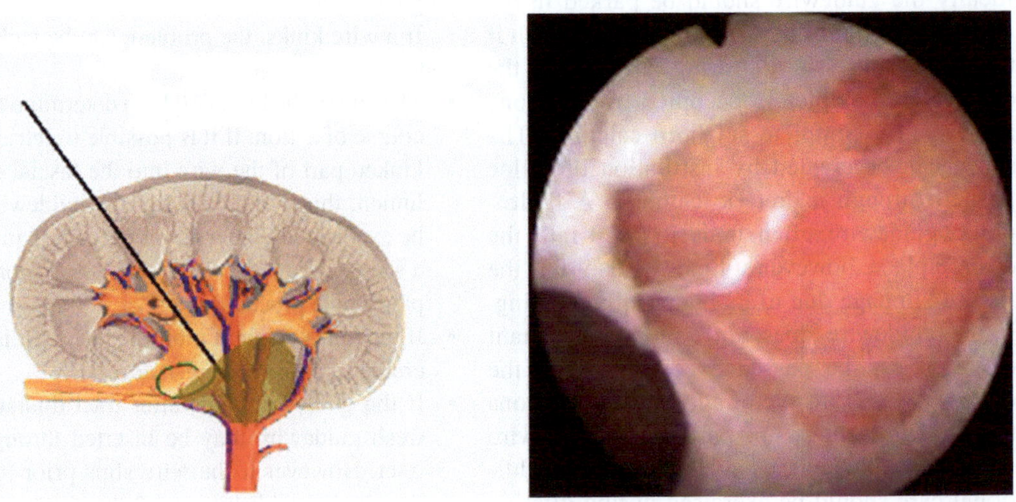

Fig. 8.4 Pelvic perforation

on the contrary if the pelvis is not dilated and the stone is in the upper ureter, a flexible nephroscope is useful. If the pelvicalyceal system is oozing and the vision is poor flexible, instrumentation does not help.
4. Wait and watch: If the stone is small enough to pass on its own (less than 4 mm), a wait-and-watch policy can be advocated.

To Stage or Not to Stage

The surgeon is likely to face this situation either preoperatively or intraoperatively.

Situation 1

In complex and complete staghorn, it is our policy to stage the procedure if the nephroscopy time exceeds 90 min. Similarly, if in the opinion of the surgeon the vision is obscuring the safe completion of the procedure, the procedure can be staged.

Situation 2

If the urine is purulent or turbid, rather than proceeding with the procedure, a tube should be placed; this helps in two ways: first, it creates a mature tract, which helps in clearance, and secondly, it clears infection. This prevents the complications related to sepsis.

Situation 3

As a policy in complex staghorn which preoperatively was planned for the stone to be cleared in stages, we place planned wires strategically into calyx of concern.

Difficulties in Special Situations

Obesity

In addition to the medical risk involved with this group of patients, technical challenges also exist. Medical morbidities such as deep vein thrombosis can be prevented with prophylaxis, with bandages, and antiplatelets and heparin. The difficulties include

- Positioning: In patients with higher body mass index, positioning is challenging. The risk involves injury to the neck and dislodgement of the endotracheal tube. This is prevented by involving adequate number of operating room personnel to perform the task. The neck is padded with cushions. An alternative to this may be to perform the procedure in a supine or modified supine position; this decreases the cardiorespiratory/anesthesia-related risk.
- Access: Due to the amount of adipose tissue in the subcutaneous space, at times the visualization of the kidney with ultrasound guidance becomes challenging. The exact distance of the kidney from the skin can be assessed preoperatively by measuring the distance from the skin to the desired calyx of access. The EchoTip needle helps in visualization of the needle path. Special instruments are required to overcome the longer distance from the skin to the desired calyx. Extra-long Amplatz sheaths/access tracts are required to access the desired calyx. The access tracts can be fixed with the help of a stitch at the site of entry to the skin. Extra-long nephroscopes or flexible nephroscopes help in clearing stones in an awkward inaccessible calyx.

Skeletal Anomalies and Anomalous Kidney

In these situations a preoperative CT scan helps to assess the relation to the surrounding structures and prevent possible injury to surrounding structures. In our opinion the considerations for these patients are

1. Preoperative CT helps to evaluate the presence of vascular and other visceral structures.
2. Adequate precautions should be taken for padding the pressure points.
3. Supine PCNL should be considered to prevent fractures and neurological postoperative problems.
4. Ultrasound-guided PCNL helps in preventing bowel injury and injury to adjacent organs.
5. Judicious use of flexible instrumentation for complete clearance in single sitting [5].

Stones in Inaccessible Calyx

After clearing the majority of the bulk, stones in inaccessible calyces can be cleared either with the help of a flexible nephroscope or an additional tract. The decision to employ a given approach depends on the situation of the calyx and the stone bulk:

- Flexible ureteroscopy: This was described to reduce the number of tracts and the resultant complications [6]. However, the major reason for failure of this modality is poor visibility. The stone once seen can be tackled either by fragmenting it or removing the stone in total with a basket.
- Additional tract: This may be done at the outset. The puncture is done in the stone-bearing calyx. The tract is dilated till 18 Fr, and a smaller nephroscope is used to remove the stone.

Bleeding

Trauma to the renal vasculature is a recognized complication of percutaneous renal surgery. The most common cause of this complication is arteriovenous fistula and pseudoaneurysm. The precautionary measures to prevent this problem are

1. Preoperatively the bleeding parameters should be checked and corrected if deranged.
2. Preoperatively patients with staghorn stones in a setting of chronic kidney disease are prone to bleed; these patients should be preoperatively worked up in close consultation with the anesthetist.
3. A perfect puncture through the cup of the calyx helps in achieving a straight access.
4. The degree and extent of dilation is dictated by the caliber of the calyx and the width of the infundibulum. An excessive dilatation leads to tearing and resultant bleeding.
5. The lateral sheering force during dilatation should be minimal. This decreases the torque.
6. While negotiating a parallel or adjacent calyx, the surgeon should make sure that the torque on the infundibulum is minimal.
7. An oozing leading to loss of vision should be an indication for staging the procedure.
8. An intraoperative event of hypotension should be an indication to stop the procedure and expect postoperative bleeding. Most of the traumatic aneurysm resolves spontaneously; those who do not respond need transarterial embolization [7].

Conclusion

The troubleshooting in rigid approach to staghorn calculus involves proper preoperative assessment with contrast-enhanced CT scan. The basic principles of endourology which include proper vision, understanding the relevant surgical anatomy, and use of proper-sized and appropriate instruments help in reducing the risks involved in this approach. Timely recognition and treatment of surgical complications help in reducing the morbidity and related mortality.

References

1. Preminger GM, Assimos DG, Lingeman JE, Nakada SY, Pearle MS, Wolfe JS. AUA guidelines on management of staghorn calculi: diagnosis and treatment recommendations. J Urol. 2005;173:1991–2000.
2. Thiruchelvam N, Mostafid H, Ubhayakar G. Planning percutaneous nephrolithotomy using multidetector computed tomography urography, multiplanar reconstruction and three dimensional reformatting. BJU Int. 2005;95:1280–4.
3. Bader MJ, Gratzke C, Seitz M, Sharma R, Stief CG, Desai M. The all-seeing needle: initial results of an optical puncture system confirming access I percutaneous nephrolithotomy. Eur Urol. 2011;59(6):1054–9.
4. Desai MR, Sharma R, Mishra S, Sabnis RB, Steif C, Bader M. Single step percutaneous nephrolithotomy (microperc): the initial clinical report. J Urol. 2011; 186(1):140–5.
5. Ganpule AP, Deasi M. Urolithiasis in kidneys with abnormal lie rotation or form. Curr Opin Urol. 2011;21(2):145–53.
6. Williams SK, Leveille RJ. Management of staghorn calculus: single puncture with judicious use of flexible nephroscope. Curr Opin Urol. 2008;18(2):224–8.
7. Skolarikos A, De la Rosette J. Prevention and treatment of complications following percutaneous nephrolithotomy. Curr Opin Urol. 2008;18:229–34.

Flexible Renal Nephroscopy: Overcoming the Difficulties

9

Joseph A. Graversen, Adam C. Mues, and Mantu Gupta

Introduction

In 1941, following an open surgery for nephrolithiasis, Rupel and Brown advanced a rigid cystoscope into the kidney through an established drainage tract to remove several obstructing calculi, effectively becoming the first to perform percutaneous nephroscopy [1]. In 1955, the field was further advanced when Goodwin and colleagues reported successful, purposeful percutaneous access into a hydronephrotic kidney [2]. However, it was not until 30 years later that percutaneous nephrostolithotomy (PCNL) would be popularized. Due to its minimally invasive nature, low morbidity, and great efficacy, PCNL has evolved into the gold standard for the treatment of large renal and proximal stones, including staghorn calculi [3].

The most common method of PCNL utilizes a specially designed offset nephroscope that is advanced into an established percutaneous tract. The modern nephroscope allows for the easy passage of a variety of large caliber instruments while maintaining a high flow of irrigant. This is important as visibility often relies on the ability to flush the upper tract free of debris throughout the case. Recent technological advancements have broadened the range of procedures in which a percutaneous approach can be utilized. Upper tract urothelial carcinoma, calyceal diverticula, stenotic infundibula, symptomatic renal cysts, and excluded calyces are but a few of the indications for percutaneous nephroscopy. While the rigid nephroscope offers many advantages, its utility is often limited by renal anatomy and complex stone formations. The advent and development of the flexible nephroscope has allowed for the urologist to perform increasingly complex procedures. This chapter will focus on basic and advanced flexible nephroscopy and overcoming the difficulties associated with complex cases.

Due to the easy accessibility and technological advancements of the modern ureteroscope, flexible nephroscopy is rarely utilized solely for the purpose of diagnosis. The majority of upper tract abnormalities are initially identified with high-quality axial imaging and further delineated using a retrograde technique. In rare instances wherein normal anatomy has been distorted, such as in urinary diversion or luminal obliteration from malignancy or stricture, flexible nephroscopy along with antegrade ureteral access can prove to be invaluable. Similarly, flexible nephroscopy is also commonly utilized with obstruction or lesions of

J.A. Graversen, M.D. (✉)
Department of Urology, University of California, Irvine, Orange, CA, 92868, USA
e-mail: jgravers@uci.edu

A.C. Mues, M.D.
Department of Urology, New York University School of Medicine,
150 E 32nd Street, 2nd Floor, New York, NY, 10016, USA
e-mail: adammues@gmail.com

M. Gupta, M.D.
Department of Urology, Columbia University,
161 Fort Washington Avenue, New York, NY, 10032, USA
e-mail: mg392@columbia.edu

A.M. Al-Kandari et al. (eds.), *Difficult Cases in Endourology*,
DOI 10.1007/978-1-84882-083-8_9, © Springer-Verlag London 2013

unclear etiology in which retrograde evaluation fails or is difficult, for example, patients with Indiana pouches or neobladders.

The majority of therapeutic indications for flexible nephroscopy are adjunctive to rigid nephroscopy, especially as it pertains to renal stone disease. However, flexible nephroscopy as a sole intervention is often utilized for very complex cases or complex anatomy. Common therapeutic indications for flexible nephroscopy include:

1. Stone disease:
   - Flexible nephroscopy is utilized to gain access to calyces not otherwise accessible by a rigid nephroscope with the purpose of retrieving residual stones and stone fragments.
   - It is less effective than rigid nephroscopy for stone comminution mainly due to limitations associated with instrumentation.
2. Upper tract urothelial carcinoma:
   - Percutaneous endoscopic resection can be utilized for the treatment of urothelial carcinoma involving the upper tract.
   - Endoscopic resection is usually performed with a standard monopolar or bipolar resectoscope.
   - Flexible nephroscopy is advantageous in its use for systematic calyceal inspection, proximal ureteroscopy, and laser ablation of smaller lesions.
3. Ureteropelvic junction obstruction:
   - Antegrade endopyelotomy/endopyeloplasty for the treatment of ureteropelvic junction (UPJ) obstruction is achieved with a balloon cutting device, Holmium:YAG laser, or a cold cutting device such as the hook knife or Sachse urethrotome.
   - Similar to endoscopic resection, flexible nephroscopy has only a limited role in the treatment of UPJ obstruction mainly due to the instruments normally utilized. However, in rare instances of distorted renal anatomy, flexible nephroscopy offers the advantage of improved accessibility over that of rigid nephroscopy.
4. Abnormal renal anatomy:
   - Obstructed calyces due to infundibular stenosis, calyceal diverticula, or excluded calyces are of special concern to the urologist due to their inaccessibility.
   - There are three methods for gaining access to such an obstructed system (retrograde, antegrade direct, or antegrade indirect):
     - In antegrade direct access, the obstructed calyx is entered directly at the time of access. This technique is usually utilized for posteriorly oriented calyces and is the preferred method.
     - Antegrade indirect access is achieved by entering the normal pelvicalyceal system and subsequently entering the obstructed calyx through the stenotic os. This technique is utilized for anteriorly located lesions and for the concomitant inspection of the remaining pelvicalyceal system.
     - Flexible nephroscopy is most often utilized during indirect access; however, it can also be used with direct access when rigid nephroscopy is incapable of navigating the abnormal renal anatomy.

Indications for Flexible Nephroscopy

The most common indication for flexible nephroscopy is to obtain access into a calyx, obstructed or otherwise, that cannot be entered with rigid nephroscopy alone. Although flexible nephroscopy can be employed for the percutaneous treatment of upper tract urothelial carcinoma, it is usually used for locating and treating nephrolithiasis. The finding of residual stones after rigid PCNL is common with rates as high as 70 % [4, 5]. Currently, the clinical significance of these residual fragments is controversial; however, as in any stone treatment, the ultimate goal is stone-free status.

Techniques vary for the identification of residual stones after PCNL. Most urologists depend on radiographic imaging, either plain film or computed tomography. However, flexible nephroscopy after PCNL is likely the most sensitive method for recognizing these residual fragments. In one study, 29 patients with preoperative stone size ≥3 cm underwent PCNL, followed by plain films, computed tomography, and lastly, flexible nephroscopy [5]. Plain films identified stones in 33 % of the patients (10/29), while computed tomography identified five more patients with residual fragments (15/29, 48 %). All 29 patients subsequently underwent flexible nephroscopy wherein an additional 5 patients were discovered to have residual stone fragments (20/29, 69 %). Moreover, upon identifying fragments, treatment was rendered without delay.

There are several treatment options available for large or complex stones within the pelvicalyceal system that cannot be removed through a single tract. Flexible nephroscopy offers the clear advantage of accessibility into the calyces without the need of new access points. Flexible nephroscopy in combination with standard rigid PCNL has demonstrated high stone-free rates despite large, complex stones [6]. The second option is the addition of multiple access tracts into the same kidney, also known as a multiperc. Stone-free rates and complications between flexible nephroscopy are similar; however, the transfusion rates and hospital stay are significantly greater with multiperc than with flexible nephroscopy [7]. A third technique that is not commonly employed involves combining PCNL with retrograde techniques [8]. Regardless of approach, the goal of therapy is stone-free status in a single procedure. In the current economic environment, the demand by both patients and healthcare will make the continued practice of multiple procedures, including multiple PCNLs soon give way to a single procedure. Time away from work after discharge will likely preclude performing even additional same day procedures such as extracorporeal shock wave lithotripsy (ESWL). Furthermore, the added hospital stay and morbidity associated with the multiperc has also engendered the popularity of flexible nephroscopy in stone patients at the time of PCNL.

A second indication for flexible nephroscopy is for the treatment of obstructed calyces and calyceal diverticula (Fig. 9.1). More commonly flexible nephroscopy is utilized for indirect entry into the obstructed system; however, acute angles or severe infundibular stenosis may necessitate the use of flexible nephroscopy during direct entry as well. For patients with calyceal diverticula with stones,

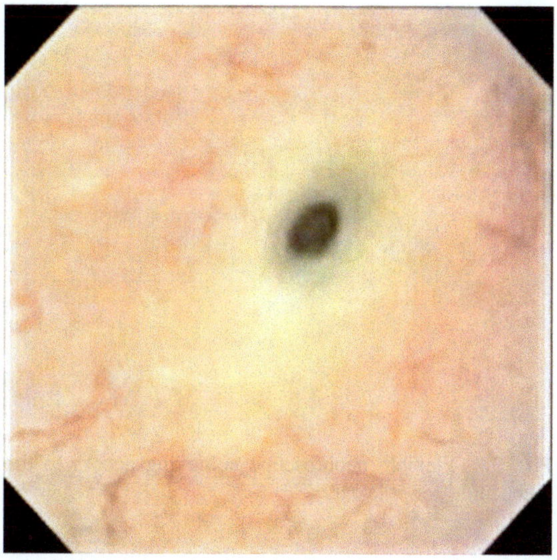

Fig. 9.1 Infundibular stenosis with tight opening during indirect access

indirect entry offers the advantage of access to the entire pelvicalyceal system and the management of additional stones therein, along with treatment for the diverticulum itself. This technique obviates the need for multiple accesses and the inherent morbidity with which they are associated. Typically, a conventional cystoscope is used to perform the flexible nephroscopy. It offers the flexibility, visualization, and familiarity that most urologists seek, with minimal compromise to the size of the working port. However, the scope's large caliber can also hinder passage through a stenotic infundibulum. To counteract this, a flexible ureteroscope can be used in lieu of the cystoscope. They are generally 7–8 Fr in size and offer better deflection than the cystoscope. Furthermore, they can easily be advanced down the ureter in antegrade fashion to retrieve stone fragments. However, ureteroscopes also have disadvantages, including loss of sturdiness, visualization, and working channel diameter. Also, the same characteristics that make the flexible ureteroscope suitable for retrograde procedures become cumbersome during antegrade procedures. The scope's length is awkward to manage with the majority of the shaft being extracorporeal, and the tight distal radius of deflection makes maneuverability within a hydronephrotic system difficult.

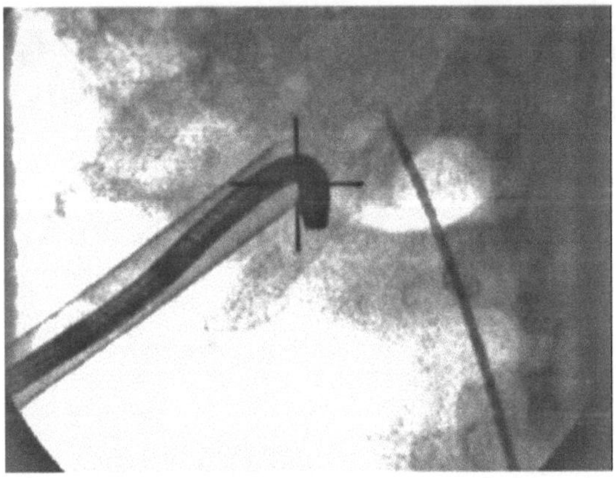

Fig. 9.2 Flexible nephroscope achieving access to the adjacent lower pole calyx

Ultimately, a combination of stone characteristics such as shape, size, and location along with PCNL access location determines the necessity of flexible nephroscopy. The most common access site for PCNL is the posterior lower pole calyx. Anterior calyx entry traverses significantly more parenchyma and risks more bleeding, and the lower pole location avoids complications from pleural injury [9, 10]. The rigid scope can subsequently be advanced into the lower pole and pelvis, but access to the upper pole and interpolar calyces can be limited without a significant amount of torque. This inaccessibility is accentuated in obese patients and low-lying renal units wherein torque is physically limited by excessive adipose tissue or the iliac crest, respectively. The rigid scope is also inadequate for passage into the ureter and adjacent lower pole calyx due to the acute angle (Fig. 9.2). If the entirety of the stone is located in the lower pole and renal pelvis, and the ureter does not require investigation, rigid nephroscopy alone may suffice, however, an upper pole or branching stone, or the need for ureteral investigation likely requires either flexible nephroscopy or a multiperc technique. Similarly, if upper pole access is obtained, there is a limited amount of torque that can be applied within the confines of the intercostal space making lower pole and posterior calyceal entry equally limited.

Preoperative Planning

All patients scheduled for PCNL should undergo standard preoperative evaluation including a complete history and physical, a basic laboratory work-up such as a complete cell blood count and basic metabolic panel, and an electrocardiogram and chest x-ray when appropriate. Patients should also stop anticoagulants 7–10 days prior to surgery with the approval of the prescribing physician. If necessary, a heparin window can be instituted in those patients that cannot stop anticoagulation for prolonged periods of time. Additionally, all patients should be type and screened and consented for blood administration.

Urine cultures should be obtained on all patients approximately 10–14 days prior to surgery and are ideally negative. However, achieving true sterility in the face of an infection stone can be difficult despite an appropriate course of culture-specific antibiotics. It is well known that the concordance between urine culture, whether positive or negative, and stone/renal pelvis culture is poor [11–13]. Data from PCNLs performed at our own institution demonstrated that urine cultures obtained from voided, intraoperative renal pelvis, and stone specimens did not correspond (Table 9.1) [14]. The obvious concern when urine culture does not predict stone/renal pelvis culture is in preoperative antibiotic choice and the postoperative choice in the event of post-PCNL fever/sepsis. For that reason, stone and renal pelvis cultures are standard for all patients.

In the early experience with PCNL, antibiotics were not uniformly prescribed [15]. Currently, however, most urologists routinely administer preoperative antibiotics. While there is no standard protocol, the authors administer a minimum of 7 days of culture-specific antibiotics for patients with positive preoperative urine cultures. All patients receive a prophylactic dose of broad spectrum antibiotics at the time of surgery followed by continuation for 24 h. Patients that develop postoperative fevers or sepsis receive culture-directed therapy.

Table 9.1 Voided, renal pelvis, and stone specimen culture concordance

Specimen (*n*)	Positive (%)	Concordance with preoperative bladder urine culture	Concordance with intraoperative renal pelvis culture
Preoperative bladder urine culture (204)	47/204 (23.0 %)	–	–
Intraoperative renal pelvis culture (204)	21/204 (10.3 %)	9/21 (42.9 %)	–
Intraoperative stone culture (204)	33/204 (16.2 %)	12/33 (36.4 %)	8/33 (24.2 %)

An emphasis should be placed on high-quality preoperative imaging. Although the preference is noncontrast axial computed tomography (CT) with coronal and sagittal reconstructions, a noncontrast axial CT alone or a high-quality intravenous pyelogram (IVP) would suffice. The goal when evaluating the film is to assess the renal anatomy, including that of the calyces, and stone characteristics such as burden, location, and shape. Adjacent structures such as the extent of the pleura and the position of the bowel and other organs should be evaluated especially as they relate to the expected tract of entry. This is especially important when the renal unit is anomalous (malrotated, horseshoe, ptotic, pelvic, ectopic, etc.). To that end, an IVP allows for renal anatomy and stone evaluation; however, a CT is far more superior for the evaluation of adjacent structures. The presence of a branching stone, multiple stones in multiple calyces, or an awkward renal position should clue the surgeon to the likely need for flexible nephroscopy. If there is doubt as to whether a stenotic infundibulum, calyceal diverticulum, or UPJ obstruction is present, the addition of contrast to the CT is advantageous. Furthermore, an angiographic phase can be performed to identify crossing vessels if an endopyelotomy is planned.

Patient Positioning

PCNL has been performed in a variety of positions under both regional and general anesthesia. However, prone with the patient under general anesthesia remains the most common. Listed below are various positions that have been described in the literature as being successful alternatives along with how they might affect attempts at flexible nephroscopy:

1. Prone:
   - The traditional method of performing PCNLs offers surgeons with familiarity and wide expanse of flank for choosing an access site.
   - Flexible nephroscopy can be performed intuitively in the prone position.
   - Incurs anesthesiological risks in the form of ventilatory, hemodynamic, and circulatory changes [16].
2. Prone split-leg [17, 18]:
   - Similar to the prone position except that the lower extremities are placed on spreader bars.
   - This modification allows for genital access so simultaneous antegrade and retrograde procedures can be performed.
   - In this position, a ureteral access sheath can also be placed to flush stone debris out of the collecting system and reduce renal pressure by functioning as a second pop-off valve.
   - Flexible nephroscopy can be performed antegrade concomitantly with retrograde ureteroscopy, although flexible retrograde access may eliminate the need for antegrade flexible nephroscopy altogether. Retrograde flexible nephroscopy, however, is further limited by the caliber of the ureteroscope.
3. Prone flexed [19]:
   - Patients are positioned in the prone position with the bed flexed approximately 30°.
   - The position maximizes the exposed flank by widening the gap between the twelfth rib and iliac crest.

- Flex position lowers the renal unit allowing for improved upper pole access.
- The ability to perform flexible nephroscopy is unlikely affected.

4. Lateral decubitus position [20–24]:
   - Described mainly in the morbidly obese and those with respiratory compromise in whom prone positioning may not be tolerated.
   - This position is used in conjunction with regional anesthesia as a means to avoid general anesthetics in the high-risk patient.
   - Likely does not affect the ability to perform flexible nephroscopy.
5. Galdakao-modified supine Valdivia position [16, 25]:
   - The patient is placed in the lithotomy position with the lower extremity ipsilateral to the stone in extension.
   - A wedge is placed under the ipsilateral flank effectively exposing it.
   - Allows for retrograde and antegrade access to the affected kidney.
   - Flexible nephroscopy can be performed in the antegrade concomitantly with retrograde ureteroscopy, although the retrograde access may eliminate the need for antegrade flexible nephroscopy altogether; however, it has the same limitations as noted previously.
6. Modified lateral position [26]:
   - Patients are positioned in a lithotomy position with the pelvis tilted on a wedge and the shoulders perpendicular to the table.
   - Allows for full genital exposure for retrograde access with maximal flank exposure for PCNL.
   - Also reduces anesthesia risks from the prone position.
   - Flexible nephroscopy can be performed antegrade concomitantly with retrograde ureteroscopy, although flexible retrograde access may eliminate the need for antegrade flexible nephroscopy altogether.
7. Reverse lithotomy [27]:
   - Mainly described for use in females, with few additional reports of this position after the initial experience.
   - Patients are placed in the prone position with legs flexed into a lithotomy-like position for genital access.
   - Flexible nephroscopy can be performed in the antegrade concomitantly with retrograde ureteroscopy, although the retrograde access may eliminate the need for antegrade flexible nephroscopy altogether.

Instrumentation

As it pertains to visualization, rigid nephroscopes are superior to flexible nephroscopes. Large working channels improve irrigant flow while also allowing for large caliber instruments to be utilized. Furthermore, with the advent of longer, digital nephroscopes with improved visualization and "chip on a stick" technology, such as the new Olympus Invisio® Smith digital nephroscope (Olympus, Gyrus ACMI, Southborough, MA), access to distant calyces is more feasible than in the past (Fig. 9.3) [28].

Similarly, the flexible nephroscope has also evolved significantly in recent years with the advent of digital cystoscopes [29, 30]. The most recent generation of flexible cystoscopes replaces the traditional fiber optics with a small charge-coupled device (CCD) located on the distal tip of the scope. The CCD converts photons to electrons, which are subsequently transmitted and translated into the image seen by the operating urologist. In head to head trials with fiber-optic scopes, the digi-

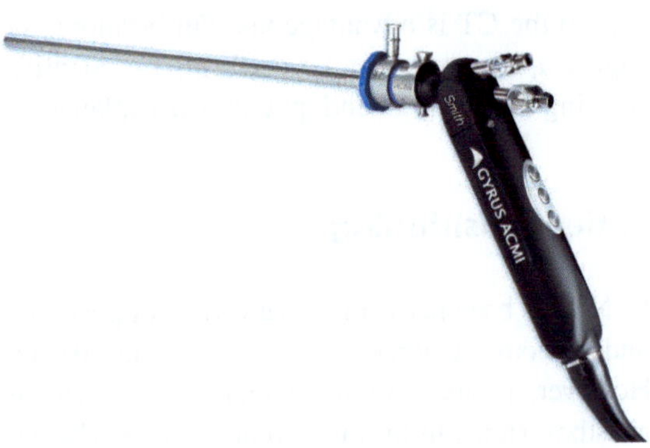

Fig. 9.3 The Invisio® Smith digital percutaneous nephroscope (Image provided courtesy of Olympus, Gyrus ACMI)

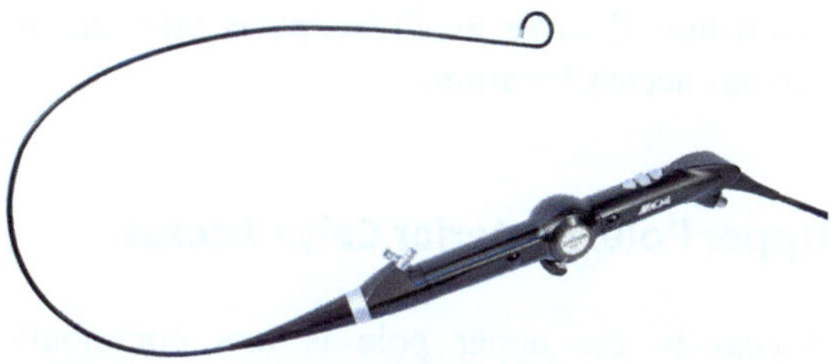

Fig. 9.4 Invisio® DUR®-D digital flexible ureteroscope (Image provided courtesy of Olympus, Gyrus ACMI)

tal scope has been shown to have improved resolution, contrast discrimination, and color recognition. Furthermore, the new generation of scopes is capable of greater deflection and withstands greater degrees of torque without loss of durability. As it pertains to flexible nephroscopy, digital scopes offer improved clarity and maneuverability within the confines of both the tight and the hydronephrotic pelvicalyceal system. This is especially important since flexible nephroscopy is often performed after rigid nephroscopy when the tissues are already traumatized and visibility is low.

Alternatively, a flexible ureteroscope can be used for nephroscopy in lieu of a cystoscope. Flexible ureteroscopes have also evolved into highly advanced digital systems. The Invisio® DUR®-D flexible ureteroscope (Olympus, Gyrus ACMI, Southborough, MA) (Fig. 9.4) utilizes 1-mm complementary metal oxide semiconductor as the distal digital sensor combined with built-in LED lights to enhance image quality over that of fiber-optic scopes. The distal tip also flexes 270° in both directions giving the ureteroscope unparalleled maneuverability (Fig. 9.5).

The primary advantage to using a flexible ureteroscope is the small caliber of the scope. At 7–8.5 Fr, flexible ureteroscopes can maneuver through the smallest infundibula. They are also capable of secondary deflection within the pelvicalyceal system, thereby improving accessibility within complex renal units. However, the smaller diameter means that there is a loss of sturdiness to the scope. One of the techniques to combat this is to pass the flexible ureteroscope through the working channel of the nephroscope. This technique gives the ureteroscope structural support along the shaft while maintaining distal flexibility (Fig. 9.6). When

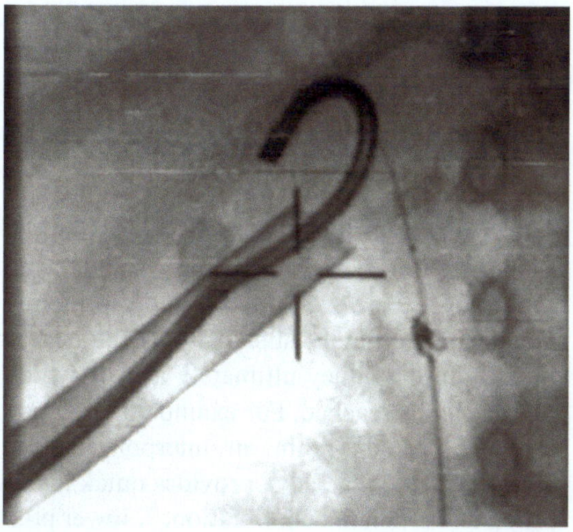

Fig. 9.5 Tight retroflexion with the flexible ureteroscope allows for access to a renal stone adjacent to PCNL sheath

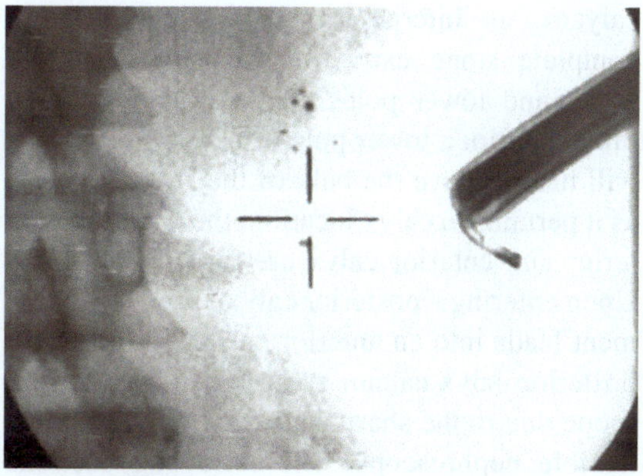

Fig. 9.6 A flexible ureteroscope has been passed through the working channel of the rigid nephroscope. The technique combines the stability of the rigid nephroscopy with the flexibility and small caliber of the flexible ureteroscope

employing this method, it is particularly useful to have two monitors displaying simultaneous images from each system (rigid and flexible). The surgeon can then use the sturdier nephroscope for the initial approach to the area in question reserving the flexible ureteroscope for the finer maneuvers.

Renal Access

The location of the initial access is the primary determinate of which calyces can be accessed. The most common access utilized is a lower pole posterior calyx. The purpose for this location is twofold. The first is to avoid the upper pole which often requires a supracostal entry site, thereby incurring the risk of pleural injury [9, 10]. The second is to avoid an anterior calyceal access which traverses significantly more renal parenchyma, thereby increasing the risk of bleeding, poor visualization, and delayed hemorrhage. However, this general principle should not be blindly abided by as the access site within the kidney ultimately affects which calyces can be reached. For example, if a single stone is located within an interpolar calyx, direct entry into that calyx provides quick localization and efficient comminution. A lower pole access in this scenario increases the difficulty of reaching the stone. However, if the stone is complex with multiple branches into several calyces, an interpolar access usually makes complete stone extraction difficult since the upper and lower poles are less accessible. In this scenario, a lower pole or upper pole access will help remove the bulk of the stone. Finally, as it pertains to calyx location, the os of the posterior and anterior calyx are directly opposed. Upon entering a posterior calyx, direct advancement leads into an anterior calyx. The adjacent posterior calyx cannot be accessed with a rigid scope due to the sharp angle and often requires flexible nephroscopy. The following sections detail how flexible nephroscopy is affected by various access locations.

Upper Pole, Posterior Calyx Access

Access to the upper pole is less commonly employed than lower pole and interpolar access due to the risk of pleural injury. If the pelvicalyceal system is moderately or severely hydronephrotic, the anterior upper pole calyx is readily accessible with a rigid scope from a posterior site. However, as the degree of hydronephrosis decreases, anterior calyceal entry becomes more difficult, especially if the posterior entry is nearer to the infundibulum than to the papilla. From the upper pole, the anterior lower pole calyces can usually be entered with a rigid scope (Fig. 9.7a); however, the sharp angle into the posterior calyces can rarely be navigated and requires flexible nephroscopy (Fig. 9.7b). The interpolar calyces, especially posteriorly, are likewise difficult to access with the rigid scope alone. From the vantage point of the upper pole, however, the renal pelvis and the ureter can be easily explored with the rigid nephroscope. Taken together, flexible nephroscopy (or multiperc) is often necessary from the upper pole to access the opposing anterior upper pole calyx in the absence of hydronephrosis, the posterior calyces in the lower

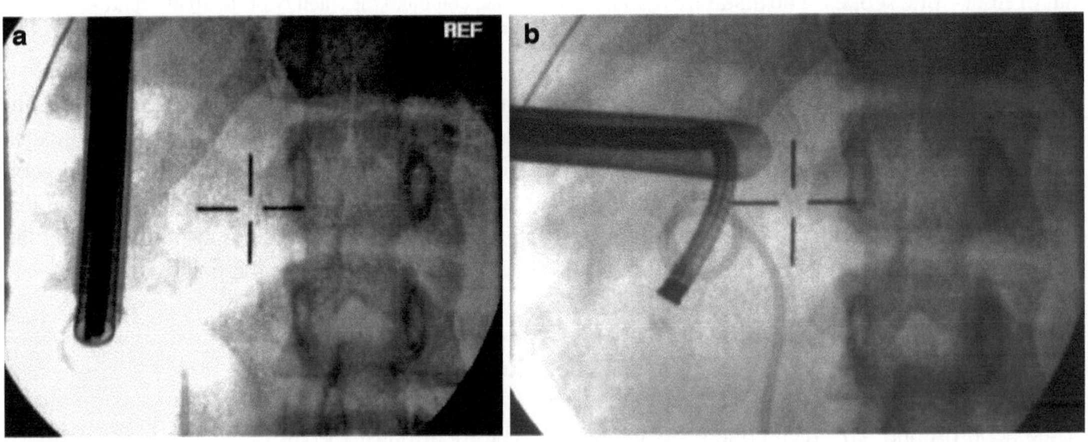

Fig. 9.7 (**a**) Rigid nephroscopy into the anterior lower pole calyx from an upper pole posterior approach. (**b**) Flexible nephroscope in the posterior lower pole from an upper pole access point

poles, and both anterior and posterior calyces in the interpolar region.

Interpolar Posterior Calyx Access

From an interpolar access point, the renal pelvis and ureter are readily explored; however, both the lower and upper poles are generally inaccessible without flexible nephroscopy. The only indications for this access are for the treatment of a solitary stone in the interpolar region, direct access into a calyceal diverticulum located there (rare), or for the treatment of renal pelvis/proximal ureteral stones.

Lower Pole, Posterior Calyx Access

The posterior lower pole access is usually the preferred access location for lower pole stones. From this site, the renal pelvis is readily accessible; however, the acute angle between the ureter and lower pole makes rigid ureteral access impossible. Additionally, upper pole and interpolar calyces can be difficult to enter without flexible nephroscopy (Fig. 9.8). Unlike for the upper pole, the anterior lower pole calyx becomes more accessible with medial (infundibular) positioning of the entry point. This can be achieved by rotating the c-arm head 20° toward the surgeon instead of 30°. In the authors' experience, this slightly more medial position is not associated with increased blood loss yet significantly impacts anterior calyx accessibility. The modified medial position is ideal for lower pole partial staghorns that do not branch into the inter- or upper pole calyces.

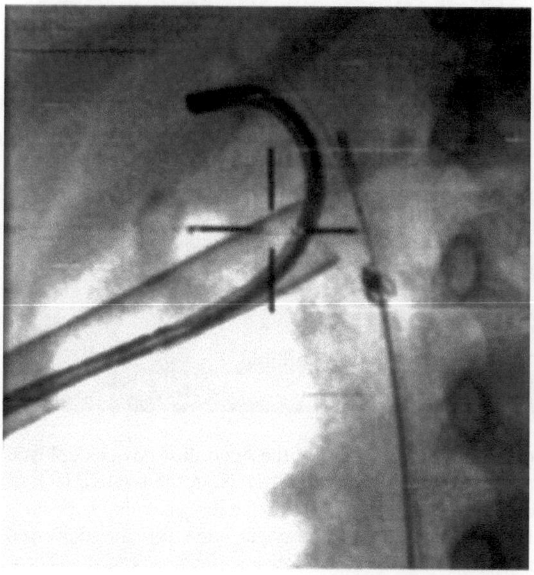

Fig. 9.8 The upper pole calyx is generally accessible from the lower pole only with a flexible nephroscope

One of the fears of PCNL, especially when operating from the lower pole, is stone migration down the ureter. To extract fragments from the ureter, the flexible nephroscope can be easily advanced antegrade into the ureter and the stones removed. However, stone migration can also be prevented during PCNL with a coaxial retropulsion device (Accordion CoAx® Stone Control Device, Percsys, Palo Alto, CA) or occlusion balloon device positioned at the UPJ (Fig. 9.9a–e) [29].

Supracostal Access

Anatomically, the extent of the parietal pleura is very low posteriorly and rises superiorly as it continues to the anterior aspect of the chest. Specifically, the pleura is located at the level of the 12th rib posteriorly, 10th rib in the midaxillary line, and 8th rib anteriorly. Supracostal PCNL access, therefore, risks injury to the pleura. Aside from the safety concerns, supracostal access also limits maneuverability by interfering with the degree of torque that can be placed on the sheath which minimizes the accessibility into other calyces. The main determinate is the distance between ribs with wide intercostal spaces providing the most maneuverability. In the majority of cases, the urologist will have to revert to flexible nephroscopy early in the case in order to achieve a stone-free status.

Tips and Tricks

Accessing the Difficult Calyx

Flexible nephroscopy is often performed after the bulk of the stone has been removed. As such,

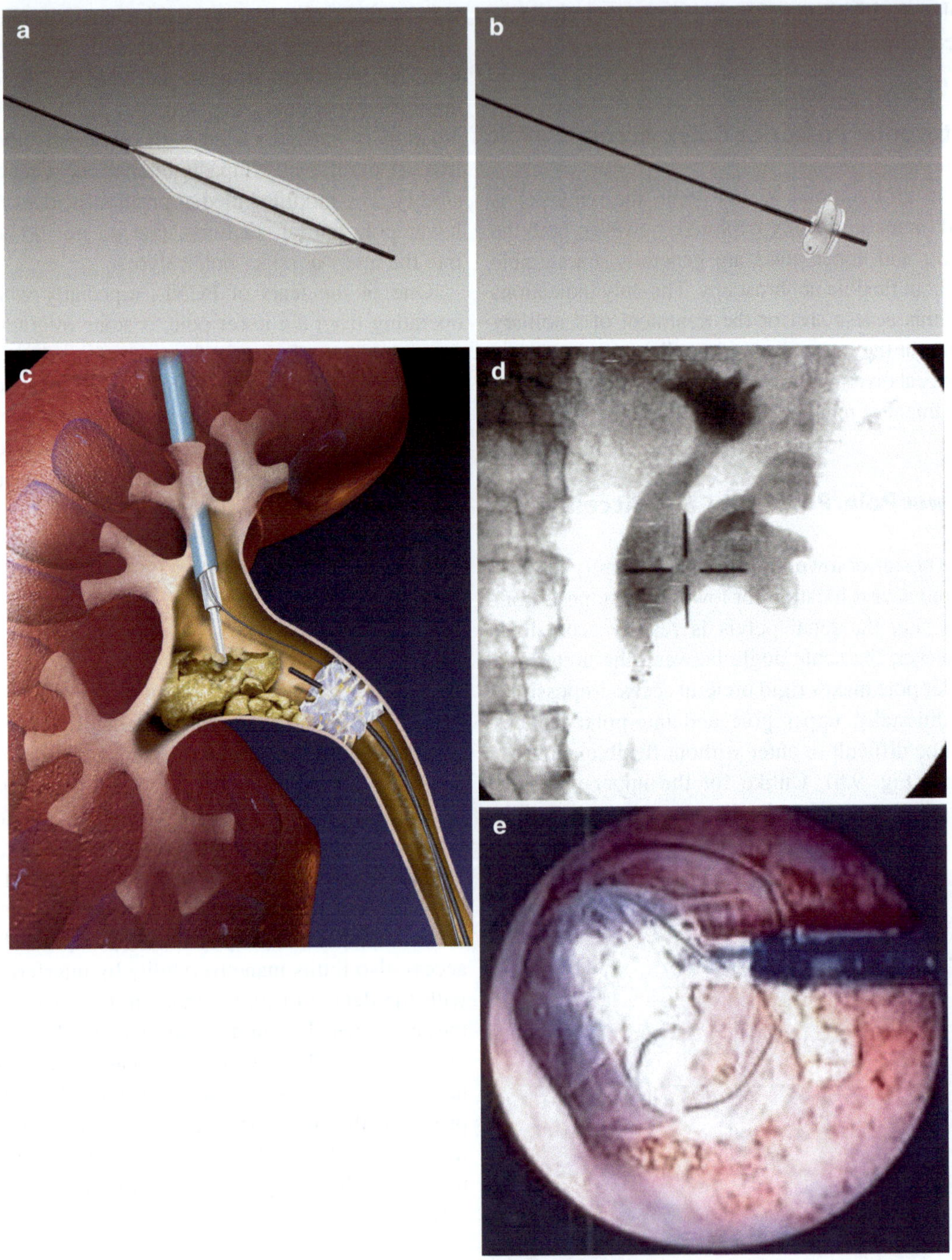

Fig. 9.9 (**a**) The Accordion CoAx® Stone Control Device prior to deployment (Image courtesy of PercSys, Palo Alto, CA). (**b**) The deployed Accordion CoAx Stone Control Device (Image courtesy of PercSys, Palo Alto, CA). (**c**) Deployed Accordion™ device during upper pole access PCNL (Image courtesy of PercSys, Palo Alto. CA). (**d**) Fluoroscopic image of the Accordion device deployed at the UPJ just prior to PCNL. Note the relative lack of contrast in the ureter distal to the device which is occluding the UPJ. (**e**) Endoscopic view of the deployed Accordion device at the UPJ

avoidance of contrast agents will improve visibility and also improve the effectiveness of fluoroscopy for identifying stones and areas of interest to be explored. The extravasation of contrast agent, especially late in the procedure when only small fragments remain, will make distinguishing stone from contrast very difficult. For this purpose, contrast agent is reserved only for use at the beginning of the case to aid in access and the end of the case to verify nephrostomy tube placement.

The flexible cystoscope is the instrument usually employed for flexible nephroscopy. This is because the cystoscope is familiar to most urologists, is durable, maintains visibility, and has a relatively large working channel. When using the scope in the pelvicalyceal system, *slow, deliberate movements* are paramount to complete visualization of the calyces. Often during calyceal exploration, small, previously unnoticed side branches can be seen. As these often harbor residual stone fragments/disease, they should also be carefully explored.

One of the advantages of rigid nephroscopy over that of flexible nephroscopy is visibility. This is in part due to better optics; however, much of the difference between the two is the higher irrigant flow of the rigid scope both with and without instruments in the working channel. Irrigation clears parenchymal bleeding, flushes out stone debris, and distends the collecting system. In this regard, the flexible cystoscope is at a disadvantage since it has a smaller working channel. However, visualization can be significantly enhanced with the *use of a pressure bag*. Because the excess flow freely drains through the nephrostomy tube, excessive pressure within the pelvicalyceal system is of minimal concern with this technique.

Occasionally when attempting to locate a particular stone or calyx, the flexible cystoscope cannot be guided by direct visualization alone. This may be due to bleeding, clot, angulation, or severe hydronephrosis. When this occurs, *interrupted periods of continuous fluoroscopy* may help position the scope in the desired location. Despite the fact that the maneuver is "blind," it is generally safe as the wide, blunt tip of the cystoscope, and the flexible nature of the shaft rarely traumatizes the urothelium significantly.

A stenotic infundibulum or a tight calyceal opening poses a unique challenge to the surgeon. The opening is uncommonly navigable by the rigid scope either due to angulation or due to the relatively large diameter of the scope. However, the rigid scope can produce the high-flow irrigation that is often necessary to distend and identify the opening; the lower flow of irrigant through the flexible scope may not be adequate. In this situation, *passing a wire through the rigid scope* and coiling it within the calyx satisfactorily identifies it with the flexible scope. The ideal wire to use is a heavy-duty J wire (Cook Urological, Spencer, IN). The J-hook tip helps deflect the wire within the calyx, helping to coil a long length of it without lacerating the calyceal wall. Additionally, the stiffness of the wire and the curved tip helps keep the wire from inadvertently dislodging. Once coiled and left in place, the flexible scope should not be passed coaxially over the wire but instead passed alongside the wire, using it as a guide. In this manner, the wire is not dislodged, the working channel of the scope remains available for instrumentation, and multiple passes can be made without the need to replace the wire.

If the infundibulum is severely stenotic and will not accommodate a flexible cystoscope, *changing to a flexible ureteroscope* may be advantageous to the surgeon. The small caliber of the flexible ureteroscope can usually gain entry into even the smallest infundibula. Unfortunately, flexible ureteroscopes also have several disadvantages, including poor irrigation, excessive length, difficult maneuverability, especially in the hydronephrotic system, and an insubstantial shaft. By itself, the flexible ureteroscope is not well suited for flexible nephroscopy. The best technique to employ is to advance the rigid nephroscope up to the stenotic os and then *pass the ureteroscope through the working channel of the rigid nephroscope*, guiding it into the calyx. Once inside, the camera can be changed to the flexible ureteroscope, or alternatively, a second tower can be used to simultaneously display images. The rigid nephroscope will provide direct access to the os, improved water flow, and will also stabilize the ureteroscope's shaft.

Stone Comminution, Retrieval, and Patient Positioning

The ability to retrieve stone fragments depends largely on the size of the stone in relation to the size of the infundibulum. While there are various techniques for stone retrieval, a grasper or basket is usually employed. Recent design changes to the stone baskets, such as the introduction of hydrophilic materials (nitinol) and tipless baskets, have improved the safety profile and efficacy of baskets. Among the recent innovations is the development of the open-tip NGage™ Nitinol Stone Extractor (Cook Urological, Spencer, IN) (Fig. 9.10).

The NGage™ offers several advantages over a traditional basket. The open-tip design allows the basket to be used in much the same way a grasper is used, "grabbing" stones end on. This is particularly useful for adherent or impacted stones and stones located against a wall or within a small calyx. When a traditional basket is deployed, stones can be grasped only with the side of the basket (side-on). The natural opening action of these baskets has the effect of pushing the basket off the wall or out of the calyx. The NGage™, however, can be positioned end-on to smaller stones, and with slight retraction of the basket during the action of opening, the tip remains in position relative to the fragment and will not push off the wall. For larger stones, the NGage™ can still be used side-on to snare the fragment. Furthermore, the open tip allows for the stone to be easily released if it is too large to be manipulated through the infundibulum or sheath.

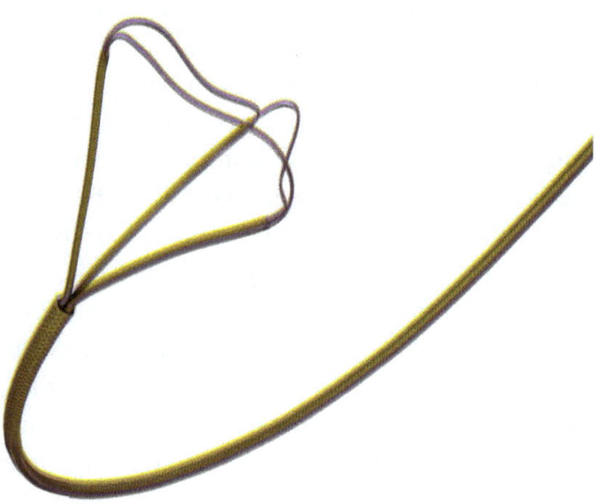

Fig. 9.10 The open tip of the NGage™ Nitinol Stone Extractor (Courtesy of Cook Medical, Inc)

In choosing the appropriate size and type of basket, several factors must be considered. If the fragments are free floating or within a ureter, then either a traditional basket or the NGage™ can be utilized using the "push-past" method, whereby the closed basket is advanced beyond the stone, opened, and then retracted ensnaring the target fragment. For impacted stones or stones within a small calyx, the NGage™ with an end-on technique is superior. The basket should be sized to meet the demands of the procedure: large enough to grasp the fragments, yet small enough to maintain irrigant flow and scope flexibility. When using the larger flexible cystoscope, a 2.4- or 3-Fr basket is adequate. However, for the smaller channeled flexible ureteroscope, a 1.8-Fr or smaller basket is preferred.

If the stone is too large to be retrieved, the urologist has several options. If the stone can be guided into the renal pelvis or some other more favorable location where it is accessible with a rigid scope, then the surgeon can proceed with rigid nephroscopy. If the stone cannot be favorably positioned, then the stone can be fragmented with the Holmium:YAG laser. Just as with baskets, the maintenance of flow and flexibility are paramount when choosing fiber size. A larger fiber can safely deliver more energy to the stone resulting in quicker fragmentation; however, the larger fiber also decreases irrigation and reduces the deflection of the scope. Usually, the flexible nephroscope can accommodate a 360-μ fiber without significantly compromising deflection or flow. The flexible ureteroscope, however, functions better which requires the use of a smaller fiber.

Choosing the laser setting largely depends on whether the surgeon intends to fragment the stone into manageable chunks that can be retrieved or to "dust" the stone into small debris that can be washed out or passed spontaneously. In order to dust the stone, a low-power (0.5 J) high-frequency (10–15 Hz) setting should be used. The periphery of the stone should be gradually painted with the laser until only the center remains, which is subsequently retrieved. The stone compositions most amenable to dusting include uric acid, calcium phosphate, and struvite stones. If the intention is to fracture and retrieve, then a high-power (1.0 J) low-frequency (5–8 Hz) setting should be used. Stones that are more durable, such as calcium oxalate monohydrate or cystine stones, are more likely to be successfully treated with this method.

Minute fragments too small to be easily basketed can be flushed from the kidney through the access sheath. A 10-cc syringe filled with saline is attached to the working port of the flexible nephroscope and forcefully expressed into the collecting system. Alternately, a shortened length of a nasogastric tube can be inserted through the sheath and the collecting system similarly flushed with saline [29]. Despite irrigation, often the stones congregate in the dependent portions of the collecting system and are resistant to flushing techniques. Rotating the bed away from the surgeon (for lateral stones), Trendelenberg (for lower pole stones) or reverse Trendelenberg (for upper pole stones) may help dislodge loose fragments. With the Accordion device in place, stone migration down the ureter can be prevented during this maneuver. Residual fragments flushed into the renal pelvis can then be retrieved. Once in the renal pelvis, the patient should remain tilted, and irrigant flow through the scope should be minimized to keep the stone fragments from being flushed back into the calyces.

Infundibular Stenosis

In infundibular stenosis, the calyceal os has been narrowed leading to a partially obstructed system. The calyx can either be dilated or nondilated, have stones, or be stone-free [31]. Infundibular stenosis can be caused by malignancy, retroperitoneal fibrosis, tuberculosis, or chronic stones or infection leading to scar tissue formation. Rarely, infundibular stenosis can be caused by a crossing segmental artery, a condition known as Fraley syndrome [32]. The end result of the partial obstruction includes pain, recurrent and chronic infections, hematuria, and deterioration of renal function in the affected area. The typical treatment of infundibular stenosis involves direct access into the affected calyx, treatment of the stones (if present), and widening of the os, usually with a Holmium:YAG laser. If the affected calyx is anteriorly located or there is some other pathology that requires investigation elsewhere in the kidney, an indirect access technique is utilized. In these instances, and even in some cases of direct access, flexible nephroscopy is necessary.

There are two main indications for treating infundibular stenosis. The first is for a true obstructed calyx. The calyx may or may not contain stones, and the system is usually dilated and is often symptomatic. Widening the infundibulum relives the obstruction and allows for access. The second indication is for a relative stenosis in a nonobstructed system. The calyx is often not dilated and may or may not contain stones. The purpose of widening the os is to gain entry for diagnostic purposes or for the treatment of a suspected pathology contained within it.

To gain access to the calyx, a heavy-duty J wire is passed through a rigid nephroscope and coiled within the calyx. The wire serves not only as a working wire, but in the event that a flap is created during treatment, the wire will also ensure continued access through the true os. If access to the calyx is lost and cannot be reestablished, the surgeon risks complete obliteration of the os and the development of a completely obstructed system. Once the wire is positioned, peanut graspers are passed through the rigid scope and used to dilate the infundibulum to a caliber that allows the passage of a flexible scope. Alternatives include balloon dilation (6 mm×4 cm) and Holmium:YAG laser incision. The appropriate technique to laser incision is to cut at the 6 and 12 o'clock positions which reduces ablation of the blood supply in the area and minimizes bleeding (Fig. 9.11) [31].

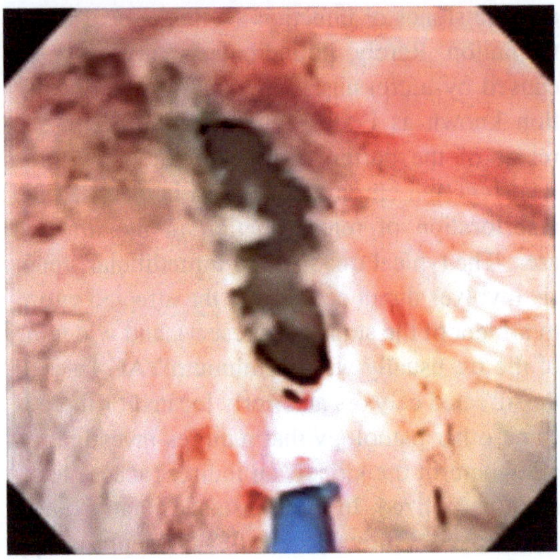

Fig. 9.11 Correct Holmium:YAG laser ablation of a stenotic infundibulum involves ablation at the 6 and 12 o'clock positions

If the os is not readily accessible with the rigid scope, then a flexible scope should be used. The scope should not be passed over the J wire as this may cause the wire to become dislodged. Once the infundibulum is well visualized, the opening can be lased at the 6 and 12 o'clock positions per standard technique. If balloon dilation is performed, the proximal end of a ureteral stent can be left within the calyx for 4–6 weeks. The size of the stent that is left in place does not affect the ultimate size of the os after healing is complete [33].

Not uncommonly, the purpose of opening the infundibulum is to treat stones located within the infundibulum. The preferred technique is to avoid stone comminution by widening the infundibulum to accommodate intact stone retrieval. In this manner, residual fragments are kept from being incorporated into the newly opened infundibular os, a situation that can lead to an increased inflammatory response and risks worsening stenosis. It follows logically to avoid fragments from elsewhere in the collecting system to become lodged in the incised os as well. If there are stones elsewhere in the collecting system, these should be removed prior to incision and all fragments and stone particles retrieved or flushed out.

The two major complications of laser incision of a stenotic infundibulum are bleeding and restenosis. Hemostasis can be achieved by increasing the distance between the tissue and the laser fiber which increases the coagulation effect. If bleeding persists, a Bugbee™ electrode (Olympus, Gyrus ACMI, Southborough, MA) (set at 20 W) can be use to electrically cauterize the tissue. When using the Bugbee, only pinpoint cauterization should be used as extensive cautery leads to ischemia and tissue contraction and ultimately increases the risk of restenosis. If these measures fail, placing a large caliber ureteral stent or a small caliber nephrostomy tube across the infundibulum should effectively tamponade the bleeding.

The Excluded Calyx

A calyx becomes excluded when it is isolated from the rest of the collecting system. This can be caused by infections, especially chronic, malignancy, and iatrogenic inflammation, usually from endoscopic surgery [34]. The diagnosis is made when a portion of the collecting system is hydronephrotic but does not fill during retrograde pyelography. The principle of treatment is to reestablish communication between the calyx and the collecting system, and as such, there are three approaches. In the retrograde approach, a ureteroscope is advanced to the area in question. Often times the infundibulum is punctate or cannot be identified altogether. In these instances, a blind directional incision is created into the calyx in the area of the expected os. Preoperative imaging is important as it will identify the location of the affected calyx. The most common site of the excluded calyx is the upper pole posterior calyx, in which case a 6 o'clock incision in the most superior portion of the upper pole renal pelvis will usually gain entry. Often, viable parenchymal tissue is also incised leading to bleeding which at times can be significant. If lasing the surface does not provide adequate hemostasis, a 2-Fr Bugbee electrode can be used. The smaller Bugbee is utilized to help avoid lowering irrigation flow.

The second technique is an indirect percutaneous approach. The indirect approach is advantageous in treating anterior excluded calyces since it is difficult to access them directly. The opposite pole of the excluded calyx offers the best angles to the infundibular os; that is, if the excluded pole is in the upper pole, a lower pole is access is better and vice versa. A needle placed into the excluded calyx under ultrasound guidance can be used to fill the calyx with contrast for easy radiographic visualization. If the os cannot be identified or if it cannot be dilated with peanut forceps, then the surgeon can proceed to laser incision. Flexible nephroscopy is often necessary with the indirect technique. The extreme torque needed to achieve adequate visualization can be obviated while the laser incision itself is not significantly compromised.

The posterior excluded calyx is usually approached with direct percutaneous access [34]. The procedure starts in the supine position with the placement of an open-ended catheter near the expected location of the infundibular os. The tip of the catheter is targeted with a needle that is passed percutaneously through the calyx and into the renal pelvis. The presence of urine leaking from the needle verifies placement in the collecting system. An Amplatz super stiff J wire is then coaxially advanced through the needle and coiled within the renal pelvis. A percutaneous balloon dilator is then passed over the wire into the renal pelvis and insufflated. The percutaneous tract that is created usually crosses the stenotic area creating a wide mouthed neo-infundibulum. Hemostasis can be achieved with a roller ball or a Bugbee electrode. To maintain the patency of the neo-infundibulum, either two 6- or 7-Fr double pigtail stents can be positioned such that the proximal end is in the excluded calyx and the distal end is in the bladder, or alternatively a Foley catheter that extends through the length of the tract into the renal pelvis can be placed. If the latter method is used, several fenestrations should be made to ensure that the excluded calyx drains appropriately. Internalized stents are preferable to the Foley nephrostomy tube since the dwell time is 4–6 weeks, making a nephrostomy tube impractical.

Symptomatic Renal Cysts (Fig. 9.12)

The majority of renal cysts are incidentally identified on computed tomography. Occasionally, a peripelvic cyst causes flank pain by compressing or distorting the infundibulum draining a calyx thereby obstructing it [35]. The treatment for the symptomatic cyst usually involves laparoscopic or percutaneous ablation. Furthermore, a renal cyst is sometimes encountered during

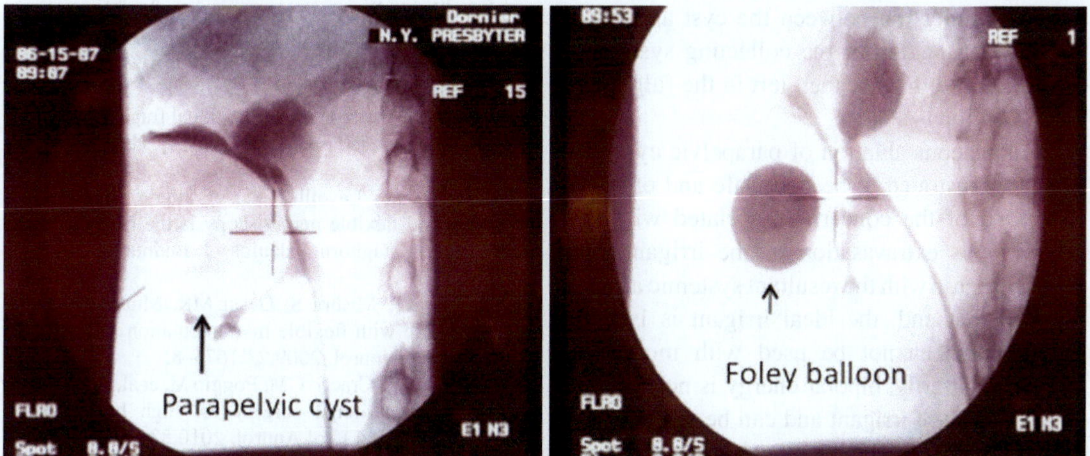

Fig. 9.12 Percutaneous ablation of parapelvic cyst

PCNL access that must be drained or traversed in order to render treatment to the targeted stone.

If the peripelvic cyst is asymptomatic but its location is complicating PCNL access, simple percutaneous needle aspiration usually suffices. If the cyst is not drained and inadvertently entered during access, the renal pelvis may subsequently be very difficult to locate. Contrarily, if the cyst is first aspirated, access into the targeted calyx can proceed without complication.

Since after needle aspiration cysts often recur, the symptomatic cyst should be ablated and not simply drained. To percutaneously ablate a cyst, first an open-ended catheter is cystoscopically advanced proximally up the ureter in retrograde fashion into the renal pelvis [36–38]. The patient is then placed in the prone position, and a retrograde pyelography is performed. Distortion of the collecting system is common and usually evident radiographically, and the location of the cyst can be inferred from the images. Direct access is then obtained by passing an 18-guage spinal needle into the cyst and coiling an Amplatz super stiff J wire within the cyst. Once the tract has been dilated, a 30-Fr Amplatz sheath is positioned. A standard resectoscope with a roller ball or standard loop connected to the Iglesias working element is then used to fulgurate the entire cyst wall including the cystic wall adjacent to the kidney. The cyst can also be marsupialized by excising a portion of the wall, thereby establishing communication between the cyst and either the retroperitoneum or the collecting system. A closed suction drain is then left in the fulgurated cystic bed for 1–2 days.

Percutaneous ablation of parapelvic cysts has been demonstrated to be both safe and effective [37]. One of the concerns associated with this procedure is extravasation of the irrigant used during the case with the resultant systemic absorption. To that end, the ideal irrigant is isotonic saline which cannot be used with monopolar energy. Contrarily, bipolar energy is not affected by the choice of irrigant and can be used for this purpose. Bipolar electrocautery has been recently popularized for transurethral prostate resection due to the ability to use isotonic saline during the procedure; it is advantageous because even after long surgical times, there is little change in the measured serum sodium [39, 40]. In the author's experience, bipolar percutaneous ablation of parapelvic and simple cysts results in fewer cases of hyponatremia. Moreover, the efficacy is unchanged from that monopolar ablation.

Summary

As the technology of the flexible cystoscope has improved, the indications for flexible nephroscopy have expanded. The modern urologist should have at his disposal a skill set that includes flexible nephroscopy. A basic understanding of advanced techniques and instruments will only improve the efficiency and the efficacy of PCNL.

References

1. Rupel E, Brown R. Nephroscopy with removal of stone following nephrostomy for obstructive calculous anuria. J Urol. 1941;46:177–82.
2. Goodwin WE, Casey WC, Woolf W. Percutaneous trocar (needle) nephrostomy in hydronephrosis. JAMA. 1955;157:891–4.
3. Preminger GM, Assimos DG, editors. Staghorn calculi. In: American Urological Association clinical guidelines; 2005. Accessed at www.auanet.org.
4. Pearle MS, Watamull LM, Mullican MA. Sensitivity of noncontrast helical computerized tomography and plain film radiography compared to flexible nephroscopy for detecting residual fragments after percutaneous nephrostolithotomy. J Urol. 1999;162:23–6.
5. Denstedt JD, Clayman RV, Picus DD. Comparison of endoscopic and radiological residual fragment rate following percutaneous nephrolithotripsy. J Urol. 145;703: 745.
6. Williams SK, Leveillee RJ. A single percutaneous access and flexible nephroscopy is the best treatment for a full staghorn calculus. J Endourol. 2008;22: 1835–7.
7. Ganpule AP, Mishra S, Desai MR. Multiperc versus single perc with flexible instrumentation for staghorn calculi. J Endourol. 2009;23:1675–8.
8. Scoffone CM, Cracco CM, Poggio M, et al. Endoscopic combined intrarenal surgery for high burden renal stones. Arch Ital Urol Androl. 2010;82:41–2.
9. Ko R, Soucy F, Denstedt JD, et al. Percutaneous nephrolithotomy made easier: a practical guide, tips and tricks. BJU Int. 2007;101:535–9.

10. Munver R, Delvecchio FC, Newman GE, et al. Critical analysis of supracostal access for percutaneous renal surgery. J Urol. 2001;166:1242–6.
11. Mariappan P, Loong CW. Mid-stream urine C&S test is a poor predictor of infected urine proximal to the obstructed ureteric stone or infected stone: a prospective clinical study. J Urol. 2004;171:2142–5.
12. Mariappan P, Smith G, Bariol SV, et al. Stone and pelvic urine culture and sensitivity are better than bladder urine as predictors of urosepsis following PCNL: a prospective clinical study. J Urol. 2005;173:1610–4.
13. Margel D, Ehrlich Y, Brown N, et al. Clinical implication of routine stone culture in percutaneous nephrolithotomy – a prospective study. Urology. 2006;67:26–9.
14. Korets R, Graversen JA, Kates M, et al. Post-PCNL systemic inflammatory response: a prospective analysis of pre-operative urine, renal pelvic urine, and stone cultures. J Urol. 2011;186(5):1899–903.
15. Charton M, Vallancien G, Veillon B, et al. Urinary tract infection for percutaneous surgery for renal calculi. J Urol. 1986;135:15–7.
16. Ibarluzea G, Scoffone CM, Cracco CM, et al. Supine Valdivia and modified lithotomy position for simultaneous anterograde and retrograde endourological access. BJU Int. 2007;100:233–6.
17. Grasso M, Nord R, Bagley DH. Prone split leg and flank roll positioning: simultaneous antegrade and retrograde access to the upper urinary tract. J Endourol. 1993;7:307–10.
18. Scarpa RM, Cossu FM, De Lisa A, et al. Severe recurrent ureteral stricture: the combined use of an antegrade and retrograde approach in the prone split-leg position without X-rays. Eur Urol. 1997;31:254–6.
19. Ray AA, Chung DG, Honey RJ. Percutaneous nephrolithotomy in the prone and prone flexed positions: anatomic consideration. J Endourol. 2009;23:1607–14.
20. Kerbl K, Clayman RV, Chandhoke PS, et al. Percutaneous stone removal with the patient in the flank position. J Urol. 1994;151:686–8.
21. Gofrit ON, Shapiro A, Donchin Y, et al. Lateral decubitus position for percutaneous nephrolithotripsy in the morbidly obese or kyphotic patient. J Endourol. 2002;16:383–6.
22. Karami H, Arbab AH, Rezai A, et al. Percutaneous nephrolithotomy with ultrasonography-guided access in the lateral decubitus flank position. J Endourol. 2009;23:33–6.
23. Karacalar S, Bilen CY, Sarihasan B, Sarikaya S. Spinal-epidural anesthesia versus general anesthesia in the management of percutaneous nephrolithotripsy. J Endourol. 2009;23:1591–7.
24. El-Husseiny T, Moraitis K, Maan Z, Papatsoris A, Saunders P, Golden B, Masood J, Buchholz NP. Percutaneous endourologic procedures in high-risk patients in the lateral decubitus position under regional anesthesia. J Endourol. 2009;23:1603–6.
25. Valdivia Uría JG, Valle Gerhold J, López JA, et al. Technique and complications of percutaneous nephroscopy: experience with 557 patients in the supine position. J Urol. 1998;160(6 Pt 1):1975–8.
26. Papatsoris AG, Zaman F, Panah A, et al. Simultaneous anterograde and retrograde endourologic access: "the Barts technique". J Endourol. 2008;22:2665–6.
27. Lehman T, Bagley DH. Reverse lithotomy: modified prone position for simultaneous nephroscopic and ureteroscopic procedures in women. Urology. 1988; 32:529–31.
28. Andonian S, Okeke Z, Anidjar M, et al. New technologies in endourology digital nephroscopy: the next step. J Endourol. 2008;22:601–2.
29. Wosnitzer M, Xavier K, Gupta M. Novel use of ureteroscopic stone entrapment device to prevent antegrade stone migration during percutaneous nephrolithotomy. J Endourol. 2009;23:203–8.
30. Panah A, Masood J, Zaman F, et al. A technique to flush out renal stone fragments during percutaneous nephrolithotomy. J Endourol. 2009;23:5–6.
31. Kim HL, Gerber GS. Use of ureteroscopy and holmium:yttrium-aluminum-garnet laser in the treatment of an infundibular stenosis. Urology. 2000;55:129–31.
32. Fraley EE. Vascular obstruction of superior infundibulum causing nephralgia: a new syndrome. N Engl J Med. 1966;275:1403–9.
33. Gupta M, Ost MC, et al. Percutaneous management of the upper urinary tract. In: Kavoussi LR, Novick AC, Partin AW, Peters CA, editors. Campbell-Walsh urology. Philadelphia: WB Saunders; 2007. p. 1526–64.
34. Mues AC, Landman J, Gupta M. Endoscopic management of completely excluded calyces: a single institution experience. J Endourol. 2010;24:1241–5.
35. Hinman Jr F. Ballottement of peripelvic cyst for operative diagnosis and localization. J Urol. 1967;97:7.
36. Kang Y, Noble C, Gupta M. Percutaneous resection of renal cysts. J Endourol. 2001;15:735–8. discussion 738-739.
37. Shah JB, Whitman C, Lee M, et al. Water under the bridge: 5-year outcomes after percutaneous ablation of obstructing parapelvic renal cysts. J Endourol. 2007;21:1167–70.
38. Kiryluk K, Gupta M. A large obstructive parapelvic cyst: challenging diagnosis and management. Kidney Int. 2007;71:955.
39. Martis G, Cardi A, Massimo D, et al. Transurethral resection of prostate: technical progress and clinical experience using the bipolar Gyrus plasmakinetic tissue management system. Surg Endosc. 2008;22: 2078–83.
40. Singh H, Desai M, Sheivastav P, et al. Bipolar versus monopolar transurethral resection of prostate: randomized controlled study. J Endourol. 2005;19: 333–8.

10 Chinese Minimally Invasive Percutaneous Nephrolithotomy (MPCNL): Overcoming the Difficulties

Zhaohui He, Guohua Zeng, and Xun Li

Introduction of Chinese MPCNL

Percutaneous nephrolithotomy (PCNL) has become the mainstay of treatment for complex renal or upper ureteral calculi over the past 30 years since it was first performed by Fernstrom and Johansson via a nephrostomy tract created specially for the purpose of stone removal in 1976 [1]. The practice of this technique was further refined over the years as technology and endoscopic equipment improved. Nowadays, PCNL has replaced open stone surgery in removing complex urinary calculi with increasing efficacy and decreasing morbidity in most institutions. Although many investigators have reported excellent outcomes with PCNL, PCNL can still be associated with significant morbidity, such as severe hemorrhage, injury to surrounding viscera, sepsis, loss of the kidney, or even death [2]. Also, in real-life clinical practice, the usual 26–34 F tract size of PCNL may be too large in pediatric kidneys and in some adult undilated kidneys. Under these conditions, some authors have modified the technique of standard PCNL by performing it with a miniature endoscope via a small percutaneous tract (11–20 F) and termed it as minimally invasive percutaneous nephrolithotomy (MPCNL) or mini-PCNL. But because of the lack of proper endoscopes and special equipment, they found that it became more difficult to maintain good endoscopic view and even more difficult to remove the stone fragments via the smaller tract. Therefore, it was concluded that MPCNL was technically feasible and could significantly decrease the risk of traditional PCNL, but it should only be used in patients with stone size less than 2 cm, or as a secondary tract to supplement standard PCNL, or in pediatric patients [3–8].

In our hospital, the first PCNL was performed in 1984. At first the procedure was performed with standard technique. Because of complex surgical procedures and high complication rate, we found that it was unacceptable and needed to be modified. In 1992, we began to modify the PCNL technique using small tract to manage all the upper urinary tract stones that need PCNL intervention. Initially, the procedure was performed in two stages. A 14–16 F percutaneous nephrostomy tract was created under X-ray, and a same size tube was placed to drain the system at stage 1. A week later, the nephrostomy tract was dilated and used for nephroscopic manipulation with an 8–9.8 F rigid ureteroscope at stage 2 [9]. In 1998,

Z. He, M.D., Ph.D. • G. Zeng, M.D., Ph.D. (✉)
Department of Urology, Minimally Invasive Surgical Center, The First Affiliated Hospital of Guangzhou Medical College, Guangdong Key Laboratory of Urology, #1 Kangda Road, Haizhou District, Guangzhou, 510230, China
e-mail: gzgyhzh@163.com; gzgyzgh@tom.com; gdgzlx@21cn.com

X. Li, M.D.
Department of Urology, Minimally Invasive Surgical Center, The First Affiliated Hospital of Guangzhou Medical College, The Fifth Affliated Hospital of Guangzhou Medical College, #1 Kangda Road, Haizhou District, Guangzhou, 510230, China

A.M. Al-Kandari et al. (eds.), *Difficult Cases in Endourology*,
DOI 10.1007/978-1-84882-083-8_10, © Springer-Verlag London 2013

the procedure was performed in one session. In 2006, we further modified the technique by using a specially designed nephroscope via the 18–20 F tract [10]. During the last 12 years, we have performed more than 13,000 MPCNL procedures for a variety of renal and upper ureteral calculi. Since 1998, this technique has been widely applied in many hospitals in mainland China, Hong Kong, and Macao districts and was named Chinese MPCNL [11]. Although some authors doubted the necessity of PCNL using a small tract, our clinical data have confirmed that Chinese MPCNL in managing all kinds of upper urinary tract calculi is safe and efficient, has decreased complications, and has better stone clearance when compared with standard PCNL [12].

Indications and Contraindication of Chinese MPCNL

Indications and contraindications of Chinese MPCNL are the same as standard PCNL. The indications include upper urinary stones that are contraindications to SWL, failure of SWL or URS associated with distal obstruction or with upper tract foreign bodies, and large or complex stones. Currently, the absolute contraindications are an irreversible coagulopathy and abnormal anatomy that precludes establishing a safe tract into the kidney. But nowadays, even with abnormal anatomy preventing creating a safe percutaneous access, PCNL still can be safely performed under the assistance of a laparoscope.

Equipment of Chinese MPCNL

Current reported MPCNL series showed that there was a lack of suitable equipment and that it took a long time to fragment and remove the broken stones. Our technique had evolved throughout the early years to overcome those difficulties. We have now standardized the use of the equipment and technique. Only one type of guidewire, a set of fascial dilator and peel-away sheath, a type of endoscope, forceps, and intracorporeal lithotripter are needed. We recommend use of 0.035 or 0.038 in. Zebra® guidewire (Boston Scientific, Natick, MA), which is hydrophilic and can be easily inserted into the puncture needle and curled into the collecting system, and the Cook fascial dilators with Peel-Away® sheath (Cook Urological, Bloomington, IN). The endoscope and forceps we mostly used are an 8.5/12.5 F nephroscope (Lixun nephroscope, Richard Wolf, Knittlingen, Germany) and a 6 F forceps (Richard Wolf, Knittlingen, Germany). When this endoscope is not available, the standard 8/9.8 F ureteroscope and the corresponding 5 F forceps can be better substitutes. See Fig. 10.1 for the instruments used in Chinese MPCNL.

Using of the pulsatile high-pressurized endoscopic perfusion pump (Fig. 10.2) to produce forceful pulse flow of irrigant to flush out the stone fragments is the character of the Chinese MPCNL. It avoids the tedious process of picking up every fragment by forceps and shortens the operative time, so the special equipment needed is the pulsatile perfusion pump. We specially designed a pulsed perfusion pump (MMC Yiyong,

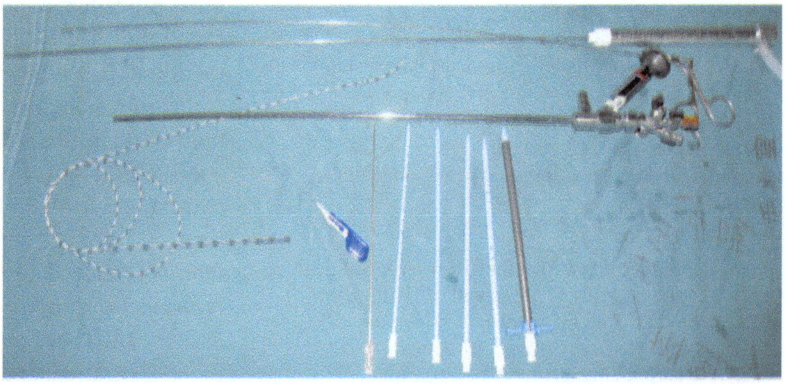

Fig. 10.1 For Chinese MPCNL, only one type of guidewire, a set of fascial dilator and peel-away sheath, a type of endoscope, forceps, and intracorporeal lithotripter are needed

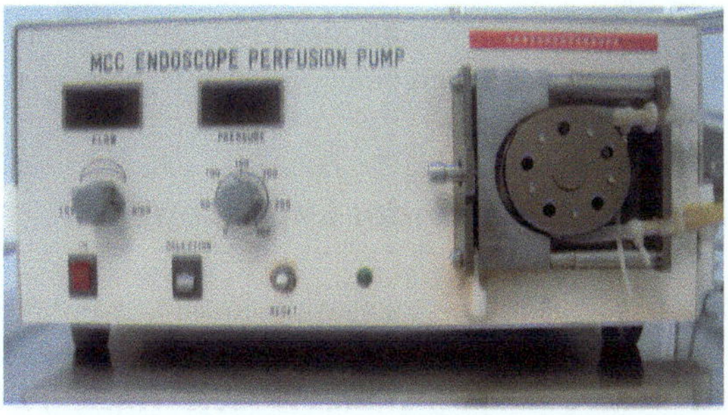

Fig. 10.2 The perfusion pump (MMC Yiyong, Guangzhou, China) can generate pressure up to 300 mmHg for about 3 s, then stop for 2 s, and then repeat the cycle

Guangzhou, China),which can generate pressure up to 300 mmHg for about 3 s, then stop for 2 s, and then repeat the cycle. When the high-pressure pulsatile pump is unavailable, some authors reported that another pressured irrigation system (Niagara® Irrigator, Cabot Medical (now Gyrus ACMI, Southborough, MA)) was a good alternative; it can provide a pressurized continuous irrigation of 300 mmHg and produce same effect as ours [11].

Surgical Technique

The surgical technique of the Chinese MPCNL has been reported in our previous published articles [9, 10, 12–15] and is presented here again.

All procedures were performed under general anesthesia or continual epidural anesthesia. The patient was first placed in a split lower limbs position, and an external 5–7 F ureteral catheter with open tip was inserted to the target ureter with the assistance of a guidewire under direct ureteroscopic vision. The placement of a ureteral catheter at the ureteropelvic junction prevented the migration of stone fragments from the renal collecting system down the ureter. In addition, the catheter allowed retrograde instillation of contrast material to facilitate renal puncture at the appropriate site and forceful retrograde normal saline flushing for stone fragment removal later on. The patients were then turned to a prone position with a pack under the abdomen to minimize lumbar lordosis; the patients with a transplanted kidney underwent MPCNL in a supine position.

Puncture

Puncture Guided by Fluoroscopy

The preoperative imaging was reviewed, and an entry calyx was selected and a 3D mental picture was constructed as to the site of the needle entry point, the needle angle in relation to the sagittal plane, and how deep the needle should go. After distension of the system by diluted contrast medium via the ureteric catheter and under the confirmation of fluoroscopy, a skin puncture site was selected. The usual skin puncture site would be in the 11th rib space bounded laterally by the posterior axillary line and medially by a line projected caudally from the lower tip of the scapula. After the skin puncture site was confirmed, a freehand puncture was performed with an 18-gauge coaxial needle, and emphasis was put on tactile feedback via the needle on going through the tissue. There will be a feeling of a giving on entry to the system, or one will feel a grinding sensation when the needle hits on the stone. The usual angle of puncture is 45–60° to the sagittal plane and perpendicular to the axis of the vertebral column. The track should take the shortest route through (straight to) the abdominal wall and the renal parenchyma to the stone or the aimed calyx, usually the middle calyx, but the actual selected calyx is tailored to the stone location and calyceal configuration. An oblique track should be avoided. With puncture as in the above method, we found that the tip of the needle most times was through the fornix of the calyx; only for the difficult cases, rotating the C-arm is needed to check the position of the actual needle tip. So the main role of fluoroscopy is to confirm the puncture, monitor the passage of a guidewire, or to guide a puncture into a specific calyx in difficult cases.

Puncture Guided by Ultrasound

Each kidney has a fibrous outer cortex, a middle layer consisting of medulla (pyramids) with surrounding cortex (columns of Bertin), and an inner renal sinus that contains the calyces and renal pelvis with larger blood vessels, lymphatics, and fatty tissue. The percutaneous access to the collecting system should be made through a renal pyramid into a calyx, thus avoiding the columns of Bertin and the larger vessels present within them [16]. On ultrasonography, the renal pyramid exhibits a low-level echo, whereas the renal column between the pyramids manifests as a high-intensity echo (echo lower than the renal sinus).

First, the ultrasonic detector should be put parallel along the long axis of kidney to identify the maximum section of kidney. From this section, by rotating the detector toward, dorsal direction, you can visualize the dorsally posterior calices, and by rotating toward ventral direction, you can visualize the anterior calices. Putting the detector vertically to the kidney, slowly moving the detector from the skin on the back to the abdomen, the calyx that is the first to be identified is the posterior calyx. With puncture guided by fluoroscopy, usually a posterior middle calyx is preferred. When the targeted calyx was seen on the ultrasonic image, the puncture-guided line of the puncture holder toward the calyx was adjusted. If the puncture holder was unavailable, the pathway of the puncture needle should be identified under the ultrasonic image. Then, under the real-time ultrasonic monitor, the needle can be seen to slowly reach the targeted calyx.

Dilation

After the fluid efflux was seen or the urine was aspirated, the diluted (30–50 %) contrast medium was injected into the collecting system to confirm the puncture. Then a 0.035-in. hydrophilic Zebra guidewire was inserted into the collecting system. Once the guidewire was inserted into the collecting system down the ureter, or coiled in the pelvis or a calyx, a 0.5–0.7-cm skin incision was made, the dilatation of the percutaneous tract was serially performed over the guidewire with a fascial dilator from 8 F, with the caliber increased gradually by progressive 2 F, until the tract was dilated to 18 or 20 F, and a same sized peel-away sheath was placed as the percutaneous access port.

Manipulation Under Endoscope

After percutaneous tract was created, an 8.5–12.5 F Lixun nephroscope was inserted to inspect the collecting system. Under direct vision, the stone was fragmented by pneumatic lithotripsy or holmium:yttrium-aluminum-garnet laser. The big fragments (0.3–0.5 cm) were extracted with forceps, and the fragments <0.3 cm were mainly pushed out with an endoscopic pulsed perfusion pump. Rapid removal of the endoscope out of the sheath synchronized with the low-flow irrigation period would create a relative vacuum within the sheath and, together with the recoil of the system from the transient high pressure from the irrigant, would flush the stone fragment out. Finally, a 4.8–6 F double-J stent was inserted in the ureter, and a same caliber nephrostomy tube (18–20 F) was left in place.

For staghorn stones where the need for multiple tracts was necessary, the secondary or third punctures were created at the outset or in same session based on the configuration of stone and collecting system and surgery condition. For bilateral upper urinary tract calculi, simultaneous bilateral MPCNL was performed if the patient's condition permitted.

Postoperative Management

KUB radiography or nephrostography was performed 24–48 h after surgery to assess the effect of surgery. For patients with a supracostal access, a chest X-ray was routinely performed the next morning. If the radiography revealed any residual stone, a second-staged MPCNL was performed 5–7 days later. A new percutaneous access tract would be created, if necessary. If a second-stage PCNL was unnecessary, the nephrostomy tube would be removed 3–5 days later when the drainage was clear, and the double-J stent would be extracted 2–3 weeks later. Before the removal the percutaneous tube, we routinely clamped it for at least 6 h.

Management of Difficult Case

Chinese PCNL for Staghorn Calculus Complicated with Spinal Deformity

Management of complex upper urinary tract calculus complicated with spinal deformity is a challenge. For anesthesiologists, the concomitant severe dysfunction of pulmonary ventilation contraindicates anesthesia. The concomitant hypermetabolism is likely to cause malignant or nonmalignant fever. The intubation under the general anesthesia may also injure the teeth and mandible [17]. Moreover, for urologists the altered anatomy of the urinary tract and the concomitant transposition of visceral organs also increase the difficulties of endoscopic therapy. Also, they must consider the risk of the bones' fragility. We report our experience of using Chinese MPCNL in treating a patient with staghorn calculi complicated with severe spinal deformity.

A 58-year-old male who complained of a 3-day history of pyuria was diagnosed with left renal complete staghorn calculi and spinal deformity and referred to our institute. The patient suffered from the impaired movement of right lower limb and right scoliosis due to polio at the age of 3 years. The IVP and CT scan identified the left renal complete staghorn calculi without hydronephrosis (Fig. 10.3a–c). No obstruction or calculus was visible in the right kidney. The lumbar column was curved to the right and angled to the left, showing a left-side scoliosis. The pulmonary function test showed a vital capacity at 75.0 % of the predicted value, a forced vital capacity at 80 % of the predicted value, and a FEV_1/FVC at 83 %, whereas the ventilation remained normal. On echocardiography, the ejection fraction was 60 %, the ratio (*E*/*A*) of early diastolic peak flow velocity (*E*) to late diastolic filling peak velocity (*E*/*A*) was 0.75, and the diasystolic function of left ventricle was mildly impaired. The blood cell analysis, hepatorenal function, arterial blood gas, and coagulation function were within the normal limits. The urine culture identified *E. coli*.

Therapeutic Process

Preoperative Preparation

The full analyses of CT, IVU, and ultrasonographic images were used to characterize the location and relation of the left kidney to neighboring organs. The left kidney was rotated medially and the hilum was projected anteriorly. The spleen was located at a lower position and visible at the level of left renal hilum where it was in close proximity to the lateral side of left kidney (Fig. 10.4a). On CT images, we could detect if puncture through the posterior calyx was safe and feasible and without the risk of injuring the adjacent viscera. Even if the puncture was through the anterior calyx, we were able to illustrate the safety range of puncture pathway beforehand (Fig. 10.4b), establishing that the percutaneous tract amid the safety margin had no risk of injury of adjacent viscera.

Because of the left kidney calculi being a complete staghorn stone, a single percutaneous tract did not allow the removal of most calculi. We prepared to establish two tracts simultaneously at outset of surgery. And because of big stone burden, a multistage procedure may be needed if the one-stage procedure fails to remove all the calculi. The anesthesiological consultation testified to the surgical tolerance and scheduled the general anesthesia with intubation due to the fact that the patient had no significant ventilation compromise or upper respiratory tract infection. The urinary tract infection was managed with sensitive antibiotics.

Surgical Procedure

Following the general anesthesia with intubation, the patient was placed in the lithotomy position. A 5 F open-tip ureteral catheter was inserted into the affected ureter. The patient was subsequently rotated to the grossly prone position in line with the spinal angle, in the presence of adequate protection, to avoid the compression of any spinal protrusion. All the joint protrusions were appropriately cushioned. The operative procedure consisted of two sessions.

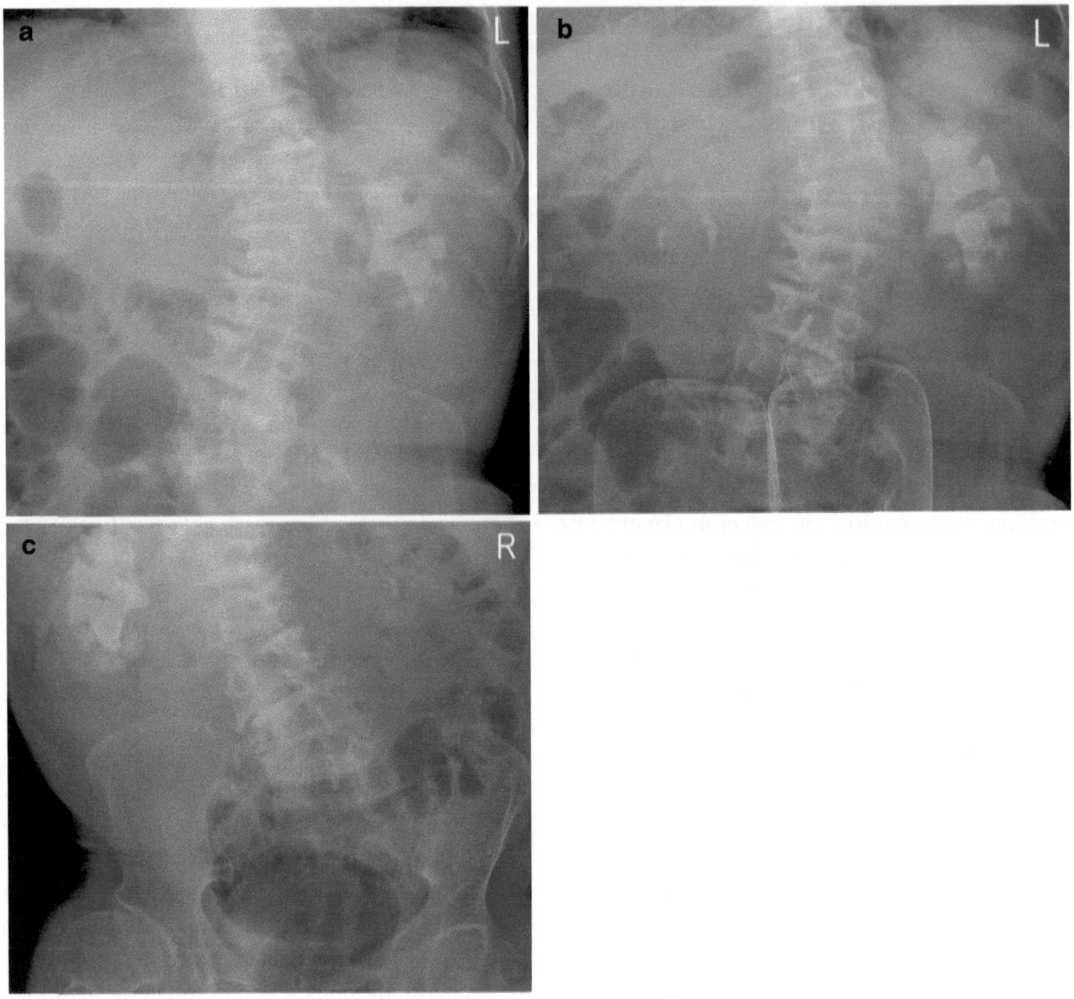

Fig. 10.3 (**a–c**) A plain abdominal film (KUB) and IVU show a complete staghorn stone in left kidney with a good function in a severe left-sided scoliosis patient

First Session PCNL

Ultrasonography and C-arm fluoroscopy were used to assist the puncture. The assistant injected normal saline through the ureteral catheter to create the artificial hydronephrosis of left kidney. Firstly, the maximum section of left kidney was identified on the ultrasonographic image. Then, the detector was slowly rotated toward the spinal column to locate the posterior calyxes. Due to the fact that the posterior calyxes were full of calculi in the patient, it was more likely to locate the posterior calyxes with the assistance of calculus echogram. After the target calyxes were identified on ultrasonic image, the puncture-guided line of the puncture holder was adjusted toward the calyx. Under the real-time monitor of ultrasonography, the middle posterior calyx and the upper posterior calyx were punctured meanwhile. After the fluid efflux was seen, the diluted (30–50 %) contrast medium was injected into the collecting system to confirm the puncture. Following the confirmation of the punctured calyxes as targets under the fluoroscopy, the Zebra guidewires were inserted, and the fascial dilator was inserted through the guidewires and used to dilate the two puncture tracts from the size 8–18 F. An 18 F peel-away sheath was maintained as the surgical access port.

An 8.5/12.5 F nephroscope (Lixun nephroscope, Richard Wolf, Knittlingen, Germany)

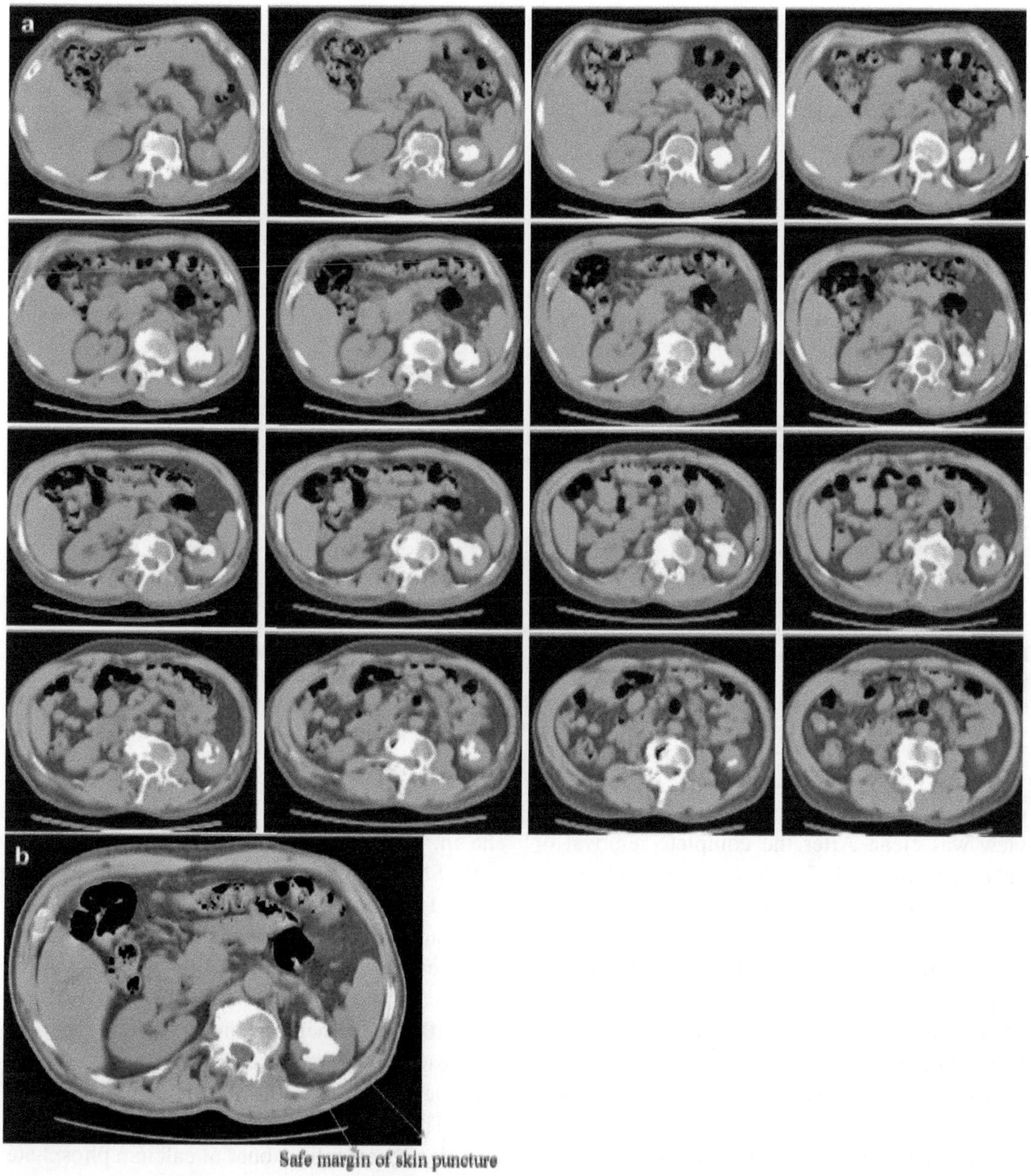

Fig. 10.4 (**a**) CT scan shows that the left kidney is malrotated and the hilum faces ventromedially. The spleen locates at a lower position and is visible at the level of left renal hilum where it is in close proximity to the lateral side of left kidney. On CT images, we could detect if puncture through the posterior calyx was safe and feasible without the risk of injuring the adjacent viscera. And even if the puncture was through the anterior calyx, we were able to illustrate the safety range of puncture pathway beforehand. (**b**) Establishing the percutaneous tract amid the safety margin had no risk of injury of adjacent viscera

was inserted through the sheath, and a pneumatic lithotriptor was used to fragment calculi. The broken stones were washed off or removed by forceps. The fragmentation and removal of calculi were conducted via the two pathways, respectively. The stone in the pelvis and between the two tracts were managed initially in order for the irrigation to flush out easily. The intraopera-

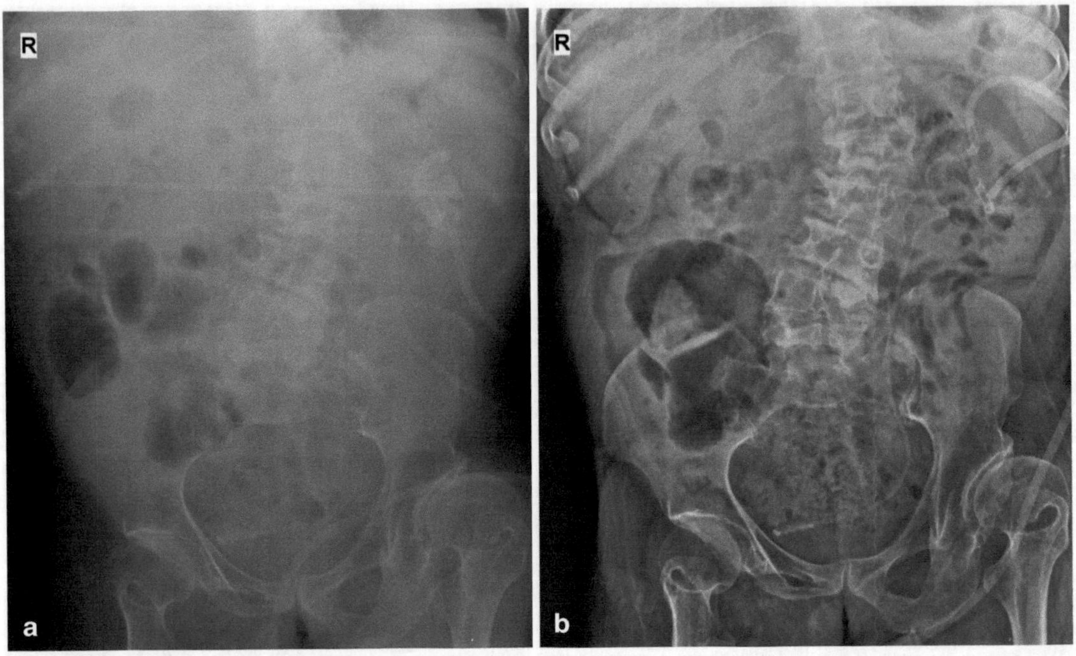

Fig. 10.5 (**a**) KUB after first session of MPCNL: the stone in pelvic and half calyxes was removed, a double-J stent was placed in the ureter, and two 18 F nephrostomy tubes were placed in the upper posterior calyx and in lower posterior calyx. (**b**) KUB after second session of MPCNL: the stone was removed completely and a ureter stent and two nephrostomy tubes were placed same as in previous KUB

tive hemorrhage was minimal and nephroscopic view was clear. After the complete removal of pelvic calculi, a 5 F double-J stent was placed in the left ureter. Due to the concern of prolonged surgical time with the bone complication, when the nephroscopic manipulation lasted approximately 90 min, we stopped the procedure and placed two 18 F nephrostomy tubes in the percutaneous tract.

The follow-up KUB radiographs were taken on postoperative day 2 (Fig. 10.5a). The follow-up routine blood test showed a decrease of hemoglobin from preoperative 14.2 g/L to postoperative 13.1 g/L. The nephrostomy tube drainage fluid remained clear, and a secondary session PCNL was conducted on postoperative day 7.

Secondary Session of PCNL

Following the general anesthesia with endotracheal intubation, the patient was placed in the prone position as above. At surgery, the Zebra guidewire was inserted through the nephrostomy tube. An 18 F fascial dilator was used to dilate the percutaneous tract along with a peel-away sheath. The sheath was maintained as the access port. Same endoscopic manipulation was performed to manage the residual stone.

Postoperative management was same as the first session. Upon the complete removal of renal calculi as confirmed by the radiography (Fig. 10.5b), the nephrostomy tube was removed on postoperative day 2 following the procedure, and the double-J stent was extracted 3 weeks later. The stone analysis showed calcium oxalate, mixed with a small amount of calcium phosphate and uric acid.

Discussion

Normal spinal column has four physiological curves on the sagittal plane, whereas no curve should be observed on the coronal plane. The curve to either side refers to scoliosis. Severe scoliosis is generally defined as a Cobb angle above 90°. The severe deformity in such patients consistently compresses neighboring organs; results in the distortion and obliqueness of chest, peritoneal cavity, and pelvis; alters the anatomical location of internal organs; and leads to dextroscoliosis or levoscoliosis. The anatomical alteration may lead to urine retention or obstruction of urinary flow which favors the formation of urinary calculi. Theoretically, the risk of urinary stone disease seems to be increased in these patients; some reported that the incidence rate of urinary calculi was up to 20 % in the case of bone dysplasia or spinal deformity. However, Vetter et al. reported that its incidence in children with osteogenesis imperfecta (OI) was 4.7–6.9 % (6/127 and 4/58, respectively), which did not appear to differ from that seen in the general population [18].

As in general patients, small-size renal calculi complicated with spinal deformity can be treated by flexible ureteroscope, and the stones with big bone deformity still require the intervention of PCNL or open procedure [19]. The difficulty of PCNL in such patients lies in establishing appropriate PCN pathway and avoidance of the adjacent organ injuries in the context of anatomical alterations. The establishment of PCN pathway with fluoroscopic monitoring alone in such patients is relatively risky or less feasible, requiring the assistance of ultrasonography or laparoscopy. The ultrasound guidance allows the safe establishment of PCN pathway in a narrow safety margin of puncture due to the anatomic alteration or abnormal anatomic structure and avoidance of injuring the neighboring organs. The experience of others' has proven that Desai et al. successfully treated nine patients with ectopic renal calculi by using ultrasonography-assisted PCNL puncture [20].

In the case of less experience in ultrasonography-assisted percutaneous renal puncture or evident space-occupying organs present around the preestablished PCN pathway, laparoscopy-assisted PCNL can be used. The laparoscope assistance allows the intentional avoidance or separation of surrounding organs, further preventing the injuries of neighboring organs. In 1985, Eshghi et al. firstly applied the technique of laparoscopy-assisted percutaneous transperitoneal nephrolithotomy (PCNL) for ectopic pelvic kidneys [21]. From then on, several authors have reported their successful experience of laparoscopy-assisted PCNL [22, 23]. Recently, Seref et al. reported using extraperitoneal laparoscopy-assisted PCNL in a patient with OI and safely removed a 11.9-mm stone at the pelvis of the right kidney [24].

In a case in which there is absence of obvious space-occupying organs around the preestablishment of PCN access, we prefer ultrasonography-assisted puncture. The use of ultrasonography-assisted puncture not only can avoid injuring the surrounding organs but also can allow accurate puncture approaching through a calyceal fornix, which reduces the intraoperative bleeding. Although the laparoscopy-assisted PCNL can be easily performed, an accurate percutaneous calyceal pathway cannot be ensured. In our center, 15 similar cases have been treated by using such procedure but exhibited no massive hemorrhage or surrounding organ injuries, suggesting the safety of such procedure.

For the complete staghorn calculi or complex calculi which obviously requires multiple tracts, we preferred to establish two or three tracts at the beginning of the surgery based on the configuration of stone and collecting system, and in most cases the secondary tract was established, but for the third puncture we only put the guidewire in the collecting system and did not dilate initially. If the surgery was smooth and surgery time was no more than 90 min, the third puncture would be dilated. We preferred establishment of multiple tracts at the outset of the surgery because there is no leak or bleeding allowing easily and accurately ultrasound-guided puncture. Obviously, the potentially intraoperative leak or hemorrhage would increase the difficulty in puncturing under the ultrasound and decrease the accuracy in establishing a new percutaneous tract. Furthermore, the simultaneous use of multiple tracts can accelerate the removal of a stone fragment and shorten the operating time, in addition to reducing the risk of urosepsis by lowering the renal pelvic pressure.

Conclusion

Complex upper urinary tract calculus complicated with spinal deformity represents a challenge to anesthetists and urologists. These patients always need PCNL intervention. The difficulty of PCNL in such patients lies in establishing appropriate PCN pathway and preventing injuries of the adjacent organ injuries. When there is no presence of obvious space-occupying organs around the preestablishment of PCN access, ultrasonography-assisted puncture can allow safe and successful establishment of PCN pathway in a narrow safety margin of puncture due to the anatomic alteration, but the operation should be performed in tertiary centers with significant experience in managing complex urolithiasis, where all the surgical equipment and specialized personnel are readily available.

References

1. Fernstrom I, Johansson B. Percutaneous pyelolithotomy: a new extraction technique. Scand J Urol Nephrol. 1976;10:257–9.
2. Michel MS, Trojan L, Rassweiler JJ. Complications in percutaneous nephrolithotomy. Eur Urol. 2007;51:899–906.
3. Helal M, Black T, Lockhart J, et al. The Hickman peel-away sheath: alternative for pediatric percutaneous nephrolithotomy. J Endourol. 1997;11:171–2.
4. Jackman SV, Hedican SP, Peters CA, et al. Percutaneous nephrolithotomy in infants and preschool age children: experience with a new technique. Urology. 1998;52:697–701.
5. Jackman SV, Docimo SG, Cadeddu JA, et al. The "mini-perc" technique: a less invasive alternative to percutaneous nephrolithotomy. World J Urol. 1998;16:371–4.
6. Chan DY, Jarrett TW. Mini-percutaneous nephrolithotomy. J Endourol. 2000;14:269–73.
7. Monga M, Oglevie S. Minipercutaneous nephrolithotomy. J Endourol. 2000;14:419–21.
8. Lahme S, Bichler KH, Strohmaier WL, et al. Minimally invasive PCNL in patients with renal pelvic and calyceal stones. Eur Urol. 2001;40:619–24.
9. Wu K, Li X, Yuan J, Guo W, Shan Z. Mini nephrostomy with ureteroscopic lithotripsy for staghorn stones. Acad J Guangzhou Med Coll. 1993;2:13–4 (article in Chinese).
10. Li X, Zeng GH, Yuan J, Wu KJ, Shan CC, Guo B, Liang ZX. Treatment of upper urinary calculi with the PCNL technique(experience of 20 years). Beijing Da Xue Xue Bao. 2004;36:124–6 (article in Chinese).
11. Li SK, Tai D, Chau L, et al. Minimally invasive percutaneous nephrolithotomy (MPCNL) according to the Chinese method. In: Baba S, Ono Y, editors. Recent advances in endourology. New York: Springer; 2006. p. 41–63.
12. Li X, He Z, Wu K, et al. Chinese minimally invasive percutaneous nephrolithotomy: the Guangzhou experience. J Endourol. 2009;23:1693–7.
13. Li X, Zeng G, Liu J, et al. Minimally invasive percutaneous nephrolithotomy in the management of complex urinary calculi: a middle calyx puncture approach. J Chin Urol. 2005;20:147–9 (article in Chinese).
14. He Z, Li X, Chen L, et al. Minimally invasive percutaneous nephrolithotomy for upper urinary tract calculi in transplanted kidneys. BJU Int. 2007;99:1467–71.
15. Guohua Z, Zhong W, Li X, et al. Minimally invasive percutaneous nephrolithotomy for staghorn calculi: a novel single session approach via multiple 14-18Fr tracts. Surg Laparosc Endosc Percutan Tech. 2007;17:124–8.
16. John NK, Jeffery AC. Surgical anatomy of the retroperitoneum, adrenals, kidneys, and ureters: kidneys. In: Alan JW, Louis RK, Andrew CN, et al., editors. Campbell-Walsh urology. Philadelphia: Elsevier; 2007. p. 22–3.
17. Karabiyik L, Parpucu M, Kurtipek O. Total intravenous anaesthesia and the use of an intubating laryngeal mask in a patient with osteogenesis imperfecta. Acta Anaesthesiol Scand. 2002;46:618–9.
18. Vetter U, Pontz B, Zauner E, et al. Osteogenesis imperfecta: a clinical study of the first ten years of life. Calcif Tissue Int. 1992;50:36–41.
19. Argyropoulos AN, Wines M, Tolley D. Case report: endourologic treatment for a ureteral stone in a patient with osteogenesis imperfecta. J Endourol. 2008;22:459–61.
20. Desai MR, Jasani A. Percutaneous nephrolithotripsy in ectopic kidneys. J Endourol. 2000;14:289–92.
21. Eshghi AM, Roth JS, Smith AD. Percutaneous transperitoneal approach to a pelvic kidney for endourological removal of staghorn calculus. J Urol. 1985;134:525–7.
22. Holman E, Toth C. Laparoscopically assisted percutaneous transperitoneal nephrolithotomy in pelvic dystopic kidneys: experience in 15 successful cases. J Laparoendosc Adv Surg Tech A. 1998;8:431–5.
23. Troxel SA, Low RK, Das S. Extraperitoneal laparoscopy-assisted percutaneous nephrolithotomy in a left pelvic kidney. J Endourol. 2002;16:655–7.
24. Seref B, Yasar O, Lutfi T, et al. Extraperitoneal laparoscopy-assisted percutaneous nephrolithotomy in a patient with osteogenesis imperfecta. Urol Res. 2010;39:73–6.

Percutaneous Renal Surgery for Renal Pelvic Tumors: Overcoming the Difficulties

11

Brian Duty, Michael Blute, Zhamshid Okhunov, Arthur D. Smith, and Zeph Okeke

Introduction

Percutaneous renal access was first employed in 1955 by Goodwin and colleagues to drain patients with hydronephrosis [1]. Fernstrom and Johansson utilized percutaneous access in 1976 to treat urolithiasis [2]. Eleven years later, Smith et al. reported the first case series of percutaneous renal pelvis tumor resection [3].

Since this initial report, numerous series have been published on percutaneous treatment of upper tract transitional cell carcinoma (UTTCC). Over time, the surgical indications for percutaneous management have expanded. This chapter will provide a general overview of UTTCC. Traditional and elective indications for endoscopic management will be detailed followed by a description of operative technique, with an emphasis on the technical nuances of the procedure that can impact the complication rate and oncologic efficacy. Lastly, the literature will be reviewed.

B. Duty, M.D. • M. Blute, M.D. • Z. Okhunov, M.D.
A.D. Smith, M.D. • Z. Okeke, M.D. (✉)
Department of Urology, Smith Institute for Urology, Hofstra North Shore – Long Island Jewish Health System, 450 Lakeville Road, New Hyde Park, NY, 11042, USA
e-mail: bduty@nshs.edu; mblute@nshs.edu; zho0616@gmail.com; asmith1@nshs.edu; zokeke@nshs.edu

Epidemiology of Upper Tract Transitional Cell Carcinoma

Urothelial tumors of the upper urinary tract account for approximately 5 % of renal malignancies and 5 % of all urothelial tumors [4]. Roughly 10 individuals/100,000 will develop the disease, with a peak incidence between the ages of 75 and 79. Men are twice as likely to be affected as women, and the disease is more common in Caucasians than African Americans [5].

Risk factors include cigarette smoking, analgesic abuse (phenacetin in particular), occupational exposure to aniline dyes and other carcinogenic compounds, chronic inflammation or infection, and prior exposure to cyclophosphamide. Tobacco use remains the most important modifiable risk factor, which increases the relative risk of UTTCC 2.5- to 7-fold. Balkan nephropathy is a degenerative interstitial nephropathy that places individuals at increased risk (100- to 200-fold) of upper tract TCC. Most tumors are low grade, but they have a tendency to be multifocal and recur. Interestingly, this condition does not place patients at heightened risk of bladder cancer. The etiology of this condition is unknown.

Roughly 1 % of patients with bladder cancer will go on to form upper tract tumors. Carcinoma in situ is a greater risk factor for upper tract recurrence than noninvasive papillary disease [6]. Thirty to fifty percent of UTTCC patients will recur within the bladder [7].

A.M. Al-Kandari et al. (eds.), *Difficult Cases in Endourology*,
DOI 10.1007/978-1-84882-083-8_11, © Springer-Verlag London 2013

Clinical Presentation

Transitional cell carcinoma of the kidney is twice as common as the ureter [8]. Ureteral tumors occur in the distal, mid, and proximal ureter approximately 70, 25, and 5 % of the time, respectively. Fifty-six to ninety-six percent of patients present with microscopic or gross hematuria [9]. Although less common, some patients present with dull flank pain due to progressive obstruction. Upper tract tumors are rarely diagnosed at the time of autopsy because most become symptomatic. Unfortunately, 60 % of upper tract tumors are invasive at the time of diagnosis, in contrast to only 15 % of bladder transitional cell carcinomas (TCC) [8]. This is believed to be a consequence of the kidney's and ureter's thinner muscle layer compared to the bladder, which allows for earlier muscle penetration. As a result, UTTCC is often associated with a poor prognosis. Up to 19 % of patients will present with metastatic disease.

Diagnosis

Computed tomographic urography (CTU) is currently the first-line diagnostic modality for patients at risk for UTTCC. The sensitivity and specificity of CTU for lesions between 5 and 10 mm in size are 96 and 99 %, respectively [10]. The sensitivity drops to 89 % for lesions between 3 and 5 mm and is only 40 % for tumors less than 3 mm in size. Magnetic resonance imaging with gadolinium is less sensitive than CTU. One study found a sensitivity of only 74 % for lesions less than 2 cm in size [11].

The differential diagnosis for a filling defect noted on contrast-enhanced imaging includes renal neoplasm (e.g., renal cell carcinoma, transitional cell carcinoma), stone, foreign body, fibroepithelial polyp, fungal ball, papillary necrosis, and/or blood clot. As a result, further workup is usually required to rule out or characterize a collecting system tumor.

Urinary cytology remains a critical component of the workup, but its performance varies dramatically by tumor grade. For high-grade lesions and carcinoma in situ, cytology's sensitivity and specificity are 90 and 98 %, respectively [12]. False positives may be due to the degenerated urothelium, human polyomavirus infection, and effects of cyclophosphamide therapy. The sensitivity of urine cytology for low-grade disease is much lower, with some series reporting it to be as low as 0 %. Consequently, urine cytology can rule in, but cannot rule out, urothelial malignancy. Saline washings and brush biopsy of the urothelium improve the diagnostic accuracy of urine cytology.

Ureteroscopy is the most important diagnostic modality in equivocal cases. The procedure begins by defining the caliceal anatomy with a retrograde pyelogram. Diagnostic ureteroscopy is then performed, which is able to visualize over 95 % of the collecting system in the majority of patients. If a lesion is identified, urine is aspirated and sent off for cytology. Saline is then injected into the collecting system and another specimen is collected. Multiple biopsies of the lesion are then obtained with either a flat-wire basket or 3-F biopsy forceps. These are pooled and sent off to the cytopathologist for interpretation.

Ureteroscopic biopsies rarely provide accurate tumor staging because of the small instrument size. However, one study showed that with repeated cold-cup biopsies, it is possible to assess for lamina propria invasion in up to 61 % of patients [13]. Ureteroscopic biopsies are able to accurately grade upper tract lesions in 78–92 % of cases [13, 14]. Fortunately, multiple studies have shown a strong correlation between tumor grade and stage for UTTCC. There is a nearly 100 % correlation between grade 1 tumors and Ta disease and 96 % association between grade 3–4 tumors and parenchymal invasion [15].

Rationale and Indications for Endoscopic Management

Radical nephroureterectomy (RNU), either via an open or laparoscopic approach, has traditionally been the treatment modality of choice for patients with pelvicaliceal TCC. Endoscopic management was initially reserved for patients with a solitary kidney, renal insufficiency, bilateral disease, and/or prohibitive medical comorbidities. Over time, the indications for endoscopic management have increased for a variety of reasons.

First, the importance of nephron preservation has been conclusively demonstrated. In a review of 1,004 patients undergoing either radical or partial nephrectomy for renal masses between 4 and 7 cm in size, the authors observed a 25 % increased risk of cardiac death in the radical nephrectomy group compared to those who underwent nephron-sparing surgery [16]. Furthermore, the life expectancy of adults on dialysis is sobering [17]. The 5-year survival rate for individuals on dialysis between 65 and 74 years of age is 19 %. This rate falls to an abysmal 10 % between the ages of 75 and 84, which is the age group containing the peak incidence of UTTCC. Furthermore, patients who develop renal insufficiency following RNU and go on to develop metastatic disease are not eligible for platinum-based chemotherapy, which is the agent of choice for TCC.

Second, clinical series have shown that patients with low-grade UTTCC do uniformly well regardless of treatment modality and individuals with high-grade lesions do poorly, even with aggressive surgical therapy. One study showed a 5-year metastasis-free survival rate following open RNU of 85 % for low-grade tumors compared to only 32 % for patients with high-grade disease [18]. Therefore, some authors have argued that RNU in the setting of high-grade disease does not significantly improve survival but subjects patients to increased morbidity and risk of renal insufficiency.

Nevertheless, RNU remains the treatment of choice in patients with UTTCC suspicious for infiltration on imaging, high-grade lesions on biopsy or cytology, and multifocal tumors [8]. Indications for conservative (endoscopic) management of UTTCC include bilateral tumors (synchronous/metachronous), predisposition to recurrence (e.g., Balkan nephropathy), solitary kidney, and/or significant medical comorbidities. Relative indications for conservative therapy include renal insufficiency and low-grade/low-stage lesions.

Percutaneous treatment is favored over the ureteroscopic approach in patients with pelvicaliceal tumors greater than 1.5 cm in size because tumor resection is more efficient and deeper biopsies can be obtained. In addition, the nephrostomy tube placed at the conclusion of the case may be utilized for adjuvant instillation therapy.

Percutaneous Resection Technique

During the informed consent process, patients must be made aware of the risks of bleeding necessitating blood transfusion and/or embolization, infection, failed access, and bowel and pleural injury. Patients considering conservative therapy must also be willing to accept a rigorous surveillance process, which includes repeated diagnostic ureteroscopy procedures.

Absolute contraindications to percutaneous TCC resection include active infection, bleeding diathesis, and uncontrolled hypertension. Morbid obesity is a relative contraindication. Extra-long instruments are available to facilitate resection, but if feasible, ureteroscopy may be more effective if tumor burden is not excessive.

Prior to induction of general anesthesia, broad-spectrum parenteral antibiotics are given and sequential compression devices are placed. The procedure begins with cystoscopy of the bladder with both a 30- and 70-degree lens to ensure no synchronous lesions are present. Access to the upper urinary tract is obtained by passing a guidewire through the ureteral orifice up into the renal pelvis under fluoroscopic control. A 5- or 6-F open-ended ureteral catheter is passed over the guidewire so that the proximal end rests within the renal pelvis. The guidewire is removed and a Foley catheter is placed. The ureteral catheter is then secured to the Foley catheter with a silk suture.

The patient is then transferred into the prone position. Morbidly obese patients who are unable to lie prone are treated in the lateral decubitus position. Foam bolsters are used to pad the face and are placed under the shoulders and pelvis to facilitate ventilation. Other pressure points such as the feet, knees, and elbows are also padded for protection. Particular attention is paid to arm positioning. The shoulders are abducted and elbows flexed less than 90° to prevent brachial plexus injury.

Attention is then turned to getting renal access. A retrograde pyelogram is obtained via the previously placed ureteral catheter, which defines the caliceal anatomy and demonstrates tumor position. With this information, the point of optimal access can be determined. If the patient has a solitary caliceal lesion, then access is obtained directly into this calyx. If the patient has multiple lesions or a tumor within the renal pelvis, then access is obtained through a posterior upper or mid pole calyx. This facilitates complete inspection of the collecting system and provides the best access to the renal pelvis and proximal ureter. If needed, access above the 12th rib is utilized.

Access is obtained using an 18-gauge diamond-tipped finder needle and biplanar fluoroscopy. Efflux of urine following removal of the needle obturator confirms positioning of the needle within the collecting system. A guidewire is then coiled in the collecting system or if possible advanced down the ureter. A second safety wire should be placed to guard against accidental loss of access. The tract is established using either a balloon dilator or sequential Amplatz dilators. The working sheath is then placed into the collecting system under fluoroscopic guidance. It is important to ensure that the access sheath remains in the collecting system at all times to prevent potential tumor seeding of the perinephric space and tract.

At this point, the rigid nephroscope is passed into the collecting system. The first task is to ensure that stable access has been obtained. This may be accomplished by either manipulating the guidewire down the ureter into the bladder or by pulling the ureteral catheter out through the nephrostomy tract to establish "through-and-through" access.

Once access has been secured, the entire collecting system is inspected to ensure all lesions have been identified. Once entirely visualized, resection is begun. The resection may be performed with a holmium laser, resectoscope, or biopsy forceps. The holmium laser should be reserved for ablating smaller satellite lesions given its inefficiency and lack of tissue for pathology. The authors prefer cold-cup biopsy forceps rather than the resectoscope because deep biopsies into the renal parenchyma carry with them a high risk of bleeding, which is difficult to control. The tumor is excised piecemeal with the cold-cup forceps. The superficial tumor specimen is pooled for analysis. The tumor base is then biopsied and sent off separately. Bleeding from the tumor bed is then controlled with either the holmium laser or loop electrocautery.

Once hemostasis has been obtained, a 24-F Malecot-type nephrostomy tube is placed under fluoroscopic guidance. The reentry tube provides large-bore collecting system drainage while minimizing parenchymal bleeding along the access tract. Its ureteral component provides secure access to the kidney and ureter. It is the authors' practice to perform second-look nephroscopy within 1 week of the initial resection. Even if no residual tumor is seen, repeat cold-cup biopsies are taken from the tumor bed. If adjuvant intrarenal instillation therapy is planned, the reentry nephrostomy tube is replaced with an 8- or 10-F pigtail nephrostomy catheter.

If the tumor is found to be unresectable, a nephroureterectomy is indicated. If resected but the final path reveals high-grade or invasive disease, a RNU is also advocated. High-grade or invasive disease, apparent on a second-look biopsy, is another indication for nephroureterectomy.

Oncologic Outcomes

The first clinical series of percutaneous UTTCC management was published by Smith et al. in 1987 [3]. Seven of the nine patients in the series were not candidates for RNU due to solitary kidney (3), poor surgical risk (2), bilateral tumors (1), and renal insufficiency (1). Five of the patients remained recurrence-free at a mean follow-up of 9.5 months.

Following this initial feasibility study, multiple series have subsequently been published on the topic. Most have been nonrandomized studies involving patients who were poor candidates for RNU. Nevertheless, what became apparent from these studies was the strong correlation between tumor grade and outcome. In general, patients with low-grade disease do uniformly well, and individuals with high-grade tumors do poorly regardless of treatment modality. This finding has expanded the use of endoscopic management techniques in select patients who would otherwise be candidates for RNU.

Review of the literature reveals a recurrence rate for patients with grade I tumors following percutaneous resection ranging from 5 to 26 %, with a mean of approximately 20 % [19–31]. Elliott and colleagues reported their experience in 21 patients treated conservatively, with a mean follow-up of 6.1 years [27]. The majority of tumors was low grade or did not appear invasive at the time of diagnostic ureteroscopy. The authors reported a local recurrence rate of 33 %. However, none of the recurrent tumors were found to have increased in grade. Eighty-one percent of patients avoided RNU. Of the 19 % that went on to nephrectomy, none experienced a deleterious effect from delayed treatment.

The reported recurrence rate for grade II tumors varies from 6 to 33 %, with an average of 26 % [19–31]. As in grade I disease, cancer-related mortality is low (<5 %). However, renal preservation is not as common, with more patients going on to RNU. In a study by Jarrett and colleagues, 6 of the 12 patients with grade II disease went on to have a RNU, three immediately and three following recurrence [19]. Jabbour et al. published a study looking exclusively at patients with grade II disease [24]. The series included 24 patients undergoing percutaneous management. Immediate RNU was performed in 4 patients due to the presence of invasive disease (2), bleeding (1), and inability to resect the whole tumor (1). Of the remaining 20 patients, 5 (20 %) went on to develop a recurrence. Three of these patients underwent delayed RNU. Disease-specific survival was 95 %.

The recurrence and cancer-related mortality rates in patients with high-grade disease are much higher. Liatsikos and colleagues published a series of 69 patients undergoing percutaneous management of UTTCC [26]. Of the 25 patients with high-grade tumors, 56 % went on to develop recurrent disease. The cancer-specific mortality rate was 36 %. The series containing the largest subset of patients with high-grade disease was published by Rastinehad et al. [31]. Of the 39 patients with grade III lesions, 38 % went on to develop a recurrence. Overall survival was 68 %.

To date, there have been two comparative studies in the urologic literature [32, 33]. Neither was randomized. The first was published by Lee and colleagues and involved 60 patients who underwent nephroureterectomy and 50 patients treated percutaneously [32]. Results were reported in terms of disease-specific survival in months. There was no significant difference between the RNU and percutaneous groups for grade I (67.8 vs. 35.9 months), grade II (53.8 vs. 53.3 months), and grade III tumors (56.7 vs. 27.8 months). It should be noted that the RNU group had a higher proportion of stage T3 tumors than the percutaneous cohort (14 vs. 3). This combined with the relatively small sample size calls into question the results of this study. Roupret et al. compared 54 patients who underwent RNU to 16 individuals treated by percutaneous resection [33]. In patients with low-grade tumors, the 5-year disease-specific survival rate was no different between those treated with RNU and percutaneous resection (84 vs. 80 %; $p=0.78$). There were not enough high-grade patients treated percutaneously to draw any meaningful conclusions.

In summary, the literature regarding the efficacy of endoscopic UTTCC management is not unequivocal given the lack of randomized controlled trials. However, the available data does support the use of endoscopic techniques in patients with low-grade disease. Although most patients with high-grade disease do poorly regardless of treatment modality, RNU remains the treatment of choice except in patients who are poor surgical candidates.

Complications

Percutaneous resection of upper tract tumors is well tolerated by most patients. As with any percutaneous renal procedure, patients are at risk of fever, urinary tract infection, collecting system stricture or perforation, hemorrhage, visceral injury, and pleural fluid collection.

Access tract tumor seeding is also a potential complication. Fortunately, the majority of clinical series have not reported a tract recurrence [19, 21, 25, 26, 31]. However, several case reports have been published. Oefelein and MacLennan described a nephrostomy tract recurrence following percutaneous resection of a T1, grade II lesion in a patient who had previously undergone radical cystectomy [34]. The patient subsequently underwent nephroureterectomy and was upstaged to T2N1M0 disease. Although the patient developed a tract recurrence, it should be noted that the patient's local disease was more significant than anticipated. Tract radiotherapy has been described to minimize the risk of recurrence [35, 36]. However, these studies are small in size and have not been randomized. Complete tumor resection with proper sheath placement throughout the case is critical to minimize this rare complication.

Adjuvant Instillation Therapy

Adjuvant therapy is traditionally done using either mitomycin-C or bacillus Calmette-Guerin (BCG). The latter is more commonly used. Adjuvant therapy may be delivered in a retrograde or antegrade fashion. Retrograde instillation may be performed through an external ureteral catheter or by relying on vesicoureteral reflux. Irie and colleagues performed cystograms on nine stented patients with carcinoma in situ and found that volumes ranging from 80 to 250 cc were required to induce reflux sufficient to reach the renal pelvis [37].

It is the authors' practice to place two ipsilateral 7-F ureteral stents at the time of the second-look percutaneous procedure. The first course of BCG is completed with the stents in place. The stents are removed at the time of the first surveillance procedure, and a ureteral meatotomy is performed. The meatotomy simplifies subsequent diagnostic ureteroscopy procedures and obviates the need for stenting during maintenance BCG courses.

Upper tract delivery is ensured via an antegrade approach. This is typically performed via a pigtail nephrostomy tube. Although well tolerated by most patients, there is an increased risk of sepsis. Therefore, many authors will hospitalize the patient overnight for observation.

Several series have evaluated the efficacy of adjuvant instillation therapy for upper tract TCC. Most have been retrospective. When stratified by tumor grade, BCG therapy has been associated with recurrence rates of 25, 27, and 35 % for grades I, II, and III tumors, respectively [21–24, 31]. Rastinehad and colleagues published the largest series evaluating adjuvant BCG therapy following percutaneous resection [31]. Of the 89 patients in the study, 50 underwent a 6-week course of BCG therapy. Compared to the 39 patients who did not undergo adjuvant therapy, the BCG group was found to have no difference in disease recurrence, interval to recurrence, and disease progression. However, because prospective comparative series are lacking, most authors still recommend adjuvant therapy in patients with known risk factors for recurrence or progression.

As with adjuvant therapy for bladder cancer, there is a risk of urinary sepsis from gram-negative organisms and disseminated BCG infection. Sharpe et al. reported one case of high-grade fever following BCG instillation in 11 patients [38]. In a larger series, Thalman and colleagues treated 37 patients with UTTCC with adjuvant BCG [39]. Two patients developed sepsis and one disseminated BCG infection.

Other reported complications include nephrostomy tube bacterial colonization and irritative voiding symptoms. Transient low-grade fevers without associated systemic infection were reported in 67 % of patients in one series [40]. Granulomas have been noted on surveillance endoscopy but are of no clinical significance [41].

Surveillance

Most recurrences appear within 3 years of initial therapy [24]. However, lifelong surveillance is required for patients treated with endoscopic resection. Up to 50 % of patients will develop a recurrence in the bladder. Cystoscopy should be performed every 3 months for the first year, biannually during the second year, and then yearly thereafter. Surveillance ureteroscopy is used to monitor the upper tracts. Chen et al. reported a sensitivity of 93 % for ureteroscopy with biopsy versus 71.7 % for retrograde pyelography alone [42]. Biannual upper tract ureteroscopy for the first 3 years and then annually thereafter is recommended.

Conclusions

Prior to the development of endoscopic management techniques, RNU was the first-line treatment modality for UTTCC. Endoscopic techniques were initially reserved for patients with a solitary kidney, bilateral disease, renal insufficiency, or who were not surgical candidates. With a greater understanding of the relationship between tumor grade and stage, the indications for conservative management have expanded to include select cases with low-grade disease. Radical nephroureterectomy remains the treatment of choice in patients with high-grade tumors who are surgical candidates. Unfortunately, these patients tend to do poorly regardless of treatment modality. Percutaneous management is well tolerated by the majority of patients. However, patients must be willing to undergo an aggressive surveillance regimen and adjuvant therapy.

References

1. Goodwin WE, Casey WC, Woolf W. Percutaneous trocar (needle) nephrostomy in hydronephrosis. J Am Med Assoc. 1955;157:891–4.
2. Fernstrom I, Johansson B. Percutaneous pyelolithotomy. A new extraction technique. Scand J Urol Nephrol. 1976;10:257–9.
3. Smith AD, Orihuela E, Crowley AR. Percutaneous management of renal pelvic tumors: a treatment option in selected cases. J Urol. 1987;137:852–6.
4. Jemal A, Tiwari RC, Murray T, et al. Cancer statistics, 2004. CA Cancer J Clin. 2004;54:8–22.
5. Greenlee RT, Murray T, Bolden S, et al. Cancer statistics, 2000. CA Cancer J Clin. 2000;50:7–33.
6. Solsona E, Iborra I, Ricos JV, et al. Upper urinary tract involvement in patients with bladder carcinoma in situ (CIS): its impact on management. Urology. 1997;49:347–52.
7. Raman JD, Ng CK, Scherr DS, et al. Impact of tumor location on prognosis for patients with upper tract urothelial carcinoma managed by radical nephroureterectomy. Eur Urol. 2010;57:1072–9.
8. Roupret M, Zigeuner R, Palou J, et al. European guidelines for the diagnosis and management of upper urinary tract urothelial cell carcinomas. Eur Urol. 2011;59(4):584–94.
9. Guinan P, Vogelzang NJ, Randazzo R, et al. Renal pelvic cancer: a review of 611 patients treated in Illinois 1975–1985. Urology. 1992;40:393–9.
10. Wang LJ, Wong YC, Chuang CK, et al. Diagnostic accuracy of transitional cell carcinoma on multidetector computerized tomography urography in patients with gross hematuria. J Urol. 2009;181:524–31.
11. Takahashi N, Kawashima A, Glockner JF, et al. Small (<2-cm) upper-tract urothelial carcinoma: evaluation with gadolinium-enhanced three-dimensional spoiled gradient-recalled echo MR urography. Radiology. 2008;247:451–7.
12. Brown FM. Urine cytology. Is it still the gold standard for screening? Urol Clin North Am. 2000;27:25–37.
13. Guarnizo E, Pavlovich CP, Seiba M, et al. Ureteroscopic biopsy of upper tract urothelial carcinoma: improved diagnostic accuracy and histopathological considerations using a multi-biopsy approach. J Urol. 2000; 163:52–5.
14. Keeley FX, Kulp DA, Bibbo M, et al. Diagnostic accuracy of ureteroscopic biopsy in upper tract transitional cell carcinoma. J Urol. 1997;157:42–3.
15. Soderdahl DW, Fabrizio MD, Rahman NU, et al. Endoscopic treatment of upper tract transitional cell carcinoma. Urol Oncol. 2005;23:114–22.
16. Weight CJ, Larson BT, Fergany AF, et al. Nephrectomy induced chronic renal insufficiency is associated with increased risk of cardiovascular death and death from any cause in patients with localized cT1b renal masses. J Urol. 2010;183:1317–23.
17. National Kidney and Urological Diseases Information Clearinghouse, National Institute of Diabetes and Digestive and Kidney Disease (NIDDK). National Institutes of Health, NIH Publication 04-3895, Feb 2004.
18. Langner C, Hutterer G, Chromecki T, et al. pT classification, grade, and vascular invasion as prognostic indicators in urothelial carcinoma of the upper urinary tract. Mod Pathol. 2006;19:272–9.
19. Jarrett TW, Sweetser PM, Weiss GH, et al. Percutaneous management of transitional cell carcinoma of the renal collecting system: 9-year experience. J Urol. 1995; 154:1629–35.
20. Plancke HR, Strijbos WE, Delaere KP. Percutaneous endoscopic treatment of urothelial tumours of the renal pelvis. Br J Urol. 1995;75:736–9.
21. Patel A, Soonawalla P, Shepherd SF, et al. Long-term outcome after percutaneous treatment of transitional

cell carcinoma of the renal pelvis. J Urol. 1996; 155:868–74.
22. Martinez-Pineiro JA, Garcia Matres MJ, Martinez-Pineiro L. Endourological treatment of upper tract urothelial carcinomas: analysis of a series of 59 tumors. J Urol. 1996;156:377–85.
23. Clark PE, Streem SB, Geisinger MA. 13-year experience with percutaneous management of upper tract transitional cell carcinoma. J Urol. 1999;161:772–5.
24. Jabbour ME, Smith AD. Primary percutaneous approach to upper urinary tract transitional cell carcinoma. Urol Clin North Am. 2000;27:739–50.
25. Jabbour ME, Desgrandchamps F, Cazin S, et al. Percutaneous management of grade II upper urinary tract transitional cell: the long-term outcome. J Urol. 2000;163:1105–7.
26. Liatsikos EN, Dinlenc CZ, Kapoor R, et al. Transitional cell carcinoma of the renal pelvis: ureteroscopic and percutaneous approach. J Endourol. 2001;15:377–83.
27. Elliott DS, Segura JW, Lightner D, et al. Is nephroureterectomy necessary in all cases of upper tract transitional cell carcinoma? Long-term results of conservative endourologic management of upper tract transitional cell carcinoma in individuals with a normal contralateral kidney. Urology. 2001;58:174–8.
28. Deligne E, Colombel M, Badet L, et al. Conservative management of upper urinary tract tumors. Eur Urol. 2002;42:43–8.
29. Goel MC, Mahendra V, Roberts JG. Percutaneous management of renal pelvic urothelial tumors: long-term followup. J Urol. 2003;169:925–9.
30. Palou J, Piovesan LF, Huguet J, et al. Percutaneous nephroscopic management of upper urinary tract transitional cell carcinoma: recurrence and long-term followup. J Urol. 2004;172:66–9.
31. Rastinehad AR, Ost MC, Vanderbrink BA, et al. A 20-year experience with percutaneous resection of upper tract transitional carcinoma: is there an oncologic benefit with adjuvant bacillus Calmette Guérin therapy? Urology. 2009;73:27–31.
32. Lee BR, Jabbour ME, Marshall FF, et al. 13-year survival comparison of percutaneous and open nephroureterectomy approaches for management of transitional cell carcinoma of renal collecting system: equivalent outcomes. J Endourol. 1999;13:289–94.
33. Roupret M, Hupertan V, Traxer O, et al. Comparison of open nephroureterectomy and ureteroscopic and percutaneous management of upper urinary tract transitional cell carcinoma. Urology. 2006;67:1181–7.
34. Oefelein MC, MacLennan G. Transitional cell carcinoma recurrence in the nephrostomy tract after percutaneous resection. J Urol. 2003;170:521.
35. Woodhouse CR, Kellett MJ, Bloom HJ. Percutaneous renal surgery and local radiotherapy in the management of renal pelvic transitional cell carcinoma. Br J Urol. 1986;58:245–9.
36. Sheperd SF, Patel A, Bidmead AM, et al. Nephrostomy track brachytherapy following percutaneous resection of transitional cell carcinoma of the renal pelvis. Clin Oncol. 1995;7:385–7.
37. Irie A, Iwamura M, Kadowaki K, et al. Intravesical instillation of bacillus Calmette-Guerin for carcinoma in situ of the urothelium involving the upper urinary tract utilizing vesicoureteral reflux created by a double-pigtail catheter. Urology. 2002;59:53–7.
38. Sharpe JR, Duffy G, Chin JL. Intrarenal bacillus Calmette-Guerin therapy for upper urinary tract carcinoma in situ. J Urol. 1993;149:457–60.
39. Thalmann GN, Markwalder R, Walter B, et al. Long term experience with bacillus Calmette-Guerin therapy of upper urinary tract transitional cell carcinoma in patients not eligible for surgery. J Urol. 2002;168:1381–5.
40. Nishino Y, Yamamoto N, Komeda H, et al. Bacillus Calmette-Guerin instillation treatment for carcinoma in situ of the upper urinary tract. BJU Int. 2000; 85:799–801.
41. Bellman GC, Sweetser P, Smith AD. Complications of intracavitary bacillus Calmette-Guerin after percutaneous resection of upper tract transitional cell carcinoma. J Urol. 1994;151:13–5.
42. Chen GL, El-Gabry EA, Bagley DH. Surveillance of upper urinary tract transitional cell carcinoma: the role of ureteroscopy, retrograde pyelography, cytology, and urinalysis. J Urol. 2000;164:1901–4.

Percutaneous Nephrolithotomy (PCNL) in the Treatment of Stones Within Horseshoe Kidneys and in Patients with Autosomal Dominant Polycystic Kidney Disease

12

Ahmed Abed, Ahmed R. El-Nahas, Ahmed M. Al-Kandari, and Ahmed A. Shokeir

Introduction

Horseshoe kidneys and adult polycystic kidneys are some of the most prevalent renal anomalies with high incidence of urolithiasis. They represent special challenges in the management of stone disease.

Horseshoe kidney is the most prevalent anomaly of renal fusion. It represents 0.25 % of the general population. The most common complications associated with horseshoe kidney necessitating surgical intervention are urolithiasis and ureteropelvic junction obstruction. Urolithiasis occurs in 20 % of horseshoe [1, 2]. Urinary stasis and the resultant recurrent urinary tract infections are the main risk factors for urolithiasis in such kidneys (up to 35 and 41 %, respectively). Stasis results from the high insertion of the ureter, its anterior course over the isthmus, and the variation in the arterial and venous vasculature [3].

Nephrolithiasis occurring in patients with autosomal dominant polycystic kidney disease (ADPKD) is 5–10 times higher than in general population. It is seen in 20–28 % of those patients, and nearly one-half of them are symptomatic. Both anatomic and metabolic factors seem to be responsible for the greater incidence of stone formation in such patients. Anatomical predisposition for stone formation results from compression of the pelvicaliceal system by the cysts leading to urinary stasis, delayed washout of crystals, and increased risk of urinary tract infections. The most common metabolic disorders contributing to stone formation include hypocitruria, aciduria, abnormal transport of ammonia, and distal acidification defects. Also low levels of urinary magnesium, phosphate, and potassium play a role in nephrolithiasis. Nephrolithiasis accelerates the onset of renal failure, as can hypertension and infection. Therefore, total clearance of the calculi is advisable, and early intervention is warranted with recurrent pain, hematuria, urinary tract infections, obstructive uropathy, and deteriorating renal function [4–8].

The most common types of stones in patients with ADPKD include uric acid stones (57 %) and/or calcium oxalate (47 %). Struvite stones were also detected with ADPKD. The high incidence of radiolucent stones in patients with ADPKD highlights the importance of the non-contrast computed tomography as an investigative tool in such patients [9, 10].

Treatment modalities for calculi in horseshoe kidneys include extracorporeal shock wave lithotripsy (SWL), flexible ureterorenoscopy, percutaneous nephrolithotomy (PNL), and open surgery.

A. Abed, M.D. • A.R. El-Nahas, M.D.
A.A. Shokeir, M.D., Ph.D., FEBU (✉)
Department of Urology, Urology and Nephrology Center, Mansoura University,
El Gomhoria Street, Mansoura 35516, Egypt
e-mail: aascor1@yahoo.com; ar_el_nahas@yahoo.com; ahmed.shokeir@hotmail.com

A.M. Al-Kandari, M.D., FRCS(C)
Department of Surgery, Kuwait University,
Jabriyah, Kuwait City 13110, Kuwait
e-mail: drakandari@hotmail.com

A.M. Al-Kandari et al. (eds.), *Difficult Cases in Endourology*,
DOI 10.1007/978-1-84882-083-8_12, © Springer-Verlag London 2013

The overall stone-free rate of all modalities for treatment of stones in horseshoe kidneys has been 53 % (range 50–79 %) [11–13].

Currently, open surgery has a limited role in management of urolithiasis in general. It is only indicated after failure of endoscopic procedures or with stones larger than applicable to less-invasive modalities [14].

Before the era of minimally invasive technology, open surgery was performed in most patients with ADPKD and nephrolithiasis [4, 15]. The introduction of minimally invasive techniques such as shock wave lithotripsy (SWL), percutaneous nephrolithotomy (PNL), and flexible ureterorenoscopy (FURS) has significantly changed the concept of treatment of these cases [8, 16, 17].

Although adequate fragmentation can be achieved by SWL, the anatomic abnormalities of horseshoe kidneys hinder the passage of the stone fragments. This leads to a higher incidence of residual fragments and also recurrent disease that may reach up to 50–86 % of patients [1, 18]. Thus, SWL is best employed for renal stones less than 20 mm. The stone-free rates after SWL in horseshoe kidneys vary between 71.4–92 % [19, 20].

For stones in patients with ADPKD, the results of SWL have been discouraging in most reports, with low stone-free rate at 25–46 % [5, 21, 22]. This may result from the obstructive effect of the cysts and the resultant urinary stasis impeding passage of the stone fragments. Grampsas et al. demonstrated a proportional relationship between the number and size of the cysts and the resultant urinary stasis and intrarenal anatomic obstruction. Also, the risk of traumatic hemorrhage into the cysts, traumatic loss of nephrons because of shock waves, and decreased clearance of the stone load should be taken into consideration [7]. On the other hand, Delakas and his colleagues reported overall stone-free rate 84.6 % [17].

The development of new instruments for retrograde intrarenal surgery (RIRS) has facilitated the use of flexible ureterorenoscope (FURS) in treatment of stones within horseshoe kidneys, especially with the help of holmium laser lithotripsy and nitinol baskets and graspers resulting in stone-free rate reaching 75 % [23, 24]. Flexible ureterorenoscope (FURS) with laser disintegration also has the advantage of having no potential to cause traumatic nephron loss and being independent of anatomic variations from the cystic disease and thus can be employed safely in ADPKD patients with bleeding diathesis, morbid obesity, and solitary kidney [25].

In this chapter, we will discuss PNL in the treatment of stones within horseshoe kidneys and patients with autosomal dominant polycystic kidney disease. Emphasis will be on the anatomical factors of each anomaly, the indications of PNL, the percutaneous access, the results, and the complications reported in each entity. Advice on how to avoid complications will also be discussed.

Percutaneous Nephrolithotomy in Treatment of Stones in Horseshoe Kidneys

Anatomical Factors

Two main anatomical factors in horseshoe kidneys should be considered during PNL. The first is that all blood vessels, except for some to the isthmus, enter the kidney from its ventromedial aspect. So percutaneous access is obtained only on the lateral aspect, far from the major arteries. The dorsal arteries to the isthmus are protected by the spine and are situated away from the nephrostomy tract. The risk of arterial bleeding is, therefore, not greater than in a normal kidney. The second factor is the orientation of the collecting system. In a horseshoe kidney, most of the calices point either dorsomedially or dorsolaterally. The calices to the isthmus lie within a coronal plane and point medially (Figs. 12.1 and 12.2). Access to the calices in the isthmus is gained across the pelvis. The anatomic situation results in a lower and more medial position of the nephrostomy tract whose orientation is more or less dorsoventral [26].

Indications of PNL in Horseshoe Kidneys

Percutaneous treatment of stones in horseshoe kidneys was indicated for large stone burden greater than 2 cm, multiple complex stones, staghorn stones, and failed SWL in 22.2, 48.9, 6.7, and 22.2 % of patients, respectively [27].

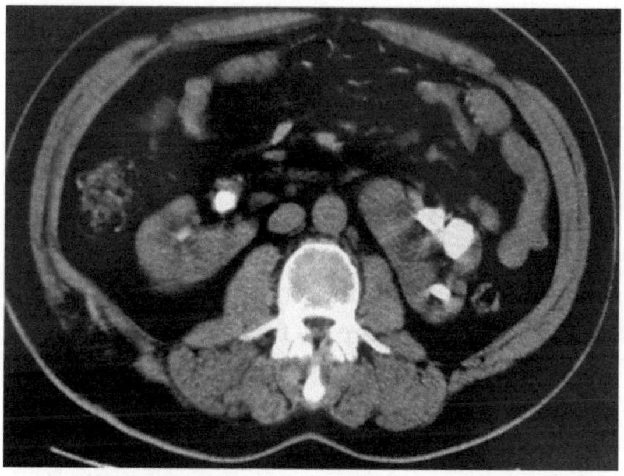

Fig. 12.1 Noncontrast CT axial view showing hyperdense stone in the renal pelvis of the right compartment and multiple stones in the left compartment of the horseshoe kidney

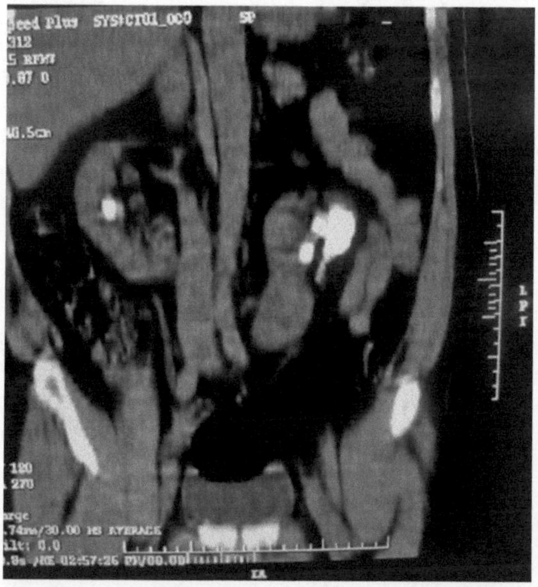

Fig. 12.2 Noncontrast CT reformatted coronal image showing stone in the renal pelvis of the right compartment and multiple stones in the upper calyx and renal pelvis of the left compartment of the horseshoe kidney

Percutaneous Access to Horseshoe Kidneys

Upper pole access is preferred to minimize nephroscope torque on renal tissue during manipulation because the long axis of the nephroscope is aligned with the long axis of the kidney, thus decreasing the blood loss (Fig. 12.3). Also, upper pole access allows access to the upper pole calices, renal pelvis, lower pole calices, pelviureteral junction, and proximal ureter [2]. Upper pole access is relatively safe in horseshoe kidney, and thus intrathoracic complications such as pneumothorax are decreased because a supracostal approach is less likely to be used than in patients with normal renal anatomy owing to the inferior displacement of the horseshoe kidney away from the pleura [2, 28].

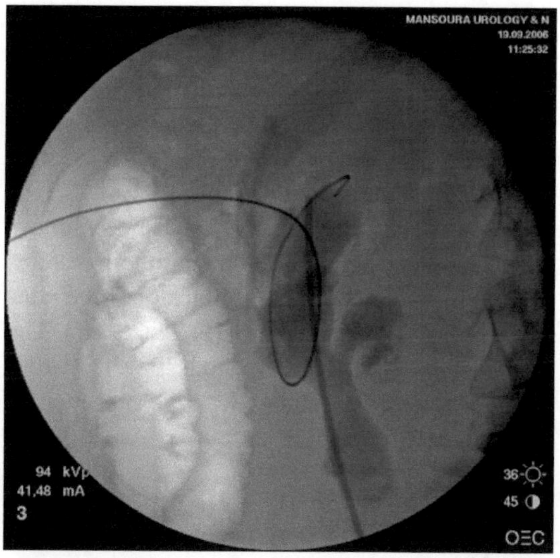

Fig. 12.3 Fluoroscopic view in prone position showing upper calyceal puncture of the left compartment of the horseshoe kidney

However, upper pole access will result in an unusually long tract, and the instruments may not reach the lower and medial calices. This problem is exacerbated in obese patients, but it can be overcome using long, rigid nephroscopes or flexible ones. Flexible nephroscope was used in 84 % of patients who underwent PNL for stones in horseshoe kidneys [2].

Upper pole access was used in 62–81 % [2, 27, 29]. In a series of 45 horseshoe kidneys, upper pole access was used in 62 % of patients. Of these patients, skin puncture was supracostal in 22 % and subcostal in 78 % [27].

Results of PNL in Horseshoe Kidneys

Few reports were published about the percutaneous management of the stones in horseshoe kidneys in the English literature. Also most of these reports include small series, with the total number hardly exceeding 100 cases. One of the largest series included 45 PNL procedures in 34 patients with stone-bearing horseshoe kidneys in a single institution [27]. The results of PNL for horseshoe kidneys are summarized in Table 12.1.

Percutaneous approach in horseshoe kidneys is adequate and safe with higher stone-free rates than ureteroscopy or SWL. Initial stone-free rates range between 72 and 87.5 % [2, 27, 29–31]. The only factor that affects the stone-free rate after PNL in horseshoe kidneys was the presence of staghorn calculus [35].

Complications of PNL in Horseshoe Kidneys

Bleeding was the most common reported complication and could be markedly reduced by proper planning of the percutaneous access to the horseshoe kidney, as previously described. Major complication rates ranged between 12.5 and 42 % [2, 27, 29–31].

Shokeir et al. reported that none of the patients with an upper pole access developed pneumothorax, compared to a rate of 6 % that was reported by Raj and coworkers [2, 28].

Colonic perforation is a rare complication of PNL. Generally the incidence ranged between 0.2 and 0.5 % [36–39]. However, horseshoe kidney is an independent risk factor for colonic perforation during PNL with incidence reaching 5.9 % [39].

The increased risk of colonic perforation could be explained by the retrorenal colonic position that is sometimes associated with horseshoe kidneys and other fusion anomalies. It results from a defect in the normal development of the lateral colic fascia combined with downward descent of the kidney. Thus, some investigators recommend CT with contrast before PNL in patients with horseshoe kidneys to avoid colonic injury. Conservative management of such cases is usually successful through withdrawal of the nephrostomy tube, temporary fixation of a ureteral stent, intravenous antibiotics, keeping the patients nil per month for a few days, and anal dilation [37, 39–41].

Percutaneous Nephrolithotomy in Treatment of Stones in Patients with Autosomal Dominant Polycystic Kidney Disease

Anatomical Factors

Percutaneous nephrolithotomy (PNL) could be a challenging procedure in treatment of stones in ADPKD. The caliceal spaces are often narrow and elongated owing to the compressive effect of multiple parenchymal cysts. This could interfere with the proper caliceal puncture and dilation. Also, the cysts can come in the way of the puncture and may need to be aspirated before a puncture is achieved. Furthermore, the patients could have varying degrees of chronic renal impairment that is commonly associated with a coagulation defect with a higher risk of bleeding during or after the procedure [5, 8, 9].

Indications of PNL in ADPKD

In published reports, PNL in ADPKD was indicated in cases with large stone burden greater than 3 cm, partial staghorn stone, lower pole renal calculi more than 2 cm, impacted stone at ureteropelvic junction or lumbar ureter, and failed SWL in 50, 15, 20, 10, and 5 %, respectively [4, 5, 8, 9].

Percutaneous Access to ADPKD

Some technical considerations could help achieve a successful approach. A proper antibiotic should be given to the patients with positive cultures to control the infection before surgical intervention. Fluoroscopy can be used to help with accurate puncture of the target calyx. Ultrasound-guided puncture could be difficult owing to the presence of multiple cysts that could interfere with accurate localization of the compressed calices. Al-Kandari et al. described a novel idea of the use of methylthioninium chloride (methyelene blue) with contrast material to assess for proper puncture and dilation that may facilitate the

Table 12.1 Results of PNL for horseshoe kidneys[a]

Series	*N*	Upper pole access	Initial stone-free rate (%)	Auxiliary procedures	Complications (%)	Secondary procedures	Stone-free rate after 2 year procedure
Jones et al. [30]	15	NR	72.3 %	NR	26 %	13.3 %	NR
Lampel et al. [31]	4	NR	75 %	25 %	25 %	NR	NR
Al-Otaibi and Hosking [29]	12	9 (75 %)	9 (75 %)	1 (8.3 %)	42 %	1 (8.3 %)	10 (83.3 %)
Lingeman, and Saw [32]	17	81 %	87.5 %	NR	29 %	33 %	NR
Raj et al. [2]	24	63 %	21 (87.5 %)	NR	3 (12.5 %)	NR	NR
Shokeir et al. [27]	45	62 %	82 %	12 (35.3 %)	6 (13.3 %)	19	NR
Gupta et al. [33]	37	33 (89.2 %)	NR	NR	3 (8.1 %)	NR	NR
Rana and Bhojwani [34]	10	9 (90 %)	6 (60 %)	4 (40 %)	NR	NR	NR
Skolarikos et al. [35]	58	100 %	65.5 %	NR	NR	NR	91 %

N number of PNL procedures, *NR* not reported
[a]Additional references for the table [32–34]

procedures in this subgroup of abnormal kidneys. This was very helpful to avoid unnecessary cyst puncture and dilation [9]. The hydrophilic-coated glidewires with a J-tip are used to negotiate the tall, narrow, and compressed caliceal neck. This will facilitate proper placement of the Teflon-coated guidewire with a J-tip without trauma to the pelvicaliceal system. The presence of multiple or large cysts causing significant narrowing of the targeted calyx could affect the approach and increase the risk of bleeding if forcible dilation is tried. In such circumstances, another wider calyx could be punctured to access most of the stone bulk and handle the remaining parts by flexible nephroscope or SWL. Therefore, the compressive effect of the cysts might be more important than the size of the cysts and their location to the target calyx. A supracostal approach may be used to achieve access in some cases [9].

Results of PNL in ADPKD

Percutaneous nephrolithotomy is a safe and effective method for the treatment of patients with autosomal dominant polycystic kidney disease and associated upper urinary tract stones. Multiple punctures may be required to make the kidney clear of stones. Also, cyst aspiration may be necessary in such cases with ADPKD if a relatively large cyst comes in the way of the puncture (reported in 5–45.5 % of cases). The overall success rate of PNL in patients with ADPKD ranges between 82 and 89.4 % with auxiliary procedures needed in 15–18 % of cases [9, 30, 37, 42–44].

Complications of PNL in ADPKD

There is no reported deleterious effect of the induced renal trauma from PNL on the renal function in patients with ADPKD, even significant improvement in the patient presented with azotemia and obstructive anuria. Generally, the incidence of complications during PNL in ADPKD has been reported in about 15 % of procedures, and the incidence of major complications does not increase in this cohort with ADPKD when compared with patients harboring normal kidneys. Acute bleeding requiring blood transfusion during or after PNL varies from 0 to 17.5 % [9, 30, 37, 42–44].

Conclusion

Percutaneous nephrolithotomy in patients with congenital and acquired renal anomalies like horseshoe kidney and adult polycystic kidneys, respectively, requires proper planning and respect of anatomical differences. PNL should be considered the treatment of choice for large kidney stones in these patients due to excellent outcomes and minimal complications. It is recommended that these procedures be done by a more experienced endourologist.

References

1. Yohannes A, Smith A. The endourological management of complications associated with horseshoe kidney. J Urol. 2002;168:5–8.
2. Raj G, Auge B, Weizer A, et al. Percutaneous management of calculi within horseshoe kidneys. J Urol. 2003;170:48–51.
3. Smith J, Van Arsdalen K, Hanno P, et al. Extracorporeal shock wave lithotripsy treatment of calculi in horseshoe kidneys. J Urol. 1989;142:683–6.
4. Torres V, Erickson S, Smith L, et al. The association of nephrolithiasis and autosomal dominant polycystic kidney disease. Am J Kidney Dis. 1988;11:318–25.
5. Torres V, Wilson D, Hattery R, et al. Renal stone disease in autosomal dominant polycystic kidney disease. Am J Kidney Dis. 1993;22:513–9.
6. Dimitrakov D, Simeonov S. Studies on nephrolithiasis in patients with autosomal dominant polycystic kidney disease. Folia Med. 1994;436:27–30.
7. Grampsas S, Chandhoke P, Fan J, et al. Anatomic and metabolic risk factors for nephrolithiasis in patients with autosomal dominant polycystic kidney disease. Am J Kidney Dis. 2000;36:53–7.
8. Ng C, Yost A, Streem S. Nephrolithiasis associated with autosomal dominant polycystic kidney disease: contemporary urological management. J Urol. 2000; 163:726–9.
9. Al-Kandari A, Shoma A, Eraky I, et al. Percutaneous nephrolithotomy for management of upper urinary tract calculi in patients with autosomal dominant polycystic kidney disease. Urology. 2009;74:273–7.
10. Nishiura J, Neves R, Eloi S, et al. Evaluation of nephrolithiasis in autosomal dominant polycystic

kidney disease patients. Clin J Am Soc Nephrol. 2009;4:838–44.
11. Baskin L, Floth A, Stoller M. The horseshoe kidney: therapeutic considerations with urolithiasis. J Endourol. 1989;3:51–4.
12. Clayman R. Effectiveness of extracorporeal shockwave lithotripsy in the management of stone-bearing horseshoe kidneys. J Urol. 1998;160:1949.
13. Gallucci M, Vincenzoni A, Schettini M, et al. Extracorporeal shock wave lithotripsy in ureteral and kidney malformations. Urol Int. 2001;66:61–5.
14. Gonzalez Enguita C, Calahorra Fernandez F, Cabrera Perez J, et al. Surgery of renoureteral lithiasis. Current indications. Actas Urol Esp. 2001;25:610–7.
15. Amar A, Das S, Egan R. Management of urinary calculus disease in patients with renal cysts: review of 12 years of experience in 18 patients. J Urol. 1981; 125:153–6.
16. Martinez Sarmiento M, Broseta R, Sanz Chinesta S, et al. Extracorporeal shock-wave lithotripsy in polycystic kidneys. Actas Urol Esp. 1994;18:35–8.
17. Delakas D, Daskalopoulos G, Cranidis A. Extracorporeal shock wave lithotripsy for urinary calculi in autosomal dominant polycystic kidney disease. J Endourol. 1997;11:167–70.
18. Kirkali Z, Esen A, Mungan M. Effectiveness of extracorporeal shockwave lithotripsy in the management of stone-bearing horseshoe kidneys. J Endourol. 1996;10:13–5.
19. Sheir K, Madbouly K, Elsobky E, et al. Extracorporeal shock wave lithotripsy in anomalous kidneys: 11-year experience with two second-generation lithotripters. Urology. 2003;62:10–6.
20. Tunc L, Tokgoz H, Tan M, et al. Stones in anomalous kidneys: results of treatment by shock wave lithotripsy in 150 patients. Int J Urol. 2004;11:831–6.
21. Cass A. Extracorporeal shock wave lithotripsy for renal stones with renal cysts present. J Urol. 1995; 153:599–601.
22. Deliveliotis C, Argiropoulos V, Varkarakis J, et al. Extracorporeal shock wave lithotripsy produces a lower stone-free rate in patients with stones and renal cysts. Int J Urol. 2002;9:11–4.
23. Andreoni C, Portis A, Clayman R. Retrograde renal pelvic access sheath to facilitate flexible ureteroscopic lithotripsy for the treatment of urolithiasis in a horseshoe kidney. J Urol. 2000;164:1290–1.
24. Weizer A, Springhart W, Ekeruo W, et al. Ureteroscopic management of renal calculi in anomalous kidneys. Urology. 2005;65:259–65.
25. Kuo R, Lingeman J, Leveillee R, et al. Lower pole II: initial results from a comparison of shock wave lithotripsy (SWL), ureteroscopy (URS), and percutaneous nephrostolithotomy (PNL) for lower pole nephrolithiasis. J Urol. 2003;169:486.
26. Janetschek G, Kunzel K. Percutaneous nephrolithotomy in horseshoe kidneys: applied anatomy and clinical experience. Br J Urol. 1988;62:117–22.
27. Shokeir A, El-Nahas A, Shoma A, et al. Percutaneous nephrolithotomy in treatment of large stones within horseshoe kidneys. Urology. 2004;64:426–9.
28. Munver R, Delvecchio F, Newman G, et al. Critical analysis of supracostal access for percutaneous renal surgery. J Urol. 2001;166:1242–6.
29. Al-Otaibi K, Hosking D. Percutaneous stone removal in horseshoe kidneys. J Urol. 1999;162:674–7.
30. Jones DJ, Wickham JEA, Kellett MJ. Percutaneous nephrolithotomy for calculi in horseshoe kidneys. J Urol. 1991;145:481–3.
31. Lampel A, Hohenfellner M, Schultz-Lampel D, et al. Urolithiasis in horseshoe kidneys: therapeutic management. Urology. 1996;47:182–6.
32. Lingeman J, Saw K. Percutaneous operative procedures in horseshoe kidneys. J Urol Suppl. 1999;161:371, abstract 1436.
33. Gupta N, Mishra S, Seth A, et al. Percutaneous nephrolithotomy in abnormal kidneys: single-center experience. Urology. 2009;73:710–5.
34. Rana A, Bhojwani J. Percutaneous nephrolithotomy in renal anomalies of fusion, ectopia, rotation, hypoplasia, and pelvicalyceal aberration: uniformity in heterogeneity. J Endourol. 2009;23:609–15.
35. Skolarikos A, Binbay M, Bisas A, et al. Percutaneous nephrolithotomy in horseshoe kidneys: factors affecting stone-free rate. J Urol. 2001;186:1894–8.
36. Segura J, Patterson D, Le Roy A, et al. Percutaneous removal of kidney stones: review of 1000 cases. J Urol. 1985;134:1077–81.
37. El-Kenawy M, El-Kappany H, El-Diasty T, et al. Percutaneous nephrolithotomy for renal stones in over 1000 cases. Br J Urol. 1992;69:470–5.
38. Gerspach J, Bellman G, Stoller M, et al. Conservative management of colon injury following percutaneous renal surgery. Urology. 1997;49:831–6.
39. El-Nahas A, Shokeir A, El-assmy A, et al. Colonic perforation during percutaneous nephrolithotomy: study of risk factors. Urology. 2006;67:937–41.
40. Skoog S, Reed M, Gaudier F, et al. The posterolateral and the retrorenal colon: implication in percutaneous stone extraction. J Urol. 1985;134:110–2.
41. Goswami A, Shrivastava P, Mukherjee A, et al. Management of colonic perforation during percutaneous nephrolithotomy in horseshoe kidney. J Endourol. 2001;15:989–91.
42. Aron M, Yadav R, Goel R, et al. Multi-tract percutaneous nephrolithotomy for large complete staghorn calculi. Urol Int. 2005;75:327–32.
43. Michel M, Trojan L, Rassweiler J. Complications in percutaneous nephrolithotomy. Eur Urol. 2007;51: 899–906.
44. Umbreit E, Childs M, Patterson D, et al. Percutaneous nephrolithotomy for large or multiple upper tract calculi and autosomal dominant polycystic kidney disease. J Urol. 2010;183:183–7.

Drainage Systems After Percutanous Renal Procedures

13

Brian Duty, Zhamshid Okhunov, Arthur D. Smith, and Zeph Okeke

Introduction

Goodwin and colleagues first described percutaneous renal access in 1955 to provide drainage in select patients with hydronephrosis [1]. This was accomplished by placement of a large finder needle into the renal pelvis followed by insertion of plastic tubing into the collecting system. The initial use of percutaneous renal access to treat urolithiasis was reported in three patients by Fernstrom and Johansson in 1976 [2]. Numerous modifications in technique and equipment have transpired, ultimately resulting in percutaneous nephrolithotomy (PCNL) becoming the treatment modality of choice for staghorn calculi and large, complex renal stones [3].

Despite the passage of more than three decades since its inception, optimal handling of the nephrostomy access tract after percutaneous renal procedures continues to be debated. The following chapter will review the myriad exit strategies available to urologists after PCNL. These include utilization of a nephrostomy tube, ureteral stent without nephrostomy tube (aka "tubeless"), or neither nephrostomy tube nor ureteral stent (aka "totally tubeless"). Potential benefits and disadvantages of each technique will be discussed followed by a review of pertinent clinical studies.

Utility of Nephrostomy Tube Drainage

A percutaneous nephrostomy tube has traditionally been placed at the conclusion of the case to drain the collecting system, tamponade the access tract, and maintain renal access. Theoretically, nephrostomy tube drainage minimizes urine extravasation from the access tract or unintentional collecting system perforations until perioperative inflammation has subsided, residual stone fragments have been cleared, and collecting system blood clots have lysed.

Proponents of nephrostomy tube placement argue that it also tamponades the access tract, thereby reducing the risk of perioperative hemorrhage. However, following the introduction of the tubeless PCNL in 1997, an increasing number of series has been published, which demonstrate minimal risk of bleeding in properly selected cases.

Approximately 20 % of patients will have residual stone fragments following PCNL for staghorn calculi [3]. Once felt to be "clinically insignificant," Streem showed that residual fragments will grow in 18 % of patients and 43 % will experience a symptomatic episode, many requiring an intervention [4]. Therefore, maintaining renal access via a nephrostomy tube is an attractive option in patients with staghorn calculi

B. Duty, M.D. (✉) • Z. Okhunov, M.D.
A.D. Smith, M.D. • Z. Okeke, M.D.
Department of Urology, Smith Institute for Urology, Hofstra North Shore – Long Island Jewish Health System, 450 Lakeville Road, New Hyde Park, NY, 11042, USA
e-mail: bduty@nshs.edu; zho0616@gmail.com; asmith1@nshs.edu; zokeke@nshs.edu

A.M. Al-Kandari et al. (eds.), *Difficult Cases in Endourology*,
DOI 10.1007/978-1-84882-083-8_13, © Springer-Verlag London 2013

or complex stones who may require a two-stage procedure to be rendered stone-free.

Types of Percutaneous Nephrostomy Tubes

A wide variety of catheters have been designed or may be adapted to drain the collecting system following PCNL. The ideal nephrostomy tube would be 100 % biocompatible, robust, resistant to obstruction and migration, and simple to place and remove. Unfortunately, no nephrostomy tube perfectly embodies all of these attributes. Each has its own set of pros and cons that must be considered when choosing a drainage tube.

General Considerations

Collecting system drainage is needed for only a short period of time in most instances, making biocompatibility a minor issue. However, biocompatibility is an important variable in cases with collecting system perforation, upper tract transitional cell carcinoma, or antegrade endopyelotomy, which require longer drainage. A variety of tube materials are available, which include silicone, polyurethane, Silitek™ (Medical Engineering Corp, Racine, WI), C-flex™ (Saint-Gobain Performance Plastics, Valley Forge, PA), and Percuflex™ (Boston Scientific Corp, Natick, MA).

Silicone has poor mechanical strength but maintains its flexibility. In contrast, polyurethane has good mechanical strength but loses its flexibility and is more likely to cause epithelial ulcerations [5]. The newer polymers, Silitek, C-flex, and Percuflex, are stronger and maintain their flexibility. Of these agents, Silitek was found to cause the greatest amount of mucosal edema [6]. A study by Tunney and colleagues found silicone to be most resistant to struvite encrustation followed by polyurethane, Silitek, Percuflex, and C-flex [7].

Nephrostomy tubes range in size from 5 to 32 F. Larger tubes are less likely to become obstructed by blood clots and stone fragments but have been shown to be less comfortable for patients, especially if adjacent to a rib [8]. Inadvertent nephrostomy tube displacement is a common problem. Tubes that do not have components extending into the ureter are more likely to be dislodged. However, a ureteral component can be a significant source of patient discomfort and irritative voiding symptoms. Securing the tube to the skin in morbidly obese patients may cause premature displacement due to movement of the patient's panus.

Pigtail Nephrostomy Tubes

Pigtail catheters vary from 5 to 14 F in size and come with and without a nylon retention string. Pigtail catheters lacking a retention string maintain their shape via the tube's inherent memory. While less complicated to place and remove, this variety of pigtail catheter is more likely to be inadvertently pulled out of the collecting system.

The most commonly used pigtail catheter with a locking mechanism is the Cope loop catheter (Cook Medical, Bloomington, IN). These catheters are made of polyurethane and come in sizes measuring 8.2–14 F and are 19.5 cm in length. Drainage is aided by a series of 15-gauge side holes. The catheter tip is connected to the last side hole via a nylon string that when placed on tension secures the catheter into a pigtail configuration to prevent dislocation. To remove the tube, the nylon string is simply taken off tension or the catheter is transected.

In general, pigtail catheters are well tolerated because of their relatively small size. This makes them ideal for pediatric patients and when long-term access is required (can stay in up to 4 months). However, their 15-G side holes are small, predisposing them to occlusion by stone debris and blood clots. Additionally, if significant bleeding is encountered during a case, the smaller size of these catheters may not effectively tamponade the access tract resulting in continued hemorrhage. Failure to release the locking mechanism prior to nephrostomy tube removal may result in parenchymal laceration and subsequent bleeding. Lastly, these tubes are difficult to place in small, nondilated collecting systems because there is not ample room to deploy the loop.

Balloon Retention Catheters

Foley, Council, and Couvelaire tip catheters are all examples of balloon retention catheters that may be utilized for collecting system drainage. They come in a variety of sizes (12–32 F), materials (latex, silastic), balloon sizes (5, 30 cc), and manufactures. Council tip catheters, which are available in sizes of 16 F or larger, are commonly used because collecting system access can be readily regained through the catheter's distal opening. Foley and Couvelaire tip catheters can be modified with either a hole punch or 14-G needle to create an opening at the catheter tip.

All three types of catheters provide large-bore drainage and are therefore appropriate in cases with substantial bleeding and/or collecting system perforation. The Couvelaire tip catheter is particularly well suited in cases with marked bleeding. Additionally, these catheters may be positioned across a stenotic infundibulum following dilation or within an ablated caliceal diverticulum.

Balloon retention catheters have several disadvantages. They lack a ureteral component predisposing them to dislodgement. The retention balloon may cause caliceal obstruction and discomfort, even in the absence of obstruction.

A type of balloon catheter that deserves special attention is the Kaye nephrostomy tamponade balloon catheter (Cook Medical, Bloomington, IN). The Kaye nephrostomy tube has a 15-cm balloon that can be inflated up to 36 F, thereby draining the collecting system while compressing the access tract. This catheter is usually reserved for cases with significant intraoperative bleeding [9].

Malecot Tubes

Malecot catheters come in a wide array of sizes (10–40 F) and are manufactured by various companies. Like the balloon retention catheters, the larger Malecot tubes provide excellent drainage of blood and stone fragments while having a built-in retention mechanism. The mushroom-style tip is less apt to cause caliceal obstruction but is more likely to become dislodged, especially in obese patients.

The reentry nephrostomy catheter (Boston Scientific, Natick, MA) is a specialized Malecot catheter made of C-flex that contains a ureteral extension [10]. The Malecot portion of the catheter is manufactured in sizes ranging from 14 to 24 F. The distal ureteral component is 17 or 18 cm in length and 6 or 8 F in diameter.

While also providing large-bore drainage of the collecting system, the reentry catheter has several advantages over standard Malecot nephrostomy tubes. The ureteral component makes displacement much less likely. By preserving ureteral access, the reentry catheter can be easily replaced should bleeding from the percutaneous access tract be noted during nephrostomy tube removal.

The catheter is ideal in complex percutaneous procedures because the reentry tube provides excellent drainage of blood and stone fragments, thereby effectively decompressing the collecting system while providing stable access. Therefore, the Malecot reentry tube should be considered in cases involving multiple punctures, moderate to severe bleeding, a large amount of residual stone debris, collecting system perforation, and staged procedures.

Endopyelotomy Stents

Percutaneous endopyelotomy stents are similar to their internal counterparts, but rather than having a proximal retention curl, they exit the access tract. These specialized nephrostomy tubes provide simultaneous wide-diameter stenting of the ureteropelvic junction/proximal ureter with externalized collecting system drainage. Their distal component tapers to a smaller diameter to prevent ureteral ischemia. They are made by multiple manufactures and come in a variety of materials (polyurethane, Percuflex, C-flex, or silicone) and sizes (proximal component 10–22 F, distal component 4.7–8.2 F).

Not surprisingly, percutaneous endopyelotomy stents provide ideal drainage following antegrade endopyelotomy. They should be considered following PCNL cases with significant UPJ trauma/inflammation and procedures requiring treatment of impacted proximal ureteral stones.

Once maximal drainage is no longer needed, the tube can be capped. This allows the ureter to remain stented while obviating the need for external drainage equipment. Should the patient develop worsening flank pain, fever, or drainage around the tube, it can be placed back to gravity drainage.

Paul and Lee reported a unique indication for this type of nephrostomy tube in patients with bladder outlet obstruction [11]. Because the ureteral component extends into the bladder, urine will reflux into the ipsilateral collecting system. As a result, patients with urinary retention following surgery may be managed by leaving the nephrostomy tube to drainage until they can void spontaneously. This avoids the need for continued Foley catheterization in patients at high risk of perioperative urinary retention.

Patients requiring stenting of the UPJ for 4–6 weeks may find the external component more uncomfortable than an internal endopyelotomy stent. Skin breakdown and irritation at the exit site is another potential disadvantage of percutaneous endopyelotomy nephrostomy tubes.

An alternative to the percutaneous endopyelotomy tube is simultaneous placement of a nephrostomy tube and endopyelotomy stent. This approach has several disadvantages as well. Discontinuing the nephrostomy tube requires fluoroscopy because the retention curls can become interlocked within the renal pelvis resulting in inadvertent endopyelotomy stent removal when pulling out the nephrostomy tube. A second procedure, cystoscopy, is required to remove the endopyelotomy stent. Lastly, endopyelotomy stents are more prone to migration than the percutaneous variety.

Circle Catheter

The circle, or loop, nephrostomy catheter is inserted through one percutaneous tract and exits via another. Circle tubes are made of silicone and come in sizes ranging from 12 to 22 F. The use of this type of nephrostomy tube was first reported in 1979 [12]. Their silicone design makes them relatively resistant to encrustation, allowing for less frequent tube changes. Unlike most other types of nephrostomy tubes, they can be used without difficulty in small, nonhydronephrotic collecting systems. Furthermore, circle catheters provide the best collecting system drainage of any nephrostomy tube because the number and location of the side holes can be tailored to the collecting system anatomy, thereby preventing caliceal obstruction. These catheters are ideal in cases with multiple access tracts.

Impact of Nephrostomy Tube Size

Case Series

Percutaneous nephrolithotomy has been traditionally performed via a 30-F access sheath. In an effort to reduce patient discomfort and decrease the risk of bleeding, Jackman and colleagues introduced the "mini-perc" technique [13]. This initial study was performed via a 13-F ureteroscope sheath in nine patients with an average stone area of 1.5 cm^2. There were no complications and the stone-free rate was 89 %.

Multiple case series have subsequently been published using access sheaths ranging from 13 to 20 F in size [14–16]. These series treated up to 21 patients, with mean stone areas ranging from 1.4 to 2.8 cm^2. Stone-free rates were between 90 and 94 %. Two patients were converted to a 26-F access tract, and one required a transfusion. Only one study objectively addressed postoperative pain following surgery.

The largest series to date included an impressive 4,760 procedures in 3,610 kidneys [17]. Staghorn stones were present in 1,240 kidneys. Lithotripsy was performed via a 20-F access sheath with either a semirigid or flexible ureteroscope. Following stone extraction, a 4.8-F double-J stent was placed along with a nephrostomy tube of the same size. The mean time to nephrostomy tube removal was 6.8 days, and the average hospital stay was 8.5 days. Multiple treatment sessions were employed in 30.3 %. The stone-free rate at postoperative day 2 was 89 %. Significant complications were encountered in only 31 patients (0.86 %), of which only 3 encountered severe bleeding.

These studies have reported stone-free rates comparable to standard PCNL. However, their results should be interpreted with caution. With the exception of the Chinese series [17], the studies included few patients with small stone burdens. More importantly, control populations were not utilized.

Comparative Series

Multiple prospective studies have been published comparing various types and sizes of nephrostomy tubes. Maheshwari managed 40 PCNL patients with either a 28-F end-hole catheter or a 9-F pigtail catheter [8]. The 20 patients in each group had comparable stone burdens. Patients receiving a pigtail catheter required significantly less parenteral narcotics and leaked urine from the access tract for a shorter period of time. Neither group required a transfusion.

In a similar study, 60 patients were randomized to either a 24-F reentry tube, an 8-F pigtail catheter, or a double-J ureteral stent [18]. The stented patients had an 18-F balloon tip catheter that was removed on the morning of postoperative day 1. Like the Maheshwari study, there was no difference in complication rates, but there was a "strong trend to less postoperative leakage" in the pigtail group compared to the patients receiving reentry tubes. In contrast to the prior study, there was no difference in analog pain scores or narcotic usage between the groups.

The same institution randomized 40 patients to either a reentry catheter or a 7-F single-J stent (bladder component of stent tapered to 3 F without a curl) with an 18-F Council nephrostomy tube [19]. Patients receiving the 18-F Council tip catheter and stent had significantly less flank drainage and less pain on an analog scale. Although not significant, there was a trend towards improved quality of life in the stented cohort as well ($p=0.09$). This group did require an additional procedure, cystoscopy, 1 week after surgery to remove the stent.

Lastly, Pietrow and associates randomized 30 patients to either a 10-F pigtail or 22-F Council tip catheter [20]. Like the previous studies, there was no difference in blood loss between the two groups. The pigtail cohort reported significantly less pain 6 h after surgery, but there was no difference beyond this time period.

In summary, the prospective randomized studies evaluating nephrostomy tube type and size have all been hampered by small sample size. Nonetheless, these studies consistently showed less tract drainage following nephrostomy removal in patients managed with smaller tubes. Although not uniformly demonstrated, patients with smaller nephrostomy tubes tended to have less postoperative discomfort. It does not appear that the size or type of nephrostomy tube impacts access tract bleeding.

Tubeless (Stented) Percutaneous Nephrolithotomy

Background

In 1984, Wickham et al. reported 250 PCNL cases [21]. The authors concluded that in select cases the access tract could be managed without a nephrostomy tube. However, 2 years later, Winfield and associates described two cases of "marked discomfort" and prolonged hospitalization attributed to not leaving a nephrostomy tube following PCNL [22].

Nephrostomy drainage subsequently became the accepted means of tract management and was not challenged until Bellman and colleagues reported 50 patients who underwent tubeless percutaneous renal surgery [23]. All 50 patients had double-J ureteral stents placed. The initial 30 patients were also managed with a Council nephrostomy tube that was removed 2–3 h after surgery. The authors showed a significant decrease in length of stay (0.6 vs. 4.6 days, $p=0.0001$), intramuscular analgesia requirement ($p=0.0001$), length of oral analgesia treatment

(5.9 vs. 11.7 days, $p = 0.0001$), and quicker return to normal activity (17.9 vs. 26.6 days, $p = 0.0004$) in the tubeless, stented group compared to a matched nephrostomy tube cohort. Additionally, they reported saving over $2000 per case in the tubeless, stented group without an increased complication rate.

Subsequent publications have validated tubeless, stented PCNL as a viable option in select patients [24–27]. This approach was initially considered only in patients with a single access tract, no significant bleeding, no evidence of collecting system perforation, and no suspicion of residual stone fragments. Over time, the indications for tubeless, stented PCNL have expanded to include patients with morbid obesity and those undergoing bilateral procedures [28, 29]. An alternative to this tubeless approach involves leaving an externalized ureteral catheter in place at the conclusion of the procedure [30]. If the patient's postoperative course is uncomplicated, the ureteral catheter is removed on postoperative day 1 and the patient is discharged home, thereby avoiding the morbidity in indwelling ureteral stent.

Randomized Studies

The earliest prospective study evaluating tubeless, stented PCNL was published by Feng et al. [31]. Thirty patients were randomized to receive a 22-F reentry nephrostomy tube (34-F tract), 22-F reentry tube (26-F tract), or double-J ureteral stent without nephrostomy tube (34-F tract). The tubeless, stented cohort was found to have a shorter length of stay, require less morphine, and had fewer procedural costs compared to both nephrostomy tube groups. However, there was no difference in postoperative pain between the three groups 1 week after surgery. None of the clinical endpoints differed between the standard PCNL (34-F tract) and "mini-perc" (26-F tract) nephrostomy tube groups.

A similar study was performed in 30 patients who were treated via a 30-F access tract and were then randomized to a "standard" 20-F nephrostomy tube, 9-F pigtail catheter, or 6-F double-J ureteral stent [32]. The stented, tubeless group had significantly less urinary leakage from the access site than either nephrostomy tube group and required less analgesic than the 20-F nephrostomy tube group. The pigtail group also had significantly less pain compared to the conventional nephrostomy tube patients. There was no difference in complications between the three groups.

Small-bore nephrostomy tube drainage compared to a tubeless, stented approach was further evaluated by Shah et al. in 65 patients [33]. Patients were randomized to receive either an 8-F pigtail nephrostomy tube or 6-F double-J ureteral stent. In contrast to the prior study, the tubeless group experienced significantly less pain and required less analgesia. Like the prior study, the tubeless group had a shorter length of stay. These results were confirmed in a study of 202 patients randomized to either a 16-F nephrostomy tube or 6-F ureteral stent [34].

Gonen and colleagues compared stented, tubeless PCNL to tubeless stone extraction with perioperative externalized ureteral catheter utilization in 46 patients [35]. Patient demographics, stone burden, operative time, number of access tracts, analgesia requirements, hospital length of stay, and complication rate did not differ between the two groups. Not surprisingly, the stented group complained of significantly more stent-related symptoms, which were mild in the majority of patients. However, two patients required the use of anticholinergic medications.

The majority of randomized studies published on tubeless, stented PCNL have concluded that in select patients it is safe to forgo nephrostomy tube drainage. Furthermore, ureteral stent morbidity appears to be superseded by increased perioperative pain and length of hospital stay in patients managed with both large- and small-bore nephrostomy tubes.

Totally Tubeless Percutaneous Nephrolithotomy

The tubeless, stented PCNL technique has several disadvantages. First, it requires a second procedure, flexible cystoscopy, to remove the ureteral stent. Second, many patients report significant discomfort and irritative voiding symptoms from ureteral stents. To avoid stent and nephrostomy tube morbidity, the feasibility of a "totally tubeless" PCNL was investigated.

Karmai and Gholamrezie published one of the earliest totally tubeless PCNL series in 30 patients [36]. The average lengths of stay and time to recovery of normal activities were 1.5 and 7 days, respectively. Their stone-free rate was 90 % with only two complications (two urinary tract infections). Abdominal ultrasonography was performed 24 h after surgery to rule out a perinephric fluid collection, which was not found in any patient. No patient required a transfusion.

Crook and colleagues subsequently published a series of 100 patients undergoing totally tubeless PCNL over a 10-year period [37]. Their stone-free rate was identical to the Karmai and Gholamrezie study. However, their length of stay was longer at 2.9 days. One patient required a blood transfusion and their overall complication rate was 6 %.

Several prospective totally tubeless PCNL studies have been performed. Kara et al. randomized 30 patients to a totally tubeless approach and 30 patients to an 18-F nephrostomy tube [38]. The length of stay was significantly shorter in the tubeless group (1.5 vs. 3.2 days, $p<0.001$) as well as the analgesia requirement ($p<0.01$). There was no difference in the complication rate, and no transfusions were needed among the 60 patients.

Although not randomized, Mandhani and colleagues prospectively evaluated 25 patients who underwent a tubeless, stented PCNL and 27 patients treated with a totally tubeless stone extraction [39]. There was no difference in length of stay or pain medication requirement between the two groups. Of note, three patients in the stent group had severe irritative symptoms, necessitating early removal of the double-J stent in one patient. The authors concluded that totally tubeless PCNL is as safe as the stented approach and avoids the added morbidity of a ureteral stent.

At present, the feasibility of the totally tubeless technique has been demonstrated in multiple small case series and several randomized studies. However, the small sample size of these studies and the risk of postoperative collecting system obstruction from blood clots and stone debris have prevented its widespread adoption.

Sealants and Other Novel Tract Treatments

A variety of adjuvant treatments have been employed to prevent bleeding from the access tract following percutaneous renal surgery. These include the use of hemostatic agents, electrocautery, and cryotherapy.

Gelatin matrix hemostatic sealant (FloSeal®, Baxter Medical, Fremont, CA) is an agent composed of bovine collagen and pooled human thrombin that in the presence of fibrinogen promotes hemostasis. The University of California, Irvine, first reported the use of FloSeal in two patients undergoing tubeless, stented PCNL [40]. Prior to FloSeal application, a ureteral occlusion catheter was inflated within the tract's adjoining calyx to prevent passage of the gelatin matrix particles into the collecting system, given the potential risk of obstruction [41]. The authors then compared ten patients treated with FloSeal to ten cases managed with a 10-F Cope loop [42]. There was no significant difference in blood loss.

Tisseel® (Baxter Healthcare, Westlake Village, CA) is composed of four products: vapor heat-treated human pooled plasma thrombin, fibrinogen, a synthetic antifibrinolytic aprotinin, and calcium chloride. It has both hemostatic and adhesive properties. Noller and colleagues evaluated the use of Tisseel in tubeless, stented PCNL [43]. Two milliliter of Tisseel was injected into the access tract without the use of an occlusion balloon in ten patients. The mean intraoperative change in hematocrit was 2.8 %. No transfusions were required. None of the patients developed urinary obstruction or a perinephric fluid collection. There was no control group.

A study out of Kaiser Permanente, Los Angeles, retrospectively compared 20 patients who underwent tubeless, stented PCNL with Tisseel to 23 cases without tract treatment [44].

The Tisseel group had a significantly shorter hospital stay (1.14 vs. 1.85 days, $p=0.019$). There was no difference in blood loss, analgesia use, or complications between the two groups.

Shah et al. performed a randomized, prospective study of Tisseel use in 63 patients undergoing tubeless, stented PCNL [45]. The two groups did not differ with regard to blood loss, length of stay, or complications, but the Tisseel group had significantly less pain ($p=0.003$) and required less analgesia ($p=0.021$). The authors postulated that tract treatment minimizes the accumulation of blood and urine within the retroperitoneum resulting in less pain. However, no imaging data was presented to support this theory.

Jou and colleagues utilized an elongated electrode probe to cauterize the access tract in 249 patients undergoing PCNL [46]. These patients were compared to 108 whose tract was not treated with electrocautery. Of the 249 electrocautery patients, 84 were managed with only a double-J ureteral stent. The remaining patients had a nephrostomy tube placed due to bleeding. The transfusion rate was significantly less in the cautery group (1.2 vs. 6.5 %, $p=0.014$).

Finally, cryotherapy has also been evaluated [47]. In this retrospective study, 30 patients underwent cryoablation of the nephrostomy tract and 31 did not. Cryoablation was performed via a 2.4-mm cryoprobe and a single 10-min freeze-thaw cycle. The cryotherapy group was managed with a double-J ureteral stent, while the control group received a 24-F reentry catheter. The mean operative time was longer in the cryotherapy group (123.9 vs. 95.2 min, $p=0.02$), but their length of stay was shorter (2.1 vs. 3.6 days, $p = 0.001$) and they had a lower incidence of delayed bleeding requiring embolization (3 vs. 13 %, $p=0.001$). The length of stay should be interpreted with caution though. The difference may have been due to the tubeless approach in the experimental group, rather than from tract cryoablation.

Conclusion

Nephrostomy tubes come in a wide array of designs and have traditionally been used following percutaneous renal procedures to tamponade the access tract, maximize collecting system drainage, and maintain access. Numerous studies have shown the feasibility of the tubeless, stented PCNL in uncomplicated cases, which minimizes patient discomfort, decreases length of stay, and leads to earlier return of normal activity. Totally tubeless PCNL has been reported but has not gained widespread acceptance given the risk of postoperative obstruction from blood clots and stone debris. Multiple institutions have evaluated the use of hemostatic agents and electrocautery to facilitate tubeless PCNL. However, their efficacy and cost-effectiveness have not been unequivocally demonstrated.

References

1. Goodwin WE, Casey WC, Woolf W. Percutaneous trocar (needle) nephrostomy in hydronephrosis. J Am Med Assoc. 1955;157:891–4.
2. Fernstrom I, Johansson B. Percutaneous pyelolithotomy. A new extraction technique. Scand J Urol Nephrol. 1976;10:257–9.
3. Preminger GM, Assimos DG, Lingeman JE, et al. AUA guideline on management of staghorn calculi: diagnosis and treatment recommendations. J Urol. 2005;173:1991–2000.
4. Streem SB, Yost A, Mascha E. Clinical implications of clinically insignificant stone fragments after extracorporeal shock wave lithotripsy. J Urol. 1996;155:1186–90.
5. Watson G. Problems with double-J stents and nephrostomy tubes. J Endourol. 1997;11:413–7.
6. Marx M, Bettman MA, Bridge S, et al. The effects of various indwelling ureteral catheter materials on the normal canine ureter. J Urol. 1988;139:180–5.
7. Tunney MM, Keane PF, Jones DS, et al. Comparative assessment of ureteral stent biomaterial encrustation. Biomaterials. 1996;17:1541–6.
8. Maheshwari PN, Andankar MG, Bansal M. Nephrostomy tube after percutaneous nephrolithotomy: large-bore or pigtail catheter? J Endourol. 2000;14:735–8.
9. Kessaris DN, Bellman GC, Pardalidis NP, et al. Management of hemorrhage after percutaneous renal surgery. J Urol. 1995;153:604–8.
10. Khasidy LR, Smith AD. The re-entry nephrostomy catheter for endourological applications. J Urol. 1985;133:165–6.
11. Paul EM, Lee BR. The use of nephrostomy tract drainage for the treatment of bladder outlet obstruction. J Endourol. 2003;17:530.

12. Smith AD, Lange PH, Miller RP, et al. Percutaneous U-loop nephrostomy. J Urol. 1979;121:355–7.
13. Jackman SV, Docimo SG, Cadeddu JA, et al. The "mini-perc" technique: a less invasive alternative to percutaneous nephrolithotomy. World J Urol. 1998; 16:371–4.
14. Chan DY, Jarrett TW. Techniques in endourology: mini-percutaneous nephrolithotomy. J Endourol. 2000; 14:269–73.
15. Monga M, Oglevie S. Minipercutaneous nephrolithotomy. J Endourol. 2000;14:419–21.
16. Lahme S, Bichler KH, Strohmaier WL, et al. Minimally invasive PCNL in patients with renal pelvic and calyceal stones. Eur Urol. 2001;40:619–24.
17. Li X, He Z, Wu K, et al. Chinese minimally invasive percutaneous nephrolithotomy: the Guangzhou experience. J Endourol. 2009;23:1693–7.
18. Marcovich R, Jacobson AI, Singh J, et al. No panacea for drainage after percutaneous nephrolithotomy. J Endourol. 2004;18:743–7.
19. Liatsikos EN, Hom D, Dinlenc CZ, et al. Tail stent versus re-entry tube: a randomized comparison after percutaneous stone extraction. Urology. 2002;59:15–9.
20. Pietrow PK, Auge BK, Lallas CD, et al. Pain after percutaneous nephrolithotomy: impact of nephrostomy tube size. J Endourol. 2003;17:411–4.
21. Wickham JE, Miller RA, Kellett MJ, et al. Percutaneous nephrolithotomy: one stage or two? Br J Urol. 1984; 56:582–5.
22. Winfield HN, Weyman P, Clayman RV. Percutaneous nephrostolithotomy: complications of premature nephrostomy tube removal. J Urol. 1986;136:77–9.
23. Bellman GC, Davidoff R, Candela J, et al. Tubeless percutaneous renal surgery. J Urol. 1997;157: 1578–82.
24. Lojanapiwat B, Soonthornphan S, Wudhikarn S. Tubeless percutaneous nephrolithotomy in selected patients. J Endourol. 2001;15:711–3.
25. Limb J, Bellman GC. Tubeless percutaneous renal surgery: review of first 112 patients. Urology. 2002;59: 527–31.
26. Shah HN, Kausik VB, Hegde SS, Shah JN, Bansal MB. Tubeless percutaneous nephrolithotomy: a prospective feasibility study and review of previous reports. BJU Int. 2005;96:879–83.
27. Abou-Elela A, Emran A, Mohsen MA, et al. Safety and efficacy of tubeless percutaneous renal surgery. J Endourol. 2007;21:977–84.
28. Yang RM, Bellman GC. Tubeless percutaneous renal surgery in the obese patients. Urology. 2004;63: 1036–40.
29. Shah HN, Kausik VB, Hedge SS, et al. Safety and efficacy of bilateral simultaneous tubeless percutaneous nephrolithotomy. Urology. 2005;66:500–4.
30. Mouracade P, Spie R, Lang H, et al. Tubeless percutaneous nephrolithotomy: what about replacing the double-J stent with a ureteral catheter? J Endourol. 2008;22:273–5.
31. Feng MI, Tamaddon K, Mikhail A, et al. Prospective randomized study of various techniques of percutaneous nephrolithotomy. Urology. 2001;58:345–50.
32. Desai MR, Kukreja RA, Desai MM, et al. A prospective randomized comparison of type of nephrostomy drainage following percutaneous nephrostolithotomy: large bore versus small bore versus tubeless. J Urol. 2004;172:565–7.
33. Shah HN, Sodha HS, Khandkar AA, et al. A randomized trial evaluating type of nephrostomy drainage after percutaneous nephrolithotomy: small bore v tubeless. J Endourol. 2008;22:1433–9.
34. Agrawal MS, Agrawal M, Gupta A, et al. A randomized comparison of tubeless and standard percutaneous nephrolithotomy. J Endourol. 2008;22:439–42.
35. Gonen M, Ozturk B, Ozkardes H. Double-J stenting compared with one night externalized ureteral catheter placement in tubeless percutaneous nephrolithotomy. J Endourol. 2009;23:27–31.
36. Karami H, Gholamrezaie HR. Totally tubeless percutaneous nephrolithotomy in selected patients. J Endourol. 2004;18:475–6.
37. Crook TJ, Lockyer CR, Keoghane SR, et al. Totally tubeless percutaneous nephrolithotomy. J Endourol. 2008;22:267–71.
38. Kara C, Resorlu B, Bayindir M, et al. A randomized comparison of totally tubeless and standard percutaneous nephrolithotomy in elderly patients. Urology. 2010;76:289–93.
39. Mandhani A, Goyal R, Vijjan V, et al. Tubeless percutaneous nephrolithotomy – should a stent be an integral part? J Urol. 2007;178:921–4.
40. Lee DI, Uribe C, Eichel L, et al. Sealing percutaneous nephrolithotomy tracts with gelatin matrix hemostatic sealant: initial clinical use. J Urol. 2004;171:575–8.
41. Uribe CA, Eichel L, Khonsari S, et al. What happens to hemostatic agents in contact with urine? An in vitro study. J Endourol. 2005;19:312–7.
42. Borin JF, Sala LG, Eichel L, et al. Tubeless percutaneous nephrolithotomy using hemostatic gelatin matrix. J Endourol. 2005;19:614–7.
43. Noller MW, Baughman SM, Morey AF, et al. Fibrin sealant enables tubeless percutaneous stone surgery. J Urol. 2004;172:166–9.
44. Mikhail AA, Kaptein JS, Bellman GC. Use of fibrin glue in percutaneous nephrolithotomy. Urology. 2003;61:910–4.
45. Shah HN, Hegde S, Shah JN, et al. A prospective, randomized trial evaluating the safety and efficacy of fibrin sealant in tubeless percutaneous nephrolithotomy. J Urol. 2006;176:2488–92.
46. Jou YC, Cheng MC, Sheen JH, et al. Electrocauterization of bleeding points for percutaneous nephrolithotomy. Urology. 2004;64:443–6.
47. Srinavasan A, Andonian S, Shapiro E, et al. Cryotherapy of the nephrostomy tract decreases the risk of hemorrhage in percutaneous renal surgery. J Endourol. 2008;22 Suppl 1:A64.

Retrograde Nephrostomy Access: Overcoming the Difficulties

14

Khalid Matar Al-Otaibi

Introduction

Percutaneous access is the most important step in the entire procedure of the percutaneous renal surgery, and this is also the portion of the procedure most often feared and often relegated to interventional radiology colleagues.

Safe and reliable percutaneous access into the renal collecting systems is the initial and most important part of a successful percutaneous intrarenal surgical procedure. Improper percutaneous entry can lead to difficulty and complications, particularly bleeding.

In 1955, Goodwin and colleagues described the use of a needle to decompress and to temporarily relieve hydronephrosis [1]. Percutaneous nephrostomy was first performed in the late 1970s, in which the primary indication was limited to diversion of urine and medical therapy in poor surgical candidates with stone disease [2, 3]. In 1976, percutaneous nephrolithotomy replaced open surgery in the management of renal calculi when the removal of a renal calculus through a percutaneous nephrostomy was described [4].

One of the most technically demanding aspects of percutaneous nephrolithotomy is the establishment of a nephrostomy tract into an appropriate calyx. The challenge is dealing with difficult situations, as nondilated collecting system, obese patients, patients with previous renal surgery, patients with horseshoe kidneys, and patients with large or impacted calculi led to difficulty in passing the guidewire down the ureter once the collecting system has been punctured [2, 3, 5]. Several techniques have been described to establish access into the collecting system [6] including ureteroscopically assisted percutaneous access [7].

Retrograde techniques for establishing a percutaneous nephrostomy tract were first described in 1983 [8, 9]. Retrograde nephrostomy is safe and involves minimal radiation exposure to the urologist. It has a short learning curve with a simpler method of establishing a percutaneous nephrostomy tract for those who do not have expertise in establishing a nephrostomy tract using conventional antegrade methods [5].

Indications

Retrograde nephrostomy access has similar indication as the antegrade percutaneous access, particularly patients with nondilated collecting system and those patients with large calculi occupying most of the collecting system [10].

Retrograde access is useful in patient with ureteropelvic junction obstruction undergoing percutaneous endopyelotomy, where the upper or middle calyx is the prober site of access.

K.M. Al-Otaibi, MBBS, FRCSC
Department of Urology, University of Dammam,
P.O. Box 40292 Khobar, 31952, Saudi Arabia
e-mail: otaibikm@yahoo.com

A.M. Al-Kandari et al. (eds.), *Difficult Cases in Endourology*,
DOI 10.1007/978-1-84882-083-8_14, © Springer-Verlag London 2013

Retrograde access is not suitable in the presence of complete ureteric obstruction, and patients should have normal lower urinary tract where the ureteric catheterization is visible.

In children, the retrograde access technique is not suitable considering the size of the ureteral catheter (7.5 F) used in the technique.

Patient Preparation

All patients undergoing retrograde access technique should have intravenous pyelogram (IVP) or CT scanning with axial urography to display a good view of the renal anatomy and function [11]. CT scan is also indicated to avoid injury to adjacent intra-abdominal organs, for instance, in patients with splenomegaly, distended colon, and horseshoe kidneys [12].

In particular cases, the retrograde access might be challenging and difficult, for instance, in obese patients in whom the upper calyx is the most proper and shortest access, in patients with previous renal surgery, and in patients with horseshoe kidneys.

Preoperative Preparation

Evaluation of patients undergoing retrograde percutaneous access should include normal bleeding profile, avoidance of any anticoagulant medication for at least 10 days, and medical clearance for those patients with medical problems, and the patient should be free of any urinary tract infection. Preoperative antibiotics based on the sensitivities of the associated organisms are indicated in infected stone cases [5]. Prophylactic antibiotics are recommended in patients with sterile urine preoperatively [13–15].

Deep general anesthesia with endotracheal tube is recommended to ensure good ventilation of both lungs particularly during the change of the patient's position to prone position during the procedure.

This kind of procedure should be performed in a facility that has full anesthesia and that has surgical, angiographic, and resuscitation services immediately available [12].

Instrumentation and Techniques

The creation of a percutaneous access tract into the renal collecting system requires imaging equipment for guidance. C-arm configuration fluoroscopy equipment is essential in the operating room where the retrograde access technique and percutaneous renal surgery are performed in one sitting. Portable ultrasonography in the operating room provides an alternative guidance system for urinary tract interventions [16, 17]. Each imaging guidance has its limitation; therefore, the availability of all these imaging guidance technologies is necessary for the broad range application of percutaneous nephrostomy access.

The retrograde nephrostomy access technique was described initially by Lawson and Hunter [8, 13]. Hosking has shared his experience and described the technique in more details [5, 18].

All procedure steps are performed in the operating room under fluoroscopic control and under general anesthesia immediately prior to the percutaneous intrarenal surgery.

Most of the equipment required for the retrograde access technique is available in kit form (Cook Urological, Spencer, IN) [5]. The kit used for this procedure (the Lawson-1 kit, 08700, Cook Urological) contains the following items:

Floppy-tipped 145-cm 0.038-in. guidewire

85-cm 7-F polyethylene (Torcon) catheter

0.045-in. deflecting guidewire with three-ring handle

0.0017-in. puncture wire and 3-F Teflon puncture wire sheath

Mitty-Pollack needle (22-gauge inner and 18-gauge outer needle)

The Lawson Retrograde Technique

Under general anesthesia, the patient is placed in the lithotomy position with the ipsilateral hemipelvis and scapula elevated using appropriate supports (Fig. 14.1). This position elevates the flank area from which the puncture wire will subsequently emerge. Posterior axillary line is our mark to which the puncture should be posterior in order to avoid any intra-abdominal organ injury.

After the patient is positioned, cystoscopy is carried out under sterile conditions. A floppy-tipped 0.038-in. guidewire is passed up the ureter into the renal pelvis under fluoroscopic control. The 7-F polyethylene catheter is passed up the ureter over the guidewire, and the guidewire is removed. Contrast material is then injected, opacifying the collecting system (Fig. 14.2a). In case of an impacted calculus, slight distention of the collecting system by contrast material may facilitate passage of the wire past an obstruction. J-tipped wire through the 7-F catheter could be used in case of tortuous ureter, and this is preferred since it is less likely to perforate the ureter or collecting system.

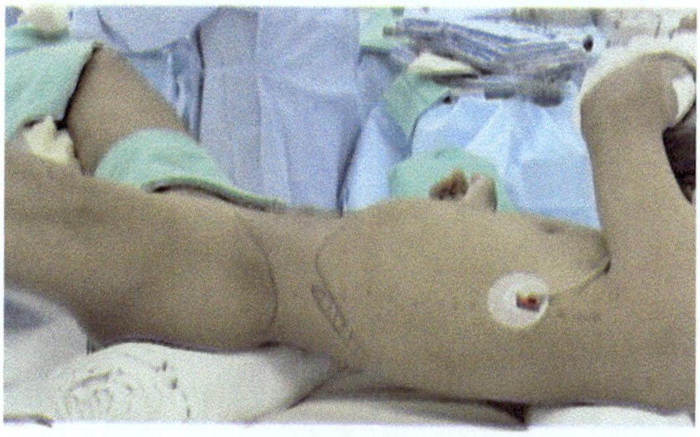

Fig. 14.1 Position for retrograde access technique

With the opacification of the collecting system, the most appropriate calyx for the nephrostomy site is selected (Fig. 14.2b). The target calyx should allow the creation of the shortest, most horizontal nephrostomy tract possible. Based on our experience, choosing the lower calyx may not be suitable for the retrograde access technique,

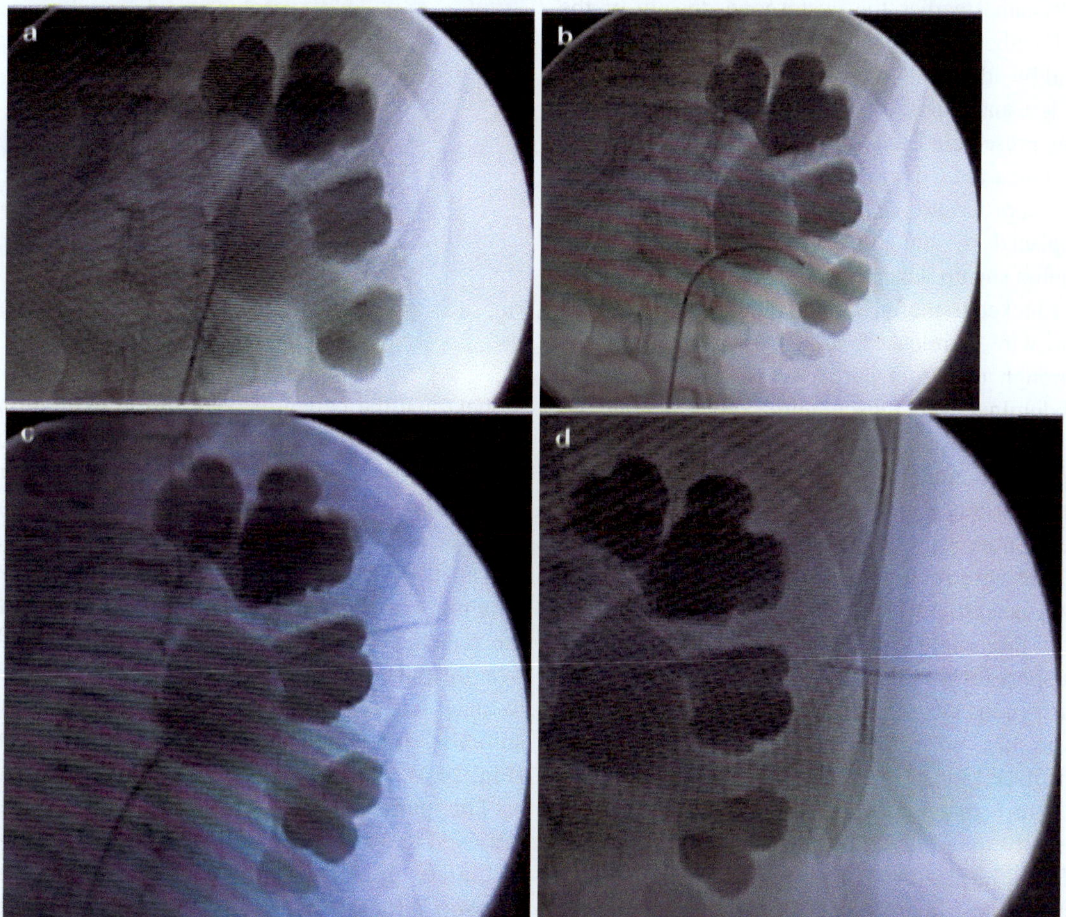

Fig. 14.2 (**a–d**) The Lawson retrograde technique steps

particularly in an obese patient and in a patient with horseshoe kidney in whom an excessively long nephrostomy tract may be created. Therefore, in some patients, the middle or upper calyx must be selected.

As long as the puncture wire exits posterior to the midaxillary line, tract dilatation is no more difficult or dangerous to neighboring viscera [14, 15, 19]. Hunter and Hosking observed that whether originating from a posterior or anterior calyx, their retrograde nephrostomy technique appeared to provide a nephrostomy tract with a posterior pathway from the posterior fornix of a calyx to the flank and allowed the nephrostomy tract to miss viscera [5, 13].

The 0.045-in.-diameter deflecting wire is passed up the 7-F polyethylene catheter and twist-locked to the base of the catheter. While an assistant steadies the cystoscope, the tip of the 7-F catheter is deflected with the deflecting wire, and by advancing the catheter/wire combination, it is usually possible to position the catheter in any preselected calyx.

Once the 7-F catheter has been positioned in an appropriate calyx, the deflecting wire is replaced by the puncture wire within its 3-F Teflon sheath. Once the puncture wire and sheath are locked to the 7-F catheter, the pin vise lock on the wire is released, and the wire is advanced through the renal parenchyma, perinephric fat, abdominal wall musculature, and subcutaneous fat until it reaches the skin (Fig. 14.2c, d). If the wire encounters a rib, it should be withdrawn a short distance and advanced once the patient's respiratory movements have changed the position of the wire relative to the rib. Occasionally you may need to advance the 7-F catheter and embed it in the renal parenchyma to provide additional support for the advancing puncture wire particularly in the case of an obese patient or in a patient who has undergone previous surgery on the involved kidney with perinephric scar tissue.

Once the puncture wire reaches the skin, it usually tents the skin rather than penetrating it (Fig. 14.3). If the wire emerges anterior to the midaxillary line, it should be withdrawn, and a different calyx should be selected for nephrostomy placement. Hosking has found it helpful to request that the patient be kept in full expiration for few seconds, which usually allows the wire to be passed just above the obstructing rib [5]. After preparing the skin over the wire, a 3- to 4-mm incision is made to allow the wire to emerge. Advance the puncture wire until 15 cm of the wire exits from the flank. With gentle traction of the puncture wire, the 7-F catheter is advanced over the puncture wire under fluoroscopic control to make sure the wire and the 7-F catheter passed smoothly till it emerges through the flank site (Fig. 14.4).

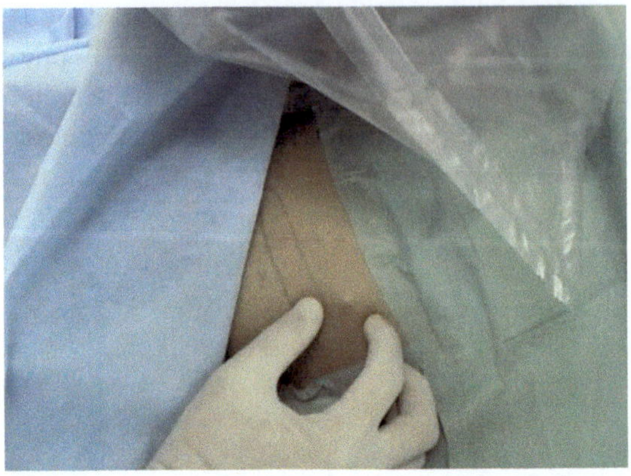

Fig. 14.3 The puncture wire tents the skin

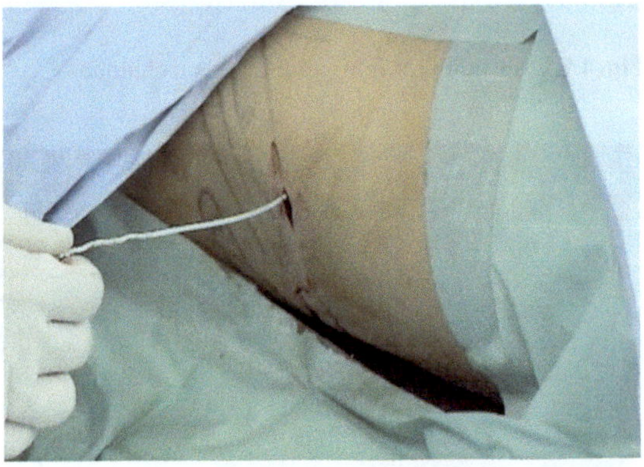

Fig. 14.4 The Lawson catheter passing through the flank site

The puncture wire and its sheet then are removed leaving behind the 7-F catheter. 0.038-in. safety guidewire is advanced through the Lawson 7-F catheter till it emerges through the cystoscope end. The cystoscope and 7-F catheter are removed, leaving the safety guidewire passing from the flank to the urethral meatus (Fig. 14.5). Clamps are placed on the guidewire at the urethral meatus end to prevent it from being displaced during subsequent tract dilatation [18].

Special Circumstances

Obese Patients

Excessive long nephrostomy tract is the concern in morbid obese patients [20]. Therefore, choosing the middle or upper calyx with retrograde access technique will create a horizontal and acceptable length of nephrostomy tract. The movement of the kidney during respiration may help in bringing the kidney near the flank site, and this will help in shortening the tract. Keeping the patient in the supine oblique position with the lithotomy position minimizes the well-known complications with the prone position particularly in such obese patients.

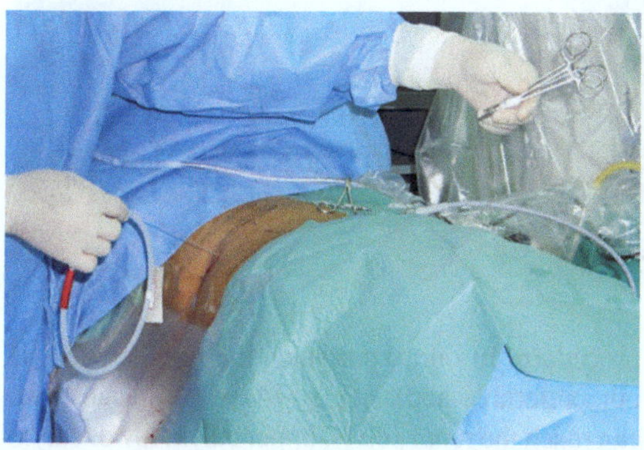

Fig. 14.5 The guidewire is through and through

Horseshoe Kidneys

Middle and upper pole access give better access to the collecting system and create short access. Because of the anatomical location and the configuration of the horseshoe kidneys, access through the lower pole leads to long access and difficulty in reaching the rest of the collecting system [21].

Supracostal Nephrostomies

Middle or upper calyx is well known to give short nephrostomy tract, but it is not unusual for the access to be above the twelfth rib and occasionally above the eleventh rib (Fig. 14.6a, b).

Postoperative pain is more with supracostal access than subcostal nephrostomies [22, 23]. The risk of other significant complications is low [24, 25]. Pneumothorax was not identified in any of the patients who underwent supracostal nephrostomy access [26]. Use of a working sheath and postoperative placement of a large-bore nephrostomy tube (24–26) appear to be important in minimizing the risk of postoperative pneumo- or hydrothorax [24, 25, 27].

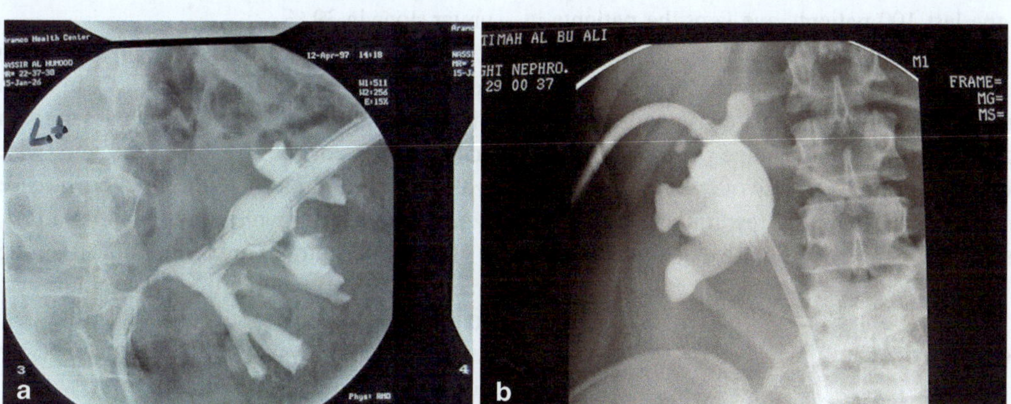

Fig. 14.6 (**a, b**) Access through the upper calyx and above the 12th rib

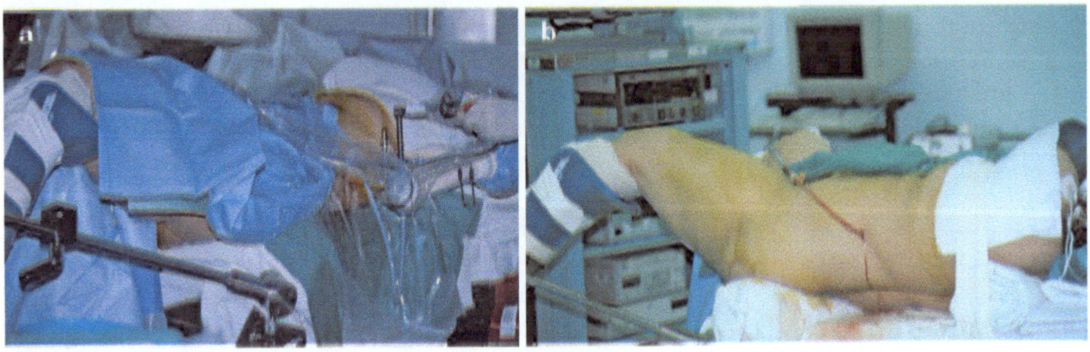

Fig. 14.7 (**a**, **b**) Supine oblique position with lithotomy position

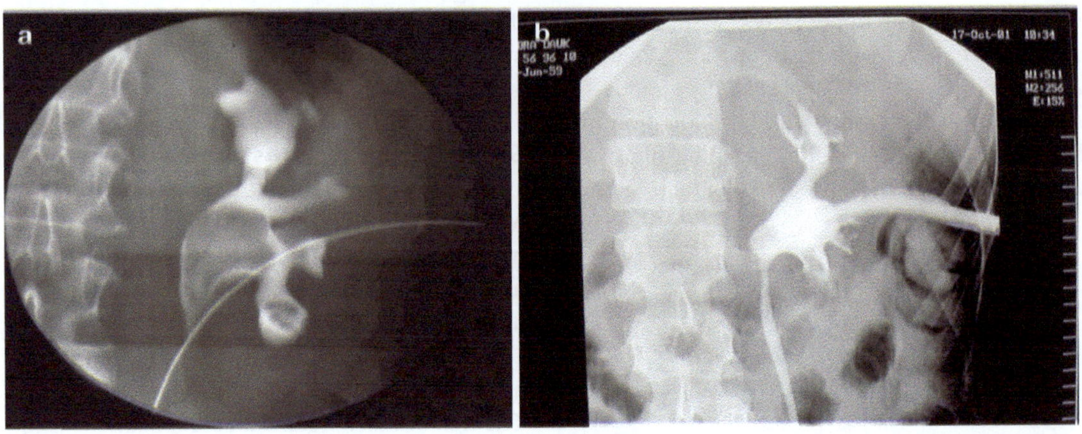

Fig. 14.8 (**a**, **b**) The retrograde access through the middle calyx

Patient Positioning

Post access creation, usually the patient is changed to prone position for nephrostomy access dilatation and percutaneous intrarenal surgery. For the last 100 patients, we kept the patients in the semidorsal lithotomy position (supine oblique position) or lateral position in a few cases with morbid obesity or complicated staghorn calculi (Fig. 14.7a, b). The advantage of the semidorsal lithotomy position is to avoid the well-known complications including respiratory and compression injury and neurologic damage.

Site Selection

It is very important to select the percutaneous nephrostomy tract that is most suited for a particular procedure. In our experience, the middle calyx is our preferable access (Fig. 14.8a, b), because we can reach the renal pelvis, upper calyx, lower calyx, and occasionally the upper ureter stone: upper calyx in 58 %, lower calyx stone in 61 %, and upper ureter stone in 39 %.

In certain circumstances, upper calyx is our second preferable access, particularly in the morbid obese patient in whom you can get the shorter access to the collecting system and good visualization for the ureteropelvic junction in case of percutaneous endopyelotomy (Fig. 14.9a, b).

Diverticular stones are best removed through a tract that directly enters the diverticulum with a stabilizing guidewire advanced into the central renal collecting system [28]. In our experience, dealing with the diverticulum from within the renal pelvis gives better visualization and direct access to the diverticulum (Fig. 14.10a, b).

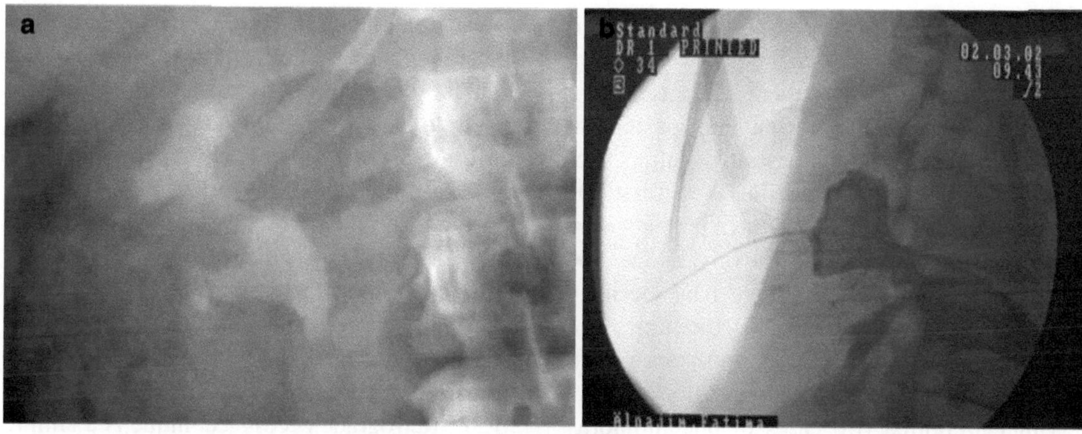

Fig. 14.9 (**a**, **b**) The retrograde access through the upper calyx in staghorn stone case

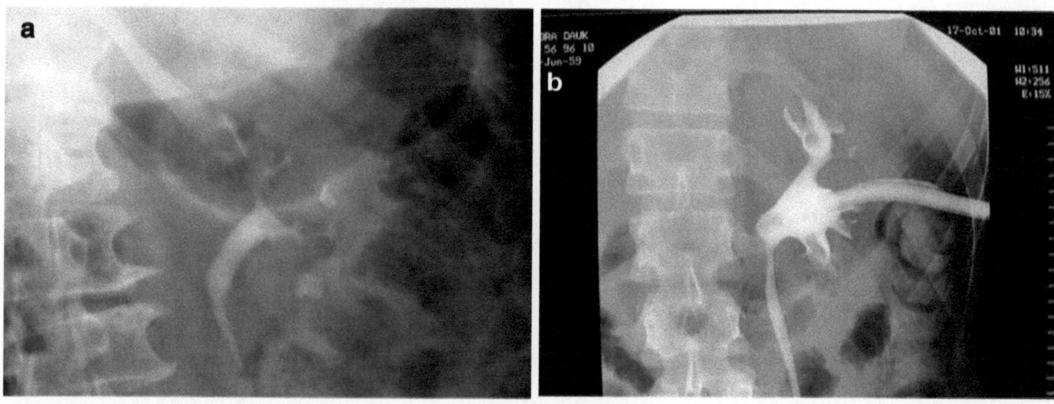

Fig. 14.10 Lower calyx diverticular stone (**a**), middle calyx access (**b**)

Results

The primary causes of access attempt failure with percutaneous access technique are the presence of nondilated renal collecting systems, small obstructing infundibular stones with minimal caliceal dilatation peripherally, impacted large stones that prevent guidewire manipulations, and obscuring of the precise location of the collecting systems by blood clot formation after initial needle insertion.

The success rate for establishing a nephrostomy tract by retrograde techniques ranges from 88 to 100 %. Hosking reported a success rate of 98 % [26]. Hawkins reported a 4 % failure rate as a result of the inability to pass a catheter into the collecting system [29]. Leal reported two failures (2.6 %): one due to a dislodged catheter from the calyx and in the other it was not possible to pass the guidewire through a tortuous ureteropelvic junction [30]. Other causes of failure included difficulty in positioning the needle in the preselected calyx, bladder neck scarring that prevented cystoscopy [13], tortuous ureter, an obstructing ureteropelvic calculus, and an obstructing infundibular calculus [10].

Complications

Hemorrhage is the major complication of percutaneous nephrostomy placement; in particular, multiple punctures, excessively medial punctures, and punctures into the kidney with abnormal anatomy are associated with an increased risk of bleeding [31, 32]. Hemorrhage is rare with the retrograde nephrostomy access technique

[26]. In the majority of cases, conservative management is generally sufficient.

Hosking reported one patient who sustained a colon perforation, and in two patients, postoperative nephrostograms demonstrated intraperitoneal leakage of contrast material, in the first 201 retrograde nephrostomies. All three patients were successfully managed conservatively. In over 300 subsequent nephrostomies, there have been no further instances of bowel perforation. Two patients developed pneumothorax postoperatively, one requiring chest tube insertion [26].

Hunter reported two cases of pneumothorax and two episodes of hemorrhage requiring blood transfusion in the first 30 patients [13]. Spirnak reported one colon perforation in 30 attempted nephrostomies [14].

The precise placement of the nephrostomy tract that the retrograde technique allows has contributed to the significant reduction of blood transfusion intraoperatively or postoperatively. Spirnak and Resnick [15] reported that none of their patients required blood transfusion and stone removal was complete in 87 % [30]. Morrisseau and Trotter reported that 1 of 71 patients required a postoperative transfusion and stone removal was successful in 86 % of their patients [33]. Hawkins reported that in his first 100 cases, 10 patients required blood transfusion. There were no cases of severe bleeding requiring embolization or nephrectomy [29]. Small collecting system perforations heal quickly with adequate urinary drainage.

Conclusion

Accurate tract creation is an essential component of successful endourologic procedures.

Needle puncture directly into the fornix of the calyx is the safest route of percutaneous entry into the renal collecting system. The complicated blood supply to the kidney makes the kidney at risk for bleeding in case of a wrong puncture site. With the retrograde nephrostomy access, the puncture needle is always directed from the inside to the outside, away from large blood vessels near the renal hilum, minimizing the risk of major hemorrhage secondary to major vessel injury at the time of tract dilatation [5]. Retrograde nephrostomy access technique does offer advantages over the more commonly used antegrade methods. Retrograde access technique provides control over both ends of the wire; this eliminates the risk of accidental wire displacement, particularly at the time of tract dilatation. Retrograde access provides a precise access, minimizes the risk of bleeding, and stabilizes the kidney during the access dilatation.

The mean procedure time for nephrostomy creation, including cystoscopy, was 27.9 min [26]. Retrograde access technique is a simple procedure and easy to learn, and the radiation exposure is significantly minimized. Access creation failures are rare, and the complication rate is low. Hawkins et al. [34] reported an average procedure time of about 30 min.

References

1. Goodwin WE, Casey WC, Woolf W. Percutaneous trocar (needle) nephrostomy in hydronephrosis. JAMA. 1955;157:891–4.
2. Almgard LE, Fernstrom I. Percutaneous nephropyelostomy. Acta Radiol Diagn. 1974;15:288–94.
3. Saxton HM. Percutaneous nephrostomy-technique. Urol Radiol. 1981;2:131–9.
4. Fernstrom I, Johanson B. Percutaneous pyelolithotomy. A new extraction technique. Scand J Urol Nephrol. 1976;10:257–9.
5. Hosking DH. Retrograde access. In: Smith AD, Badlani GH, Kavoussi LR, et al., editors. Smith's textbook of endourology. St. Louis: Quality Medical; 1996. p. 211–23.
6. Kidd CR, Conlin MJ. Ureteroscopically assisted percutaneous renal access. Urology. 2003;61:1244–5.
7. Grasso M, Lang G, Taylor FC. Flexible ureteroscopically assisted percutaneous renal access. Tech Urol. 1995;1:39–43.
8. Lawson RK, Murphy JB, Taylor AJ, Jacobs SC. Retrograde method for percutaneous access to kidney. Urology. 1983;22:580–2.
9. Hunter PT, Nanni G, Hawkins IF, Senior D, Finlayson B. Hawkins-Hunter retrograde transcutaneous nephrostomy: a new technique. Urology. 1983;22:583–7.
10. Bloom LS, Nieh PT. Retrograde nephrostolithotomy in management of complex renal calculi. J Urol. 1991; 145:706–9.
11. LeRoy AJ. Diagnosis and treatment of nephrolithiasis: current perspectives. AJR Am J Roentgenol. 1994;163:1309–13.

12. LeRoy AJ. Percutaneous access. In: Smith AD, Badlani GH, Kavoussi LR, et al., editors. Smith's textbook of endourology. St. Louis: Quality Medical; 1996. p. 211–23.
13. Hunter PT, Finlayson B, Drylie DM, Leal J, Hawkins IF. Retrograde nephrostomy and percutaneous calculus removal in 30 patients. J Urol. 1985;133:369–74.
14. Spirnak JP. Retrograde percutaneous nephrostolithotomy: an acceptable alternative to antegrade techniques. J Urol. 1987;137:841–4.
15. Spirnak JP, Resnik MI. Retrograde percutaneous stone removal using modified Lawson technique. Urology. 1987;30:551–3.
16. Pedersen JF. Percutaneous nephrostomy guided by ultrasound. J Urol. 1974;112:157–9.
17. Juul N, Nielsen V, Top-Pedersen S. Percutaneous balloon catheter nephrostomy guided by ultrasound. Scand J Urol Nephrol. 1985;19:291–4.
18. Hosking DH. Retrograde nephrostomy: experience with two techniques. J Urol. 1986;135:1146–9.
19. Sprinak JP, Resnike MI. Retrograde percutaneous nephrostomy. Urol Clin North Am. 1988;15:393–7.
20. Nguyen TA, Belis JA. Endoscopic management of urolithiasis in the morbidly obese patient. J Endourol. 1998;12:33–5.
21. Al-Otaibi K, Hosking DH. Percutaneous stone removal in horseshoe kidneys. J Urol. 1999;162:674–7.
22. Carson CC. Complications of percutaneous stone extraction: prevention and treatment. Semin Urol. 1986;4:161–9.
23. Coleman CC, Castaneda-Zuniga W, Miller R, Lange P, Clayman R, Reddy P, Hunter D, Hulbert JC, Salomonowitz E, Lund G, Amplatz K. A logical approach to renal stone removal. AJR Am J Roentgenol. 1984;143:609–15.
24. Forsyth MJ, Fuchs EF. The supracostal approach for percutaneous nephrostolithotomy. J Urol. 1987;137: 197–8.
25. Hulbert JC. Percutaneous extraction of difficult renal stones. Semin Urol. 1986;4:139–47.
26. Hosking DH, Reid RI. The evaluation of retrograde nephrostomy in over 200 procedures. In: Walker VR, Sutton RAL, Cameron ECB, Pak CYC, Robertson WG, editors. Urolithiasis: proceeding of the sixth international symposium on urolithiasis. New York: Plenum Press; 1989.
27. Narasimham DL, Jacobsson B, Vijayan P, Bhuyan BC, Nyman U, Holmquist B. Percutaneous nephrolithotomy through an intercostals approach. Acta Radiol. 1991;32:162–5.
28. Bellman GC, Silverstein JI, Blickensderfer S, Smith AD. Technique and follow-up of percutaneous management of caliceal diverticula. Urology. 1993;42: 21–5.
29. Hawkins IF. Retrograde percutaneous nephrostomy. Crit Rev Diagn Imaging. 1987;27:153–65.
30. Leal JJ. Percutaneous removal of renal and ureteral stones with and without concomitant transurethral manipulation by a urologist using antegrade and retrograde techniques without a radiologist assistance. J Urol. 1988;139:1184–7.
31. Sampaio FJB. Surgical anatomy of the kidney. In: Smith AD, Badlani GH, Kavoussi LR, et al., editors. Smith's textbook of endourology. St. Louis: Quality Medical; 1996. p. 153–84.
32. Martin X, Tajra LC, Gelet A, et al. Complete staghorn stones: percutaneous approach using one or multiple percutaneous accesses. J Endourol. 1999;13:367–8.
33. Morrisseau PM, Trotter SJ. Retrograde percutaneous nephrolithotomy: urological treatment of a urological problem. J Urol. 1988;139:1163–5.
34. Hawkins IF, Hunter P, Leal G, Nanni G, Hawkins M, Finlayson B, Senior D. Retrograde nephrostomy for stone removal: combined cystoscopic/percutaneous technique. AJR Am J Roentgenol. 1984;143: 299–304.

Percutaneous Nephrolithotomy (PCNL): The Supine Approach – Overcoming the Difficulties

15

Francisco Pedro Juan Daels

Introduction

Urinary stone disease is a recurrent condition. This stimulated the development of new minimally invasive techniques, especially after the 1970s, in order to obtain the same therapeutic results of traditional open surgery while reducing the aggressiveness and postoperative complications of traditional open surgery.

That was the concept that determined the emergence of percutaneous nephrolithotomy (PCNL), ureteroscopy, extracorporeal shock wave lithotripsy, and laparoscopic surgery. All these therapeutic options became the gold standard to treat and solve most of the urinary stone cases, thereby reducing the size of incision, analgesic requirements, transfusion necessity, hospitalization, and recovery time.

Each one of these methods has its own indications and limitations depending on the stone's size, location and composition, the anatomic and functional features of the patient's urinary tract, and the demographic and socioeconomic context in which the procedure is being performed. Considering all these factors, PCNL is today accepted as the first-choice technique when managing complex renal stones. Nevertheless, despite being the procedure with best results, residual stones postoperatively are encountered in between 5 and 29 % of the cases [1]. Simultaneous combination of minimally invasive procedures seems to be the next necessary step in order to improve results.

The Prone Position

In order to make this solution feasible in a rational way, some redefinitions are necessary. An overview of the decubitus approach for PCNL might be useful. The percutaneous approach to the kidney must fulfill two requirements:

1. Achieve good access to the renal pelvis and calyx
2. Be harmless to the neighboring structures

The kidney is a retroperitoneal organ in close contact with the psoas muscle, half intrathoracic, and half intra-abdominal. Regarding its relationship with the other organs, the anterior face of the right kidney is close to the right adrenal, the duodenum, the liver, and the hepatic angle of the colon. The anterior face of the left kidney is close to the left adrenal, the spleen, the stomach, the pancreas, the jejunum, and the splenic angle of the colon. The posterior face of the kidneys shows both upper poles close to the pleura. When taking into consideration the retroperitoneal position of the kidney, its relationship with other organs, and its own particular vascular distribution, it seems that the safest access to the urinary tract is through

F.P.J. Daels, M.D.
Department of Urology, Instituto Universitario del Hospital Italiano de Buenos Aires,
Hospital Italiano de Buenos Aires Peron 4190, Buenos Aires, C1181ACH, Argentina
e-mail: pedro.daels@hiba.org.ar

A.M. Al-Kandari et al. (eds.), *Difficult Cases in Endourology*,
DOI 10.1007/978-1-84882-083-8_15, © Springer-Verlag London 2013

a posterior calyx papilla [2]. Hence, the access will always be through the lumbar area of the patient. This is the main reason why we have all been taught to access the kidney with the patient in the *prone position*. The *prone position* has two recognized advantages:

1. It allows good access to the whole lumbar puncture surface.
2. Puncture, tract dilation, and endoscopic instrumentation are always downward. This guarantees safe, comfortable, and precise maneuvers.

We cannot forget that proper access requires correct urinary tract visualization. Despite the fact that the puncture can be made under ultrasound guidance, the dilation requires radiographic control.

Therefore, the first step in PCNL consists of a retrograde ureteral catheterization to visualize the urinary collecting system. Once under anesthesia, the patient is placed initially in a traditional lithotomy position. A genital surgical field is then created; a cystoscopy is performed, and the ureteral catheter is introduced. After these steps, the ureteral catheter is fixed to a bladder catheter; the surgical field is withdrawn, and only then the patient is placed in *prone decubitus* (Fig. 15.1) [3–6].

Positioning a patient that is asleep and relaxed is not an easy task. Placing him in the correct prone position is only achieved after moving the flaccid body considerably, which requires taking good care to avoid extreme extensions and flexions that may hurt the neck or shoulders. At least four or five persons are required to perform this coordinated and risky body up-down movement. The prone decubitus may harm the forehead, eyes, nose, elbows, knees, and toes. All these structures must be carefully padded in order to avoid harming them. Complete blindness, forehead necrosis, nose deformity, and injuries to the cervical and brachial plexus and peripheral nerve compression, among others, are described in the literature [7–15].

Prone decubitus produces significant changes in blood distribution, breathing movements, and lung perfusion. The fact that the thorax is lying on the surface of the operating table restricts respiratory movements. Due to this, intermittent positive pressure ventilation is necessary to bear the weight of the chest. This results in an increased intrathoracic pressure which decreases the venous backflow from the legs. These disadvantages are much more significant in obese and elderly patients. Air tract control and resuscitation maneuvers are also difficult in this position.

The Supine Position and Further Evolutions

More than 25 years ago, Valdivia from Zaragoza, Spain, demonstrated the feasibility and convenience of performing the percutaneous approach with the patient in *supine decubitus* (*Valdivia's position*) (Fig. 15.2) [16, 17]. As in the previous case, a ureteral catheter is placed in the patient in lithotomy position. Compared to the traditional prone position, the supine one shows some interesting differences: In order to place the patient in a *supine position*, an empty 3-l water bag which has been blown up with air is placed under the

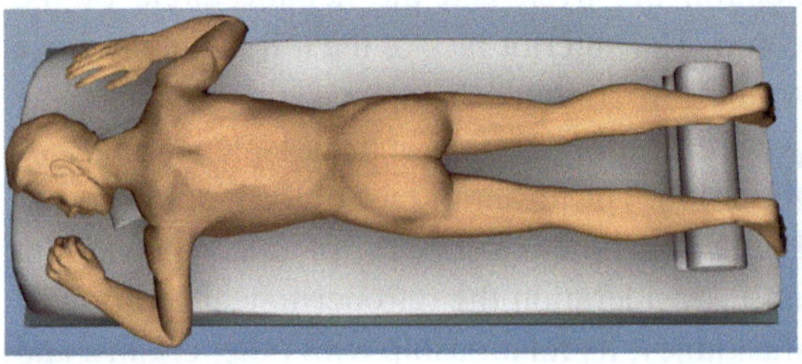

Fig. 15.1 The prone decubitus position (Copyright © 2011 Tatú Studios)

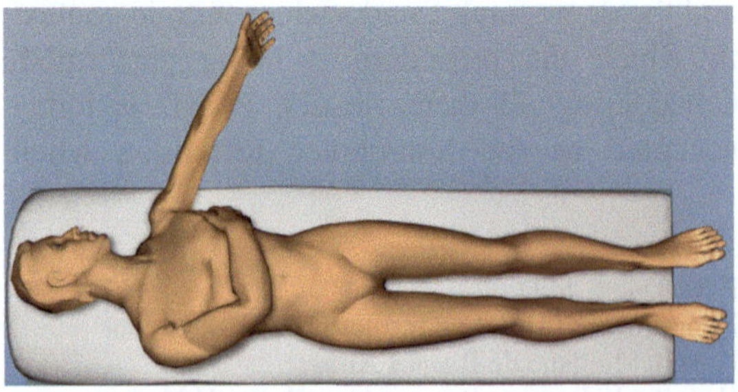

Fig. 15.2 The supine decubitus position (Valdivia's position) (Copyright © 2011 Tatú Studios)

lumbar area of the side that is to be treated. Then, the thorax is rotated 45°, and the ipsilateral arm is folded across the chest. Good exposure of the posterior axillary line is obtained (puncture site). Placing the patient like this is much easier than in the prone decubitus. Only a few persons are needed to place the patient in the final position.

Due to the body being barely moved, hyperextensions and hyperflexions are avoided. The chance of injuring the joints and the neck in particular is clearly diminished. Also, there is less risk of unintended extubation. There is no chance of injuring the forehead, eyes, nose, elbows, knees, and toes because there is no contact with the operating table. There is no impairment to the venous circulation: The rib cage is not restricted. In case of an emergency, the anesthesiologist has better access to assist the patient. Furthermore, the bowel slips away from the puncturing site, lowering the risk of an undesired injury [18]. In order to clear this issue, we compared the distance between the colon and the end of the 12th rib in 20 patients placed in *prone and supine decubitus*, confirming that the colon slips away an average of 2.5 cm from the puncture area, measured with spiral CT scan [19].

Despite these clear advantages, *supine position* presents some drawbacks:

1. It forces us to puncture upward which tends to be less comfortable and accurate.
2. The access to the safe lumbar puncture area is smaller, decreasing the possibilities of an easy approach to the upper calyx.

Fortunately, this *supine decubitus* (or *Valdivia's position*) was meant to keep evolving. Ibarluzea (Bilbao, Spain) introduced the *Valdivia-Galdakao decubitus*, a variation of the *supine decubitus* [20, 21]. In the *Valdivia-Galdakao decubitus* (Fig. 15.3), the patient is placed in supine decubitus with extension of the homolateral lower limb and flexion of the contralateral at 90°. It preserves all the pros and cons of the *supine decubitus*, but it provides some other significant advantages that are worth mentioning:

1. Once under general anesthesia, the patient is placed in the *Valdivia-Galdakao decubitus*. A single lumbar and genital sterile surgical field is created, allowing the retrograde endoscopic placement of ureteral catheter and the lumbar percutaneous puncture at the same time, *without the need of patient repositioning*. This reduces significantly the operative time.
2. Antegrade and retrograde simultaneous endoscopic access is possible, increasing the efficiency and safety of the endourological procedures.
3. Endourologic and laparoscopic simultaneous access is possible, allowing intra- and extraluminal combined visualization and instrumentation of the affected organs.

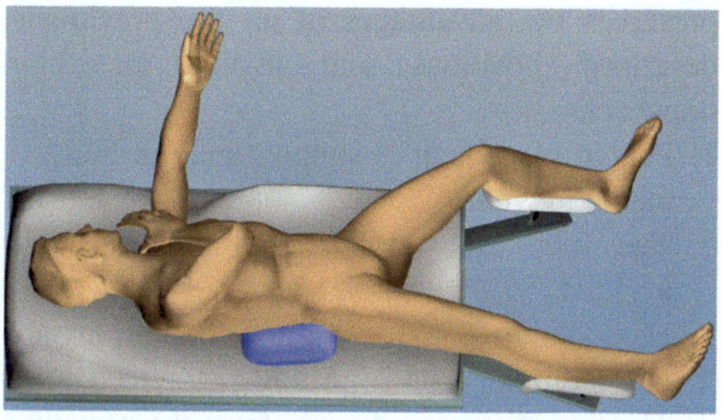

Fig. 15.3 The Valdivia-Galdakao decubitus position (Copyright © 2011 Tatú Studios)

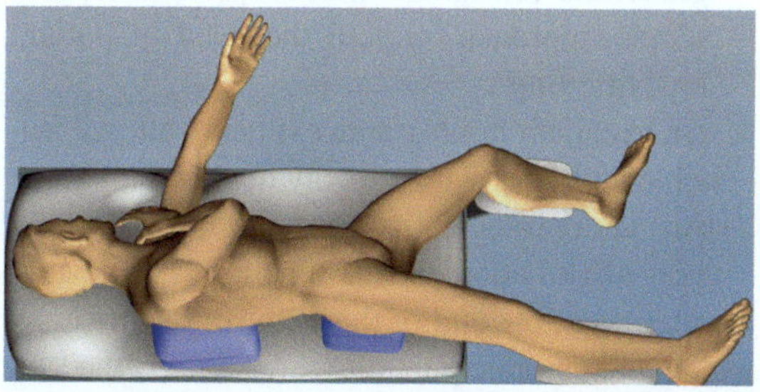

Fig. 15.4 The intermediate supine decubitus position (Copyright © 2011 Tatú Studios)

Despite these considerable improvements, there is still another better patient position which we have adopted since April 2006 in our department: the *intermediate supine decubitus* (Fig. 15.4). The *intermediate supine decubitus* is a variation of the *Valdivia-Galdakao decubitus* in which the patient is placed a little more sideways. Instead of putting a bag under the lumbar area of the patient, it is placed under the hip. This simple detail improves the *Valdivia-Galdakao decubitus* in many ways. The *intermediate supine decubitus* preserves the advantages of all the previously described positions and avoids all their drawbacks:

1. Patient placement is simple, and the body is barely moved.
2. The joint and pressure point lesions are avoided.
3. Hemodynamic and respiratory conditions are preserved; air tract control is guaranteed.
4. The bowel is moved away from the puncture site.
5. There is the possibility of simultaneous antegrade and retrograde endoscopic and laparoscopic approach without the need of patient repositioning.
6. An excellent lumbar area exposure allows feasible and easy access to any desired calyx.
7. An endourologically friendly horizontal or even slightly descendent puncture is achieved.

Furthermore, the end of the 12th rib results in an excellent anatomic puncture reference: If the kidney is located in its normal position, the puncture performed 2 cm below and behind the end of the 12th rib never harms the colon and reaches the kidney via its posterior face in 98 % of cases.

Since 1985, almost 1,800 percutaneous nephrolithotomies have been performed in our department. *Prone decubitus* was used in the first 585 patients. In 1998, we adopted the *supine decubitus* (*Valdivia's decubitus*), performing it on 695 patients. Since April 2006, we adopted the *intermediate supine decubitus*, performing it until today on more than 500 cases.

Case History 1 (Fig. 15.5a–f)

- A 56-year-old woman is suffering from pain in the left lumbar region.
- A renal pelvic stone measuring 28 mm was found.
- Hepatosplenomegaly caused by myelofibrosis was present.
- In order to treat the case, a combined percutaneous and laparoscopic access was decided upon.
- The patient was positioned in intermediate supine decubitus.
- A ureteral catheter was inserted. The transperitoneal laparoscopic access was carried out, and the spleen was displaced cephalically enabling a safe percutaneous access to the kidney, thus achieving the nephrolithotomy.

Case History 2 (Fig. 15.6a–e)

- A 58-year-old woman has a solitary right kidney. She was suffering from pain in the right lumbar region and a urinary infection due to multiresistant Acinetobacter.
- The excretory urogram and computed tomography (CT) scan show five stones in five different calyces: 6 mm in the upper major calyx, 6 mm in the lower major calyx, 12 mm in the lower middle calyx, 13 mm in the upper minor calyx, and 12 mm in the lower minor calyx. The calyceal necks were narrow.
- A double-J stent was put in place.
- A combined ureteral and percutaneous treatment was decided upon.
- The patient was positioned in intermediate supine decubitus.
- The percutaneous access was used to treat the stones in the posterior middle calyx and the anterior lower calyx. The retrograde flexible ureteroscopic approach was used to remove the remaining calyceal stones that were unaccessible to the nephroscope.
- Following the procedure, the patient was stone-free and had no urinary infection.

Conclusions

Intermediate supine decubitus is demonstrated to be simpler, safer, and more versatile for PCNL. It is our first choice when simple percutaneous nephrolithotomies are to be performed and becomes essential when confronting complex cases since this position allows for a rational minimally invasive combined approach.

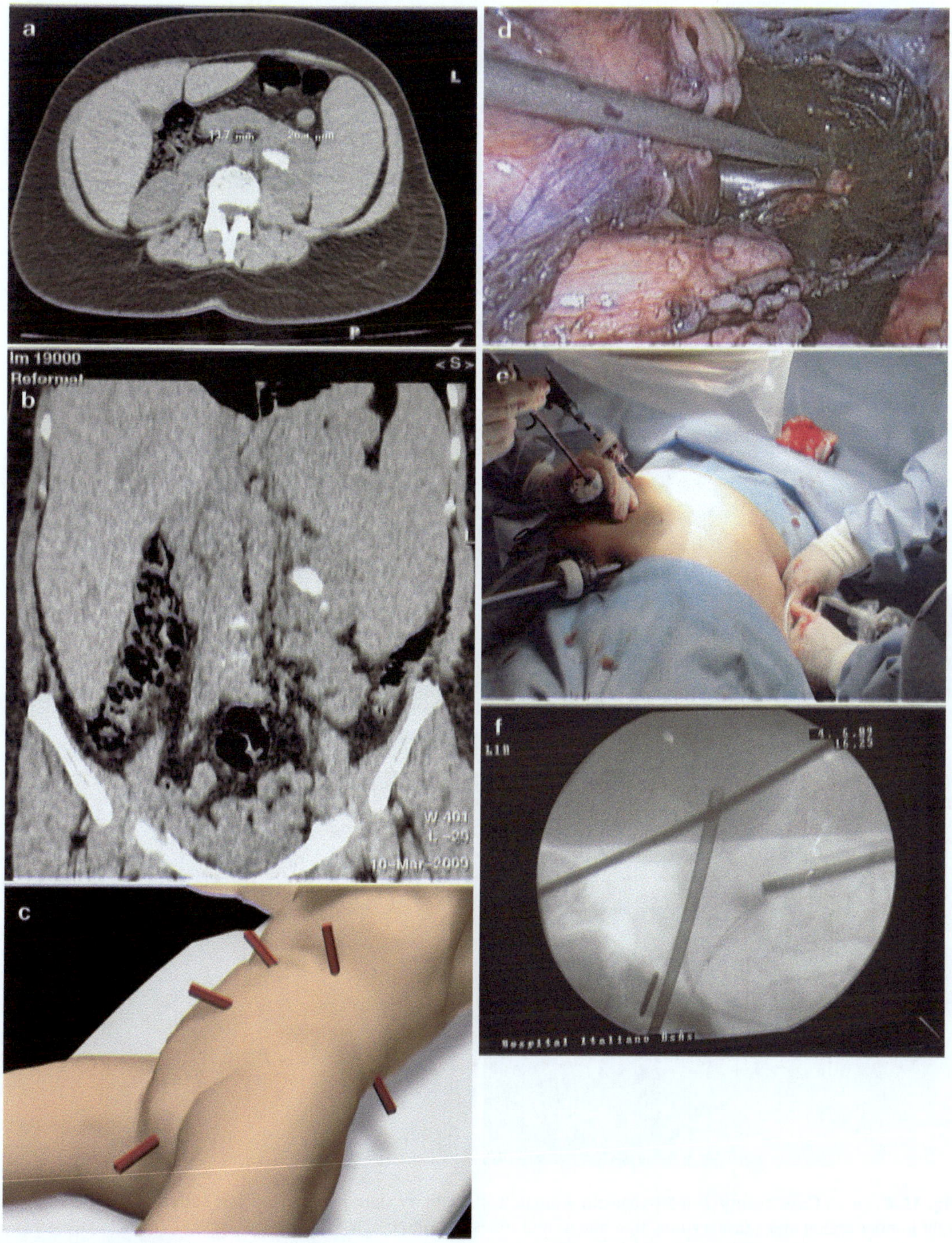

Fig. 15.5 (a–f) Case history 1: a 56-year-old woman is suffering from pain in the left lumbar region

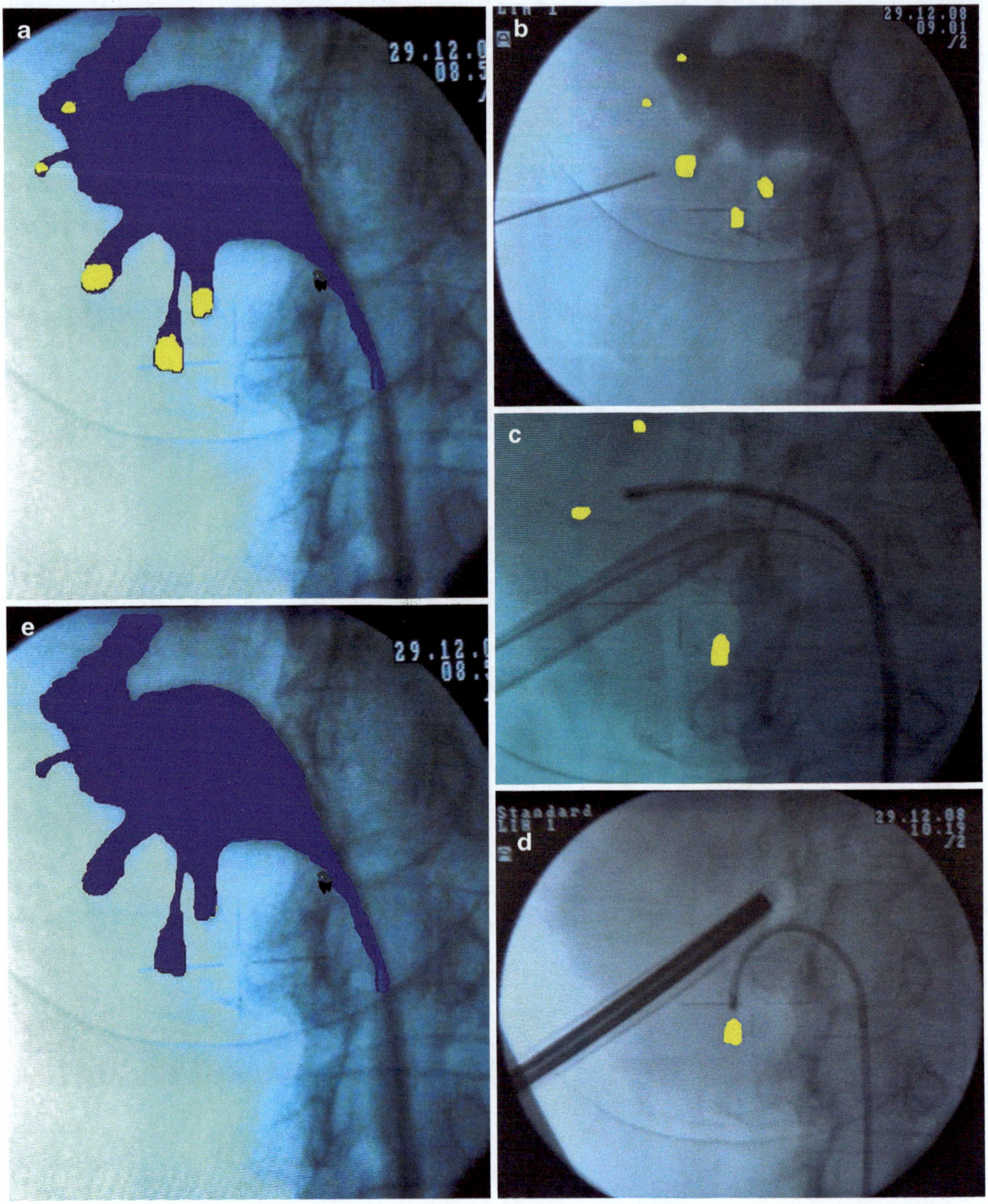

Fig. 15.6 (**a–e**) Case history 2: a 58-year-old woman has a solitary right kidney. She was suffering from pain in the right lumbar region and a urinary infection due to multiresistant Acinetobacter

References

1. Wen CC, Nakada SY, Wen CC, Nakada SY. Treatment selection and outcomes: renal calculi. Urol Clin North Am. 2007;34(3):409–19.
2. Sampaio FJB. Anatomía renal: consideraciones endourológicas. Urol Clin North Am. 2000;4:623–42.
3. Deane LA, Clayman RV. Advances in percutaneous nephrostolithotomy. Urol Clin North Am. 2007;34:383–95.
4. Preminger GM, Assimos DG, Lingeman JE, et al. AUA guideline on management of staghorn calculi: diagnosis

and treatment recommendations. J Urol. 2005;173: 1991–2000.
5. Segura J, Smith J. Percutaneous lithotripsy. J Urol. 1983;130(6):1051–4.
6. Preminger GM, Assimos DG, Lingeman JE, Nakada SY, Pearle MS, Wolf Jr JS. Chapter 1: AUA guideline on management of staghorn calculi: diagnosis and treatment recommendations. J Urol. 2005;173:1991.
7. Edgcombe H, Carter K, Yarrow S. Anaesthesia in prone position. Br J Anaesth. 2008;100(2):165–83.
8. Singer MS, Salim S. Bilateral acute angle-closure glaucoma as a complication of facedown spine surgery. Spine J. 2010;10(9):e7–9.
9. Goepfert CE, Ifune C, Tempelhoff R. Ischemic optic neuropathy: are we any further? Curr Opin Anaesthesiol. 2010;23(5):582–7.
10. Sestoft B, Larsen B, Erlandsen M, Hansen ES. Positioning injuries among patients undergoing spine surgery. Ugeskr Laeger. 2009;171(7):518–21.
11. Grisell M, Place HM. Face tissue pressure in prone positioning: a comparison of three face pillows while in the prone position for spinal surgery. Spine. 2008;33(26):2938–41.
12. Atwater BI, Benumof JL Wahrenbrock E, Mazzei WJ. Pressure on face while in the prone position: prone view versus prone positioner. J Clin Anesth. 2004; 16(2):111–6.
13. Jeon YT, Park YO, Won Hwang J, Lim YJ, Oh YS, Park HP. Effect of head position on postoperative chemosis after prone spinal surgery. J Neurosurg Anesthesiol. 1991;19:1–4.
14. Nikolaev AP, Svetlov VA. Spinal operations performed in prone position: pulmonary gas exchange, hemodynamics, and possible complications. Anesteziol Reanimatol. 2004; Sep-Oct (5):32–7.
15. Stambough JL, Dolan D, Werner R, Godfrey E. Ophthalmologic complications associated with prone positioning in spine surgery. J Am Acad Orthop Surg. 2007;15(3):156–65.
16. Valdivia Uria JG, Valle Gerhold J, Lopez Lopez JA, et al. Technique and complications of percutaneous nephroscopy: experience with 557 patients in the supine position. J Urol. 1998;160:1975–8.
17. Valdivia Uria JG, Valle J, Villarroya S. Why is percutaneous nephroscopy still performed with patient prone? J Endourol. 1990;4:269–72.
18. LeRoy Aj, Williams Jr HJ, Bender CE, et al. Colonic perforation following percutaneous nephrostomy and renal calculus removal. Radiology. 1985;155:83–5.
19. Gonzalez MS, Billordo Peres N, Daels P et al. Colon position in ventral and intermédiate dorsal decubitus (Valdivia). In: World congress endourology, Munich, 2009. Abstract N° MP4-19.
20. Ibarluzea G, Scoffone CM, Cracco CM, et al. Supine Valdivia and modified lithotomy position for simultaneous anterograde and retrograde endourological access. BJU Int. 2007;100:233–6.
21. Daels F, Gonzalez MS, García Freire F, et al. Percutaneous lithotripsy in Valdivia-Galdakao decubitus position: our experience. J Endourol. 2009; 23(10):1615–20.

Percutaneous Nephrolithotomy (PCNL) in Obese Patients: Overcoming the Difficulties

16

Soroush Rais-Bahrami and Arthur D. Smith

Introduction

Increasing Prevalence of Obesity

The prevalence of obesity has significantly increased over recent decades in the United States and other developed western countries. Obesity is often termed a contemporary "epidemic" with evidence that greater than 30 percent of American adults are currently obese and this rate continues to rise [1]. Overweight and obese status have been defined based upon body mass index (BMI) ranges of 25–29.9 kg/m^2 and greater than 30 kg/m^2, respectively, where BMI is an objective measure equal to weight in kilograms divided by height in meters squared [2].

Obesity and Nephrolithiasis

Population-based studies have demonstrated a correlation between weight gain and increased risk of nephrolithiasis [3, 4]. With the rates of obesity and rates of nephrolithiasis rising in parallel, there is a suggestion that the two processes share a common pathophysiology [5]. Although the exact processes explaining this association have not been defined, this linked relationship has been largely attributed to the alterations in metabolism and urinary metabolite excretion in obese patients [6]. Also, urinary pH which is one of the influenceable factors of stone formation has been found to be inversely related to BMI [7, 8].

Obesity presents numerous challenges to the clinician. Diagnosis and imaging must be properly tailored to this patient population. Furthermore, this state of altered metabolism and lifestyle behaviors in overweight and obese individuals poses a challenge to the urologist employing medical management of renal stone disease [9]. Additionally, obese stone formers have been shown to have high stone recurrence rates after treatment compared to nonobese patients with nephrolithiasis [10].

There are also surgical hurdles of increased anesthetic risk and physical limitations of positioning and instrumentation for both endoscopic retrograde and percutaneous antegrade approaches to clearing renal stone burden. Surgical management of nephrolithiasis in obese individuals may be more laborious, may require additional procedures to achieve similar results, and may pose a higher risk of procedural morbidity to the patient.

Obesity and Percutaneous Nephrolithotomy

Percutaneous nephrolithotomy (PCNL) was first performed in 1976 [11]. Since its inception, PCNL has largely replaced open nephrolithotomy and

S. Rais-Bahrami, M.D.(✉) • A.D. Smith, M.D.
The Arthur Smith Institute for Urology, Hofstra North Shore - Long Island Jewish School of Medicine,
450 Lakeville Road, New Hyde Park, NY 11042, USA
e-mail: soroushraisbahrami@gmail.com;
asmith1@nshs.edu

A.M. Al-Kandari et al. (eds.), *Difficult Cases in Endourology*,
DOI 10.1007/978-1-84882-083-8_16, © Springer-Verlag London 2013

offers a minimally invasive approach for the treatment of stones larger than 2 cm, staghorn calculi, stones with concomitant ureteropelvic junction obstruction, stones within calyceal diverticuli, and anatomical aberrancies including ectopic kidneys [12]. Indications for PCNL have expanded to treatment of very complex stones and anatomic variants which challenge the urologist, driving the development of novel instrumentation and modified techniques to overcome these difficulties [13]. Herein, we present clinical scenarios of how an obese patient can complicate PCNL and suggest various techniques to overcome these challenges.

Challenges Faced with PCNL in Obese Patients

Overall Surgical and Anesthetic Risk

Obesity can be considered a surrogate for other medical comorbidities which commonly place patients at increased surgical and anesthetic risk [14]. Interestingly, rates of stone clearance and postoperative complications have been shown in multiple studies to be comparable in patients undergoing PCNL stratified by weight and body mass index [15–17]. Criticism of these findings questions the effects of selection bias of the obese patients that were counseled to undergo PCNL. Furthermore, these studies represent experienced centers well versed and equipped to overcome the technical challenges encountered with this patient population.

General anesthetic concerns arise for cases of PCNL in obese patients due to compromised cardiopulmonary status. Obese patients inherently have increased restriction of their chest wall due to increased body weight, and restricted chest expansion can lead to inadequate ventilation, particularly when performed in the prone position, traditionally used for PCNL. Hence, some anesthesiologists prefer flank or supine positioning to facilitate more effective ventilation [18–20].

Percutaneous Access

Challenges with obtaining percutaneous access in overweight and obese patients are threefold. Primarily, limitations with the penetration of ultrasound and fluoroscopy alter the effectiveness of real-time, intraoperative imaging. Compromised resolution or positioning due to the patient body habitus limits the ease with which an accurate, well-targeted calyceal puncture can be achieved.

The limitations of imaging are multiple. Ultrasonographic examination of the kidney loses resolution due to energy attenuation. In cases of obese patients requiring CT-guided nephrostomy tube insertion, weight limitations of the CT table as well as girth limitations of the CT scanner gantry can restrict morbidly obese patients from using this imaging modality [19]. The use of biplanar fluoroscopy can be used in the operating room setting with only a slightly decreased resolution suffering from increased absorption and scatter of the radiation penetrance. With any imaging modality selected for guidance of the percutaneous puncture, there are challenges with obtaining access in a precise manner due to the body habitus of most obese patients undergoing PCNL.

Secondly, the distance between the skin and the targeted stone is greater due to the girth of the patient. This in turn makes puncture, tract dilation, and securing a working sheath more difficult than in a nonobese patient with a shorter skin-to-stone distance.

Lastly, once obtained and secured, maintaining access presents added difficulty due to the limitations on the length of working sheaths, nephroscopes, working instruments, and lithotriptors that are routinely available. At times, due to the increased girth and skin-to-stone distance, the access sheath is commonly more susceptible to be advanced under the surface of the skin into the subcutaneous tissues or, at times, may be withdrawn from the renal collecting system.

Strategies to Overcome Challenges Encountered

Operative Positioning

Since its inception, PCNL has been performed with the patient in the prone position to achieve access through a nearly avascular plane into the renal collecting system. Presented with the challenges of providing general anesthesia and ventilation of obese patients in the customarily employed prone position, anesthesiologists and urologists may prefer either a modified-flank or supine positioning to facilitate ventilation throughout the operation [18, 21]. PCNL in the supine position was first described by Valdivia and colleagues in 1987 [22]. This approach has also been reported for unique PCNL cases including treatment of stones in patients with ectopic pelvic kidneys or renal allograft recipients [23, 24]. Its use was widely expanded to include PCNL for morbidly obese patients or those with other high-risk cardiopulmonary features [20]. However, some groups report that these modified approaches increase the length of the percutaneous nephrostomy tract used and alter the anatomy which may decrease maneuverability of the nephroscope during the case resulting in a slightly lower stone-free rate [25].

A meta-analysis comparison of PCNL done in the prone versus supine position revealed that supine PCNL provided an effective approach without significantly altering the safety profile of the procedure compared to the traditional prone position [26]. This meta-analysis evaluated rates of stone clearance, complications, transfusions, and postoperative fevers, although prior analyses by de la Rosette and colleagues showed a lower stone-free rate with the supine technique [25].

Awake Intubation

Awake endotracheal intubation and patient self-positioning have been reported as a mechanism to reduce potential challenges with ventilating obese patients in the prone position [27]. This procedure has also been described specifically for obese patients undergoing PCNL [28]. Following patient preparation with premedication with antisialogogues and sedatives, the airway is numbed with either topical anesthesia or laryngeal nerve blocks, and fiber-optic, awake intubation is performed (Fig. 16.1). This allows the patients to then position themselves into a comfortable prone position lessening the chances for positional nerve injuries. Furthermore, as per routine, rolls are positioned to support the chest, shoulders, and pelvis, and all pressure points are padded. Comfort and the need for additional padding can be confirmed with the awake, conscious patient, and adjustments can be made as necessary. Also, from an anesthetic perspective, the patient continues spontaneous respiration in the prone position as a test of ventilation adequacy prior to induction of general anesthesia.

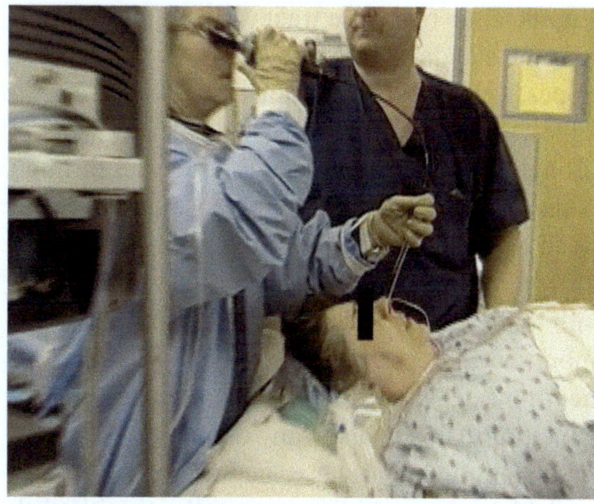

Fig. 16.1 Awake fiber-optic endotracheal intubation with sedated but cooperative patient

Modified Access Technique

A case report described a unique modification to conventional PCNL to allow for a shortened percutaneous operative tract to overcome limitations of standard access sheaths, rigid nephroscopes, and working instruments [29]. A fascial cutdown technique was reported with an incision through the skin and subcutaneous tissues through to the level of the underlying fascia. This provided a shortened tract for the sheath to traverse allowing for access into the collecting system with standard Amplatz dilators and sheaths, important in obese patients prior to the development of extra-long dilators, sheaths, and instrumentation. It is also an essential technical modification when these newer tools are not available or in morbidly obese patients with girth too large for the extra-long sheaths.

Specialty Sheaths and Instrumentation

Limitations on the length of standard dilators, working sheaths, and instruments are challenges faced when attempting PCNL in obese patients. Challenges resulting from obtaining and maintaining access in obese patients require appropriate instrumentation to facilitate a safe and effective PCNL procedure which may not be routinely available. However, with appropriate preoperative imaging and assessment of the skin-to-stone distance, one can ensure that the appropriate equipment is available and ready for these specific cases. Modified extra-long Amplatz dilators and access sheaths have been developed to facilitate the creation and maintenance of the working tract. These longer sheaths also have a slightly larger bore up to 32 Fr to allow for use of longer and larger-bore nephroscopes measuring up to 30 Fr.

The standard nephroscope is only slightly longer than standard Amplatz sheaths and therefore cannot be used with extra-long sheaths. The use of gynecologic laparoscopes as extra-long nephroscopes and bronchoscopic grasping forceps has been reported for percutaneous access to kidney stones in obese patients in order to overcome the increased skin-to-stone distance [30]. This provides a rigid nephroscope with extended reach and instruments tailored to use through this elongated scope.

Also, employing a flexible cystoscope or ureteroscope as a nephroscope can overcome limitations of conventional rigid nephroscopes in reaching passed a lengthened skin-to-stone distance. Furthermore, as in the case of using flexible nephroscopy for full staghorn calculi, this technical approach can minimize the number of percutaneous tracts necessary to address complex stones minimizing the torque and manipulation. This is of added importance in obese individuals whereby a larger body habitus would additionally challenge the ability to safely manipulate a rigid nephroscope for management of stones involving multiple calyces.

Sheath Retrieval

Despite the use of specialty percutaneous access sheaths and instrumentation, PCNL in the setting of obese patients can present challenges throughout the operation. Commonly, through manipulation of the nephroscope and working instruments through the nephroscope, the access sheath can be inadvertently advanced and, in obese patients, may be lost under the level of the skin within the subcutaneous tissues. There are a number of reported methods of overcoming the challenges of sheath retrieval in these situations. Classically, the sheath can be manipulated, and attempts of retrieval can be made using a clamp (Fig. 16.2).

To help prevent losing access or providing a retrieval mechanism, the working sheath can be secured to the skin surface or in cases of fascial cutdown to the fascia. This presents an added risk of skin tears if the sheath is aggressively manipulated. Thus, our group prefers tagging the working sheath with sutures placed solely through the sheath, at opposing sides, to provide retrieval ties for instances when the sheath migrates deep to the level of the skin (Fig. 16.3a–c) [31]. In addition to preemptive suture placement in the working sheath, retraction of the sheath can be accomplished using the open jaws of the grasping forceps passed through the sheath (Fig. 16.4). Also, under fluoroscopic guidance, a council-tipped Foley catheter can be advanced through the sheath over a wire into the collecting system.

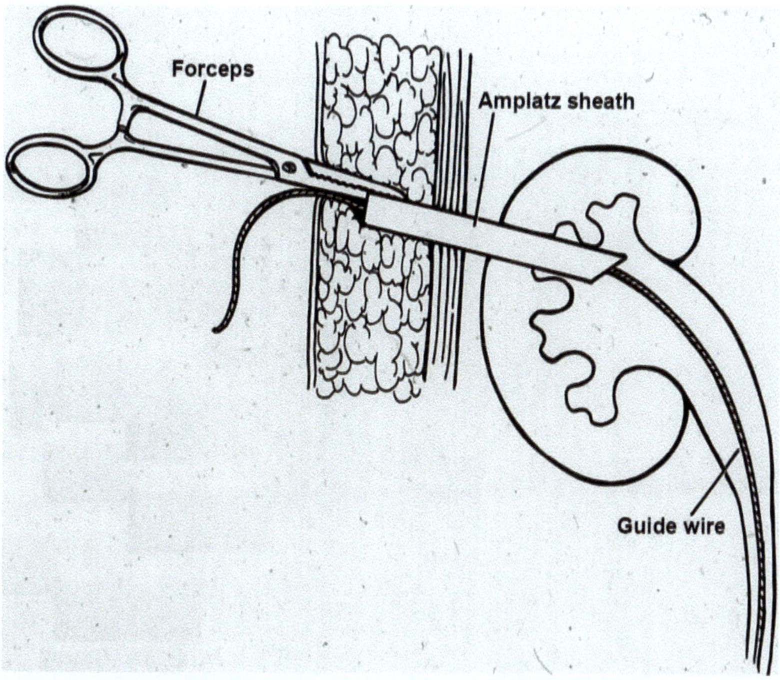

Fig. 16.2 Attempted retrieval of working sheath with a clamp

The balloon can then be inflated to a diameter greater than the sheath, and then the catheter can serve as a retractor with safe distal control of the sheath (Fig. 16.5). Bugeja and colleagues have described using a 10-cc syringe barrel to facilitate retrieval of migrated Amplatz access sheaths during PCNL in obese patients [32].

These techniques are essential preventative measures necessary to have in a urologist armamentarium when performing PCNL on obese patients. The described measures allow for minimally invasive measures to prevent or rectify situations in which the sheath migrates deep to the skin or muscle fascia. In more dramatic cases of sheath migration with loss of percutaneous access when these techniques are not employed, laparoscopic retrieval may be necessary [33].

Nephrostomy Tube Drainage

The ideal strategy for renal drainage following PCNL is a topic of continued controversy and innovation. Traditionally, externalized drainage via a nephrostomy tube is accepted practice following PCNL. The use of different nephrostomy tubes has been reported, including Foley catheters, Malecot catheters, reentry nephrostomy tubes, endopyelotomy tubes, Cope loops, self-retaining pigtail catheters, and circle nephrostomy tubes. Secondary to optimizing drainage, nephrostomy tubes have been used to maintain access for reentry for staged procedures, allow antegrade nephrostography, and provide a theorized mechanism for tamponade in the nephrostomy tract.

The heightened risk of tube dislodgement is of specific concern in the obese population. Repositioning at the culmination of the case in cases of prone PCNL and instances of bed transfers, especially in the obese patient population, increases the risk of the tube to migrate from its ideal position. When secured to the skin, as customarily done, the tube may dislodge due to a large pannus during patient repositioning [34]. Hence, it is suggested that reentry nephrostomy tubes may provide a more secure drainage mechanism since they provide a longer component in the collecting system with a Malecot in the pelvis and extension of the tube into the proximal ureter. Also, in cases where dislodgement is a concern after repositioning or patient transfer, an antegrade

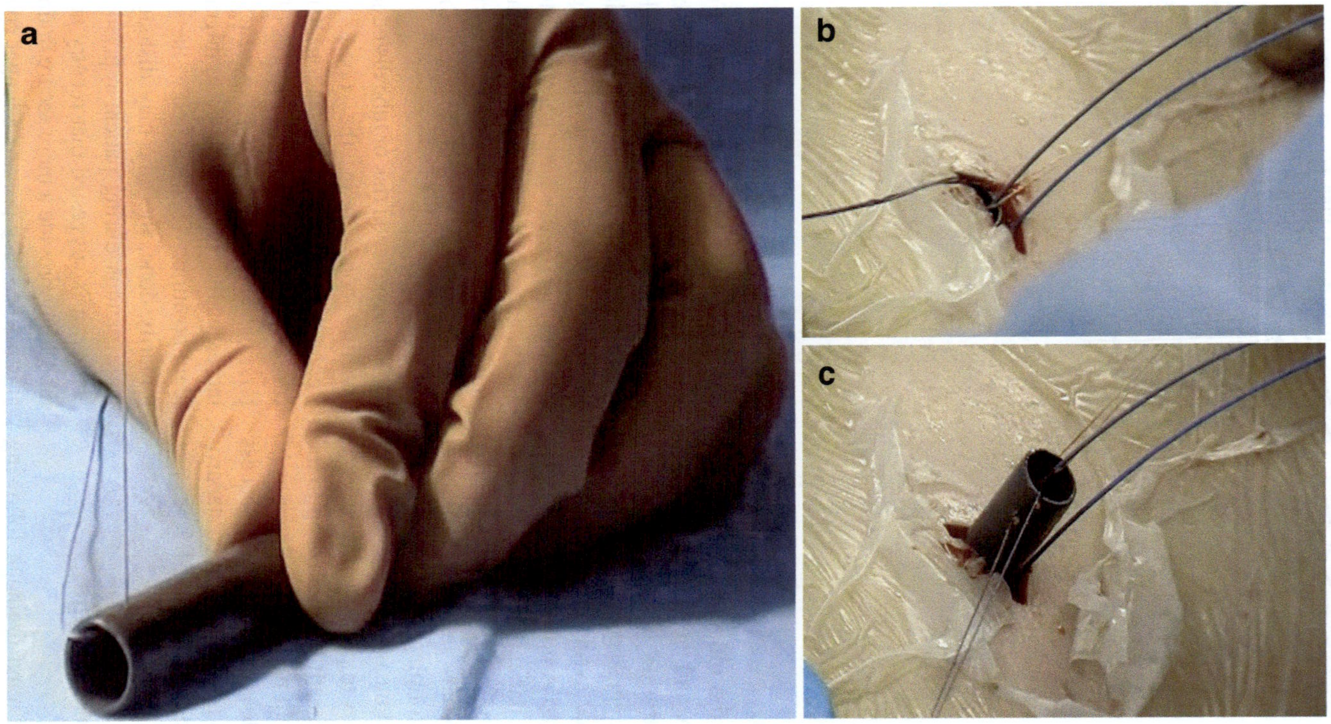

Fig. 16.3 (**a**) Preoperative placement of drawstring sutures in working access sheath. (**b**) Working sheath advanced under the level of the skin in an obese patient. (**c**) Using suture drawstrings to withdraw working sheath from under the level of the skin and subcutaneous tissues in an obese patient

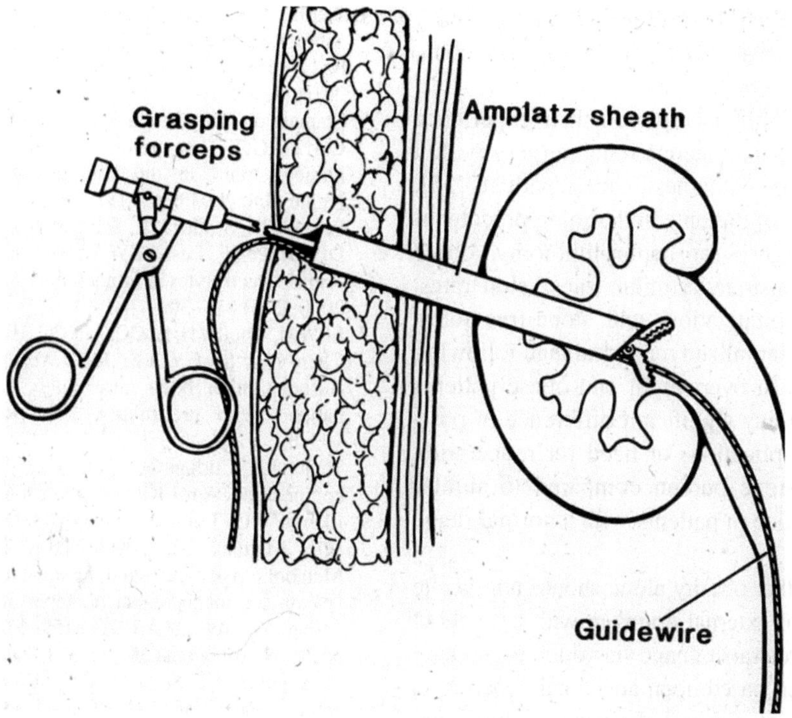

Fig. 16.4 Use of open stone grasping forceps to withdraw working sheath that has advanced deep to the surface of the skin

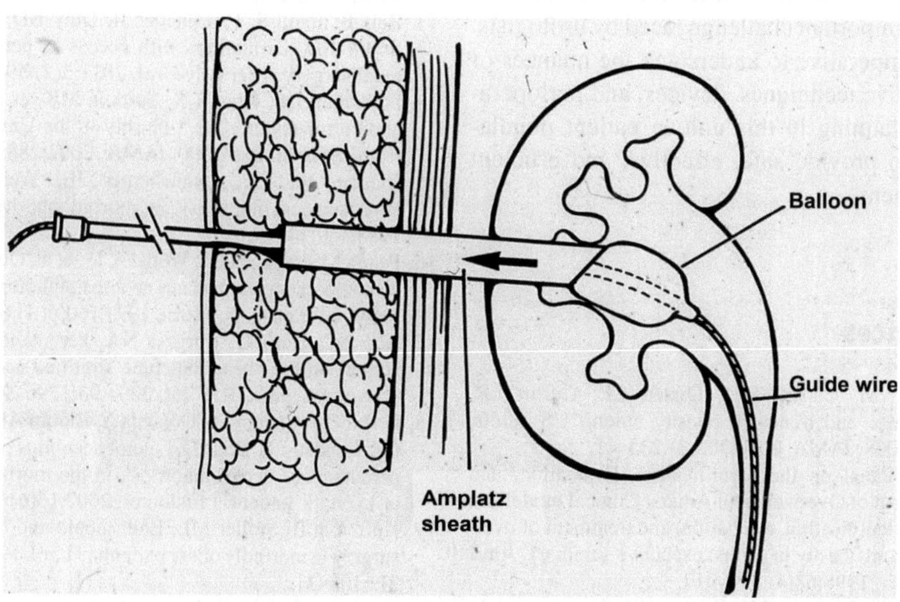

Fig. 16.5 Use of a council-tipped catheter with inflated balloon to withdraw working sheath that has advanced deep to the surface of the skin

nephrostogram can be performed, and a reentry tube may be repositioned more easily than some other drainage tubes.

Yang and Bellman reported their experience with tubeless percutaneous renal surgery with a specific focus on outcomes in obese patients [35]. In their subset of patients undergoing percutaneous renal surgery for nephrolithotomy, obese patients demonstrated similar transfusion rates, length of hospitalization, and stone-free rates. The lack of externalized renal drainage following the procedure in overweight and obese patients did not reveal any significant difference in postoperative complications or need for reoperation for residual stone burden compared to similar drainage practice in patients with a normal range BMI.

It appears that obesity alone should not dictate the decision of external drainage with or without internalized ureteral drainage via a double-J ureteral stent. However, based upon anecdotal experience, certain forms of external drainage nephrostomy tubes may provide more secure drainage in overweight and obese patients who are at risk of dislodgement.

Conclusions

PCNL in morbidly obese patients is an ever-more important challenge faced by urologists. It is imperative to understand the nuances of operative techniques, devices, and perioperative planning in this unique patient population to provide safe, effective, and efficient treatment.

References

1. Flegal KM, Carroll MD, Ogden CL, Curtin LR. Prevalence and trends in obesity among US adults, 1999–2008. JAMA. 2010;303(3):235–41.
2. Expert Panel on the Identification, Evaluation, and Treatment of Overweight in Adults. Clinical guidelines on the identification, evaluation, and treatment of overweight and obesity in adults: executive summary. Am J Clin Nutr. 1998;68(4):899–917.
3. Taylor EN, Stampfer MJ, Curhan GC. Obesity, weight gain, and the risk of kidney stones. JAMA. 2005;293(4):455–62.
4. Semins MJ, Shore AD, Makary MA, Magnuson T, Johns R, Matlaga BR. The association of increasing body mass index and kidney stone disease. J Urol. 2010;183(2):571–5.
5. Stamatelou KK, Francis ME, Jones CA, Nyberg LM, Curhan GC. Time trends in reported prevalence of kidney stones in the United States: 1976–1994. Kidney Int. 2003;63(5):1817–23.
6. Powell CR, Stoller ML, Schwartz BF, Kane C, Gentle DL, Bruce JE, Leslie SW. Impact of body weight on urinary electrolytes in urinary stone formers. Urology. 2000;55(6):825–30.
7. Li WM, Chou YH, Li CC, Liu CC, Huang SP, Wu WJ, Chen CW, Su CY, Lee MH, Wei YC, Huang CH. Association of body mass index and urine pH in patients with urolithiasis. Urol Res. 2009;37(4):193–6.
8. Taylor EN, Curhan GC. Body size and 24-hour urine composition. Am J Kidney Dis. 2006;48(6):905–15.
9. Ekeruo WO, Tan YH, Young MD, Dahm P, Maloney ME, Mathias BJ, Albala DM, Preminger GM. Metabolic risk factors and the impact of medical therapy on the management of nephrolithiasis in obese patients. J Urol. 2004;172(1):159–63.
10. Nishio S, Yokoyama M, Iwata H, Takeuchi M, Kamei O, Sugamoto T, Seike Y, Ochi K, Kin M, Aoki K, Nabeshima S, Takeda H, Takei S. Obesity as one of the risk factors for urolithiasis. Nippon Hinyokika Gakkai Zasshi. 1998;89(6):573–80.
11. Fernström I, Johansson B. Percutaneous pyelolithotomy. A new extraction technique. Scand J Urol Nephrol. 1976;10(3):257–9.
12. Skolarikos A, Alivizatos G, de la Rosette JJ. Percutaneous nephrolithotomy and its legacy. Eur Urol. 2005;47(1):22–8.
13. Rais-Bahrami S, Friedlander JI, Duty BD, Okeke Z, Smith AD. Difficulties with access in percutaneous renal surgery. Ther Adv Urol. 2011;3(2):59–68.
14. Freedman DS, Khan LK, Serdula MK, et al. Trends and correlates of class 3 obesity in the United States from 1990 through 2000. JAMA. 2002;288:1758–61.
15. Carson 3rd CC, Danneberger JE, Weinerth JL. Percutaneous lithotripsy in morbid obesity. J Urol. 1988;139:243–5.
16. Pearle MS, Nakada SY, Womack JS, et al. Outcomes of contemporary percutaneous nephrostolithotomy in morbidly obese patients. J Urol. 1998;160(pt 1):669–763.
17. Koo BC, Burtt G, Burgess NA. Percutaneous stone surgery in the obese: outcome stratified according to body mass index. BJU Int. 2004;93:1296–9.
18. Gofrit ON, Shapiro A, Donchin Y, Bloom AI, Shenfeld OZ, Landau EH, Pode D. Lateral decubitus position for percutaneous nephrolithotripsy in the morbidly obese or kyphotic patient. J Endourol. 2002;16(6):383–6.
19. Hofmann R, Stoller ML. Endoscopic and open stone surgery in morbidly obese patients. J Urol. 1992;148(pt 2):1108–11.
20. Manohar T, Jain P, Desai M. Supine percutaneous nephrolithotomy: effective approach to high-risk and morbidly obese patients. J Endourol. 2007;21(1):44–9.

21. Kerbl K, Clayman RV, Chandhoke PS, Urban DA, De Leo BC, Carbone JM. Percutaneous stone removal with the patient in a flank position. J Urol. 1994;151(3):686–8.
22. Valdivia Uría JG, Lachares Santamaría E, Villarroya Rodríguez S, Taberner Llop J, Abril Baquero G, Aranda Lassa JM. Nefrolitectomía percutánea: Técnica simplificada (nota previa). Arch Esp Urol. 1987;40(3).
23. Desai MR, Jasani A. Percutaneous nephrolithotripsy in ectopic kidneys. J Endourol. 2000;14(3):289–92.
24. Francesca F, Felipetto R, Mosca F, Boggi U, Rizzo G, Puccini R. Percutaneous nephrolithotomy of transplanted kidney. J Endourol. 2002;16(4):225–7.
25. de la Rosette JJ, Tsakiris P, Ferrandino MN, Elsakka AM, Rioja J, Preminger GM. Beyond prone position in percutaneous nephrolithotomy: a comprehensive review. Eur Urol. 2008;54(6):1262–9.
26. Liu L, Zheng S, Xu Y, Wei Q. Systematic review and meta-analysis of percutaneous nephrolithotomy for patients in the supine versus prone position. J Endourol. 2010;24(12):1941–6.
27. Swerdlow BN, Brodsky JB, Butcher MD. Placement of a morbidly obese patient in the prone position. Anesthesiology. 1988;68(4):657–8.
28. Wu SD, Yilmaz M, Tamul PC, Meeks JJ, Nadler RB. Awake endotracheal intubation and prone patient self-positioning: anesthetic and positioning considerations during percutaneous nephrolithotomy in obese patients. J Endourol. 2009;23(10):1599–602.
29. Curtis R, Thorpe AC, Marsh R. Modification of the technique of percutaneous nephrolithotomy in the morbidly obese patient. Br J Urol. 1997;79(1):138–40.
30. Giblin JG, Lossef S, Pahira JJ. A modification of standard percutaneous nephrolithotripsy technique for the morbidly obese patient. Urology. 1995;46(4):491–3.
31. Nguyen TA, Belis JA. Endoscopic management of urolithiasis in the morbidly obese patient. J Endourol. 1998;12:33–5.
32. Bugeja S, Zammit P, German K. Use of a modified syringe barrel to ensure control of the amplatz sheath during percutaneous nephrolithotomy in obese patients. J Endourol. 2009;23:1817–9.
33. Castillo OA, Metrebian E, Vitagliano G. Laparoscopic retrieval of a migrated Amplatz sheath. JSLS. 2007;11(1):116–8.
34. Srinivasan AK, Herati A, Okeke Z, Smith AD. Renal drainage after percutaneous nephrolithotomy. J Endourol. 2009;23(10):1743–9.
35. Yang RM, Bellman GC. Tubeless percutaneous renal surgery in obese patients. Urology. 2004;63(6):1036–40.

17 Percutaneous Nephrolithotomy (PCNL) for Calyceal Diverticulum: An Egyptian Experience

Ahmed Mohamed Elshal, Ahmed M. Shoma, and Ahmed A. Shokeir

Introduction

Calyceal diverticulum is a urine-containing cavity within the renal parenchyma, lined by transitional epithelium and surrounded by a layer of muscularis mucosae. It may be congenital which results from failure of regression of the ureteric bud or acquired in the form of hydrocalyces secondary to blunt renal trauma or obstruction of calyceal infundibulum [1].

In intravenous pyelograms (IVP), it occurs in 0.21–0.45 % of patients; of these, only 3 % are bilateral [1].

Two types of calyceal diverticulum can be distinguished: type I is situated at the upper pole and communicates with a minor calyx; it is most common, while type II communicates with either the renal pelvis or a major calyx [2].

Diagnostic Approach

Calyceal diverticulum is asymptomatic in most of the cases. Once symptomatic, patients complain of flank pain, hematuria, recurrent urinary tract infections (UTIs), or stone formation. Laboratory investigations including routine urine analysis, serum creatinine, and calcium (ionized calcium or total calcium plus albumin) are usually unremarkable. UTIs could be suspected by a positive dipstick test and confirmed by urine culture [3, 4]. Auge et al. reported at least one metabolic abnormality, such as hypercalciuria, hyperuricosuria, hypocitraturia, or hyperoxaluria in all patients with calyceal diverticula. The most common abnormality was low urine volume (less than 2,000 ml/day) in 11 out of 12 patients in the study group [5]. Imaging is the cornerstone in diagnosis. Renal ultrasound (US) is diagnostic in about 80 % of cases [6]. The diverticulum may appear as a cyst-like lesion, indistinguishable from a simple cyst (Fig. 17.1). On IVP, most calyceal diverticula will opacify owing to the connection with the collecting system. This occurs later in the examination, since the diverticulum is filled in a retrograde fashion from its connecting calyx or the renal pelvis [7] (Fig. 17.2). Computed tomogram urography (CTU) may be utilized for better delineation of the diverticulum especially when intervention is warranted (Figs. 17.3 and 17.4). When the neck of a calyceal diverticulum is obstructed, it will not opacify, making it impossible to distinguish between a renal cyst and calyceal diverticulum on preoperative imaging [8]. If calyceal diverticula are suspected during management of associated pathology, a retrograde pyelogram is recommended.

A.M. Elshal, M.D. (✉) • A.M. Shoma, M.D.
A.A. Shokeir, M.D., Ph.D., FEBU
Department of Urology, Urology and Nephrology Center, Mansoura University, El Gomhoria Street, Mansoura 35516, Egypt
e-mail: elshalam@hotmail.com; ahmedshoma@hotmail.com; ahmed.shokeir@hotmail.com

A.M. Al-Kandari et al. (eds.), *Difficult Cases in Endourology*,
DOI 10.1007/978-1-84882-083-8_17, © Springer-Verlag London 2013

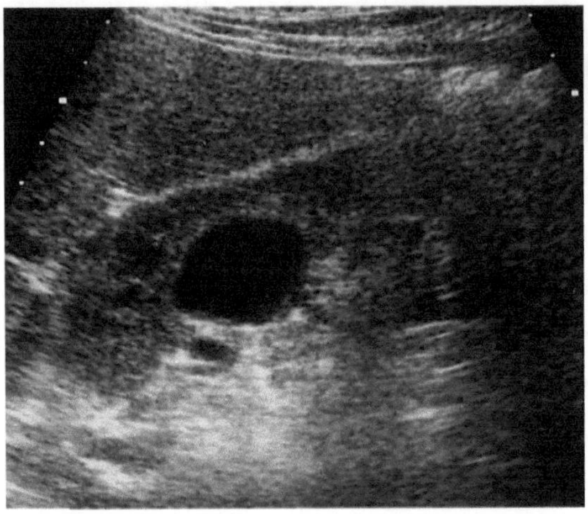

Fig. 17.1 US appearance of calyceal diverticulum

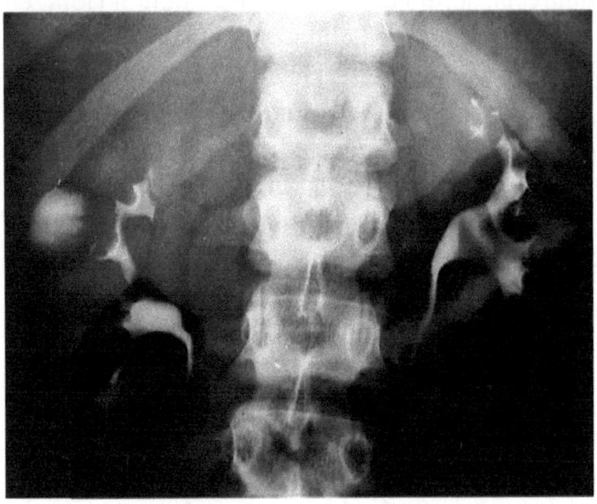

Fig. 17.2 IVU appearance of calyceal diverticulum

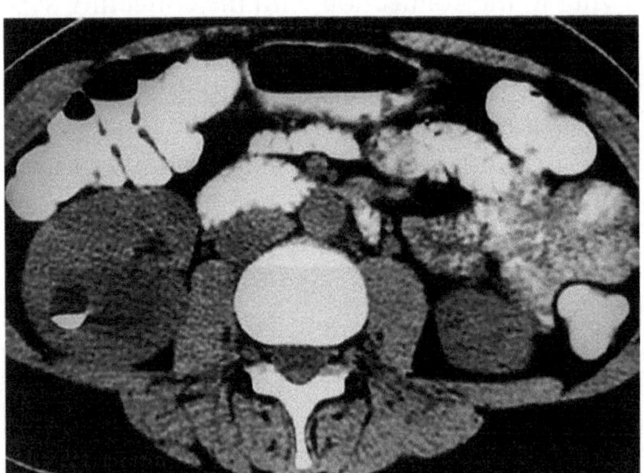

Fig. 17.3 Contrast enhanced CT in supine position, right-sided calyceal diverticulum

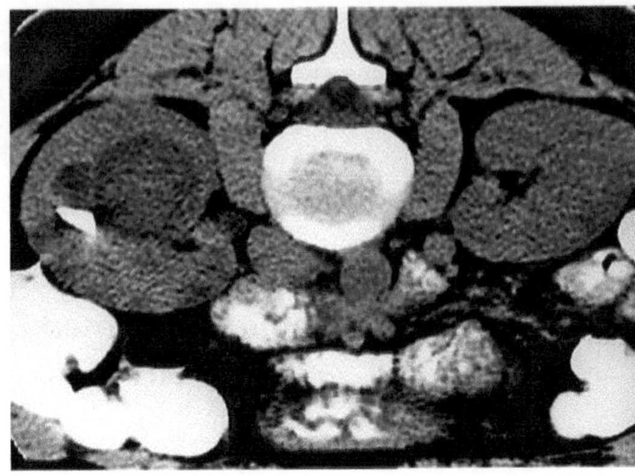

Fig. 17.4 Contrast enhanced CT in prone position, right-sided calyceal diverticulum

Calyceal Diverticulum Stone

The incidence of stone formation in calyceal diverticula is rather high, with a rate of 9.5–39 % [9, 10]. The etiology of calyceal diverticular calculi is controversial; both urinary stasis and underlying metabolic abnormalities were implicated as causative factors [11, 12]. If left untreated, stones in calyceal diverticulum may cause recurrent UTIs in 25 % of cases and obstruction of the diverticular neck which may lead to sepsis, abscess formation, or hypertension in rare instances [13]. Once a patient is symptomatic, investigations should follow the same diagnostic approach for stone disease with few added laboratory investigations to detect any associating metabolic abnormality. Imaging should be done with interest to opacify and delineate the diverticulum and its communication with pelvicalyceal system.

Treatment Approach for Calyceal Diverticulum Stone

Some patients do not need further treatment but continue to receive follow-up care to check for the presence of infections and calculi. Indications for treatment include chronic or recurrent pyelonephritis, pain, gross hematuria, and renal damage [14]. Treatment options include extracorporeal shock wave lithotripsy (ESWL), retrograde intrarenal surgery (RIRS), percutaneous nephrolithotomy (PCNL), or surgical extraction through laparoscopic or open surgical approach. Many factors will influence the choice for treatment modality, including location of the diverticulum: anterior or posterior and upper, middle, or lower pole. The overlying parenchymal thickness, the stone size, and the width of the diverticular neck also have a role.

ESWL

The narrow neck of a diverticulum hinders free passage of stone fragments. Caution should be exercised in the treatment of stone-containing calyceal diverticula by ESWL. It should be reserved for selected cases with small symptomatic diverticulum containing calculi less than 1 cm with a large infundibulum and patients wishing for noninvasive treatment [15]. ESWL is of limited value in any other case due to inadequate passage of stone fragments through the tight diverticular neck, lack of eradication of the existing anatomical defect, and repeat symptomatology due to UTIs [16]. Turna et al. reported on ESWL for 38 calyceal diverticulum stones: stone-free rate of 21 %, symptom-free rate of 61 %, and the need for reendoscopic treatment in 32 % of cases [15].

Retrograde Intrarenal Surgery (RIRS)

The use of flexible ureteroscope and the tipless stone basket has extended the role of RIRS in the management of calyceal diverticula. In combination with either holmium:YAG or thulmium:YAG lasers to incise the stenotic infundibulum, stone clearance and prevention of recurrence may be achieved. One problem that occurs when using this approach is identification of the diverticular neck [8]. However, ureteroscopic management yielded poor results with regard to stone-free rate (19–58 %), symptom-free rate (35–69 %), and diverticular obliteration status (approximately 20 %) with highest success rate in upper pole diverticula [17, 18].

PCNL

Percutaneous approach should be considered the primary treatment modality in calyceal diverticula [17]. Detailed information about the role of percutaneous management of calyceal diverticular stones will follow.

Laparoscopic Approach

Laparoscopic approach is either utilized for laparoscopic nephrolithotomy or laparoscopic-assisted PCNL. Laparoscopic access using retroperitoneal or transperitoneal approach is done. Gerota's fascia is incised to identify and mobilize the kidney, followed by complete examination of its surface. If the calyceal diverticulum cannot be directly visualized, retrograde injection of indigo carmine (turning the diverticulum blue), intraoperative fluoroscopy, or intraoperative laparoscopic US to identify the calculus is done. Once identified, a perpendicular incision through the parenchyma or along the avascular plane of Brodel's line at the posterior lateral aspect of the kidney is performed with electrosurgical scissors or J-hook electrocautery. The calculus or calculi are extracted and placed within an endoscopy bag [19, 20]. Laparoscopic-assisted PCNL technique is used for particular indications. This technique addresses the unusual combination of an anterior calyceal diverticulum together with large stone burden or a stenotic orifice. The anterior location of the diverticulum precluded treatment with PCNL, while the stone burden and stenotic orifice precluded management with ESWL [21, 22]. Brunet et al. reported on three cases of laparoscopic-assisted PCNL that became symptom-free without complications and with obliteration of the diverticular cavity in two patients [22].

Open Surgery

There remains a small role for open surgery in those cases in which stones cannot be removed by a reasonable number of extracorporeal, percutaneous, or endoscopic procedures, in which anatomic considerations exclude their use or when these techniques have simply failed [23].

PCNL for Calyceal Diverticulum Stone

Technique

Percutaneous treatment of symptomatic calyceal diverticular calculi involves renal access, stone removal, dilation of the diverticular communication, treating the diverticular neck, and placement of a nephrostomy tube.

Renal Access

Direct puncture onto a well-opacified diverticulum after opacification of the collecting system either by retrograde pyelography or by IVU until the calyceal diverticulum is well outlined. If the diverticulum failed to opacify, direct puncture onto the radioopaque stones or US-guided access is utilized [13]. Three-dimensional CT-guided puncture of the collecting system to ensure correct access may be utilized [24]. New PC-based software that simulates percutaneous access has been introduced [25]. When the puncture is made directly into the calyceal diverticulum itself, a hydrophilic-coated guide wire may successfully pass through the neck of the diverticulum, but more often the neck is not blindly accessible and the wire must be coiled in the diverticular cavity. If the diverticulum is large enough to accommodate a second wire, a safety wire is also placed before dilatation of the tract [26].

Dilatation of the Tract

For dilation, balloon catheter may be preferable [10]. Dilating the tract with sheath dilators is more difficult and may result in an anterior false passage of the diverticulum (Fig. 17.5). Amplatz sheath is placed into the diverticulum, after which the rigid nephroscope is introduced [26].

Stone Extraction

Any calculus present is treated by either intact removal or after disintegration [26]. For stone disintegration, the holmium:YAG laser has the advantage of being utilized with rigid and flexible nephroscope; also it may be used to fulgurate the wall of the diverticular cavity and the infundibular neck [13]. Both pneumatic and US lithotripter may be utilized; the pneumatic lithotripter seems to be more cost effective, while US lithotripter has a major advantage of combining stone fragmentation and simultaneous fragment removal [27].

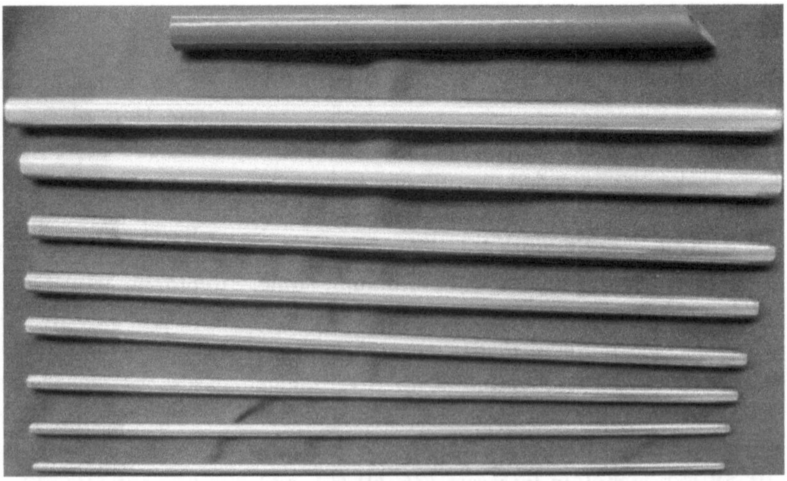

Fig. 17.5 Metal dilators and Amplatz sheath

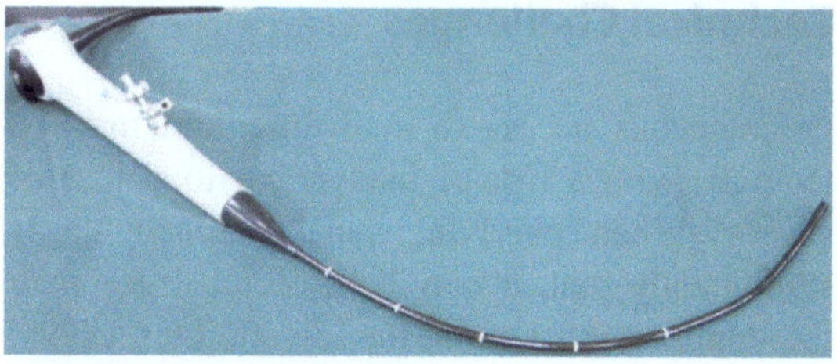

Fig. 17.6 Flexible nephroscope

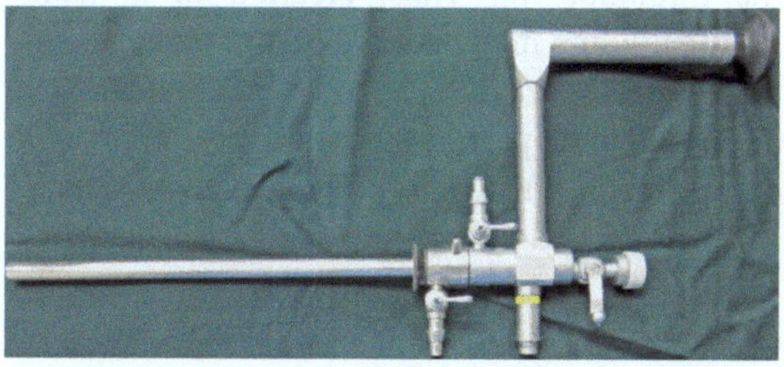

Fig. 17.7 Rigid nephroscope (KarlStorz, Tuttlingen, Germany)

Treating the Diverticular Neck

The connection between the diverticulum and the collecting system is either enlarged or ablated [13].

Examination of the interior of the diverticulum using rigid or flexible nephroscope, with or without retrograde instillation of indigo carmine or room air, is performed (Figs. 17.6 and 17.7). Once the neck of the diverticulum is visualized, a guide wire can be passed across the neck of the diverticulum and coiled in the renal pelvis. Next, balloon dilation of the neck of the diverticulum with a 4-cm-long ureteral dilating balloon is carried out (Fig. 17.8). The neck of the diverticulum is incised under direct vision with cold knife, electrosurgical probe, or holmium:YAG laser. Several shallow incisions (2–4 mm) are made in the neck of the diverticulum in a radial fashion (12, 3, 6, and 9 o'clock). A solitary deep cut into the diverticular neck should be avoided because this may result in significant hemorrhage [17]. After the neck of the diverticulum is opened, a large-bore (22-Fr) nephrostomy tube is placed such that its shaft traverses the diverticulum and the tip of the catheter lies in the renal pelvis. The nephrostomy tube can be removed as early as 3 days after the procedure [28]. In the case of an anterior calyceal diverticulum, the neck will likely never be seen, or in cases in which the stenotic infundibulum cannot be traversed with a guide wire, either creation of neoinfundibulotomy or fulguration of the diverticulum will be the alternative [13].

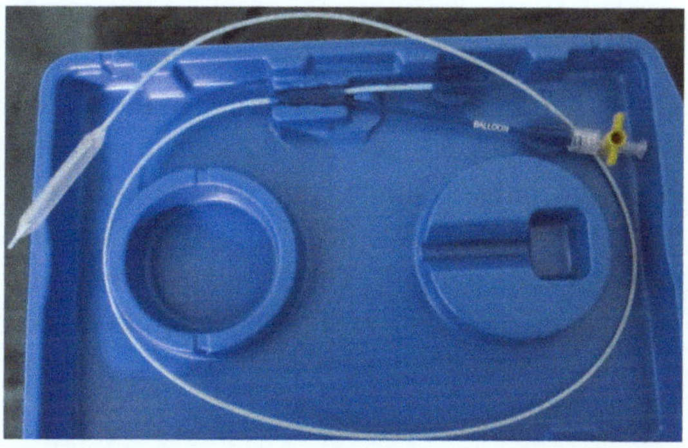

Fig. 17.8 Balloon ureteral dilator

Creation of a neoinfundibulotomy may permit a secure access to the collecting system while providing effective results. If guide-wire passage is unsuccessful after several attempts, the needle is advanced directly through the diverticulum wall into the renal pelvis. The wire is then manipulated down the ureter. After a second (safety) wire is placed through a two-wire introducer, the neoinfundibulotomy tract is dilated to 30 F with a standard fascial dilating balloon. The sheath is advanced under fluoroscopic guidance into the renal pelvis, and nephroscopy is performed. This approach has the advantage of extraction of other renal pelvis stone through the same track [17]. Fulguration of the diverticulum is a faster and perhaps simpler alternative not to identify the diverticular neck. Instead, the entire surface of the diverticulum, including the area of the unidentified diverticular neck, is thoroughly fulgurated using rollerball electrode on a transurethral resectoscope (50-W pure coagulation) or holmium laser (15 J, 10 Hz) [13]. If electrocautery is utilized, the safety wire should be insulated with an open-ended catheter to prevent inadvertent transmission of current down the ureter. Care should be taken to limit fulguration to the lining of the diverticulum to avoid injury to the underlying parenchyma. A 22-Fr drainage catheter is placed only to tamponade the percutaneous tract; the tip of the catheter thus resides in the calyceal diverticulum. The "calycostomy" tube is removed on the following morning, provided that there is no drainage [29].

Outcome

Stone-free rate is ranging from 78 to 100 % [13, 30], and symptom-free rate is ranging from 85 to 88 % [30, 31].

Complete diverticular obliteration has been evaluated with follow-up CT, as IVP or retrograde pyelography is rarely accurate at demonstrating calyceal diverticula, with complete diverticular obliteration ranging from 61 to 100 % at 3-month follow-up [13, 17, 24]. Minor complications during percutaneous ablation and calculus removal include hemorrhage, pneumothorax, persistent urinary extravasation, and mild extravasation of irrigant [32].

Major complications include renal pelvis perforation with urinoma formation, pneumothorax or hemothorax requiring tube thoracostomy, and massive hemorrhage requiring angiographic intervention; these are relatively uncommon (0–9.5 %) [17, 32].

Technical Challenges

Percutaneous access to a diverticulum may be tenuous, with a risk of inadvertent total loss of access. When overlying renal parenchyma is significantly thin, it may be difficult to stabilize the guide wire within the diverticular cavity. Furthermore, a large calculus within the cavity may make it more difficult to coil a wire or traverse the infundibulum. Thus, creation of a neoinfundibulotomy may permit a secure percutaneous transureteral access to the collecting system [30].

In addition, percutaneous ablation of a wide calyceal neck is frequently difficult, potentially leading to prolonged postoperative urinary leakage.

Summary of Treatment

Treatment options for symptomatic calyceal diverticulum stone include PCNL as a first option with certain circumstances that open the door for other treatment options. Laparoscopic nephrolithotomy is applicable with thin overlying parenchyma; laparoscopic-assisted PCNL for anteriorly located calyceal diverticula and upper pole calyceal diverticular small stones can be managed with either RIRS or ESWL. Open surgical approach remains the last resort with failed or complicated procedures by other means. An algorithm for management of calyceal diverticulum stone is illustrated in Fig. 17.9.

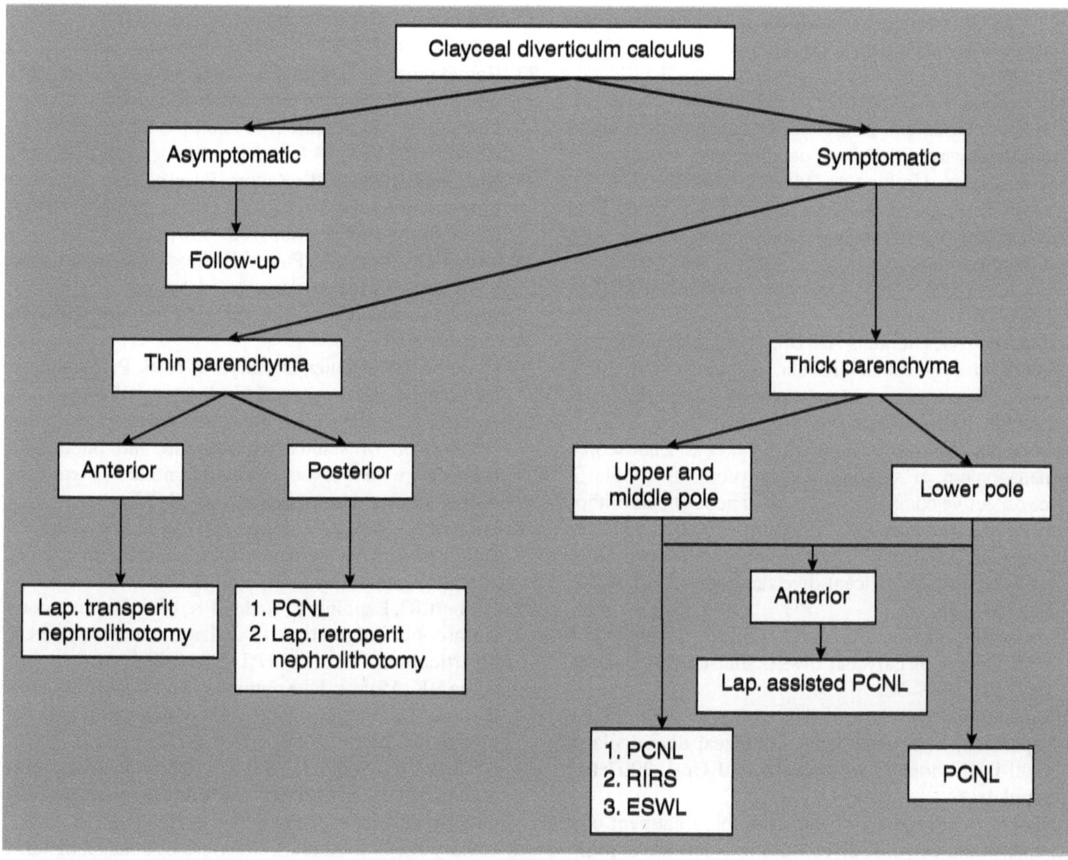

Fig. 17.9 Algorithm for management of calyceal diverticulum stone

References

1. Hulbert JC, Reddy PK, Hunter DW, Castaneda-Zuniga W, Amplatz K, Lange PH. Percutaneous techniques for the management of caliceal diverticula containing calculi. J Urol. 1986;135:225–7.
2. Wulfsohn MA. Pyelocaliceal diverticula. J Urol. 1980; 123:1–8.
3. Argyropoulos A, Farmakis A, Doumas K, Lykourinas M. The presence of microscopic hematuria detected by urine dipstick test in the evaluation of patients with renal colic. Urol Res. 2004;32:294–7.
4. Kobayashi T, Nishizawa K, Mitsumori K, Ogura K. Impact of date of onset on the absence of hematuria in patients with acute renal colic. J Urol. 2003;170: 1093–6.
5. Auge BK, Maloney ME, Mathias BJ, et al. Metabolic abnormalities associated with calyceal diverticular stones. Br J Urol. 2006;97:1053–6.
6. Rathaus V, Konen O, Werner M, et al. Pyelocalyceal diverticulum: the imaging spectrum with emphasis on the ultrasound features. Br J Radiol. 2001;74: 595–601.
7. Matlaga BR, Kim SC, Watkins SL, et al. Preper cutaneous nephrolithotomy opacification for calyceal diverticular calculi. J Endourol. 2006;20: 175–8.
8. Traxer O, Sebe P, Chambade D, et al. How to identify the neck of a calyceal diverticulum in flexible ureterorenoscopy. Prog Urol. 2005;15:100–2.
9. Jones JA, Lingeman JE, Steidle CP. The roles of extracorporeal shock wave lithotripsy and percutaneous nephrostolithotomy in the management of pyelocaliceal diverticula. J Urol. 1991;146:724–7.
10. Grossa AJ, Herrmann RWT. Management of stones in calyceal diverticulum. Curr Opin Urol. 2007;17: 136–40.
11. Hsu TH, Streem SB. Metabolic abnormalities in patients with caliceal diverticular calculi. J Urol. 1998;160:1640–2.
12. Liatsikos EN, Bernardo NO, Dinlenc CZ, Kapoor R, Smith AD. Caliceal diverticular calculi: is there a role for metabolic evaluation? J Urol. 2000;164:18–20.

13. Canales B, Monga M. Surgical management of the calyceal diverticulum. Curr Opin Urol. 2003;13(3): 255–60.
14. Kriegmair MM, Schuller J, Schmeller N, et al. Diverticular calculi of the kidney calices: extracorporeal shockwave lithotripsy, percutaneous extraction or open surgery. Urologe A. 1990;29:204–8.
15. Turna B, Raza A, Moussa S, Smith G, Tolley DA. Management of calyceal diverticular stones with extracorporeal shock wave lithotripsy and percutaneous nephrolithotomy: long-term outcome. BJU Int. 2007;100:151–6.
16. Hendrikx AJ, Bierkens AF, Bos R, et al. Treatment of stones in calyceal diverticula: extracorporeal shock wave lithotripsy versus percutaneous nephrolitholapaxy. Br J Urol. 1992;70:478–82.
17. Auge BK, Munver R, Kourambas J, et al. Endoscopic management of symptomatic calyceal diverticula: a retrospective comparison of percutaneous nephrolithotripsy and ureteroscopy. J Endourol. 2002;16:557–63.
18. Batter SJ, Dretler SP. Ureterorenoscopic approach to the symptomatic caliceal diverticulum. J Urol. 1997; 158:709–13.
19. Miller SD, Ng CS, Streem SB, Gill IS. Laparoscopic management of calyceal diverticular calculi. J Urol. 2002;167:1248–52.
20. Ramakumar S, Gaston KE, Fabrizio MD, et al. Laparoscopic management of calyceal diverticula: a multi-institutional study [abstract]. J Urol. 2002;167 Suppl 4:18.
21. Ruckle HC, Segura JW. Laparoscopic treatment of a stone-filled, calyceal diverticulum: a definitive, minimally invasive therapeutic option. J Urol. 1994;151: 122–4.
22. Brunet P, Meria P, Mahe P, Danjou P. Laparoscopically assisted percutaneous nephrolithotomy for the treatment of anterior calyceal diverticula. BJU Int. 2000; 86(9):1088–9.
23. Ramakumar S, Segura JW. Laparoscopic surgery for renal urolithiasis: pyelolithotomy, calyceal diverticulectomy, and treatment of stones in a pelvic kidney. J Endourol. 2000;14:829–32.
24. Matlaga BR, Shah OD, Zagoria RJ, et al. Computerized tomography guided access for percutaneous nephrostolithotomy. J Urol. 2003;170:45–7.
25. Traxer O, Osorio A, Pasqui F. A new PC based software using a reality augmented system to simulate percutaneous nephrolithotomies. J Endourol. 2004;18 (Suppl):A151.
26. Clayman RV, Hunter D, Surya V, et al. Percutaneous intrarenal electrosurgery. J Urol. 1984;131:864–7.
27. Auge BK, Lallas CD, Pietrow PK, et al. In vitro comparison of standard ultrasound and pneumatic lithotrites with a new combination intracorporeal lithotripsy device. Urology. 2002;60:28–32.
28. Hulbert JC, Reddy PK, Hunter DW, et al. Percutaneous techniques for the management of caliceal diverticula containing calculi. J Urol. 1986;135:225–7.
29. Hulbert JC, Lapointe S, Reddy PK, et al. Percutaneous endoscopic fulguration of a large volume caliceal diverticulum. J Urol. 1987;138:116–7.
30. Auge BK, Munver R, Kourambas J, et al. Neoinfundib ulotomy for the management of symptomatic caliceal diverticula. J Urol. 2002;167:1616–20.
31. Shalhav AL, Soble JJ, Nakada SY, et al. Long-term outcome of calyceal diverticula following percutaneous endosurgical management. J Urol. 1998;160:1635–9.
32. Landry JL, Colombel M, Rouviere O, et al. Long term results of percutaneous treatment of caliceal diverticular calculi. Eur Urol. 2002;41:474–7.

18 Endourological Management of Urological Complications Following Renal Transplantation

Ahmed S. El-Hefnawy, Mohamed M. Elsaadany, Shady A. Soliman, Yasser Osman, Ahmed M. Shoma, and Ahmed A. Shokeir

Introduction

The most commonly reported complications after renal transplantation are ureteral obstruction and urinary leakage. Post renal transplantation ureteral complications can also present as vesicoureteral reflux (VUR), urolithiasis, or lymphocele.

Urological complications after renal transplantation are not uncommon and may cause significant morbidity that could seriously affect both graft and patient survival. For a long time, open surgical intervention has been considered a traditional option for management of urological complications after renal transplantation. However, technical difficulties related to perigraft adhesions render any reconstructive attempt to be a hazardous step.

With the evolution of instruments and accumulated experience of techniques, endourological intervention has emerged as a safe, effective, and minimally invasive treatment option for transplantation urological complications. Unfortunately, the variety of endourological techniques and the small sizes of patient series conspire to make the assessment of these endourological procedures difficult. In addition, the wide range of reported success rates for the same procedure may reflect inadequacy of careful patient selection for each specific technique.

In this chapter, the various endourological techniques used for treatment of urological complications after renal transplantation have been discussed. In addition, comparison between different endourological options, optimization of patient selection, and criteria of success of these minimally invasive procedures are provided.

Materials and Methods

The database of PubMed and the Cochrane Database were searched through May 2011 without time limit. The following keywords were used: renal transplant, urological complications, urinary leakage, stricture, reflux, urolithiasis, and endoscopy. A total of 500 publications were retrieved. In this chapter, leader studies with good design and adequate follow-up were included in the analysis of data. Studies of high level of evidence (level I and II) together with large retrospective studies (level III) were included in our review.

Ureteral Obstruction

Incidence and Etiology

Ureteral obstruction (UO) represents the most common complication after renal transplantation

A.S. El-Hefnawy, M.D. • M.M. Elsaadany, M.D., M.Sc.
S.A. Soliman, M.D. • Y. Osman, M.D. • A.M. Shoma, M.D.
A.A. Shokeir, M.D., Ph.D., FEBU (✉)
Department of Urology, Urology and Nephrology Center, Mansoura University, El Gomhoria Street, Mansoura 35516, Egypt
e-mail: a_s_elhefnawy@yahoo.com; elsaadany@windows.live.com; shady_tx@yahoo.com; y_osman99@yahoo.com; ahmedshoma@hotmail.com; ahmed.shokeir@hotmail.com

A.M. Al-Kandari et al. (eds.), *Difficult Cases in Endourology*,
DOI 10.1007/978-1-84882-083-8_18, © Springer-Verlag London 2013

Table 18.1 Causes of ureteral obstruction after renal transplantation

Usual causes	Unusual causes
1. Narrowing of ureterovesical junction secondary to ischemia or rejection	1. Papillary necrosis causing hydronephrosis
2. Technical error in ureteroneocystostom	2. Ureteropelvic junction compression caused by crossing vessels of renal allograft
3. Kinking of the ureter	3. Postural ureteral obstruction
4. Calculi	4. Vesical wall acting as valve causing obstruction to the lower end of the ureter
5. Fungus balls	5. Ureteral torsion
6. Clots	6. Sliding hernia containing the ureter
7. Extrinsic compression by fluid collections	7. Urothelial ureteric lesions due to rejections
	8. Ovarian tumor
	9. Cytomegalovirus (CMV) ureteritis
	10. Extrinsic scar of abdominal wound causing fibrosis and compression

Modified with permission from Shivde et al. [6]

with reported incidence varying between 2 and 10 % [1–4]. The obstruction may be intrinsic or extrinsic. Most of the obstructions (80 %) involved the distal ureter or vesicoureteral junction [5]. Early postoperative UO is not common and occurs mainly as a result of technical errors such as narrow antireflux tunnel and external compression by hematoma or lymphocele [6]. While late UO is more frequent and mostly related to ureteral stenosis [7], damage to the ureteral blood supply during graft harvest or transplantation may result in ureteral ischemia and subsequent obstruction [8]. Variations in vascular anatomy, immunosuppressive therapy, and allograft rejection episodes are all implicated [3, 9]. In a recent review, Shivde and colleagues have enlisted other rare causes which have been incriminated in UO after renal transplantation [6] (Table 18.1). In a series of 1,688 consecutive renal transplantation patients, male recipient, African male recipient, and "U"-stitch technique were identified as independent risk factors for urinary complications after renal transplantation [2]. Ureteral stricture was an independent risk factor for graft loss. Shokeir et al. found primary urinary continuity as the only risk factor that affected the incidence of surgical complications among pediatric and adolescent live-donor renal transplantation, with the extravesical technique of Lich-Gregoir providing the best results [1]. Interestingly, neither patient nor graft survival was affected in that series. In a sequential double-blind random trial with 170 kidney transplant recipients, patients who had ureteral spatulation length ≥10 mm had significant less complications compared to those who had spatulation ≤10 mm ($P < 0.05$) [10].

Diagnosis

Early detection of UO after transplantation is of paramount importance. Obstruction of renal allograft should be suspected in any patient with an unexplained decrease in urine output, an enlargement or tenderness of the allograft, and a rising in serum creatinine. Routine use of renal ultrasound (US) in the early postoperative period and during the evaluation of progressive azotemia allows early identification of this complication. Renal hydronephrosis is not always present. Low grade dilatation of the collecting system in the early postoperative period may occur with vigorous diuresis or edema at the anastomosis [11]. Elevated resistive index (RI) is an early alarming sign [12]. Diuretic renogram (DR) is useful in equivocal cases. Additional radiographic studies such as computed tomography (CT) [8] or magnetic resonance urography (MRU) may be of assistance in some cases. Further evaluation involves intravenous, retrograde, or antegrade pyelography. Insertion of a percutaneous

Table 18.2 Results of endoscopic procedures used for management of ureteral obstruction after renal transplantation

Series	Endoscopic procedure	Success/total number of cases	Follow-up (months)
Voegeli et al. [17]	Antegrade balloon dilatation	11/13	29
Yong et al. [18]	Antegrade balloon dilatation and ureteric stent	8/9	22
Juaneda et al. [15]	Antegrade balloon dilatation and stent	20/45	78
Aytekin et al. [19]	Antegrade balloon dilatation and stent	Initial 19/19 Late 8/19	34.3
Basiri et al. [18]	Retrograde balloon dilatation	4/10	–
Conrad et al. [20]	Cold-knife endoureterotomy	Initial 10/11 Late 9/11	26
Siddins et al. [21]	Cold-knife endopyelotomy	1/1	–
Katz et al. [22]	PCN and transurethral electrocautery incision	13/14	8
Bahayani et al. [23]	Acucise endoureterotomy	2/3	21
Schwartz et al. [24]	Acucise endoureterotomy (balloon cautery endoureterotomy)	5/6	27
Yossef et al. [25]	Acucise endoureterotomy	3/3	16
Kristo et al. [5]	Antegrade balloon dilatation with or without holmium: YAG laser endoureterotomy	9/9	24
He et al. [26]	Antegrade or retrograde diathermic incision or holmium: YAG laser incision	5/8	16
Gdor et al. [27]	Six combined balloon dilatation and laser	4/6	52

nephrostomy (PCN) and antegrade pyelography is preferred because they avoid intravenous contrast administration and potential difficulties in retrograde access to the transplant ureteral orifice. Antegrade pyelography allows definitive visualization of the site and length of UO, whereas temporary diversion with the PCN aids in the resolution of the azotemia [13].

Management

The treatment of ureteral stenosis has traditionally been operative reconstruction [14], although such intervention may be associated with serious complications, including graft loss and even perioperative mortality [15]. More recently, endourological treatment has been proposed due to its low morbidity. An antegrade approach is used to treat transplant ureteral stenosis. However, if the transplant ureteral orifice is accessible, a retrograde approach may be used [14, 16]. Many endourological techniques have been utilized for management of UO resulting from stricture after renal transplantation including balloon dilation, holmium laser endoureterotomy, Acucise® (Applied Medical, Rancho San Marita, CA), endoureterotomy, and electrocautery. In addition, rigid or flexible ureteroscopy was utilized for management of other causes of UO via either antegrade or retrograde routes. Table 18.2 summarizes the results of endoscopic procedures used for management of UO after renal transplantation.

Endourological Management of UO Owing to Ureteral Stricture

Antegrade Balloon Dilatation

Since Barbaric and Thompson described the first successful PCN in four patients with transplant ureteral stenosis in 1978 [28], there have been many reports of successful percutaneous antegrade balloon dilatation of transplant ureteric stenosis. The procedure usually starts with PCN fixation. Dilatation of stenotic segment is then carried out with high-pressure balloon catheter, 5- to 8-mm balloon size, at a pressure of 8–15 atm for 5–10 min [19]. Following successful dilatation, internal stents could be left in situ for a variable period. Figure 18.1a–c

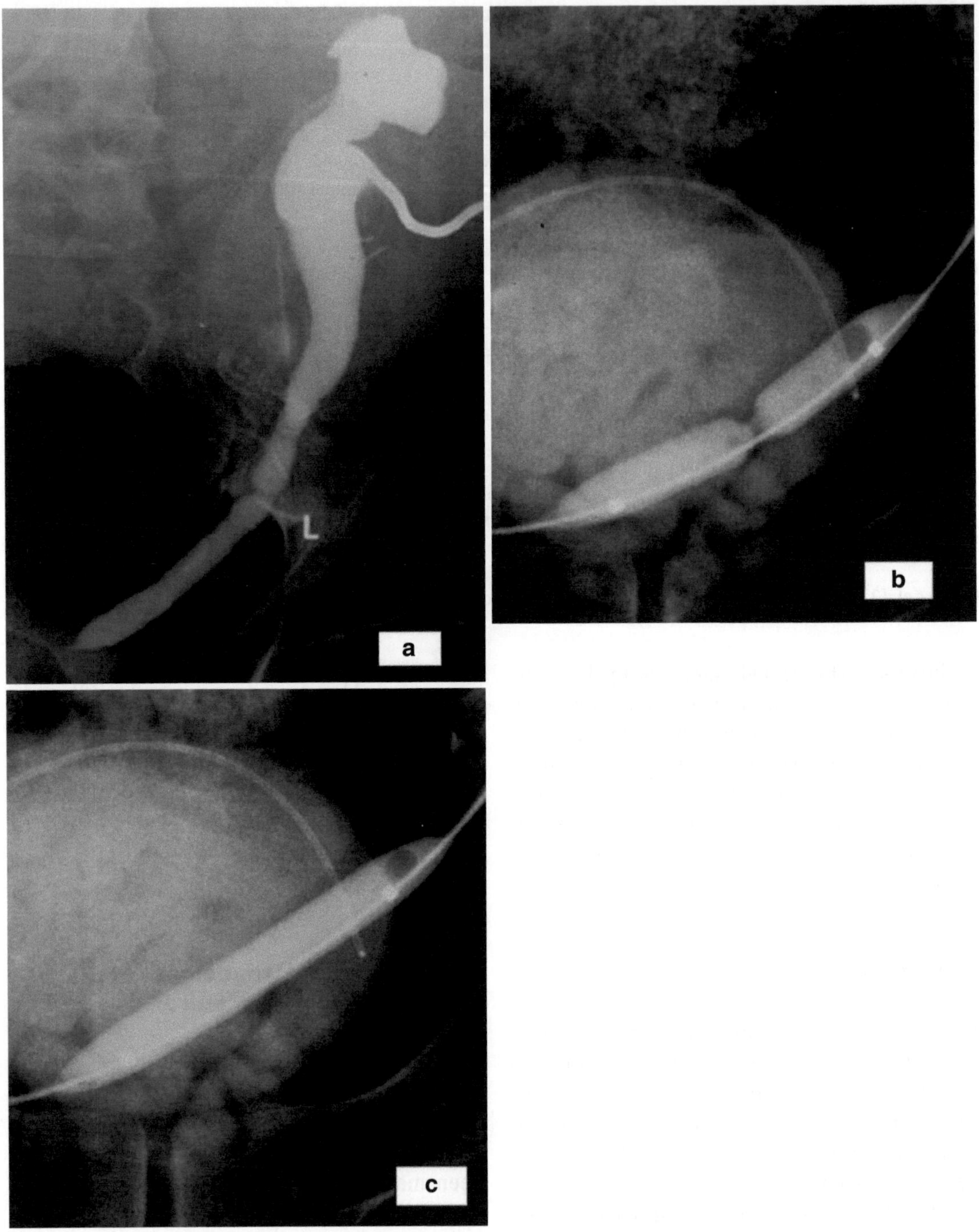

Fig. 18.1 Antegrade balloon dilatation and ureteric stenting for distal transplant ureteral obstruction. (**a**) Antegrade pyelogram showing stricture at the ureteroneocystostomy. (**b**) Balloon catheter is inflated for dilatation of the stricture. (**c**) Successful dilatation with obliteration of the balloon waist

represent a case scenario of successful management of distal ureteral stenosis by antegrade balloon dilatation.

The incidence of success ranges from 30 to 100 %, dependent on the site and nature of the stricture and the time interval following transplantation

[15, 17–19]. Several reports have demonstrated that early obstructions (which are usually secondary to technical factors) have the most favorable outcome, but late obstructions resulting from ischemia have a relatively poor prognosis [6, 15, 18, 19]. On the other hand, other reports have shown that the timing of the obstruction does not affect the success rate [29, 30]. Jauneda et al. found that presence of previous acute rejection episodes was a good prognostic factor for the endourological solution [15]. Eytkin et al. [19] have recommended repetition of balloon dilatation in severe cases of ureteral obstruction, yet neither maximum number of trials nor definition of severity was clear.

Retrograde Balloon Dilatation

To avoid the possible complications of antegrade approach, Basiri and coworkers advocated retrograde ureteroscopy in management of ureteral stenosis with results comparable with antegrade balloon dilation and low morbidity [14, 31]. The main difficulties encountered included finding the ureteral orifice and negotiating the ureter through the intramural part. Critical analysis of their results showed that dilatation was successful only in four out of ten patients. All of those four cases had incomplete obstruction, so that they were able to pass a guide-wire, and the length of the stenosis was 5–8 mm. In 28 patients with different pathologies including ureteral stricture, retrograde access was successfully obtained in 59 and 100 % of patients using the Lich-Gregoir and Politano-Leadbetter methods, respectively.

Endoureterotomy

Balloon dilatation causes multiple tears at the stenotic segment which results in significant periureteral fibrosis which may be a contributing factor for the reported high recurrence rates. To avoid the disadvantages of balloon dilatation, some authors recommended endoureterotomy (incision of the obstructed segment), prolongation of the stent, or utilization of combined techniques.

Cold-Knife Endoureterotomy/ Endopyelotomy

Conrad and colleagues reported that 9 out of 11 ureters incised with a cold knife had long-term success [20]. The complication of hemorrhage requiring blood transfusion has been reported after allograft endopyelotomy under fluoroscopic guidance [20, 21]. Seddins and coworkers reported safe use of cold-knife endopyelotomy in transplant kidneys under guidance of intrarenal Doppler ultrasonography probe [21]. According to authors' opinion, the cost of the probe is justified by greater security in avoiding vascular injury.

Electrocautery

Electrocautery incision for transplant ureteral stricture has been reported with successful outcome [22, 26, 32]. The procedure could be accomplished via antegrade or retrograde techniques and followed by routine ureteral stenting for 6–8 weeks. He and coworkers found no statistical significant results of endoscopic incision of obstructed vesicoureteral anastomosis in transplanted kidneys compared with laser endoureterotomy [26]. For economic reasons, laser endoureterotomy is preserved for cases with stricture more than 10 mm or when obstruction is complete.

Acucise® Endoureterotomy

Endoureterotomy with the Acucise® device (Applied Medical, Rancho San Marita, CA), which incorporates an electrocautery wire and a low-pressure balloon, is another alternative, with reports in series of 1–6 patients and a short-term success rate of 76–100 % [23–25, 32–34].

It was first introduced into clinical practice by Chandhoke and coworkers [34]. The treatment of renal-transplant ureteral stenosis with balloon cautery endoureterotomy has so far been investigated in only a small number of patients [24]. To improve long-term patency of treated ureters, some authors suggest that patient selection is important before operation, i.e., the interval between the appearance of the stricture and the primary operative trauma should be at least 6 months, the length of the stricture should not exceed 1.5 cm, and the function of the obstructed kidney should not be less than 25 % of the total renal function [32]. Bleeding is one of the most feared complications. Additionally, the cost of the device is considerable.

Laser Endoureterotomy

The coagulative and precise incisional properties of Ho: YAG laser, minimal collateral damage and easy manipulation of laser fibers through small caliber flexible ureteroscopy, make it an appealing option in the treatment of transplant ureteral stricture. In 2003, Kristo et al. reported on the first use of Ho: YAG laser endoureterotomy in ureteral stricture after transplantation. In three out of nine patients presented with late-onset ureterovesical strictures (median 7 months), Ho: YAG laser was carried out concomitantly with antegrade balloon dilatation. After a median follow-up of 24 months, the ureteral patency and graft function rates were both 100 % without perioperative complications. Noteworthy, in those three cases, stricture length was 2.5–5 mm [5].

The importance of adding Ho: YAG laser endoureterotomy to balloon dilatation is further supported by others [27]. Authors found recurrence of two out of three cases with strictures less than 10 mm treated with balloon only, compared with 100 % success in combined technique. Overall success rate of combined technique was 67 % (four out of six cases); in all of them, the length of stricture was less than 10 mm. In the same series, three patients with pelviureteral junction obstruction had been treated with laser endopyelotomy with a success rate of 100 %.

Endoscopic Management of Other Causes of Obstruction

In Basiri study, ureteroscopy was successful in retrieval of seven out of nine patients (78 %) with upwardly migrated ureteral stents [14]. In the study of Del Pizzo et al., double pigtail stents had migrated in three cases. In that study, all of the migrated stents could be seen, and all but one were retrieved [35]. Intraluminal obstacles (stone, blood clot, debris) or ureteral compression due to adjacent fluid collection (lymphocele, hematoma, urinoma) also can result in obstruction. However, these complications can be handled easily with percutaneous methods [19]. Figure 18.2a–c represent a case profile of posttransplant UO due to a stone in the distal part of the transplanted ureter.

Role of Stents in Transplant Obstructed Ureter

Routine intraoperative insertion of ureteral stents during renal transplantation to prevent possibility of ureteral leakage and obstruction is a matter of controversy [36]. Debates of this issue are beyond the focus of this chapter. However, routine insertion of ureteral stents after endoscopic management of transplant UO is nearly universally reported. To avoid hazards associated with antegrade maneuvers, retrograde stenting is preferred. Although the reported complications after extravesical Lich-Gregoir technique is much less than Politano-Leadbetter ureteroneocystostomy, it is associated with greater failure of retrograde urgent stent placement [37].

Double J stent has been employed. However, double J stents have several associated problems, namely, encrustation, pain, infection, and migration [38]. In small case series involving three patients with recurrent transplant UO and one patient with complete ureteral occlusion, Memokath 051 stents (a tightly coiled wire of nickel and titanium alloy) were placed via antegrade route [39]. Patients were followed for 18–21 months. During follow-up, one stent migrated within 10 days after stent insertion and was removed cystoscopically. Another stent had to be removed in the 14th month due to resistant infection and was replaced with a new Memokath 051 stent which remained patent for another 8 months. The other two stents were fully patent at the 18th and 21st month of follow-up, respectively.

More recently, Olsburgh et al. described the use of silicone-polytetrafluoroethylene (PTFE)-bonded extra-anatomic urinary tract stent for urinary tract drainage in two cases with failed endoscopic and open surgical reconstruction [40]. The technique was carried out via open cystostomy.

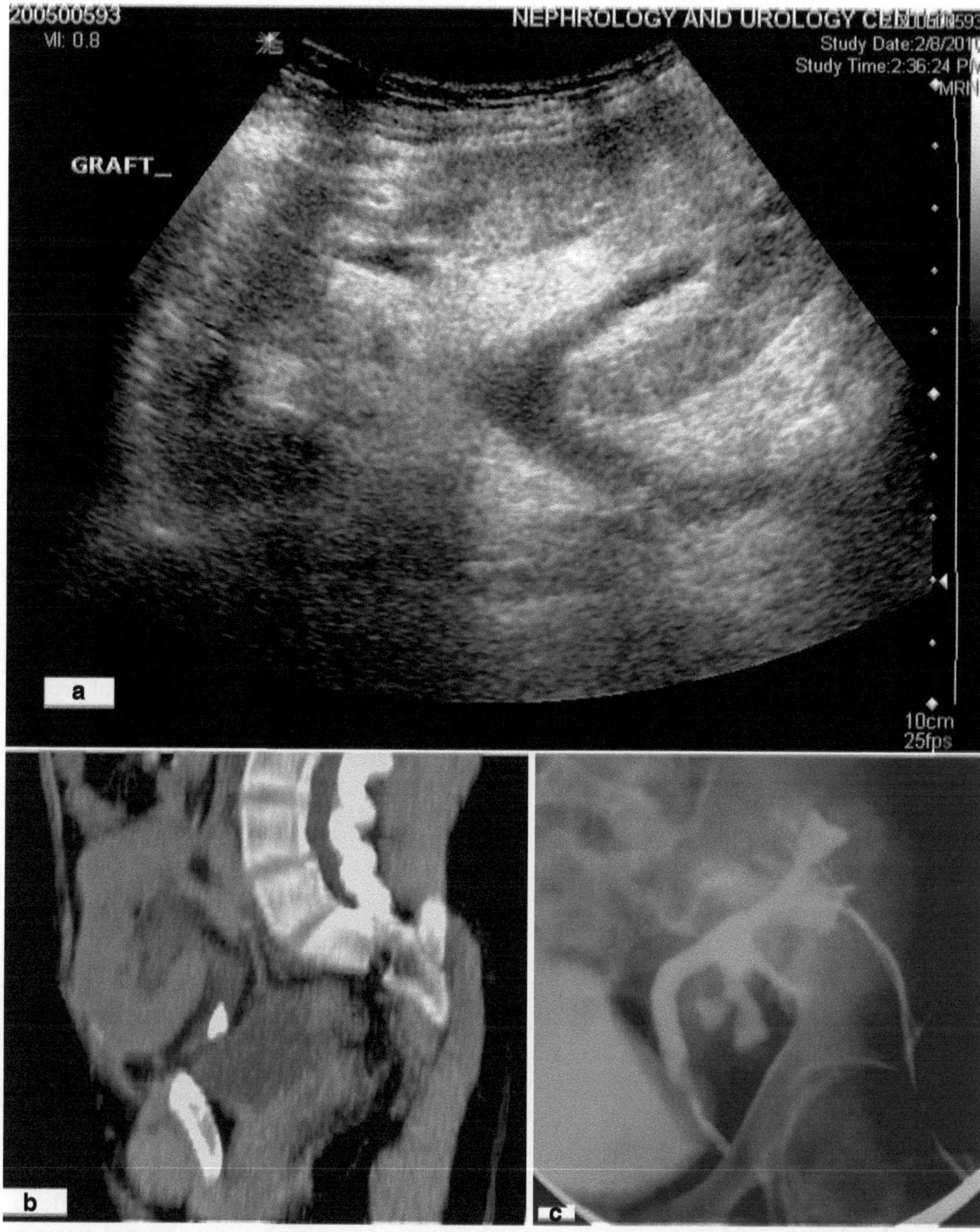

Fig. 18.2 A 27-year-old male presented with dysuria and rising serum creatinine, 4 years after renal transplantation. (**a**) Ultrasonography showing mild hydronephrosis and dilated upper ureter. (**b**) Reconstructed computed tomography showing stone at lower part of transplanted ureter. (**c**) Antegrade study showing filling defect of stone with narrowing of transplanted ureter distal to the stone

Guidelines for Management of Transplant UO

Variability of outcome after endourological management of UO might be a logical finding in the light of the heterogeneity of underlying pathophysiology, variability of patient selection, and variability of techniques involved. Based on aforementioned studies, successful endourological treatment of transplant UO is solely affected by the site and length of the stricture as well as the duration from transplantation. Early UO seems to respond better to endourological management when compared with late UO. Also, distal ureteral strictures near or at the ureterovesical anastomosis respond best to endourological management. Regardless of the endourological technique used, internal or external stent should be used for 4–6 weeks.

The recommended plan for management of transplant intrinsic or mural causes of UO usually starts with fixation of PCN for purpose of drainage and confirmation of diagnosis. Shokeir and colleagues found that use of graft PCN in the initial management of ureteral complications including stricture had many advantages, including allowance resolution of azotemia, enhancement of treatment of infection, and enabled better definition of the site of UO [41]. In addition, it significantly improves the graft survival and function, diminishes the hospital stay, and reduces the incidence of posttreatment complications. According to antegrade study, the treatment decision is determined. Figure 18.3 provides an algorithm for management of posttransplant ureteral stricture. In case of migrated stents or small ureteral stones, flexible ureteroscopy is recommended starting with retrograde route.

Urinary Leakage

Incidence and Etiology

The reported incidence of urinary leakage varies between 1.2 and 8.9 % [4, 42, 43]. In pediatric and adolescent group, the reported rate is 4 % [1]. Urinary leakage is generally evident early after transplantation and commonly caused by vascular insufficiency secondary to inadvertent damage to the vessels that supply the ureter during organ harvesting. Preservation of accessory arteries to the lower pole of the kidney and periureteral fat is important, as they may constitute the blood supply of the collecting system or the ureter. Their ligation may lead to necrosis and ureteral leak [44].

It may also occur as a result of technical problems during ureteroneocystostomy, particularly with transvesical procedures. The rate is slightly higher in patients who received kidneys from living donors than in those who received organs from cadavers [45, 46]. This is presumably a result of more extensive hilar dissection required during harvesting from the living donor, with the attendant risks of injury to the blood supply of the ureter [42]. With the early learning curve of laparoscopic live-donor nephrectomy, the incidence of ureteral complications was significantly higher in comparison to open live-donor nephrectomy [47–49]. The higher incidence of ureteral complications with laparoscopic nephrectomy was attributed to extensive dissections close to the wall of the ureter. With the current knowledge of the necessity for a meticulous preparation of the ureter and its surrounding fatty tissue, the proportion of ureteral complications no longer differs between laparoscopic and open live-donor nephrectomy [50]. Some authors even describe fewer ureteral complications with the laparoscopic approach [2, 47, 51].

Diagnosis

The clinical presentation of urinary fistulas after renal transplantation includes unexplained pain, perigraft swelling, ipsilateral lower limb edema, rising serum creatinine, decreasing urine output, or urinary leakage from the draining tube. For accurate diagnosis, graft US, ascending cystography, and CT scan may be helpful [13]. Determining the nature of the fluid collecting around the graft or leaking from the wound is paramount. A quantitative estimation of the creatinine content of this fluid differentiates between urine and

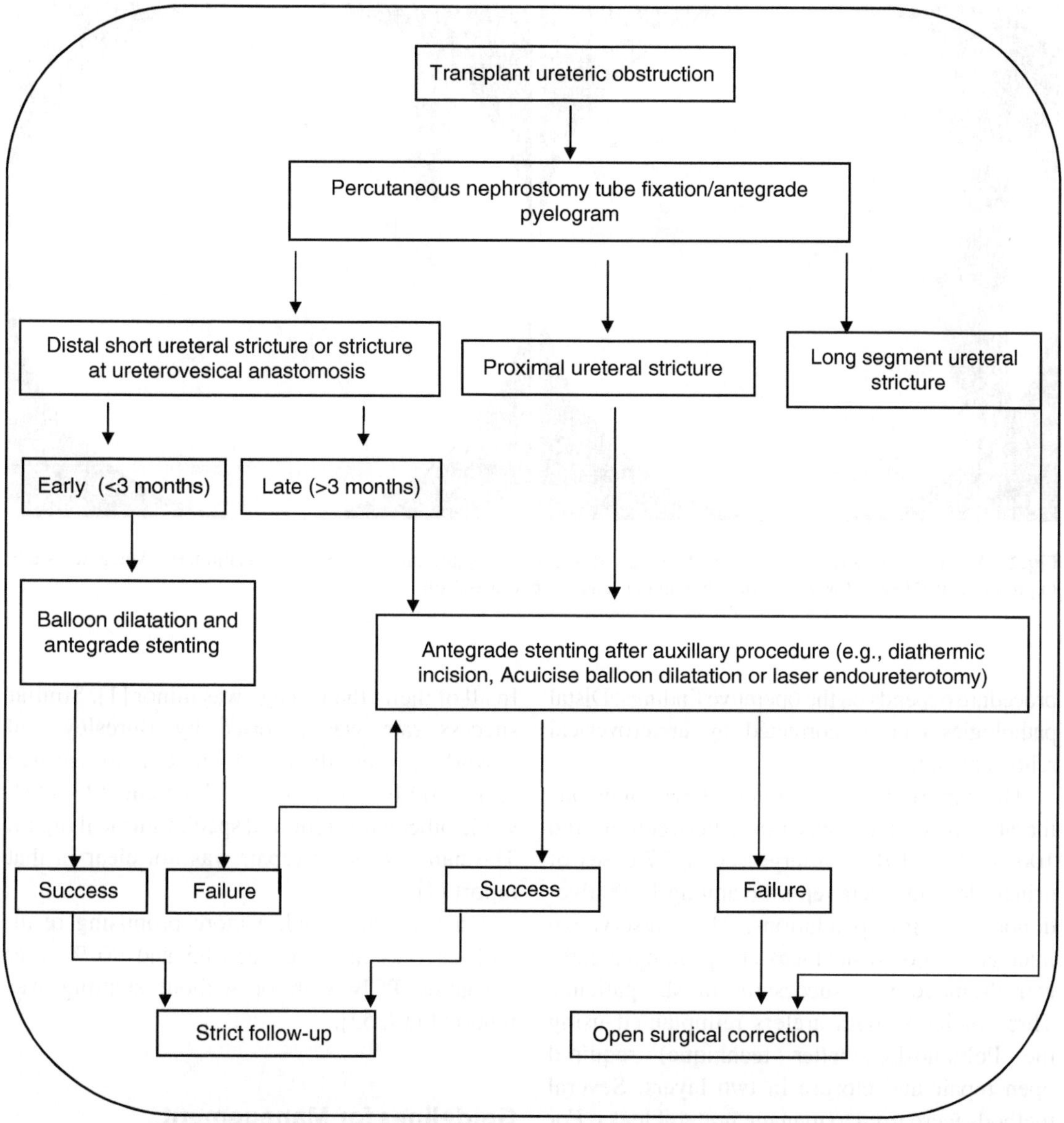

Fig. 18.3 Algorithm for management of ureteral stricture after renal transplantation

lymph. If urine leakage is diagnosed, its possible sources could be either the site of the ureterovesical anastomosis or a ureteral fistula [42].

Management

A few days of watchful waiting with proper drainage of the wound and the bladder usually result in cessation of the urine leak if its source is the bladder. However, if urine continues to leak, then a ureteral fistula is suspected. The diagnosis is usually confirmed by fixation of a graft PCN and antegrade study. Subsequently, ureteral stent should be fixed via antegrade route. If there is urine collection, percutaneous tube drain should be fixed under US or CT guidance. Figure 18.4a, b represent a case scenario of successful management of ureteral leak through graft PCN and antegrade fixation of ureteral stent.

Open surgical revision can be used subsequently if this fails. The choice of the reconstructive

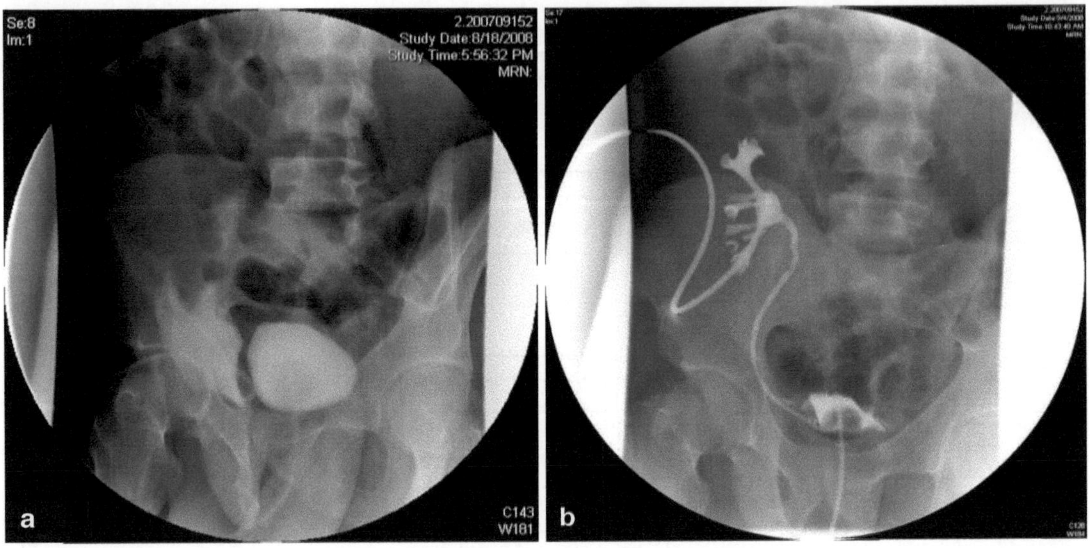

Fig. 18.4 Urinary leakage in a 35-year-old male. (**a**) Ascending cystogram showing extravasation. (**b**) Antegrade study in presence of DJ stent few days after showing absence of extravasation

procedure depends on the operative findings. Distal pathologies can be corrected by ureterovesical reimplantation.

The reported success rates of percutaneous therapy for ureteral leak range between 30 and 100 % [1, 4, 19]. In a large series, 37 cases of urinary leakage were reported among 1,200 live-donor renal transplantations. The conservative management of vesical leaks by prolonged catheter drainage was successful in six patients. Three patients (with ureters reimplanted using the Politano-Leadbetter technique) required open repair and closure in two layers. Several methods were used to manage ureteral leaks. For minor leaks at the vesicoureteral junction, definitive treatment by PCN drainage was attempted in 14 patients. Two patients required subsequent reconstructive procedures. Open surgical revision was required in 16 patients [43]. In a more recent study, Shokeir and coworkers reported ten cases of urinary leakage among 250 adolescent and pediatric patients. In those special categories of patients, the same protocol was followed by initial management using conservative and endourological treatment. Antegrade fixation of JJ stent for 6–8 weeks was sufficient to control such a situation in four cases (40 %). In all of them, the leakage was minor [1]. Similar success rate was reported by Buresley and coworker, where the conservative treatment was successful only in 5 out of 15 patients (33.3 %), while other cases required special surgical repair. The nature of such repair was not clear in that report [4].

On the other hand, a more promising result with success rates between 85 and 90 % after antegrade PCN with or without stenting was reported [19, 52].

Guidelines for Management of Ureteral Leakage

Conservative management of ureteral leak is recommended as an initial step by prolongation of urethral catheter in case of vesical leakage or fixation of PCN ± ureteral stenting. Figure 18.5 provides an algorithm of management of urinary leakage following renal transplantation. However, such measures are not effective in cases of extensive ureteral necrosis where early surgical management is mandatory. Figure 18.6a, b are an example of failure of endourological management of ureteral leakage following renal transplantation.

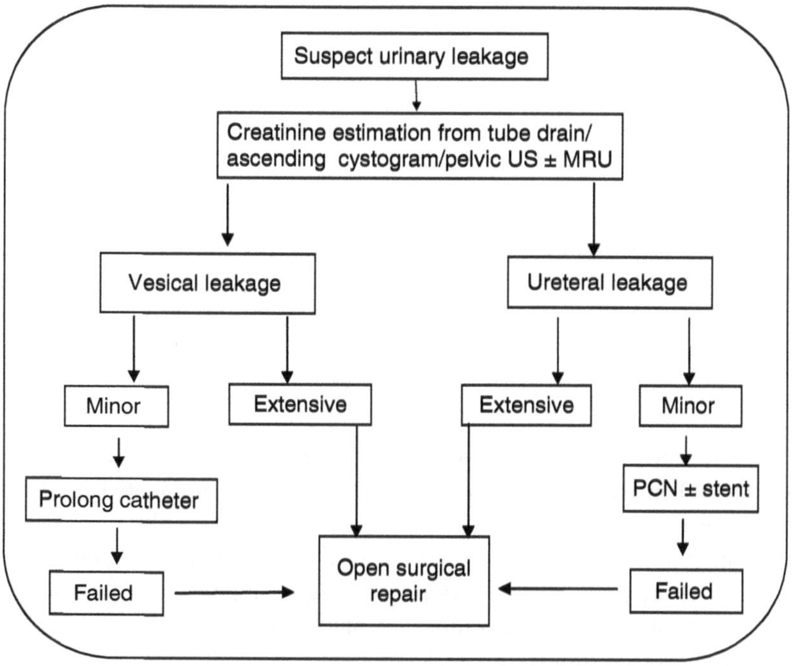

Fig. 18.5 Algorithm of management of urinary leakage after renal transplantation

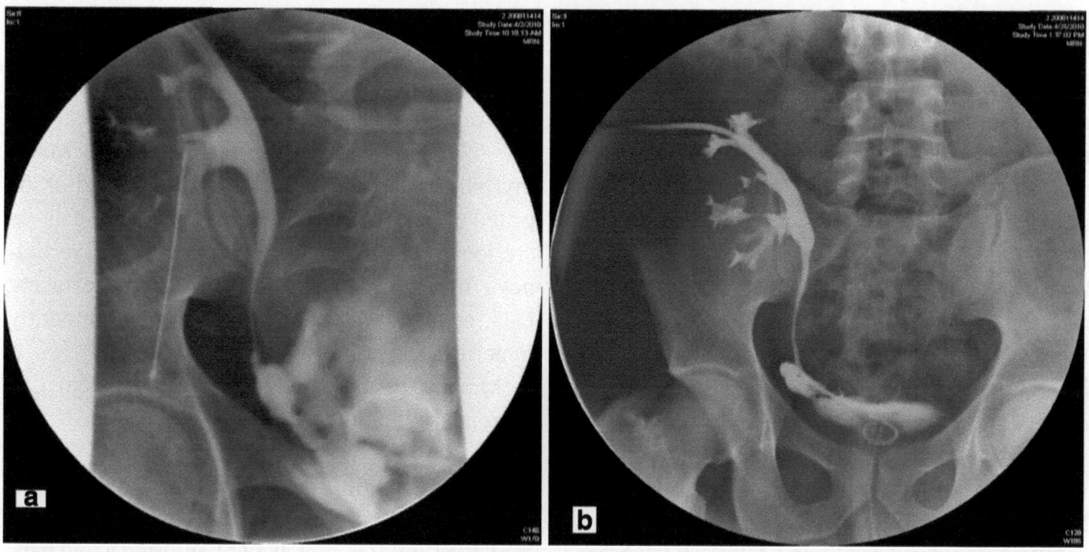

Fig. 18.6 Urinary leakage in a 27-year-old male. (**a**) Antegrade study showing extensive leakage from the lower part of the ureter of the transplanted kidney. (**b**) Antegrade study of the same patient a few days after drainage of the graft by PCN showing persistence of extravasation in spite of presence of DJ stent. Therefore, open revision of ureteroneocystostomy was carried out

Vesicoureteral Reflux (VUR)

The incidence of posttransplantation VUR ranges between 1 and 86 % [51]. VUR occurs mainly due to technical errors as a result of short antireflux tunnel or too wide ureterovesical anastomosis with the fear of obstruction. Some authors do not consider VUR an important issue

Table 18.3 Results of various bulking agents used in management of posttransplant vesicoureteral reflux

Series	Bulking agents	Success/total number of cases	Remarks
Cloix et al. [56]	Polytetrafluoroethylene	7/21	
Mallet et al. [57]	Polytetrafluoroethylene	10/15	
Latchamsetty et al. [58]	Collagen	0/7	
Ozok et al. [60]	NA Dx/HA	24/29	Better in low grade reflux
Seifert et al. [59]	NA Dx/HA	4/4	Reinjection in two cases
Vemulakonda et al. [61]	NA Dx/HA	6/11	Case series in children
Yucel et al. [51]	NA Dx/HA	14/26	Better in low grade reflux

NA Dx/HA nonanimal dextranomer/hyaluronic acid copolymer

in absence of outflow obstruction and urinary tract infection (UTI). When VUR is complicated by recurrent UTI, it may cause premature graft loss in adults and children [53, 54]; however, this applies only to 4.5 % of recipients who develop symptomatic UTI necessitating hospitalization. Since open re-ureteroneocystostomy may be difficult with relatively high morbidity [55], endoscopic management of such a case could be helpful in such a situation. Several bulking agents with variable success rates have been described, including polytetrafluoroethylene, collagen, and nonanimal dextranomer/hyaluronic acid copolymer (NA Dx/HA) [51, 56–61]. Table 18.3 summarizes the results of various bulking agents used in the management of posttransplantation VUR.

In a retrospective study, Yucel and colleagues have not found any difference between intraureteral and subureteral injection techniques. Interestingly, success rate was very high (90 %) in nondilating reflux compared with 31.5 % in dilating reflux regardless the technique or the volume of injection [51]. In contrast, Kirsch et al. found that intraureteral injection technique with higher injected material volume led to better results particularly in dilated VUR [62]. A second injection trial with a large volume of bulking agents has been recommended in failed cases [59]; however, this was found not effective by others [51]. Moreover, it might be complicated with obstruction [63] and add more significant periureteral reaction which might complicate later surgical intervention.

It seems that the nature of the bulking agent has the only impact on success. Literature has shown that injection treatment is more successful in a previously implanted ureter with antireflux procedures [64, 65]. Low grade nondilated VUR has a better response to such treatment [51]. The technique, number, and dose of injection are still a matter of controversy.

Urolithiasis

In 1975, Rattiazzi et al. reported the first calculus in a renal transplantation [66]. The current reported rates vary between 0.2 and 1.7 % [67–69]. The risk factors are mainly hyperparathyroidism and nonabsorbable sutures and graft-gifted lithiasis [70]. Other predisposing factors are identical to those of patients with native kidneys including obstructive uropathy, recurrent UTI, or metabolic abnormalities (predominantly hyperuricosuria) [69, 70].

Most patients with calculi of <1.5 cm can be rendered stone-free with ESWL [71]. If this failed, flexible ureterorenoscopy and holmium laser fragmentation, although technically difficult in these kidneys, can be attempted. Del Pizzo et al. [35] and Basiri et al. [14] reported a low incidence of complications for retrograde endoscopy. The complexity of the transplant ureteral orifice, which is iatrogenically ectopic and anterior, and a large stone size appear to be the limitations of this technique. It is important to determine where the transplant ureteral orifice is located or whether the distal native ureter was used. For larger stones or technical difficulties with retrograde route, percutaneous nephrolithotomy (PNL) gives the

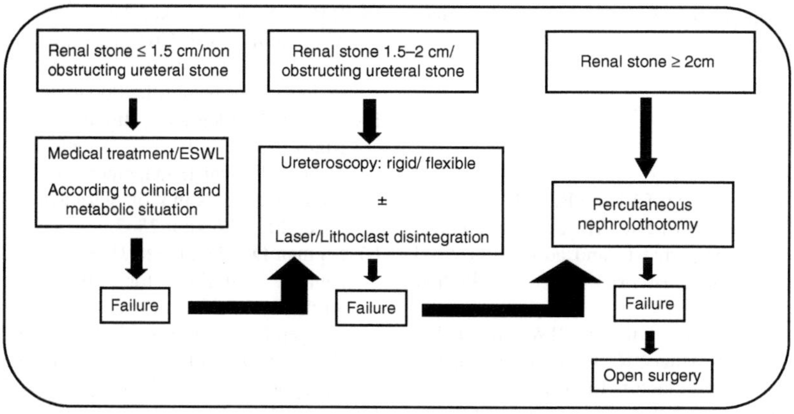

Fig. 18.7 Algorithm of management of urolithiasis after renal transplantation

best chance of complete stone clearance [69–71]. Figure 18.7 provides an algorithm for management of urolithiasis after renal transplantation.

Percutaneous removal of calculi from transplanted kidneys was first described in 1985 by Hulbert et al. [72] and has been proven to be a safe procedure. In a recent study, Rifaioglu et al. reported a 100 % stone-free rate after PNLs that were carried out in 15 patients without any reported complications or need for blood transfusion [69].

There are some technical points that should be raised when dealing with PNL in a transplanted kidney. US guidance is recommended for percutaneous access to aid in direct caliceal puncture and to avoid potential injury to overlying bowel [73]. Alternatively, preoperative CT could be performed to exclude overlying bowel and to help plan the appropriate percutaneous renal access [69]. In contrast to PNL in normal kidneys, during which access is normally directed toward a posterior calix with the patient in the prone position, percutaneous access into a transplanted kidney is done with the patient in the supine position and into an anterior calix. This is a result of the anterior location of the transplanted kidney in the true pelvis, as well as the change in the axis of the kidney. After dilatation, owing to the orientation of the transplanted kidney, antegrade flexible ureteroscopy can also be required [74]. The availability of a laser system can facilitate use of flexible endoscopy and lithotripsy of those stone-bearing calices that cannot be reached with rigid instrumentation [75].

Conclusion

A vast majority of, but not all, urological complications after renal transplantation are amenable to endourological intervention. Early diagnosis and careful patient selection for specific endourologic techniques are the mainstays of successful outcome.

Major urological complications following renal transplantation are ureteral leakage and stricture resulting mainly from technical errors. Initial management of obstructed ureters by PCN may improve graft survival and provide better access for diagnosis and intervention. Regardless of the technique of management of ureteral stricture, postoperative ureteral stenting for 6–8 weeks is mandatory. Minimal urinary leakage is an encouraging factor for applying conservative treatment by prolonged urethral catheterization in case of vesical leakage or PCN ± ureteral stent for ureteral leakage; otherwise, early open surgical reconstruction is recommended. Endoscopic intraureteral or subureteral injection of bulking agents seems to be a plausible alternative treatment to correct VUR posttransplant ureters, particularly in nondilating VUR. Meticulous and careful trials of stone disintegration and extraction by flexible ureteroscopy should be attempted before making a decision to proceed to PNL.

References

1. Shokeir AA, Osman Y, Ali-El-Dein B, El-Husseini A, El-Mekresh M, Shehab-El-Din AB. Surgical complications in live-donor pediatric and adolescent renal transplantation: study of risk factors. Pediatr Transplant. 2005;9(1):33–8.
2. Englesbe MJ, Dubay DA, Gillespie BW, Moyer AS, Pelletier SJ, Sung RS, Magee JC, Punch JD, Campbell Jr DA, Merion RM. Risk factors for urinary complications after renal transplantation. Am J Transplant. 2007;7(6):1536–41.
3. Yigit B, Tellioglu G, Berber I, Aydin C, Kara M, Yanaral F, Titiz I. Surgical treatment of urologic complications after renal transplantation. Transplant Proc. 2008;40(1):202–4.
4. Buresley S, Samhan M, Moniri S, Codaj J, Al-Mousawi M. Postrenal transplantation urologic complications. Transplant Proc. 2008;40(7):2345–6.
5. Kristo B, Phelan MW, Gritsch HA, Schulam PG. Treatment of renal transplant ureterovesical anastomotic strictures using antegrade balloon dilation with or without holmium: YAG laser endoureterotomy. Urology. 2003;62(5):831–4.
6. Shivde SR, Date J, Dighe TA, Joshi PM. Unusual causes of obstruction to transplant ureter. Saudi J Kidney Dis Transpl. 2010;21(2):310–3.
7. Karam G, Hétet JF, Maillet F, Rigaud J, Hourmant M, Soulillou JP, Giral M. Late ureteral stenosis following renal transplantation: risk factors and impact on patient and graft survival. Am J Transplant. 2006;6(2):352–6.
8. Taylor RJ. Ureteral complications following renal transplantation. In: Graham SD, Glann JF, Keane TE, editors. Glenn's urological surgery. 6th ed. Phila delphia: Lippincott Williams & Wilkins; 2004. p. 103–7. Chapter 12.
9. Nane I, Kadioglu TC, Tefekli A, Koçak T, Ander H, Köksal T. Urologic complications of extravesical ureteroneocystostomy in renal transplantation from living related donors. Urol Int. 2000;64(1):27–30.
10. Asadpour A, Molaei M, Yaghoobi S. Management of ureteral complications in renal transplantation: prevention and treatment. Saudi J Kidney Dis Transpl. 2011;22(1):72–4.
11. Gritsch HA, Vivas CA, Jordan ML. Complications of renal transplantation. In: Taneja SS, Smith RB, Ehrich RM, editors. Complications of urologic surgery prevention and management. 3rd ed. Philadelphia: W.B. Saunders; 2001. p. 342–53. Chapter 28.
12. Shokeir AA, Abubieh EA, Dawaba M, el-Azab M. Resistive index of the solitary kidney: a clinical study of normal values. J Urol. 2003;170(2 Pt 1):377–9.
13. Hobart MG, Streem SB, Gill IS. Renal transplant complications. Minimally invasive management. Urol Clin North Am. 2000;27(4):787–98.
14. Basiri A, Nikoobakht MR, Simforoosh N, Hosseini Moghaddam SM. Ureteroscopic management of urological complications after renal transplantation. Scand J Urol Nephrol. 2006;40(1):53–6.
15. Juaneda B, Alcaraz A, Bujons A, Guirado L, Díaz JM, Martí J, de la Torre P, Sabaté S, Villavicencio H. Endourological management is better in early-onset ureteral stenosis in kidney transplantation. Transplant Proc. 2005;37(9):3825–7.
16. Sigman DB, Del Pizzo JJ, Sklar GN. Endoscopic retrograde stenting for allograft hydronephrosis. J Endourol. 1999;13(1):21–5.
17. Voegeli DR, Crummy AB, McDermott JC, Jensen SR. Percutaneous dilation of ureteral strictures in renal transplant patients. Radiology. 1988;169(1):185–8.
18. Yong AA, Ball ST, Pelling MX, Gedroyc WM, Morgan RA. Management of ureteral strictures in renal transplants by antegrade balloon dilatation and temporary internal stenting. Cardiovasc Intervent Radiol. 1999;22(5):385–8.
19. Aytekin C, Boyvat F, Harman A, Ozyer U, Colak T, Haberal M. Percutaneous therapy of ureteral obstructions and leak after renal transplantation: long-term results. Cardiovasc Intervent Radiol. 2007;30(6): 1178–84.
20. Conrad S, Schneider AW, Tenschert W, Meyer-Moldenhauer WH, Huland H. Endo-urological cold-knife incision for ureteral stenosis after renal transplantation. J Urol. 1994;152(3):906–9.
21. Siddins M, Kanchanabat B, Rao MM. Intraoperative vascular localization to facilitate endopyelotomy after renal transplantation. ANZ J Surg. 2001;71(8):485–6.
22. Katz R, Pode D, Gofrit ON, Shenfeld OZ, Landau EH, Golijanin D, Shapiro A. Transurethral incision of ureteroneocystostomy strictures in kidney transplant recipients. BJU Int. 2003;92(7):769–71.
23. Bhayani SB, Landman J, Slotoroff C, Figenshau RS. Transplant ureter stricture: acucise endoureterotomy and balloon dilation are effective. J Endourol. 2003; 17(1):19–22.
24. Schwartz BF, Chatham JR, Bretan P, Goharderakhshan R, Stoller ML. Treatment of refractory kidney transplant ureteral strictures using balloon cautery endoureterotomy. Urology. 2001;58(4):536–9.
25. Youssef NI, Jindal R, Babayan RI, Carpinito GA, Idelson BA, Bernard DB, Cho SI. The acucise catheter: a new endourological method for correcting transplant ureteric stenosis. Transplantation. 1994; 57(9):1398–400.
26. He Z, Li X, Chen L, Zeng G, Yuan J, Chen W, Zhang C. Endoscopic incision for obstruction of vesico-ureteric anastomosis in transplanted kidneys. BJU Int. 2008;102(1):102–6.
27. Gdor Y, Gabr AH, Faerber GJ, Wolf Jr JS. Holmium:yttrium-aluminum-garnet laser endoureterotomy for the treatment of transplant kidney ureteral strictures. Transplantation. 2008;85(9):1318–21.
28. Barbaric ZL, Thomson KR. Percutaneous nephropyelostomy in the management of obstructed renal transplants. Radiology. 1978;126(3):639–42.

29. Peregrin J, Filipová H, Matl I, Vítko S, Làcha J. Percutaneous treatment of early and late ureteral stenosis after renal transplantation. Transplant Proc. 1997;29(1–2):140–1.
30. Bachar GN, Mor E, Bartal G, Atar E, Goldberg N, Belenky A. Percutaneous balloon dilatation for the treatment of early and late ureteral strictures after renal transplantation: long-term follow-up. Cardiovasc Intervent Radiol. 2004;27(4):335–8.
31. Basiri A, Simforoosh N, Nikoobakht M, Hosseini Moghaddam MM. The role of ureteroscopy in the treatment of renal transplantation complications. Urol J. 2004;1(1):27–31.
32. Hsiao HL, Li CC, Chang TH, Wu WJ, Chou YH, Shen JT, Jang MY, Huang CH. Treatment of transplant ureteral stricture with Acucise endoureterotomy: case report and literature review. Kaohsiung J Med Sci. 2007;23(5):259–64.
33. Gross AJ, Seseke F, Lorf T, Ringe B, Ringert RH. Treatment of transplant ureteral stenosis with Acucise endoureterotomy. Transpl Int. 1998;11(4):316–9.
34. Chandhoke PS, Clayman RV, Stone AM, McDougall EM, Buelna T, Hilal N, Chang M, Stegwell MJ. Endopyelotomy and endoureterotomy with the acucise ureteral cutting balloon device: preliminary experience. J Endourol. 1993;7(1):45–51.
35. Del Pizzo JJ, Jacobs SC, Sklar GN. Ureteroscopic evaluation in renal transplant recipients. J Endourol. 1998;12(2):135–8.
36. Osman Y, Ali-El-Dein B, Shokeir AA, Kamal M, El-Din AB. Routine insertion of ureteral stent in live-donor renal transplantation: is it worthwhile? Urology. 2005;65(5):867–71.
37. Tillou X, Raynal G, Demailly M, Hakami F, Saint F, Petit J. Endoscopic management of urologic complications following renal transplantation: impact of ureteral anastomosis. Transplant Proc. 2009;41(8):3317–9.
38. Arya M, Mostafid H, Patel HR, Kellett MJ, Philp T. The self-expanding metallic ureteric stent in the long-term management of benign ureteric strictures. BJU Int. 2001;88(4):339–42.
39. Boyvat F, Aytekin C, Colak T, Firat A, Karakayali H, Haberal M. Memokath metallic stent in the treatment of transplant kidney ureter stenosis or occlusion. Cardiovasc Intervent Radiol. 2005;28(3):326–30.
40. Olsburgh J, Dorling A, Tait P, Williams G. Extraanatomic stents for transplant ureteric stenosis. Br J Radiol. 2007;80(951):216–8.
41. Shokeir AA, el-Diasty TA, Ghoneim MA. Endourologic management of ureteric complications after live-donor kidney transplantation. J Endourol. 1993; 7(6):487–91.
42. Ghoneim MA, Shokeir AA. Emergencies following renal transplantation. In: Hohenfellner M, Santucci RA, editors. Emergencies in urology. Berlin/Heidelberg: Springer; 2007. p. 451–83. Chapter 18.4.1.
43. El-Mekresh M, Osman Y, Ali-El-Dein B, El-Diasty T, Ghoneim MA. Urological complications after living-donor renal transplantation. BJU Int. 2001;87(4): 295–306.
44. Karam G, Maillet F, Parant S, Soulillou JP, Giral-Classe M. Ureteral necrosis after kidney transplantation: risk factors and impact on graft and patient survival. Transplantation. 2004;78(5):725–9.
45. Loughlin KR, Tilney NL, Richie JP. Urologic complications in 718 renal transplant patients. Surgery. 1984;95(3):297–302.
46. Cimic J, Meuleman EJ, Oosterhof GO, Hoitsma AJ. Urological complications in renal transplantation. A comparison between living-related and cadaveric grafts. Eur Urol. 1997;31(4):433–5.
47. Ratner LE, Fabrizio M, Chavin K, Montgomery RA, Mandal AK, Kavoussi LR. Technical considerations in the delivery of the kidney during laparoscopic live-donor nephrectomy. J Am Coll Surg. 1999;189(4):427–30.
48. Rawlins MC, Hefty TL, Brown SL, Biehl TR. Learning laparoscopic donor nephrectomy safely: a report on 100 cases. Arch Surg. 2002;137(5):531–4, discussion 534–5.
49. Shokeir AA. Open versus laparoscopic live donor nephrectomy: a focus on the safety of donors and the need for a donor registry. J Urol. 2007;178(5):1860–6.
50. Genc V, Ozgencil E, Orozakunov E, Can OS, Yilmaz AA, Ozsay O, Cipe G, Oztuna D, Cakmak A, Tuzuner A, Hazinedaroglu SM. Pure laparoscopic versus open live donor nephrectomy: evaluation of health survey and graft functions. Transplant Proc. 2011;43(3): 791–4.
51. Yucel S, Akin Y, Celik O, Erdogru T, Baykara M. Endoscopic vesicoureteral reflux correction in transplanted kidneys: does injection technique matter? J Endourol. 2010;24(10):1661–4.
52. Matalon TA, Thompson MJ, Patel SK, Ramos MV, Jensik SC, Merkel FK. Percutaneous treatment of urine leaks in renal transplantation patients. Radiology. 1990;174(3 Pt 2):1049–51.
53. Mastrosimone S, Pignata G, Maresca MC, Calconi G, Rabassini A, Butini R, Fandella A, Di Falco G, Chiara G, Caldato C, et al. Clinical significance of vesicoureteral reflux after kidney transplantation. Clin Nephrol. 1993;40(1):38–45.
54. Vianello A, Pignata G, Caldato C, Di Falco G, Calconi G, Fandella A, Rabassini A, Maresca MC. Vesicoureteral reflux after kidney transplantation: clinical significance in the medium to long-term. Clin Nephrol. 1997;47(6):356–61.
55. Krishnan A, Swana H, Mathias R, Baskin LS. Redo ureteroneocystostomy using an extravesical approach in pediatric renal transplant patients with reflux: a retrospective analysis and description of technique. J Urol. 2006;176(4 Pt 1):1582–7, discussion 1587.
56. Cloix P, Gelet A, Desmettre O, Cochat P, Garnier JL, Dubernard JM, Martin X. Endoscopic treatment of vesicoureteric reflux in transplanted kidneys. Br J Urol. 1993;72(1):20–2.
57. Mallet R, Game X, Mouzin M, Sarramon JP, Vaessen C, Malavaud B, Rischmann P. Symptomatic vesicoureteral reflux in kidney transplantation: results of endoscopic injections of Teflon and predictive factors for success. Prog Urol. 2003;13(4):598–601.

58. Latchamsetty KC, Mital D, Jensik S, Coogan CL. Use of collagen injections for vesicoureteral reflux in transplanted kidneys. Transplant Proc. 2003;35(4): 1378–80.
59. Seifert HH, Mazzola B, Ruszat R, Muller A, Steiger J, Bachmann A, Sulser T. Transurethral injection therapy with dextranomer/hyaluronic acid copolymer (Deflux) for treatment of secondary vesicoureteral reflux after renal transplantation. J Endourol. 2007; 21(11):1357–60.
60. Ozok U, Eroglu M, Imamoglu A, Bakirtaş H, Güvence N, Kiper A. Subureteral dextranomer/hyaluronic acid copolymer injection for vesicoureteral reflux in transplant candidates. J Endourol. 2005;19(10):1185–7.
61. Vemulakonda VM, Koyle MA, Lendvay TS, Risk MC, Kirsch AJ, Cheng EY, Cisek LJ, Campbell JB. Endoscopic treatment of symptomatic refluxing renal transplant ureteroneocystostomies in children. Pediatr Transplant. 2010;14(2):212–5.
62. Kirsch AJ, Perez-Brayfield M, Smith EA, Scherz HC. The modified sting procedure to correct vesicoureteral reflux: improved results with submucosal implantation within the intramural ureter. J Urol. 2004;171(6 Pt 1):2413–6.
63. Seifert HH, Mazzola B, Zellweger T, Ruszat R, Muller A, Burkhalter F, Steiger J, Sulser T, Bachmann A. Ureteral obstruction after dextranomer/hyaluronic acid copolymer injection for treatment of secondary vesicoureteral reflux after renal transplantation. Urology. 2006;68(1):203.e17–9.
64. Perez-Brayfield M, Kirsch AJ, Hensle TW, Koyle MA, Furness P, Scherz HC. Endoscopic treatment with dextranomer/hyaluronic acid for complex cases of vesicoureteral reflux. J Urol. 2004;172(4 Pt 2):1614–6.
65. Jung C, DeMarco RT, Lowrance WT, Pope 4th JC, Adams MC, Dietrich MS, Brock 3rd JW. Subureteral injection of dextranomer/hyaluronic acid copolymer for persistent vesicoureteral reflux following ureteroneocystostomy. J Urol. 2007;177(1):312–5.
66. Rattiazzi LC, Simmons RL, Markland C, Casali R, Kjellstrand CM, Najarian JS. Calculi complicating renal transplantation into ileal conduits. Urology. 1975;5(1):29–31.
67. Lu HF, Shekarriz B, Stoller ML. Donor-gifted allograft urolithiasis: early percutaneous management. Urology. 2002;59(1):25–7.
68. Klingler HC, Kramer G, Lodde M, Marberger M. Urolithiasis in allograft kidneys. Urology. 2002;59(3): 344–8.
69. Rifaioglu MM, Berger AD, Pengune W, Stoller ML. Percutaneous management of stones in transplanted kidneys. Urology. 2008;72(3):508–12. Epub 2008 Jul 23.
70. Francesca F, Felipetto R, Mosca F, Boggi U, Rizzo G, Puccini R. Percutaneous nephrolithotomy of transplanted kidney. J Endourol. 2002;16(4):225–7.
71. Challacombe B, Dasgupta P, Tiptaft R, Glass J, Koffman G, Goldsmith D, Khan MS. Multimodal management of urolithiasis in renal transplantation. BJU Int. 2005;96(3):385–9.
72. Hulbert JC, Reddy P, Young AT, Hunter DW, Castaneda-Zuniga W, Amplatz K, Lange PH. The percutaneous removal of calculi from transplanted kidneys. J Urol. 1985;134(2):324–6.
73. Gupta M, Lee MW. Treatment of stones associated with complex or anomalous renal anatomy. Urol Clin North Am. 2007;34(3):431–41.
74. Rhee BK, Bretan Jr PN, Stoller ML. Urolithiasis in renal and combined pancreas/renal transplant recipients. J Urol. 1999;161(5):1458–62.
75. Deane LA, Clayman RV. Advances in percutaneous nephrostolithotomy. Urol Clin North Am. 2007;34(3): 383–95.

19 Difficult Situations in Percutaneous Nephrolithotomy (PCNL) for Solitary Kidney and Renal Failure

Arvind P. Ganpule, Amit Satish Bhattu, and Mahesh Desai

Background

The management of stones in patients with chronic kidney disease requires coordination between the treating nephrologists, the urologist, and the anesthetist.

For safe, quick, and efficacious completion of the procedure, the treating physicians must employ risk reduction strategies that involve preoperative, intraoperative, and postoperative considerations. In this chapter, we cover all the aspects with regard to the principles that should be followed from surgical, anesthesia, and nephrology standpoints. Particular reference is made to the troubleshooting and the remedial measures one should employ.

In the setting of chronic kidney disease, deobstruction of the obstructed system should be the first line of management. CT scan offers the advantage in planning treatment in this group of patients. The method of access is a matter of surgeon preference. Proper surgical training is the key to gain adequate and precise surgical access.

A.P. Ganpule, M.S., DNB, MNAMS (✉)
A.S. Bhattu, M.S. • M. Desai, M.S., FRCS
Department of Urology, Muljibhai Patel Urological Hospital, Dr. Virendra Desai Road, Nadiad 387001, Gujarat, India
e-mail: doctorarvind1@gmail.com; amitmpuh@gmail.com; mrdesai@mpuh.org

Introduction

Kidney stones and chronic kidney disease (CKD) are common, affecting 5 and 13 % of the adult population, respectively. The workgroup of the US National Kidney Foundation, Kidney Disease Outcomes Quality Initiative Advisory Board, recommended that "chronic kidney disease" should be defined as sustained kidney damage greater than 3 months resulting in a GFR of less than 60 mL/min/1.73 m^2. Among the various treatment options available, PCNL is the most effective. We describe the technique and troubleshooting for PCNL in this subgroup of patients.

Preoperative Planning

In patients with obstructed upper tracts in a solitary kidney and obstructing ureteric stones in the setting of CKD, our policy is deobstructing the dilated upper tracts. The issues that need to be addressed on initial presentation are:

1. Does the patient need to be dialyzed prior to surgical deobstruction?
2. Is a preoperative percutaneous nephrostomy (PCN) or a double J stent the modality of deobstruction?
3. What are the predictors of recoverability of renal function?
4. Anesthesia consideration for percutaneous nephrolithotomy (PCNL)

A.M. Al-Kandari et al. (eds.), *Difficult Cases in Endourology*,
DOI 10.1007/978-1-84882-083-8_19, © Springer-Verlag London 2013

5. Role of imaging in managing stones in patients with CKD

Does the Patient Need to Be Dialyzed Prior to Surgical Deobstruction?

On physical examination, if the patient is breathless with signs of fluid overload such as pitting pedal edema and bilateral lower lung zone crepitations, the patient might require a session of hemodialysis prior to deobstruction. The biochemical parameters "on presentation" are the best predictors of dialysis need and recoverability from a long-term perspective. If the patient has hyperkalemia and acidosis on serum biochemistry, the patient should undergo a session of hemodialysis prior to surgical deobstruction.

Is a Preoperative Percutaneous Nephrostomy (PCN) or a Double J Stent the Modality of Deobstruction?

As a policy, we prefer deobstruction of the dilated upper tracts with a percutaneous nephrostomy (PCN). The advantages of a PCN are that it can be done under local anesthesia, is a quick procedure, and requires minimal radiation. In addition, a PCN, if strategically placed, forms a mature tract which can be utilized for PCNL once the general condition of the patient improves. In our opinion, a percutaneous nephrostomy is more comfortable than a double J stent for the patient; it also helps to assess the split function and perform creatinine clearance of a given renal unit. PCN is the choice of deobstruction when the contents in the pelvicalyceal system are turbid or thick pus.

The indication for placing a double J stent for deobstruction is a small lower ureteric stone in a solitary kidney or bilateral lower ureteric obstruction due to a small non-impacted lower ureteric calculus. However, if an attempt is made to pass a stent in a patient with impacted stone and it is likely to fail, percutaneous nephrostomy is the treatment of choice in such a situation.

Table 19.1 Predictors of recoverability of renal function

Preoperative
Age <15 years
Duration of symptoms
Solitary functioning kidney
Coexisting hypertension and diabetes
Stone burden
Atrophic renal cortex(<5 mm parenchymal thickness)
Intraoperative
No. of tracks
Postoperative
Residual fragments
Recurrent infection
Proteinuria (>300 mg/day)
Recurrence of calculus

Adapted with permission from Kukreja et al. [1]

What Are the Predictors of Recoverability of Renal Function?

After placement of PCN tube, the recoverability of renal function can be predicted depending on the nadir creatinine reached after deobstruction. Factors predicting recoverability of renal function are good cortical thickness and normal echogenecity of kidney on sonography and absence of infection or any other pre-existent medical condition like diabetes mellitus or hypertension. The risk factors and the predictors of recoverability are listed in Table 19.1.

After placement of PCN, the planning for percutaneous removal of stone is done when nadir serum creatinine value is achieved; this is considered to be when there is no further exponential fall in creatinine value for 2–3 days.

Anesthesia Consideration for Percutaneous Nephrolithotomy (PCNL)

Preoperative Risk in CKD Patients (Patient Specific, Procedure Specific, and Anesthesia Specific)

Major risk factors for cardiac event in patients with CKD are active ischemia, poor left ventricular function, and baseline ventricular arrhythmia [2]. Preoperative cardiac testing is indicated in patients with established ischemia, ventricular arrhythmias, and abnormal left ventricular ejection fraction [2]. CKD patients with chronic obstructive pulmonary disease, active asthma, or current infection are at high risk for pulmonary complications. CKD patients with diabetes mellitus should achieve optimal control (<200 mg/dL) before surgery. Drugs which can worsen outcome in CKD patients are ACE inhibitors, NSAIDs, radiographic contrast media, cyclooxygenase-2 inhibitors, and aminoglycosides [2].

Intraoperative Considerations

Local Anesthesia/General Anesthesia: What Is Preferred?

General anesthesia is associated with a greater than normal risk in patients with chronic renal disease as it is associated with increased complications such as intraoperative hypertension, hypotension, blood loss, tachycardia, hypoxia, myocardial depression, and acute kidney injury.

PCNL can also be done under local anesthesia. This is particularly important for patients who have associated comorbidities such as morbid obesity, spinal deformity with kyphoscoliosis ischemic heart disease, and unstable -medical conditions which make them very high risk for general anesthesia, or for patients who cannot be put into supine or prone positions. PCNL in local anesthesia can be done in supine or Valdivia position; these positions have better control of cardiovascular and respiratory parameters. For PCNL under local anesthesia, generally strategically preplaced PCN is necessary. This track can be used during PCNL and will cause less pain and less bleeding. It is to be kept in mind that PCNL in local anesthesia is absolutely contraindicated in noncompliant patients, and the patient has to be completely aware of the nature and details of the procedure preoperatively.

Role of Imaging in Managing Stones in Patients with CKD

A plain X-ray helps as the first imaging modality. However, in the setting of CKD, a multislice CT scan offers a wealth of information. A multislice CT is helpful in the following situations:

1. TCC: There are instances in which transitional cell carcinoma may be associated with renal calculi. These may be missed on conventional plain X-ray KUB and ultrasonography. Multislice CT has a potential to diagnose these.
2. Three-dimensional (3D) reconstruction: The 3D reconstruction CT scan helps in preoperative planning for PCNL, for example, for planned calyx for puncture, and it gives a better idea about the surrounding structures of the kidney (bowel and major vessels). CT scan also allows the analysis of stone morphometry which helps in planning PCNL and can predict the number of stages and tracks required for complete clearance of stones which is particularly relevant in staghorn stones. This has critical impact on incidence of possible complications, number of days of hospital stay, and hence on cost of treatment.
3. Radiolucent stone: CT urography or plain CT KUB is the investigation of choice in radiolucent calculus.

Position of Patient

Prone Position

Conventional position for PCNL is a prone position. However, it may not be possible to do PCNL in prone position in all the CKD patients as this position is associated with relatively poor ventilator control. The prone position is associated with a decrease in the cardiac index and an increase in pulmonary functional residual capacity. Prone position has the advantage of easy access to all the calyces and theoretical decreased risk of bowel injury. The PCNL in this position also has the disadvantage of need for changing the position after ureteric catheterization.

Supine Position

An increased risk of liver and spleen injury exists for upper pole puncture with the patient in the supine position. The supine position decreases surgeon radiation exposure and promotes spontaneous stone drainage during the procedure.

This position saves time as it does not require change of position after ureteric catheter insertion. In patients with CKD and other associated comorbidities, this is a more comfortable position from an anesthesia standpoint. However, all centers may not be well versed with the puncture technique in the supine position [3].

Valdivia Position

The Valdivia position is an intermediate dorsal decubitus with extension of its homolateral lower limb and flexion of the contralateral. This position preserves cardiovascular and ventilatory dynamics and allows a better access to the respiratory tract. In this position, the bowel slips away from the puncture area, lowering the risk of its damage. A single lumbar and genital sterile surgical field is created, allowing antegrade and retrograde simultaneous endoscopic and even laparoscopic access, increasing efficiency and safety of the minimally invasive procedures [4]. This method may have advantages particularly in patients with chronic kidney disease.

Methods of Gaining Percutaneous Access

Ultrasound

The principles for gaining perfect access include a straight tract (it should be the shortest possible tract from the skin to the desired calyx), and preferably, the tract should go from the skin through the cup of the calyx, papilla, and finally the desired calyx. Ultrasound offers the advantage of perfect access.

Difficulties in Ultrasound Access

The key to perfect access is the ability to visualize the needle throughout the tract. The problems encountered in ultrasound-guided puncture are:

1. *Not being able to see the needle in the path*: The possibilities are poor resolution machine and intervening bowel, leading to lack of adequate window to visualize the needle. These problems can be overcome by:
   (a) Using a new needle or special echotip needle. The echo-reflective nature of this needle helps in proper visualization of these needles.
   (b) A gentle jiggle on the needle helps in "seeing" the needle on the needle path.
   (c) The skin, the cup of the calyx, and the stone should be visualized along the same path.
   (d) A high-frequency probe helps in visualizing the needle.
2. *No egress of urine*: The possibilities include improper position of the needle and presence of turbid urine or blood clots in the pelvicalyceal system. If the kidneys are poorly functioning, the urine is unlikely under pressure; as a result, after initial puncture, there will be no egress of urine. The dilemma can be overcome by the following:
   (a) The position of the needle in relation to the stone or a contrast-filled calyx can be ascertained by noting the position in zero degree and 30°.
   (b) A glide (hydrophilic) wire can be passed into the pelvicalyceal system; the form of the wire helps in knowing the position of the needle.
   (c) A small amount of contrast may be injected to show the position of the needle. Although a useful technique at times, it may be counterproductive because if the needle is not in the system the contrast will extravasate, making the procedure cumbersome.

Difficulties in Nephroscopy

The stone fragmentation should proceed in a systematic way. The fragments should not be too small, as they tend to migrate into a distant calyx. In the case of a fragment migration into a distant calyx, the management depends on the size of the fragment and the calyceal anatomy. The options available include:

1. Flexible instrumentation: For clearance of stone in distant calyx with awkward anatomy, flexible instrumentation is found to be useful. Use of flexible instruments for PCNL decreases

number of tracts required for complete clearance and, hence, decreases incidence of complication while also having a favorable impact on recoverability of renal function [5, 6]. This is particularly relevant in patients with chronic renal disease.
2. Puncture wash: Puncture wash is a useful technique when small stone is in calyx which is not accessible from the tract created for major bulk stone clearance. In this case, a puncture is done in the calyx that has small stone and gentle wash is given through the puncture needle. This will push the stone into the pelvis, and then, it can be removed from the existing tract. This is not possible in conditions when the infundibulum is narrow, generally narrower than 24 Fr, that is, 8 mm, and for similar reason, stone larger than this size will be obviously not be suited for the puncture wash technique.
3. Wait and watch: For small calculi, generally smaller than 5 mm in size, and if intraoperative time is increasing or patient has high comorbidities, then a wait-and-watch policy may be observed for residual gravel.

Pelvic Perforation (Fig. 19.1)

The management of percutaneous surgery complicated with a pelvic perforation depends on the following factors:

1. Stage at which the perforation is detected
2. Stone burden
3. Size of the perforation
4. Expertise and instrumentation.

Postoperative Considerations

Patients with CKD have a higher chance of having medical and surgical complications in the postoperative period. Due to the deranged platelet function in CKD, the incidence of post-PCNL bleeding complication is high. The postoperative course is also associated with electrolyte imbalance. Careful fluid and electrolyte management and meticulous, measured intrarenal manipulation during PCNL may reduce these complications.

Bleeding

The role of transarterial embolization of renal pseudoaneurysm or arteriovenous malformation in case of post-PCNL bleeding is very important. With advances in this technique, it is possible to perform angiography and selectively embolize the feeding vessel. This option should always be kept in mind as it is not only lifesaving but also renal sparing [7]. See Fig. 19.2.

Serum Creatinine Does Not Decrease After PCN

There are situations in which serum creatinine does not decrease despite adequate decompression with PCN. In this situation, it first needs to be evaluated whether the PCN is in pelvicalyceal system (whether it is in a decompressing pelvicalyceal system completely). Whether the acute

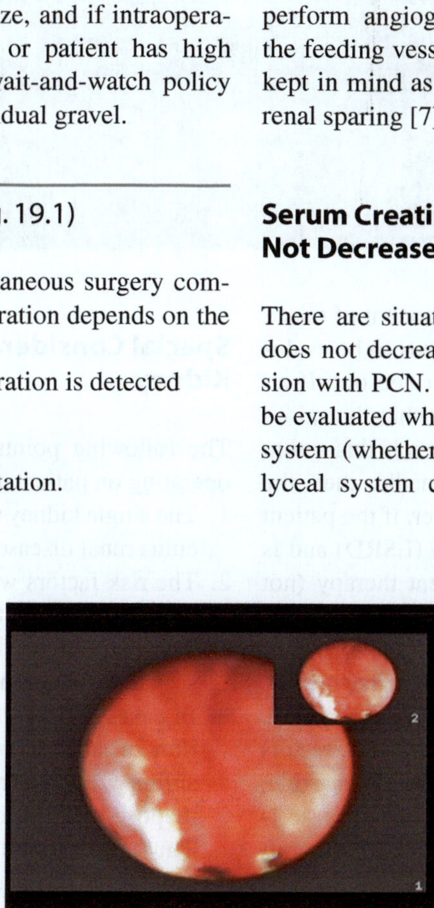

Fig. 19.1 Pelvic perforation

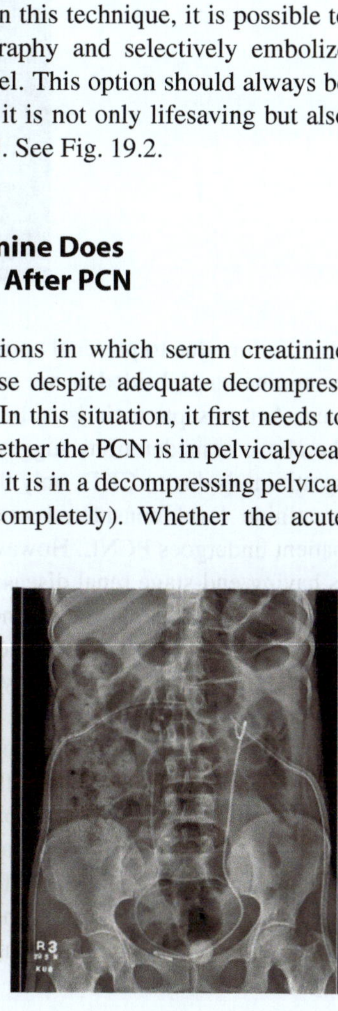

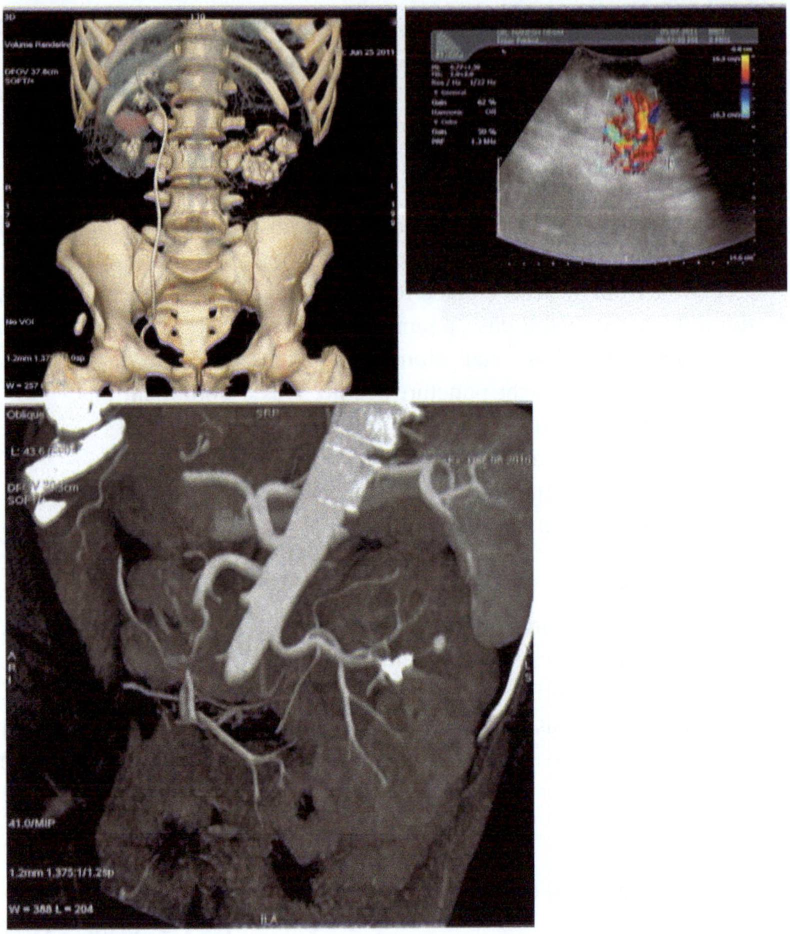

Fig. 19.2 AV fistula post PCN puncture

renal failure due to prerenal component of raised creatinine has subsided or not needs to be evaluated. Active septicemia is to be ruled out. If all the above considerations suggest that the raised creatinine is due to CKD, only then is this serum creatinine level considered as nadir; then the patient undergoes PCNL. However, if the patient is having end-stage renal disease (ESRD) and is on maintenance renal replacement therapy (not transplantation), then management of renal stone disease is complex. Generally speaking, if a patient is asymptomatic and has no active urinary infection, then active intervention is not required. If renal function is very poor, the PCNL results may be poor as kidney may not be salvageable. Active intervention for renal calculus disease is required in patients considered for renal allograft transplantation; intervention should be decided based on residual renal function.

Special Considerations in Solitary Kidney

The following points need consideration when operating on patients with single kidney:

1. The single kidney which is CKD is having calculus renal disease.
2. The risk factors which affected the other kidney are also affecting the residual single kidney (except in the situation of congenital solitary functioning kidney).
3. In cases of infection or any other complication intraoperatively or postoperatively, the solitary functioning kidney may be more predisposed to acute or chronic renal failure. Thus, the possibility of the need of perioperative renal replacement therapy is greater in such cases of a solitary functioning kidney.

However, PCNL is safe and has an acceptably low complication rate in patients with solitary kidneys. At long-term follow-up, renal function had stabilized or improved in more than 90 % of patients with a solitary kidney after PCNL [8, 9].

Factors predicting good outcome after PCNL in solitary functioning kidney [9] are:

1. Female gender
2. Early dietary modification to renal diet
3. Glomerular filtration rate

In summary, even in patients with solitary functioning kidney with CKD, PCNL is a safe and effective treatment that will help to preserve or rather improve renal function provided it is done with care and full understanding of the possible complications.

Conclusion

In the setting of chronic kidney disease, deobstruction of the obstructed system should be the first line of management. CT scan offers the advantage in planning treatment in this group of patients. The method of access is a matter of surgeon preference. Proper surgical training is the key to gain adequate and precise surgical access.

The management of this group of patients is challenging. The PCNL should be done, adhering to all risk reduction strategies. While treating the patient, efforts should be made to clear the stone and make the renal unit stone-free. Stone eradication by PCNL delays deterioration of renal function and delays the onset and requirement for dialysis and subsequent renal replacement. Percutaneous renal surgery offers the best results with good stone clearance rates and low morbidity.

References

1. Kukreja R, Desai M, Patel SH, Desai MR. Nephrolithiasis associated with renal insufficiency: factors predicting outcome. J Endourol. 2003;17(10):875–9.
2. Oldfarb DA, Nally Jr JV, Schreiber Jr MJ. Chapter 41: etiology, pathogenesis, and management of renal failure. In: Campbell-Walsh urology. 9th ed. Philadelphia: WB Saunders; 2007.
3. Manohar T, Jain P, Desai M. Supine percutaneous nephrolithotomy: effective approach to high-risk and morbidly obese patients. J Endourol. 2007;21(1):44–9.
4. Daels F, González MS, Freire FG, Jurado A, Damia O. Percutaneous lithotripsy in Valdivia-Galdakao decubitus position: our experience. J Endourol. 2009;23(10):1615–20.
5. Wong C, Leveillee RJ. Single upper-pole percutaneous access for treatment of ≥5-cm complex branched staghorn calculi: is shockwave lithotripsy necessary? J Endourol. 2002;16:477–81.
6. Williams SK, Leveillee RJ. A single percutaneous access and flexible nephroscopy is the best treatment for a full staghorn calculus. J Endourol. 2008;22:1835–8.
7. Jain V, Ganpule A, Vyas J, Muthu V, Sabnis RB, Rajapurkar MM, Desai MR. Management of non-neoplastic renal hemorrhage by transarterial embolization. Urology. 2009;74(3):522–6.
8. Akman T, Binbay M, Tekinarslan E, Ozkuvanci U, Kezer C, Erbin A, Berberoglu Y, Yaser-Muslumanoglu A. Outcomes of percutaneous nephrolithotomy in patients with solitary kidneys: a single-centre experience. Urology. 2011;78(2):272–6.
9. Canes D, Hegarty NJ, Kamoi K, Haber GP, Berger A, Aron M, Desai MM. Functional outcomes following percutaneous surgery in the solitary kidney. Urology. 2009;181(1):154–60.

Percutaneous Nephrolithotomy (PCNL) and Other Simultaneous Procedures

20

Ravindra B. Sabnis, Raguram Ganesamoni, and Amit Doshi

Introduction

The 1980s saw inventions that revolutionized stone management. Percutaneous nephrolithotomy (PCNL) was first described by Fernstrom and Johansson in 1976 [1]. In a few years, Arthur Smith and Peter Alken presented their initial experiences [2, 3]. Around the same time, Christian Chaussy described the use of shockwave lithotripsy for treating renal calculi [4]. The first patient was treated on February 7, 1980, in Munich, using Dornier HM1 lithotripsy machine [5]. This started the era of noninvasive treatment of stones. By then, ureteroscopy had been already conceptualized and was in practice.

Since then, in the last 35 years, many more advances have been made in all these modalities. Optics have become much better, imaging systems have improved, and energy sources have become better and better. Mini PCNL, flexible nephroscopy, flexible ureteroscopy, and various disposables have become important tools in the armamentarium of urologists treating urinary stones. All these inventions have resulted in improved success rate, reduced rate of complications, and less morbidity and negligible mortality. Several prospective, randomized, controlled trials have rationalized the treatment options involving PCNL, SWL, URS, flexible URS, etc. Over the period of years, it has been also realized that all these modalities are complementary and not competing with each other. Hence, we have evolved combination treatments like PCNL combined with SWL, URS combined with PCNL, flexible URS combined with PCNL, etc. Typically, these procedures are done in different sittings. However, some procedures can be done simultaneously in the same sitting under single anesthesia.

It is necessary to understand that simultaneous procedures are not easy and should be undertaken only by experienced surgeons. The objectives of the simultaneous procedures are:

1. To reduce hospital stay
2. To reduce morbidity
3. To achieve better success rates (stone clearance rate)
4. To reduce complication rates
5. To increase the overall safety of the procedure
6. To reduce the cost of treatment

PCNL is done to remove stones from the kidney. However, along with kidney stones, patient may have various other conditions such as PUJ obstruction, ureteric stones, calyceal stenosis, calyceal diverticulum, etc. All these conditions can be treated simultaneously with PCNL. There are some situations such as bilateral renal stones and multiple calyceal stones which can be treated along with PCNL by carrying out the other procedure simultaneously to achieve

R.B. Sabnis, M.S., MCH (✉) • R. Ganesamoni, M.S., MRCS, MCh • A. Doshi, MBBS, M.S.
Department of Urology, Muljibhai Patel Urological Hospital,
Dr. Virendra Desai Road, Nadiad 387001, Gujarat, India
e-mail: rbsabnis@gmail.com; dr_raguramg@yahoo.co.in; dr.doshiamit@rediffmail.com

A.M. Al-Kandari et al. (eds.), *Difficult Cases in Endourology*,
DOI 10.1007/978-1-84882-083-8_20, © Springer-Verlag London 2013

the above-mentioned objectives. Ectopic kidney PCNL poses a challenge, and it can be tackled by combining it with laparoscopy. In this chapter, we give an overview of all such procedures done simultaneously with PCNL in same sitting and under the same anesthesia.

Bilateral PCNL

Conventionally in bilateral renal stones, one side is treated completely and then the other side is tackled. However, in several centers, stones on both sides are treated in one single anesthesia in one sitting. This can be done especially in those stones that are relatively easy to treat and in one for which one does not anticipate any complications. Typically, renal pelvic stones or solitary calyceal stones which are hard or in awkwardly placed angulated calyces are classic indications for bilateral simultaneous PCNL.

The technique for this procedure is like any conventional PCNL. The patient is placed in a prone position after ureteric catheter placement on both sides. Once one side is finished, then either the table is turned or the C-arm unit is moved and the other side is tackled, like in any other PCNL. This technique has the following advantages:

1. It is much safer, as the other side is tackled only after the first side is finished uneventfully.
2. The procedure is still economical as it is done under single anesthesia and in the same admission.

Bilateral PCNL has several advantages as stated earlier. If one side is simple stone and the other side contains large or complex stone (needing two stages), then the simpler side can be cleared and the first stage on the other side can be combined, thus avoiding one extra stage. Preoperative factors that may preclude a simultaneous approach, for example, patients with a large stone burden (i.e., >1,000 mm^2 on any one side) complex calyceal anatomy, age > 50 years, American Society of Anesthesiologists class > 1, preoperative serum hemoglobin level < 12 g/dL, morbid obesity (body mass index > 40 kg/m^2), and patient refusal [6]. Most series report good outcomes for bilateral PCNL, including high stone-free rates (95–97 %), low complication rates (9–12 %), short length of hospital stay (0.4–6 days), and blood transfusion rates (2–7 %) similar to those reported in series of unilateral PCNL [6]. Cost analysis has revealed a significant cost advantage for synchronous versus staged bilateral PCNL with direct cost savings of $5,126 (37 %) and $4,374 (30 %), respectively [7].

PCNL with Ureteroscopy

Many patients have renal as well as ureteric stones. Choices of management options depend upon their individual merit. If ureteric stone is to be treated by ureteroscopy and renal stone by PCNL, then both these procedures can be combined. Ureteroscopy is done in lithotomy position, once fragmentation is complete, and then ureteric catheter is placed. The patient is then turned to a prone position, and PCNL is completed. Those surgeons who are familiar with PCNL in a supine position can perform both ureteroscopy and PCNL in Galdakao-modified supine Valdivia position [8]. This avoids changing position to prone. The advantage of combining URS with PCNL is that one does not have to worry about migration since even if whole stone or a few fragments migrate, they can be removed during PCNL. Upper ureteric stone can to be pushed back into the kidney by placing ureteric catheter/dilator and gently flushing with saline. If this succeeds, it avoids ureteroscopy. Large ureteric stone takes a longer time to fragment completely. Hence, when you are combining URS with PCNL, instead of fragmenting ureteric stone fully in ureter, attempts should be made to push the stone back into the kidney. By ureteroscopy, the periphery of stone can be broken so as to disimpact it and allow it to migrate. PCNL with ureteroscopy has now become a standard simultaneous treatment option. Care should be taken not to prolong the duration of surgery beyond the allowable limit, which is usually 2 h.

Flexible Ureteroscopy with PCNL (Passing the Ball)

Indications for simultaneous Flex URS and PCNL are:

1. Multiple calyceal stones, typically larger bulk (>1 cm) and relatively hard.
2. After the first stage of PCNL for staghorn stone, if the remaining stones are of significant bulk, scattered in different calyces, and seem unlikely to be approachable by flexible nephroscopy, then this procedure is done.

The patient is placed in Galdakao-modified supine Valdivia position. PCNL is performed by adopting the standard steps (appropriate calyx puncture, tract dilatation, placing Amplatz sheath, carrying out nephroscopy). Simultaneously, another surgeon passes a flexible ureteroscope into the pelvicalyceal system. Calyceal stones are visualized, caught into the basket, and brought to the pelvis. Here, they are released from the basket. They are then removed by nephroscope. In this way, whatever fragments scattered in different calyces can be removed. Several advantages of this procedure are:

1. Large bulk stones take longer time to fragment by flex URS. This method avoids that.
2. Large stones can be removed through the PCNL tract, which is a larger tract.
3. Scattered calyceal stones may not be amenable to flexible nephroscopy, especially if they are at an acute angle and in parallel calyces.
4. It avoids another tract if stone is not approachable by PCNL (including flexible nephroscopy).

The limitations of the technique are:

1. It needs two sets of instruments and two experienced urologists.
2. Galdakao-modified supine Valdivia position is not as comfortable as prone position, and one has to get used to it.

Combined use of flexible ureterorenoscopy and PCNL has been shown to be a safe, effective, and highly versatile procedure with a high single-stage stone-clearance rate, with definite anesthesiological advantages, and without additional procedure-related complications [8].

PCNL with Endopyelotomy/ Endopyeloplasty

PUJ obstruction with stones is not an uncommon condition. Stones can be removed by PCNL, and PUJ obstruction can be treated by endopyelotomy or endopyeloplasty.

Open-ended ureteric catheter is placed in ureter, and prone position is assumed. Pelvicalyceal system is accessed through appropriate calyx so as to have straight access to PUJ. The tract is dilated and all the stones are removed. Usually these are small round secondary stones. Once stones are cleared completely, ureteric catheter is pulled out from the tract. This pull causes a little invagination of PUJ and ureter into the pelvis and thus helps in identifying posterolateral aspect on which cut is made, either by cold knife or hot current. Once adequate incision is made, endopyelotomy stent is kept along with nephrostomy.

In endopyeloplasty, incised ureteric mucosa is sutured to the cut end of pelvis. This suturing is done by an endoscopic suturing device (EndoStitch™, AutoSuture USSC, Norwalk, CN) inserted through nephroscope [9]. Typically, 2–3 sutures are taken with 3-0 Vicryl. Since there is approximation of cut ends of ureteric and pelvis mucosa, it is supposed to yield better results.

If stones are larger, then PCNL is done in first stage, and later endopyelotomy is done.

Success rate of endopyelotomy is approximately 70 % as compared to 95–97 % for laparoscopic pyeloplasty [10]. During laparoscopic pyeloplasty, stones can be removed by using laparoscopic graspers, giving wash and flushing the stones out of the kidney or by flexible ureteroscope, which can be passed through one of the ports to remove stones. If stones are multiple and scattered, there is always chance of missing some stones during laparoscopy. In such situations, PCNL can be combined with laparoscopic pyeloplasty [11]. First PCNL is done, and all stones are cleared; then, laparoscopic pyeloplasty is done in the same anesthesia. During pyeloplasty, fluid can be injected from nephrostomy to make pelvis full for easy dissection during pyeloplasty. The only precaution to be taken during PCNL is to avoid any extravasations and finish the procedure as quickly as possible.

PCNL and Calyceal Diverticulotomy

Calyceal diverticular stones can be treated by various methods. The objective is to remove the stones as well as widen the mouth of diverticulum. This can be done by PCNL combined with diverticulotomy.

After placing ureteric catheter and assuming a prone position, puncture is done, targeting the stone directly. Usually, there is not enough space for a guidewire to coil up. Dilatation is done very carefully, and a nephroscope is passed. Once stone is broken and fragments are evacuated, the diverticular mouth opening is searched. At this point, contrast and methylene blue are injected through the ureteric catheter to help identify the mouth. This can be widened by using laser or cautery (Bugbee™ Electrode, Gyrus ACMI, Southborough, MA). Then, nephrostomy or DJ stent is kept across the widened opening. Sometimes the diverticulum is small and its opening is very narrow and not visualized. In such situation, whole urothelium of the diverticulum can be fulgurated by bugbee electrode. Stone removal and fulguration of the diverticulum without dilation of the opening has been shown to have 87.5 % resolution rate of diverticulum [12, 13].

Some patients have calyceal stone with narrow infundibulum. They are also treated in the same manner.

Laparoscopy-Guided PCNL

PCNL for a large stone in pelvic ectopic kidney is now a standard procedure. During puncture, there is always a risk of bowel injury. To avoid this, laparoscopy is done simultaneously with PCNL.

Ureteric catheter is placed. The supine position (with a little tilt toward the opposite side to ensure that bowel moves away from kidney) is assumed. Puncture is made under fluoroscopic guide, and a guidewire is passed. Puncture can be done by ultrasound guide, which ensures that there is no bowl or other important structures between the skin and the renal parenchyma. Once the guidewire is properly placed, pneumoperitoneum is created and a trocar is inserted through the umbilical incision. Inspection is done to check whether the guidewire has gone through the bowel. If yes, it is removed, and repuncture is attempted and reconfirmed by laparoscopy by deflating gas but keeping the trocar in position. Once puncture is achieved without going through the bowel, the rest of the procedure is carried out in the same way as standard PCNL. During tract dilatation and nephroscopy, gas is completely removed. At the end, laparoscopic inspection is done once again to check for any extravasation or intraperitoneal spillage of fluid. Tube drain can be placed through the trocar site along with nephrostomy. Zafar and Lingeman [14] reported the use of intracorporeal suturing of the nephrotomy with placement of a ureteral catheter, thereby achieving hemostasis and eliminating the need for a nephrostomy tube. An extraperitoneal approach has been reported using a balloon dissector to open the extraperitoneal space [15]. Simultaneous laparoscopy with PCNL has made ectopic kidney PCNL safe.

Case 1: Bilateral Simultaneous PCNL

A 54-year-old female presented with a history of nausea, vomiting, and bilateral flank pain. She had hypertension and hypothyroidism. On examination, she was obese with a BMI of 34.2. On evaluation, she was diagnosed to have 24-mm right renal pelvic calculus and two calculi in the left kidney (size 12 mm each) (Fig. 20.1). She underwent bilateral simultaneous PCNL. Complete stone clearance was obtained without any complication (Figs. 20.1 and 20.2). Thus, the morbidity associated with multiple anesthesia and the extra cost associated with multiple procedures were reduced.

Careful patient selection and good expertise in PCNL are the keys to successful performance of bilateral PCNL in single setting. The more symptomatic and more endangered kidney should be tackled first. If both sides are similar in these respects, then it is wiser to operate on the side with the smaller stone burden to maximize

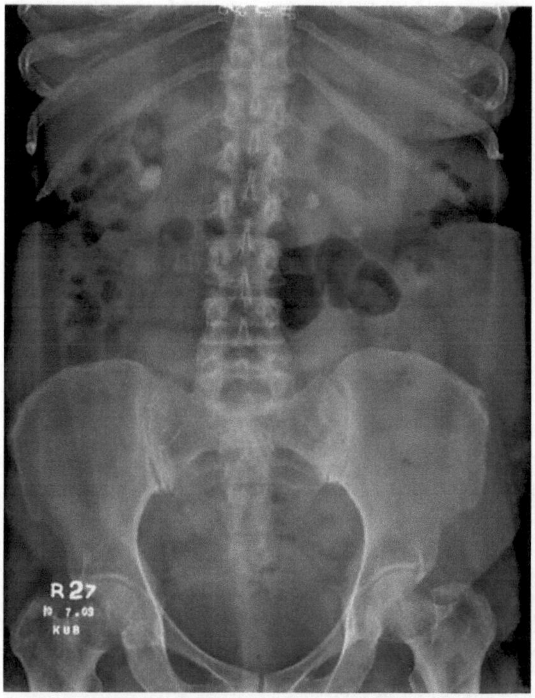

Fig. 20.1 X-ray KUB showing single renal pelvic calculus in right side and two renal calculi in left side

the chance of completing both procedures in same sitting.

Case 2: Passing the Ball

A 25-year-old male with recurrent stone former presente d with left flank pain. X-ray KUB and CT scan revealed multiple small bladder calculi, left lower ureteric calculi, and multiple left renal calculi (Fig. 20.3). The patient underwent cystolithotripsy, left URS, and left PCNL with simultaneous flexible ureteroscopy. Superior calyceal puncture was made and calculi in superior calyx were removed percutaneously (Fig. 20.4 a, b). Using flexible ureteroscopy, middle and inferior calyceal calculi were caught in a basket and "passed" onto the rigid nephroscope for retrieval via the percutaneous tract (Fig. 20.4 c, d). Thus, complete stone clearance was obtained in a single stage by the combined use of PCNL and flexible ureteroscopy.

Passing the ball technique can be judiciously used to reduce the number of tracts and stages in PCNL. Careful positioning of the patients and appropriate handling of instruments are essential to avoiding complications related to technical errors.

Case 3: PCNL with Endopyeloplasty

A 25-year-old male presented with right flank pain for 6 months. On evaluation, he was diagnosed with having right PUJ obstruction with secondary calculi (Fig. 20.5). He underwent right PCNL with simultaneous endopyeloplasty (Figs. 20.6, 20.7, 20.8, and 20.9 a, b).

PCNL with endopyeloplasty is a good alternative to laparoscopic pyeloplasty with pyelolithotomy. Anyone who is well versed in PCNL can be easily trained in endopyeloplasty as compared to the steep learning curve associated with laparoscopic pyeloplasty. Furthermore, PCNL is associated with a better stone clearance rate compared to laparoscopic pyeloplasty with pyelolithotomy.

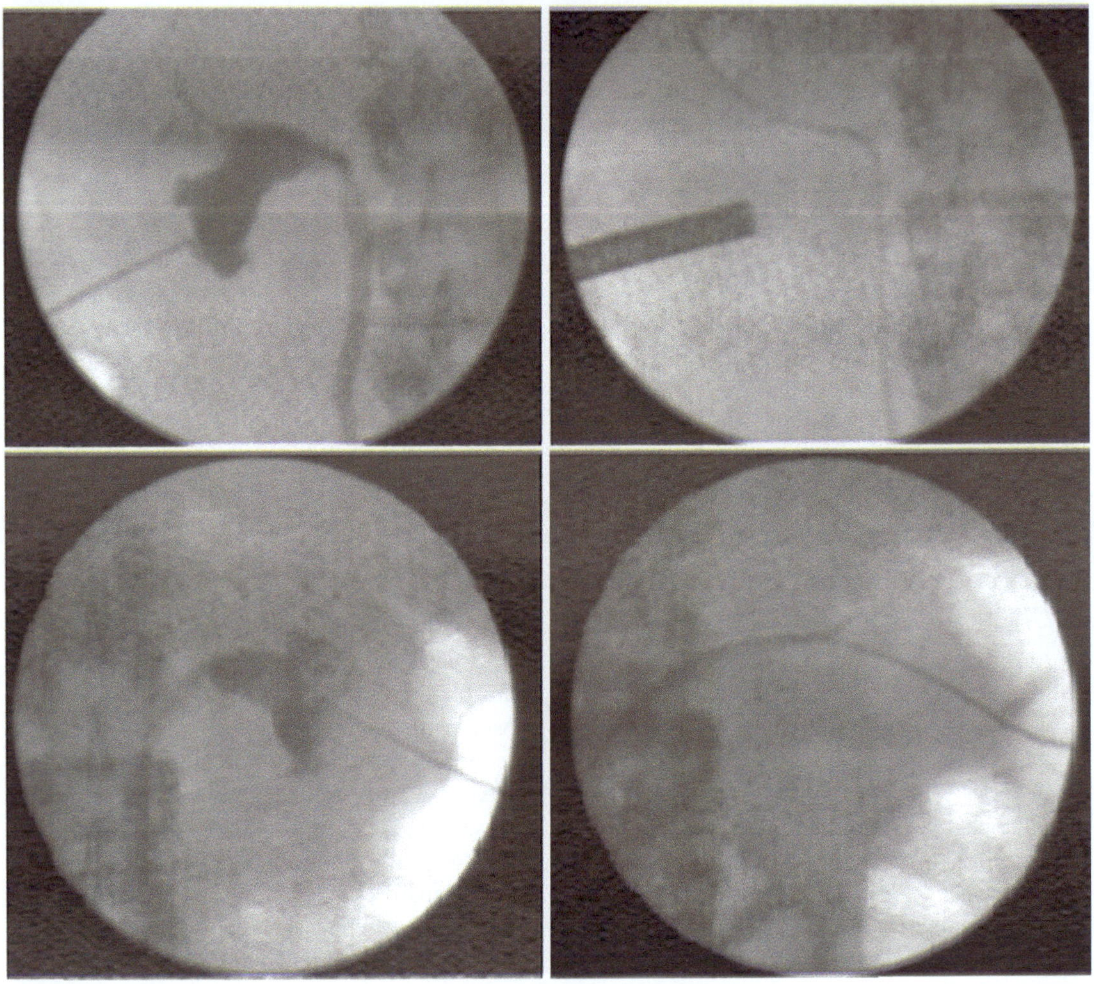

Fig. 20.2 Left followed by right side PCNL was done with complete stone clearance

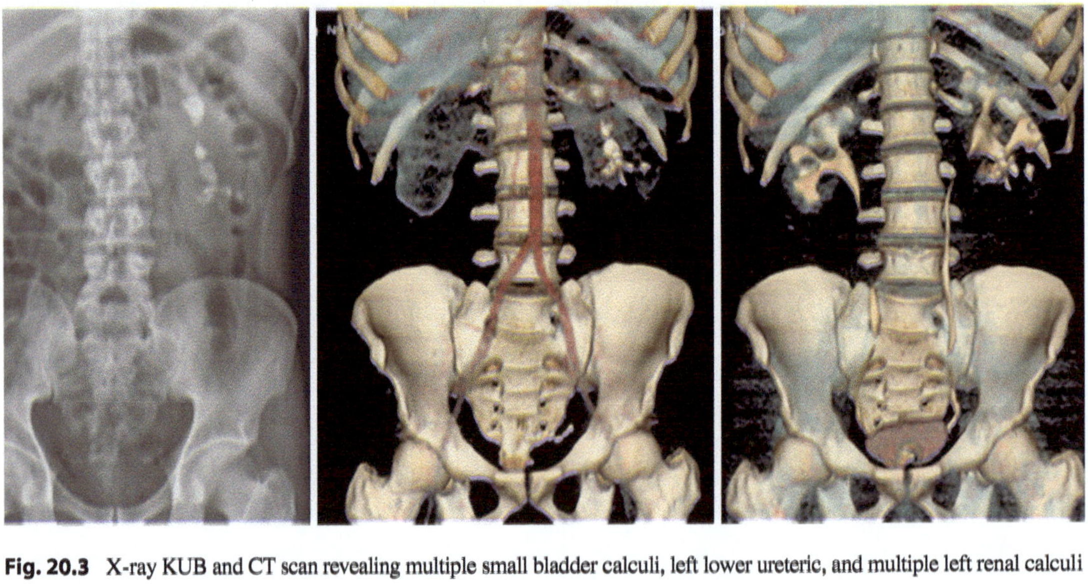

Fig. 20.3 X-ray KUB and CT scan revealing multiple small bladder calculi, left lower ureteric, and multiple left renal calculi

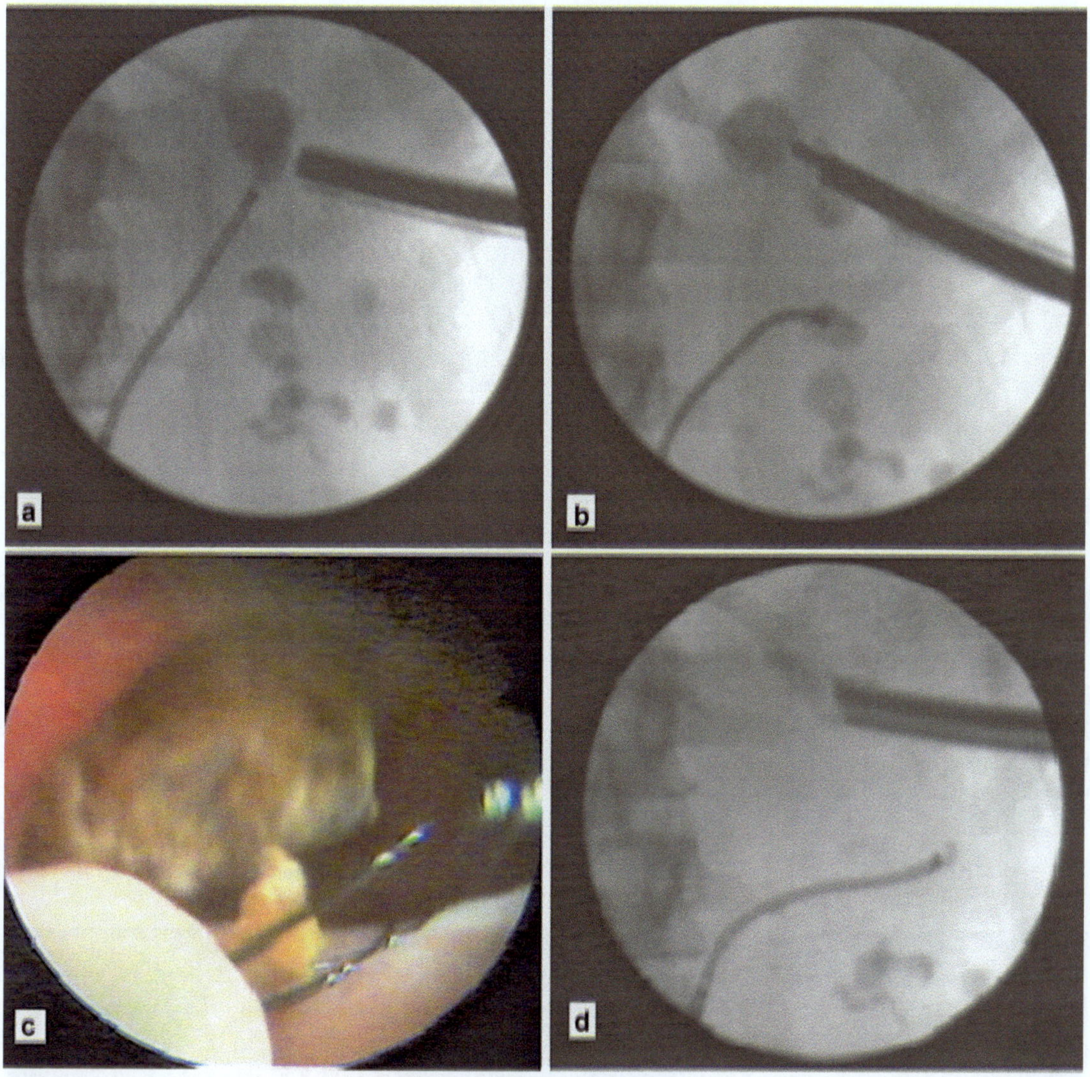

Fig. 20.4 Superior calyceal puncture has been made and calculi in superior calyx removed percutaneously (**a, b**). Using flexible ureteroscopy, middle and inferior calyceal calculi were caught in basket and "passed" onto the rigid nephroscope for retrieval via percutaneous tract (**c, d**)

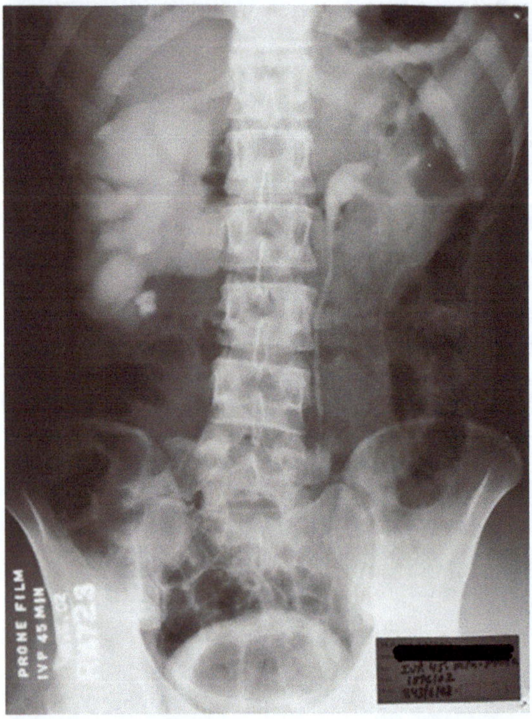

Fig. 20.5 Preoperative IVU showing right PUJ obstruction with secondary renal calculi

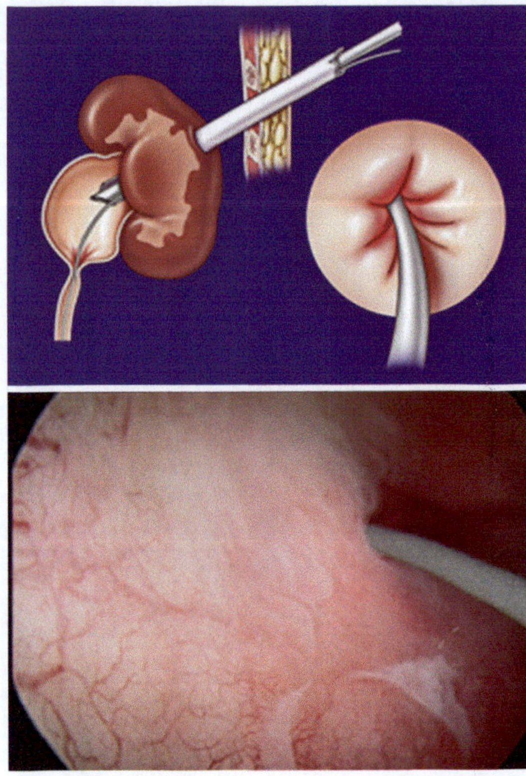

Fig. 20.6 Antegrade access with slight pull on the guidewire to make the pelvic side of PUJ prominent (*Left illustration* used with permission of Desai et al. [9])

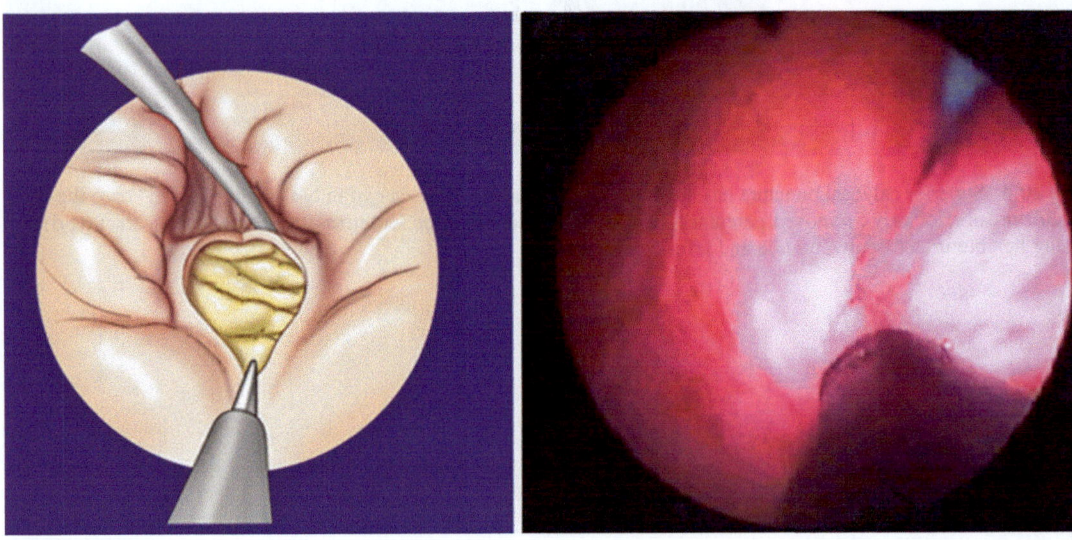

Fig. 20.7 Following endopyelotomy, the upper end of ureter is dissected out and spatulated (*Top and bottom left* illustrations used with permission from Desai et al. [9])

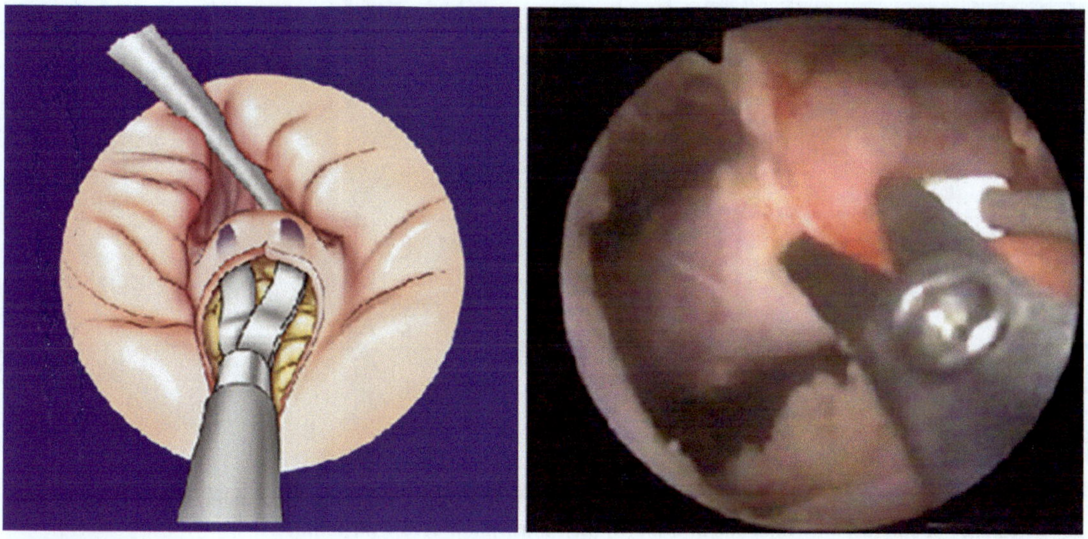

Fig. 20.7 (continued)

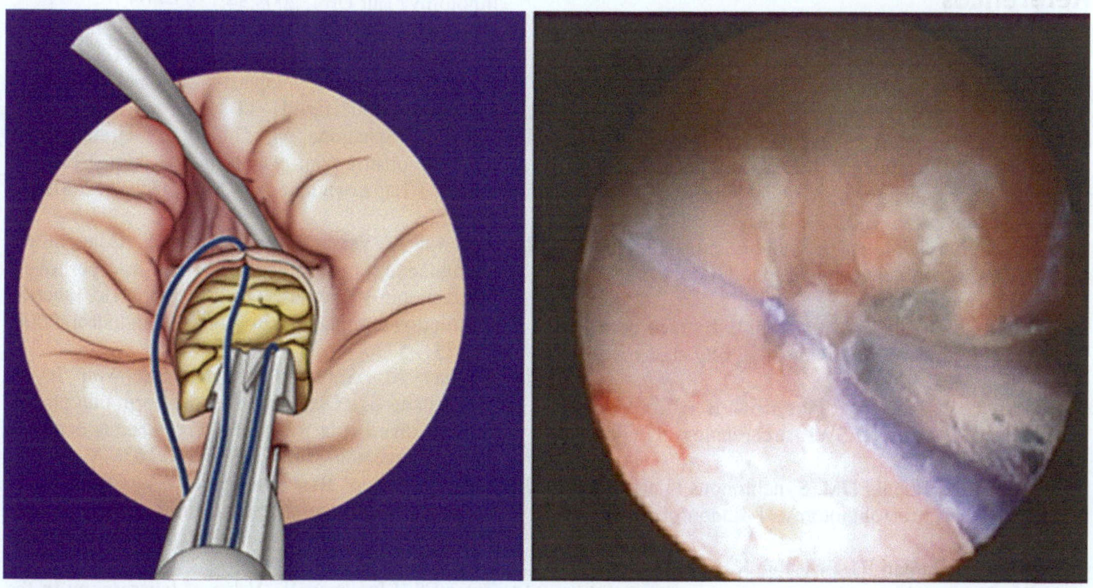

Fig. 20.8 Upper end of spatulated ureter is sutured to pelvis using Endostitch™ device (AutoSuture USSC, Norwalk, CT) (*Left illustration* used with permission from Desai et al. [9])

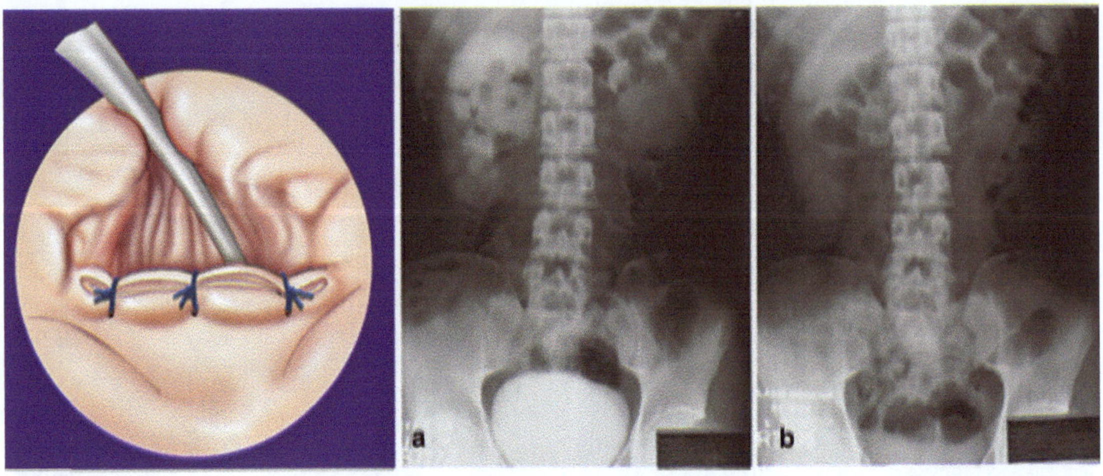

Fig. 20.9 Final appearance after suturing. Postoperative IVU showing adequately functioning right kidney (**a**) and good clearance of contrast after injection of lasix (**b**) (*Left illustration* used with permission from Desai et al. [9])

References

1. Fernstrom I, Johansson B. Percutaneous pyelolithotomy. A new extraction technique. Scand J Urol Nephrol. 1976;10:257–9.
2. Castaneda-Zuniga WR, Clayman R, Smith A, Rusnak B, Herrera M, Amplatz K. Nephrostolithotomy: percutaneous techniques for urinary calculus removal. AJR Am J Roentgenol. 1982;139:721–6.
3. Alken P, Hutschenreiter G, Günther R, Marberger M. Percutaneous stone manipulation. J Urol. 1981;125:463–6.
4. Chaussy Ch, Brendel W, Schmiedt E. Extracorporeally induced destruction of kidney stones by shock waves. Lancet. 1980;2:1265–8.
5. Chaussy C, Eisenberger F, Forssmann B. Extracorporeal shockwave lithotripsy (ESWL): a chronology. J Endourol. 2007;21:1249–53.
6. Williams SK, Hoenig DM. Synchronous bilateral percutaneous nephrostolithotomy. J Endourol. 2009;23:1707–12.
7. Bagrodia A, Raman JD, Bensalah K, Pearle MS, Lotan Y. Synchronous bilateral percutaneous nephrostolithotomy: analysis of clinical outcomes, cost and surgeon reimbursement. J Urol. 2009;181:149–53.
8. Scoffone CM, Cracco CM, Cossu M, Grande S, Poggio M, Scarpa RM. Endoscopic combined intrarenal surgery in Galdakao-modified supine Valdivia position: a new standard for percutaneous nephrolithotomy? Eur Urol. 2008;54:1393–403.
9. Desai MM, Gill IS, Carvalhal EF, Kaouk JH, Banks K, Raju R, Raja SS, Meraney AM, Sung GT, Sauer J. Percutaneous endopyeloplasty: a novel technique. J Endourol. 2002;16:431–43.
10. Gallo F, Schenone M, Giberti C. Ureteropelvic junction obstruction: which is the best treatment today? J Laparoendosc Adv Surg Tech A. 2009;19:657–62.
11. Agarwal A, Varshney A, Bansal BS. Concomitant percutaneous nephrolithotomy and transperitoneal laparoscopic pyeloplasty for ureteropelvic junction obstruction complicated by stones. J Endourol. 2008;22:2251–5.
12. Shalhav AL, Soble JJ, Nakada SY, Wolf Jr JS, McClennan BL, Clayman RV. Long-term outcome of caliceal diverticula following percutaneous endosurgical management. J Urol. 1998;160:1635–9.
13. Kim SC, Kuo RL, Tinmouth WW, Watkins S, Lingeman JE. Percutaneous nephrolithotomy for caliceal diverticular calculi: a novel single stage approach. J Urol. 2005;173:1194–8.
14. Zafar FS, Lingeman JE. Value of laparoscopy in the management of calculi complicating renal malformations. J Endourol. 1996;10:379–83.
15. Troxel SA, Low RK, Das S. Extraperitoneal laparoscopy-assisted percutaneous nephrolithotomy in a left pelvic kidney. J Endourol. 2002;15:655–7.

Adult Endopyelotomy Overcoming the Difficulties

21

Zhamshid Okhunov, Brian Duty, Zeph Okeke, and Arthur D. Smith

Introduction

During the last two decades, open surgery for ureteropelvic junction obstruction (UPJO) has been gradually replaced by laparoscopic and endoscopic procedures [1]. First introduced by Anderson and Hynes, the open dismembered pyeloplasty has been considered the "gold standard" treatment for UPJO with success rates of over 90 % [2–4]. The first report of percutaneous pyelolisis by Wickham and colleagues brought into question the need for open pyeloplasty [5]. Shortly thereafter, Smith and colleagues described the antegrade endopyelotomy (EP) using a cold knife in 31 patients [6]. The same group showed in a larger cohort that the procedure could be associated with long-term efficacy, while significantly reducing the morbidity of UPJO surgery [7].

Since its inception, multiple reports have been published evaluating risk factors associated with adverse outcomes following EP. The importance of careful patient selection and a variety of technical nuances became apparent [8–10]. In this chapter, we will discuss risk factors associated with treatment failure following EP, as well as technical considerations to help mitigate these hurdles.

Z. Okhunov, M.D. • B. Duty, M.D.
Z. Okeke, M.D. (✉) • A.D. Smith, M.D.
Department of Urology,
Smith Institute for Urology,
Hofstra North Shore – Long Island
Jewish Health System,
450 Lakeville Road, New Hyde Park, NY 11042, USA
e-mail: zho0616@gmail.com; bduty@nshs.edu;
zokeke@nshs.edu; asmith1@nshs.edu

Prognostic Factors and Patient Selection

Preoperative evaluation should begin with a complete patient assessment, which includes gender, age, duration of symptoms, prior interventions at the ureteropelvic junction (UPJ), and known medical comorbidities. The degree of hydronephrosis, stricture length, ipsilateral renal function, and presence of stones are well-known prognostic factors that play important role in EP outcomes [11–13]. It is of paramount importance to consider these clinical factors when choosing the optimal treatment modality for patients with UPJO.

Degree of Hydronephrosis

Lam and colleagues evaluated the impact of hydronephrosis severity on endoscopic UPJO treatment results [11]. The authors stratified patients by the degree of hydronephrosis and found that subjects with massive hydronephrosis were less likely to have successful EP. Of patients who underwent an EP, 18 had massive, 26 had severe, 14 had moderate, and 6 had mild hydronephrosis, with a success rate of 66.7, 80.8, 92.6, and 100 %, respectively. Antegrade EP, however, was more successful than retrograde EP in patients

A.M. Al-Kandari et al. (eds.), *Difficult Cases in Endourology*,
DOI 10.1007/978-1-84882-083-8_21, © Springer-Verlag London 2013

with massive hydronephrosis demonstrating 66.7 versus 20.0 % success rate. Similarly, in a study by Van Cangh and colleagues, the risk of treatment failure was significantly increased by high-grade compared to low-grade hydronephrosis. Their final success rate decreased from 81 to 54 % when high-grade hydronephrosis was present [9]. Berkman et al. classified patients into mild, moderate, severe, and massive hydronephrosis [14]. Patients with massive or severe hydronephrosis had a significantly lower success rate (70 %) compared to patients with low and moderate hydronephrosis (87 %). Our own experience supports these previous studies. In our series of 22 patients with massive hydronephrosis, the success rate was only 50 %, compared to 96 % in individuals with low or moderate hydronephrosis [13]. In our practice, we carefully select patients based up on their degree of hydronephrosis. We exclude patients with severe and massive hydronephrosis.

Crossing Vessels

The effect of crossing vessels on UPJO pathogenesis and treatment outcomes remains controversial [13, 15, 16]. Van Cangh and colleagues [9] demonstrated that high-grade hydronephrosis and the presence of a crossing vessel on preoperative digital subtraction angiography DSA were significant independent factors in lowering the success rate of percutaneous endopyelotomy. Long-term success rate was 39 % when both factors were identified versus 95 % when neither factor was present. In a later study from the same institution, the authors found that the presence of a crossing vessel lowered the success rate from 82 to 33 % [17]. It should be noted that only 33 % of patients in the study had a crossing vessel and their overall success rate (65 %) was lower than in most other antegrade endopyelotomy studies.

We believe crossing vessels have little impact on UPJO formation and treatment outcomes. Gupta et al. reported 54 patients who underwent open UPJO repair following failed antegrade EP [13]. The presence of an obstructing crossing vessel was noted in only 13 of the 54 cases (24 %). These 54 patients were drawn from a series of 401 consecutive percutaneous EP procedures performed over a 12-year period. Thus, treatment failure due to the presence of a crossing vessel, at most, accounted for 4 % (13 of 401) of patients undergoing percutaneous EP in this population [13]. The most common finding at exploration for endopyelotomy failure was severe intrinsic or extrinsic fibrosis, suggesting failure of the Davis intubated ureterotomy principle (i.e., adequate smooth muscle regeneration following a transmural ureteral incision). Other studies have demonstrated a higher incidence of crossing vessels at the time of exploration for endopyelotomy failure [18]. However, these series were small, and no distinction was made between vessels that appeared to be incidental versus those that were clearly causing obstruction [10]. It is important to notice that the presence of a vessel is not sufficient to confirm that the vessel is causing obstruction. Lastly, Sampaio identified vessels at the UPJ in more than 70 % of patients without UPJ obstruction, while only 44 % of patients with UPJ obstruction were noted to have crossing vessels [19].

Renal Function

Renal function has been shown to be a significant prognostic factor [11, 20]. Patients with ipsilateral renal impairment are at higher risk of surgical failure. In a study of 205 patients that underwent endoscopic excision of UPJO, patients were stratified into three groups based upon preoperative differential renal function [13]. Based on renal scintigraphy results, renal function was considered good, moderate, and poor if the kidney contributed greater than 40, 25–40 %, and less than 25 % of total renal function, respectively. Patients with good, moderate, and poor renal function demonstrated success rates of 92, 80, and 54 %, respectively [13]. Similarly, Berkman et al. reported a success rate of 62 % in patients with poor baseline renal function compared to 80 % in patients with moderate renal insufficiency [14].

Primary Versus Secondary UPJO

EP was initially introduced to manage obstruction after failed primary intervention. However, subsequent studies reported successful use of EP in patients with primary UPJO [13, 21, 22]. Nowadays, UPJO is a well-studied phenomenon in terms of its etiology. With regard to secondary obstruction, Hoeing and colleagues evaluated the role secondary UPJO etiology has on treatment outcomes [22]. The study included 24 patients who had failed laparoscopic or open pyeloplasty and 11 patients who developed a recurrence following EP. All patients underwent subsequent antegrade or retrograde EP using the Acucise® (Applied Medical, Rancho Santa Margarita, CA) device. Success rates were higher in patients who had failed pyeloplasty than EP. In particular, the subjective success rate of secondary EP was 88 and 71 % in patients who underwent prior pyeloplasty and EP, respectively. The objective success rate in the failed-pyeloplasty group was 71 % compared to 55 % in the prior EP group.

The presence of concomitant ipsilateral stone disease presents a confounding variable into the understanding of this entity. As we have discussed previously, an important controversy remains regarding stones at the UPJ obstruction, whether the stone results in the UPJO or vice versa. In the report of Hulbert and colleagues, the success rate of EP was significantly decreased when a stone was involved during the initial operative procedure [23]. They concluded that a stone in the presence of UPJ obstruction may worsen the prognosis by increasing the amount of inflammation in the ureteral wall. Motola and colleagues performed microscopic analysis of UPJO in a failed EP in which deposition of both collagen and crystalline material was observed [7]. Although it was not noted whether a stone was present in their case report, it is possible that some patients with lithogenic urine may be predisposed toward intramural crystal formation within the healing UPJ, resulting in exuberant scarring. Thus, the presence of a stone at the UPJ may worsen the degree of obstruction and potentially exacerbate an already compromised renal unit.

In our series of secondary UPJO to renal stones, it consisted of 48 patients. Simultaneous PSE and EP are considered if the calculi in the pelvicalyceal system are mobile and there is no evidence of UPJ edema. In patients with significant inflammation at the UPJ, the presence of obstruction should be reevaluated several weeks after PSE to avoid the risk of injury to the inflamed UPJ and unnecessary EP. In contrast, if no inflammation is noted and the UPJ is found to be stenotic at the time of stone removal, then EP is performed during the PSE. Several patients with stones and obstruction at the UPJ had resolution of the obstruction without endopyelotomy. With a mean follow-up of 52 months, only two (4.7 %) patients in this subset were found to have persistent obstruction. Our results are supported by the literature. Berkman et al. reported a 90 % success rate in a group of patients with concomitant kidney stones treated simultaneously with EP [14]. Similarly, Shalhav and colleagues reported their single institution experience with EP in 149 patients [21]. The authors stratified the results by primary or secondary UPJO, calculi-related obstruction, high ureteral insertion, and presence of impaired renal function [21]. Subjective results were evaluated on an analog pain scale. Objective results determined by renal scan, excretory urography, or Whitaker test. Patients with UPJO secondary to stone disease showed the highest success rates of 93 %. Patients with a high ureteral insertion were treated successfully in 70 % of cases. Clearly, endopyelotomy is feasible and may be considered a primary treatment option in the management of UPJO in patients with stone disease.

Length of Stricture

Length of stricture is an important consideration in preoperative decision-making. Strictures greater than 2 cm or complete obliterations are obvious contraindications for EP. There is clear evidence that failure in patients with longer strictures at UPJ is significantly higher [7, 24, 25]. Patients with these features are recommended for open or laparoscopic pyeloplasty.

Surgical Technique

The procedure is performed under general anesthesia following parenteral delivery of appropriate antibiotic prophylaxis and sequential compression device placement. The procedure begins with the patient in the lithotomy position. Cystoscopically, with the use of fluoroscopic guidance, a Teflon-coated guidewire is placed through the ureteral orifice up the ureter into the renal pelvis followed by a 6-F open-end ureteral catheter. The guidewire is removed, and a Foley catheter is placed. The ureteral catheter is then secured to the Foley catheter with a silk suture.

The patient is then transferred into the prone position. A foam pillow is used to pad the face and facilitate ventilation. Bolsters are placed under the shoulders and pelvis to reduce resistance to breathing. Additionally, pressure points such as the feet, knees, and elbows are also padded to prevent compression and stretch injuries. Following proper positioning, the ipsilateral flank is prepped and draped in a sterile fashion.

The collecting system is then opacified with contrast material via the previously placed ureteral catheter. Thorough assessment of the renal collecting system anatomy allows for optimal access. Access should be obtained through either an upper- or mid-pole posterior calyx to provide optimal exposure to the UPJ. Entry through a posterior calyx minimizes parenchymal injury, thereby reducing the risk of bleeding.

Once an appropriate calyx has been selected, the C-arm is rotated 30° toward the surgeon. This fluoroscopy beam angle visualizes most posterior calices end-on and facilitates proper needle alignment. The finder needle is then advanced toward the selected calyx. Needle depth is monitored with the C-arm in the 90° position, while continuing to advance the needle at the previously chosen angle. When the tip of the needle appears to be within the collecting system, the needle trocar is removed, leaving only the needle cannula in place. To confirm placement within the collecting system, sterile water is injected through the needle cannula. Dispersion of contrast should be noted fluoroscopically. Alternatively, aspiration of urine also confirms the needle's intraluminal position.

Puncture of the renal collecting system with an 18-gauge diamond-tip needle permits the introduction of a 0.038-in. guidewire into the collecting system. A Teflon-coated wire is advanced carefully across the caliceal infundibulum. A 1-cm skin incision is made around the needle with a No. 10 blade, and the needle is removed. A 30-F access tract is then established with either serial dilators or with a balloon dilator. A rigid nephroscope is then used to bring the previously placed ureteral catheter out through the nephrostomy tract. A 0.038-in. super stiff wire is advanced through the catheter, thereby establishing secure access.

The UPJ is then prepared for incision. An 8-F Teflon catheter is advanced across the UPJ and into the ureter. Under fluoroscopic guidance, a 12-F dilator is advanced down the UPJ over the 8-F catheter. A resectoscope with a hook-shaped cold knife is used to make a posterolateral full-thickness incision in the UPJ until periureteral fat is visible and the UPJ appears wide open. Direct vision allows prevention of crossing a vessel incision at this point. The incision must be extensive enough to allow visualization of the previously obscured proximal ureter.

Alternatively, scissors may be used to cut the UPJ. With the scissors closed, a full-thickness puncture is made 1 cm away from the UPJ through the renal pelvis into the perirenal space posterolaterally. The perinephric space is inspected for crossing vessels. The scissors are then opened, and the posterolateral UPJ incision is continued down to the proximal ureter. Lastly, a holmium laser may also be used to open the UPJ.

Multiple exit strategies may be utilized. The Smith endopyelotomy tube that is constructed of polyurethane has both an internal and external component. The nephrostomy portion of the tube is 14 F and exits via the access tract. The distal component tapers to 8.2 F and has a curl that rests within the bladder. Percutaneous EP tubes provide optimal drainage and maintain percutaneous access, while both the nephrostomy tract and UPJ incision heal.

Another option is to place an endoureterotomy stent and Council catheter nephrostomy. The nephrostomy tube is usually removed within 48 h. Our major concern with the EP stent has always been that it is relatively inaccessible, which is problematic if the stent becomes obstructed following nephrostomy tube removal. Furthermore, the proximal coil can migrate outside the EP site and into the retroperitoneum.

A nephrostogram is performed 48 h after the procedure either through the EP tube or the Council catheter. If no extravasation is evident, the EP tube is capped, or the Council tip catheter is removed, and the patient is discharged from the hospital.

Antegrade Versus Retrograde

Two approaches have been developed for EP: antegrade and retrograde. Experience with antegrade EP is quite large, and the results have been excellent. However, management of the nephrostomy tract and increased patient discomfort resulting in longer hospitalizations are the main drawbacks to the antegrade approach.

Tolley and colleagues developed a new retrograde ureteroscopic technique for EP [26]. They reported their initial experience with ureteroscopic EP in ten patients with five primary and five secondary UPJO. Procedure was performed using a 3- or 5-F Greenwald cutting electrode passed through a 12-F rigid, 10.8-F flexible, or 9.8-F flexible deflectable ureteronephroscope. Although less invasive, this approach was technically complex resulting in longer operative times and a high incidence of ureterovesical stenosis [27, 28]. However, subsequent technical modifications overcame many of these challenges [29]. Retrograde endopyelotomy has reported success rates ranging from 60 to 87.5 % [30–34]. Matin and colleagues have reported a 65 % symptomatic and radiographic success rate in their series of 46 retrograde EP with a mean follow-up of 23 months [8]. Antegrade endopyelotomy has reported success rates ranging from 61 to 89 % [11, 14, 22]. Knudsen et al. have recently presented an overall 67 % success rate in their series of 80 antegrade endopyelotomy after a mean follow-up of 55 months [35]. In our series, after a mean follow-up of 44.7 months, the overall success rate of antegrade endopyelotomy was 90.3 %. Further retrospective studies demonstrated that antegrade EP was statistically more successful than retrograde EP in the setting of massive hydronephrosis [11, 21, 36].

Antegrade EP may be more successful in certain clinical setting such as severe and massive hydronephrosis because it allows for direct visualization of the UPJO so a more precise incision can be performed. Additionally, in patients with concomitant kidney, calculi stones can be extracted at the time of EP [21].

Chandhoke and colleagues first reported the use of a ureteral cutting balloon device, the Acucise catheter, to treat UPJO [37]. The Acucise catheter is a 7-F catheter with a 2.8 cm long, 150 μ wide electrosurgical cutting wire mounted on an 8-mm balloon. The entire assembly at the broadest point is 13 F. The procedure is performed ureteroscopically. Since its first introduction, it has been embraced by many urologists. Later in 1996, the same group reported long-term efficacy in 28 patients [38]. Over 60 % of patients had a favorable response with 36 % totally free of pain and 25 % markedly improved. Of these 28 patients with objective follow-up, 81 % had a patient ureteropelvic junction based on a diuretic renal scan with a half time of less than 10 min or a normal Whitaker test. Subsequently, numerous studies have reported their experience with Acucise catheter. The success rates range from 70 to 100 % [38–42]. However, currently this procedure is not commonly performed due to a significant bleeding associated with this modality [39, 43].

Complications

Endopyelotomy is a minimally invasive procedure well tolerated by the majority of patients. Nevertheless, the potential for various complications is present. The complications associated with EP are similar with those occurred during percutaneous stone extraction. Most common complications include hemorrhage due to vascular injury, ureteral injury with urinary tract perforation, pulmonary injury, and sepsis [39, 44, 45].

Hemorrhage

Hemorrhage is the most common and worrisome complication associated with percutaneous access [46–48]. The reported rate of hemorrhage after percutaneous surgery requiring transfusion ranges from 1 to 11 % [49]. Significant bleeding can occur during initial needle passage, tract dilation, and while incising the UPJ.

Frequently, bleeding is associated with renal parenchymal trauma or perinephric vessel injury. Anterior and posterior segmental arteries are most commonly injured vessels [50]. Sampaio and colleagues studied renal vascular anatomy using polyester resin endocasts at the time of autopsy [19]. The study demonstrated that 71 % of kidneys have crossing vessels within 1.5 cm of the UPJ. Over 90 % of these vessels are located anterior to the UPJ, and the remainders are posterior. The UPJ should be carefully inspected for pulsations prior to making the incision. It is recommended that endoscopic incisions be directed posterolaterally to avoid the injury to a vessel crossing the UPJ. Preoperative imaging such as helical computerized tomography may also help to identify crossing vessels [51–54]; however, we do not think that it is indicated routinely. Conservative and surgical management of bleeding such as tamponade catheters, angioembolization, cryoablation of the nephrostomy tract, and use of different sealant materials have been thoroughly evaluated in previous studies [55–57].

Postoperative Care and Follow-Up

At our institution, we perform a nephrostogram on postoperative day 2. If no extravasation is noted and the endopyelotomy tube is in good position, it is capped and the patient is sent home. If an EP stent and nephrostomy tube were placed, then the nephrostomy tube is pulled and the patient is discharged. Patients are sent home on prophylactic antibiotics until all tubes are removed.

The EP tube has traditionally been left in place for 6 weeks [58, 59]. As suggested by Oppenheimer and Hinman [59], a 6-week period is necessary for regeneration of the muscular wall of the ureter. At this point, the percutaneous EP tube or EP stent is removed in clinic.

Follow-up imaging is obtained 4–6 weeks later and generally includes a CT or renal scintigraphy [60]. If the patient remains asymptomatic, the degree of caliectasis has decreased, and the renogram T1/2 is less than 15 min, then the treatment is considered a success. Reevaluation is performed at 6- and then 12-month intervals for at least 2 year.

Conclusions

Endopyelotomy remains a viable treatment modality for UPJO. Most of the literature presented on success rates of endoscopic treatment of UPJO includes studies published more than a decade ago, without a knowledge of risk factors resulting in poor patient selection. Used in the proper setting (mild hydronephrosis, stricture less than 2 cm in length, and no significant ipsilateral renal insufficiency), antegrade EP has excellent success rates that are comparable to pyeloplasty. It is particularly suitable in patients who have secondary UPJO.

References

1. Yong D, Albala DM. Endopyelotomy in the age of laparoscopic and robotic-assisted pyeloplasty. Curr Urol Rep. 2010;11(2):74–9.
2. Anderson JC, Hynes W. Retrocaval ureter; a case diagnosed preoperatively and treated successfully by a plastic operation. Br J Urol. 1949;21(3):209–14.
3. Braga LH, Lorenzo AJ, Skeldon S, Dave S, Bagli DJ, Khoury AE, et al. Failed pyeloplasty in children: comparative analysis of retrograde endopyelotomy versus redo pyeloplasty. J Urol. 2007;178(6):2571–5, discussion 5.
4. Bauer JJ, Bishoff JT, Moore RG, Chen RN, Iverson AJ, Kavoussi LR. Laparoscopic versus open pyeloplasty: assessment of objective and subjective outcome. J Urol. 1999;162(3 Pt 1):692–5.
5. Wickham JE, Kellet MJ. Percutaneous pyelolysis. Eur Urol. 1983;9(2):122–4.
6. Badlani G, Eshghi M, Smith AD. Percutaneous surgery for ureteropelvic junction obstruction (endopyelotomy): technique and early results. J Urol. 1986;135(1):26–8.
7. Motola JA, Badlani GH, Smith AD. Results of 212 consecutive endopyelotomies: an 8-year follow-up. J Urol. 1993;149(3):453–6.
8. Matin SF, Yost A, Streem SB. Ureteroscopic laser endopyelotomy: a single-center experience. J Endourol. 2003;17(6):401–4.
9. Van Cangh PJ, Wilmart JF, Opsomer RJ, Abi-Aad A, Wese FX, Lorge F. Long-term results and late recurrence after endoureteropyelotomy: a critical analysis of prognostic factors. J Urol. 1994;151(4):934–7.

10. Van Cangh PJ, Nesa S. Endopyelotomy. Prognostic factors and patient selection. Urol Clin North Am. 1998;25(2):281–8.
11. Lam JS, Cooper KL, Greene TD, Gupta M. Impact of hydronephrosis and renal function on treatment outcome: antegrade versus retrograde endopyelotomy. Urology. 2003;61(6):1107–11, discussion 11–2.
12. Chow GK, Geisinger MA, Streem SB. Endopyelotomy outcome as a function of high versus dependent ureteral insertion. Urology. 1999;54(6):999–1002.
13. Gupta M, Tuncay OL, Smith AD. Open surgical exploration after failed endopyelotomy: a 12-year perspective. J Urol. 1997;157(5):1613–8, discussion 8–9.
14. Berkman DS, Landman J, Gupta M. Treatment outcomes after endopyelotomy performed with or without simultaneous nephrolithotomy: 10-year experience. J Endourol. 2009;23(9):1409–13.
15. Danuser H, Ackermann DK, Bohlen D, Studer UE. Endopyelotomy for primary ureteropelvic junction obstruction: risk factors determine the success rate. J Urol. 1998;159(1):56–61.
16. Van Cangh PJ, Jorion JL, Wese FX, Opsomer RJ. Endoureteropyelotomy: percutaneous treatment of ureteropelvic junction obstruction. J Urol. 1989; 141(6):1317–21, discussion 21–2.
17. Van Cangh PJ, Nesa S, Galeon M, Tombal B, Wese FX, Dardenne AN, et al. Vessels around the ureteropelvic junction: significance and imaging by conventional radiology. J Endourol. 1996;10(2):111–9.
18. Renner C, Frede T, Seemann O, Rassweiler J. Laser endopyelotomy: minimally invasive therapy of ureteropelvic junction stenosis. J Endourol. 1998;12(6): 537–44.
19. Sampaio FJ, Favorito LA. Ureteropelvic junction stenosis: vascular anatomical background for endopyelotomy. J Urol. 1993;150(6):1787–91.
20. Amon Sesmero JH, del Valle Gonzalez N, Rodriguez Toves LA, Conde Redondo C, Rodriguez Tesedo V, Martinez-Sagarra Oceja JM. Long-term follow-up of antegrade endopyelotomy. Factors that influence the outcome. Actas Urol Esp. 2009;33(1):64–8.
21. Shalhav AL, Giusti G, Elbahnasy AM, Hoenig DM, McDougall EM, Smith DS, et al. Adult endopyelotomy: impact of etiology and antegrade versus retrograde approach on outcome. J Urol. 1998;160(3 Pt 1): 685–9.
22. Hoenig DM, Shalhav AL, Elbahnasy AM, McDougall EM, Smith D, Clayman RV. Impact of etiology of secondary ureteropelvic junction obstruction on outcome of endopyelotomy. J Endourol. 1998;12(2): 131–3.
23. Hulbert JC, Hunter D, Castaneda-Zuniga W. Classification of and techniques for the reconstitution of acquired strictures in the region of the ureteropelvic junction. J Urol. 1988;140(3):468–72.
24. Perez LM, Friedman RM, Carson 3rd CC. Endoureteropyelotomy in adults. Review of procedure and results. Urology. 1992;39(1):71–6.
25. Rodrigues Netto Jr N, Ikari O, Esteves SC, D'Ancona CA. Antegrade endopyelotomy for pelviureteric junction obstruction in children. Br J Urol. 1996;78(4): 607–12.
26. Inglis JA, Tolley DA. Ureteroscopic pyelolysis for pelviureteric junction obstruction. Br J Urol. 1986; 58(3):250–2.
27. Meretyk I, Meretyk S, Clayman RV. Endopyelotomy: comparison of ureteroscopic retrograde and antegrade percutaneous techniques. J Urol. 1992;148(3):775–82, discussion 82–3.
28. Clayman RV, Basler JW, Kavoussi L, Picus DD. Ureteronephroscopic endopyelotomy. J Urol. 1990; 144(2 Pt 1):246–51, discussion 51–2.
29. Thomas R. Rigid ureteroscopy: pitfalls and remedies. Urology. 1988;32(4):328–34.
30. Gerber GS, Kim JC. Ureteroscopic endopyelotomy in the treatment of patients with ureteropelvic junction obstruction. Urology. 2000;55(2):198–202, discussion 202–3.
31. Giddens JL, Grasso M. Retrograde ureteroscopic endopyelotomy using the holmium: YAG laser. J Urol. 2000;164(5):1509–12.
32. Conlin MJ, Bagley DH. Ureteroscopic endopyelotomy at a single setting. J Urol. 1998;159(3):727–31.
33. Geavlete P, Georgescu D, Mirciulescu V, Nita G. Ureteroscopic laser approach in recurrent ureteropelvic junction stenosis. Eur Urol. 2007;51(6):1542–8.
34. Tawfiek ER, Liu JB, Bagley DH. Ureteroscopic treatment of ureteropelvic junction obstruction. J Urol. 1998;160(5):1643–6, discussion 6–7.
35. Knudsen BE, Cook AJ, Watterson JD, Beiko DT, Nott L, Razvi H, et al. Percutaneous antegrade endopyelotomy: long-term results from one institution. Urology. 2004;63(2):230–4.
36. Minervini A, Davenport K, Keeley Jr FX, Timoney AG. Antegrade versus retrograde endopyelotomy for pelvi-ureteric junction (PUJ) obstruction. Eur Urol. 2006;49(3):536–42, discussion 42–3.
37. Chandhoke PS, Clayman RV, Stone AM, McDougall EM, Buelna T, Hilal N, et al. Endopyelotomy and endoureterotomy with the acucise ureteral cutting balloon device: preliminary experience. J Endourol. 1993;7(1):45–51.
38. Nadler RB, Rao GS, Pearle MS, Nakada SY, Clayman RV. Acucise endopyelotomy: assessment of long-term durability. J Urol. 1996;156(3):1094–7, discussion 7–8.
39. Kim FJ, Herrell SD, Jahoda AE, Albala DM. Complications of acucise endopyelotomy. J Endourol. 1998;12(5):433–6.
40. Preminger GM, Clayman RV, Nakada SY, Babayan RK, Albala DM, Fuchs GJ, et al. A multicenter clinical trial investigating the use of a fluoroscopically controlled cutting balloon catheter for the management of ureteral and ureteropelvic junction obstruction. J Urol. 1997;157(5):1625–9.
41. Faerber GJ, Richardson TD, Farah N, Ohl DA. Retrograde treatment of ureteropelvic junction obstruction using the ureteral cutting balloon catheter. J Urol. 1997;157(2):454–8.
42. Gelet A, Combe M, Ramackers JM, Ben Rais N, Martin X, Dawahra M, et al. Endopyelotomy with the

Acucise cutting balloon device. Early clinical experience. Eur Urol. 1997;31(4):389–93.
43. Wagner JR, D'Agostino R, Babayan RK. Renal arterioureteral hemorrhage: a complication of acucise endopyelotomy. Urology. 1996;48(1):139–41.
44. Dobry E, Usai P, Studer UE, Danuser H. Is antegrade endopyelotomy really less invasive than open pyeloplasty? Urol Int. 2007;79(2):152–6.
45. Walz J, Lecamus C, Lechevallier E, Barriol D, Bretheau D, Albert P, et al. Complications of "Acucise" balloon endopyelotomy. Prog Urol. 2003;13(1): 39–45.
46. de la Rosette J, Assimos D, Desai M, Gutierrez J, Lingeman J, Scarpa R, et al. The Clinical Research Office of the endourological society percutaneous nephrolithotomy global study: indications, complications, and outcomes in 5803 patients. J Endourol. 2011;25(1):11–7.
47. Akman T, Binbay M, Sari E, Yuruk E, Tepeler A, Akcay M, et al. Factors affecting bleeding during percutaneous nephrolithotomy: single surgeon experience. J Endourol. 2011;25(2):327–33.
48. Kurtulus F, Fazlioglu A, Tandogdu Z, Karaca S, Salman Y, Cek M. Analysis of factors related with bleeding in percutaneous nephrolithotomy using balloon dilatation. Can J Urol. 2010;17(6):5483–9.
49. Gallucci M, Fortunato P, Schettini M, Vincenzoni A. Management of hemorrhage after percutaneous renal surgery. J Endourol. 1998;12(6):509–12.
50. Richstone L, Reggio E, Ost MC, Seideman C, Fossett LK, Okeke Z, et al. First prize (tie): hemorrhage following percutaneous renal surgery: characterization of angiographic findings. J Endourol. 2008;22(6): 1129–35.
51. Cassis AN, Brannen GE, Bush WH, Correa RJ, Chambers M. Endopyelotomy: review of results and complications. J Urol. 1991;146(6):1492–5.
52. Mitterberger M, Pinggera GM, Neururer R, Peschel R, Colleselli D, Aigner F, et al. Comparison of contrast-enhanced color Doppler imaging (CDI), computed tomography (CT), and magnetic resonance imaging (MRI) for the detection of crossing vessels in patients with ureteropelvic junction obstruction (UPJO). Eur Urol. 2008;53(6):1254–60.
53. Sauer B, Flocquet M, Batch T, Blum A, Hubert J. Vascular renal anatomy and the ureteropelvic junction: preoperative multidetector CT scanning with split-bolus injection as a predictor of laparoscopic findings. J Endourol. 2008;22(1):13–8.
54. Herts BR. Helical CT and CT angiography for the identification of crossing vessels at the ureteropelvic junction. Urol Clin North Am. 1998;25(2): 259–69.
55. Li R, Louie MK, Lee HJ, Osann K, Pick DL, Santos R, et al. Prospective randomized trial of three different methods of nephrostomy tract closure after percutaneous nephrolithotripsy. BJU Int. 2011;107(10): 1660–5.
56. Okeke Z, Andonian S, Srinivasan A, Shapiro E, Vanderbrink BA, Kavoussi LR, et al. Cryotherapy of the nephrostomy tract: a novel technique to decrease the risk of hemorrhage after tubeless percutaneous renal surgery. J Endourol. 2009;23(3): 417–20.
57. Lee DI, Uribe C, Eichel L, Khonsari S, Basillote J, Park HK, et al. Sealing percutaneous nephrolithotomy tracts with gelatin matrix hemostatic sealant: initial clinical use. J Urol. 2004;171(2 Pt 1):575–8.
58. Davis DM, Strong GH, Drake WM. Intubated ureterotomy; experimental work and clinical results. J Urol. 1948;59(5):851–62.
59. Oppenheimer R, Hinman Jr F. Ureteral regeneration: contracture vs. hyperplasia of smooth muscle. J Urol. 1955;74(4):476–84.
60. Albani JM, Yost AJ, Streem SB. Ureteropelvic junction obstruction: determining durability of endourological intervention. J Urol. 2004;171(2 Pt 1): 579–82.

Ureteroscopy for Upper Ureteral Stones: Overcoming the Difficulties of the Rigid Approach

22

Tamer S. Barakat, Ahmed R. El-Nahas, Ahmed M. Shoma, and Ahmed A. Shokeir

Introduction

Traditionally, rigid ureteroscopy (URS) has been the favored approach for the surgical treatment of mid and distal ureteral stones, while shock wave lithotripsy (SWL) has been preferred for the less accessible proximal ureteral stones [1]. With the development of smaller caliber semirigid URS and the improvement of instrumentation, URS has evolved into a safer and more efficacious modality for treatment of stones in all locations in the ureter with increasing experience worldwide [2].

Indication of URS for Proximal Ureteral Calculi

Ureteroscopy is indicated mainly for large (>1 cm) or impacted proximal ureteric stones, bleeding diathesis as in patients with anticoagulant treatment, and morbid obesity [3–5]. All are considered as contraindication for SWL treatment. Failure of conservative management or SWL disintegration is also considered as indication for ureteroscopic intervention. Other indications include patients with multiple ureteral stones [6], those with bilateral ureteral stones in need of simultaneous URS [7], and pregnant women after failure of conservative management [8–10].

T.S. Barakat, M.D. (✉) • A.R. El-Nahas, M.D.
A.M. Shoma, M.D. • A.A. Shokeir, M.D., Ph.D., FEBU
Department of Urology,
Urology and Nephrology Center, Mansoura University,
El Gomhoria Street, Mansoura 35516, Egypt
e-mail: drtamerbarakat@gmail.com;
ar_el_nahas@yahoo.com; ahmedshoma@hotmail.com;
ahmed.shokeir@hotmail.com

Instruments and Equipment

The list of instruments used for rigid URS includes guidewires, dilation devices, semirigid URS, lithotripsy devices, stone extraction devices, and ureteric occlusion devices.

Guidewires

Guidewires are used to gain access to the ureter, which is the initial step in ureteroscopic surgeries. Guidewires differ with respect to size, flexibility, and coating material. Wire diameter ranges from 0.018 to 0.038 in.. Guidewire length ranges from 145 to 260 cm. Generally, the ones commonly used are a 145-cm, 0.035- and 0.038-in. guidewire. Calibrated guidewires are now available which are marked to help identify length during ureteroscopic procedures.

Guidewire surface is generally coated with polytetrafluoroethylene (PTFE) or a hydrophilic material to create a frictionless surface. The hydrophilic guidewires are best used to navigate tight strictures or impacted stones. However, they may become displaced more easily; therefore, we generally prefer to replace them with PTFE-coated wires whenever possible. Guidewires have

A.M. Al-Kandari et al. (eds.), *Difficult Cases in Endourology*,
DOI 10.1007/978-1-84882-083-8_22, © Springer-Verlag London 2013

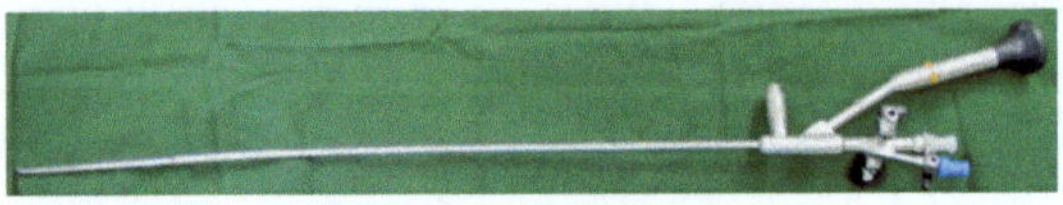

Fig. 22.1 Semirigid ureteroscope

various tip designs including standard straight-tipped and angled tips (J-tip) which help to navigate tortuous or narrow ureteral segments, as well as bypass impacted stones [11].

Ureteral Dilation Devices

Mechanical dilation is the oldest mechanism of ureteral dilation. Balloon dilating systems are now the most commonly used with URS. With the introduction of small-caliber ureteroscopes, ureteral dilation is needed only in selected ureteroscopic procedures as to treat a ureteric stricture, to allow the URS to be advanced through the tight intramural ureter, and with large ureteral stones when disintegration and extraction of multiple stone fragments is required via repeated introduction of the URS [12].

Semirigid URS

Semirigid URSs (Fig. 22.1) have the advantage of good image transmission through fiberoptic techniques and larger working channels. For this reason, they are ideal for calculus extraction using a variety of URS instruments, such as forceps and baskets. They are also more easily used by a single operator because the instruments can be manipulated using the other hand. Most semirigid URSs offer a beveled tip sheath, designed to reduce trauma to both the ureter and to the ureteral orifice while introducing the URS [11].

Proximal ureteral stones are better treated by flexible URS [13]. However, it is not used in many hospitals worldwide [14, 15] because of financial reasons or lack of experience in these hospitals. Therefore, semirigid URS is still used in many places because it is less expensive and more durable with better vision, and its small diameter allows its passage into the proximal ureter [16].

Lithotripsy Devices

Several types of intracorporeal lithotriptors exist for the management of calculi, including pneumatic lithotriptors (PLs), laser lithotriptors (LLs), electrohydraulic lithotriptors (EHLs), and ultrasonic lithotriptors (ULs). It is advisable to use holmium laser for proximal ureteral calculi because of its higher safety and efficacy profile and the minimal chance of stone migration [2, 17].

Pneumatic Lithotripsy (PL)

Pneumatic lithotriptors fragment calculi through the transfer of mechanical energy to the stone. One major advantage of PLs lies in their wide margins of safety, which is significantly better than the margins of safety for other types; also, some new versions of PLs have the ability to suck stone fragments as well. But there is higher rate of migration of fragments into more proximal parts of the urinary tract which decreases the stone-free rate [18].

Laser Lithotripsy (LL)

Since its first use in lithotripsy, laser technology has been significantly refined, and the holmium:yttrium-aluminum-garnet (Ho:YAG) laser (Fig. 22.2) using a photothermal mechanism is currently the most commonly used laser in the treatment of urinary calculi. Laser fiber must have contact with stone surface. It can disintegrate all types of stones regardless of their chemical composition and provides less stone migration than the pneumatic probes [19].

Ultrasonic Lithotripsy (UL)

Ultrasonic lithotripsy is based on the generation of ultrasonic vibrations to fragment urinary calculi. Its major advantage is its ability to combine stone fragmentation with removal, which is accomplished through an aspiration port of the lithotriptor probe. The probes have the disadvantage of associated significant ureteral injury. So ultrasound lithotripsy is less commonly used currently with URS [20].

Electrohydraulic Lithotripsy (EHL)

Electrohydraulic lithotriptors fragment calculi through energy produced following an underwater

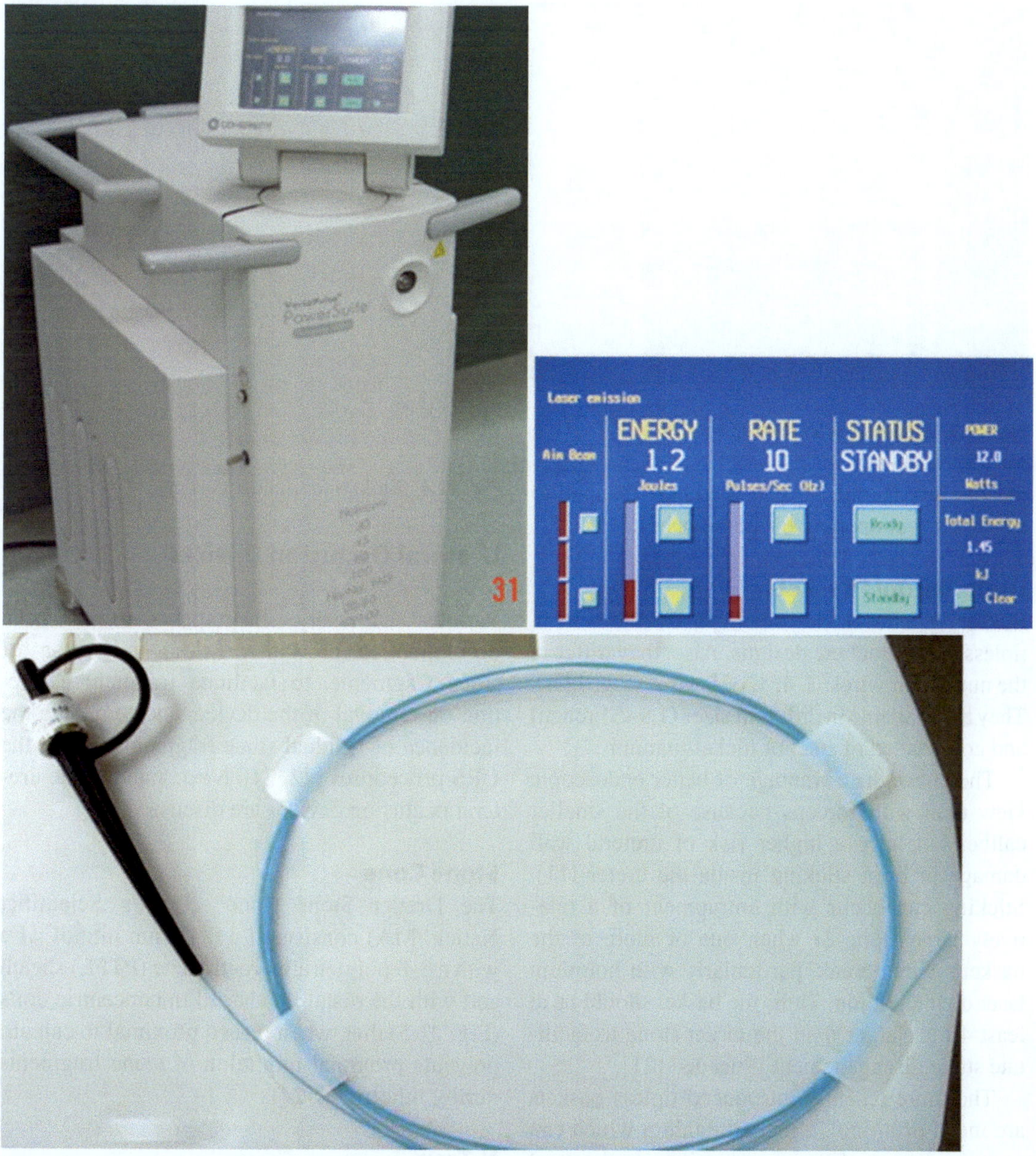

Fig. 22.2 Holmium laser machine, screen shot, and fibers (Courtesy of VersaPulse PowerSuite, Luminus® Surgical, Germany GmbH)

discharge of electrical current. They have the advantage of flexible probes, which allow for the treatment of more proximal stones. But, electrohydraulic lithotriptors also may cause significant ureteral injuries; thus, it is currently rarely used with URS as a result of the development of better lithotripsy devices [20].

Stone Extraction Devices

Endoscopic Graspers and Forceps

Endoscopic graspers and forceps are available in two- or three-pronged types and may be retracting or nonretracting [11] (Fig. 22.3). The forceps must be pushed until the whole opening

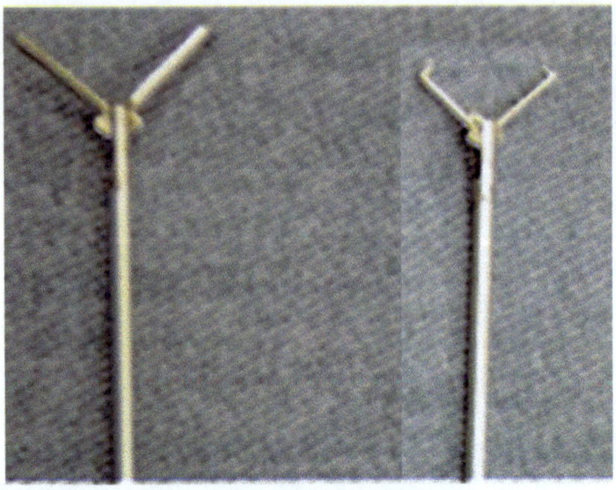

Fig. 22.3 Stone extraction forceps

mechanism is out of the working channel to assure correct opening of the branches.

Ureteroscopic Baskets

Basket varieties include helical, double-helical, tipless, and parachute designs. Also, they differ in the number of wires: 3, 4, 5, or 6 wires (Fig. 22.4). They are available in different sizes (1.9–5 French) and constructed of steel or nickel/titanium.

They have the advantage of better endoscopic view than with forceps because of the smaller caliber but have a higher risk of ureteral wall damage or even sticking inside the ureter [11]. Sticking can occur with entrapment of a relatively large stone or when one or more of the basket's wires break, particularly with holmium laser disintegration. Thus, the basket should be at least 4 mm larger than the target stone to facilitate stone disengagement if needed [21].

The more recently introduced tipless baskets are made of nitinol, a nickel/titanium which can overcome most of the shortcomings of the steel wire baskets because of the tipless design and the soft "springy" nature of the wires (increased flexibility) which allows the basket to reach the upper ureter to capture a stone with less tissue injury. Stone disengagement is another advantage of the tipless over the tip basket.

European Association of Urology (EAU) and American Urological Association (AUA) guidelines for the management of ureteral calculi stated that stone extraction with a basket without endoscopic visualization of the stone (blind basketing) should not be performed [2].

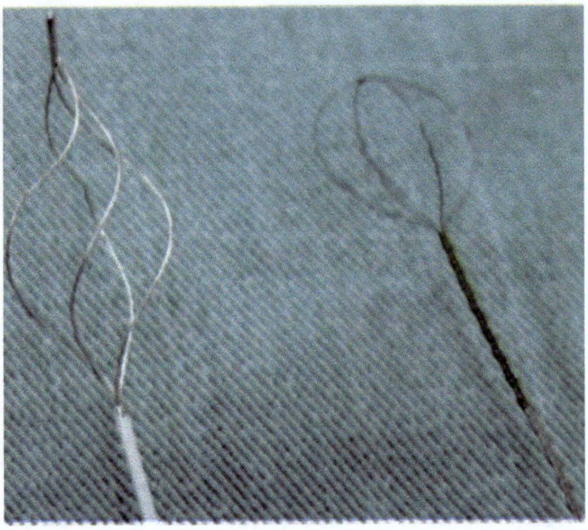

Fig. 22.4 Baskets for stone extraction

Ureteral Occlusion Devices

Various accessory instruments have been developed to prevent proximal migration of stone fragments, to facilitate fragment extraction on removal of the device, and to reduce the incidence of residual stone fragments during the URS procedures [22, 23]. Next, some of the ureteral occlusion devices are discussed.

Stone Cone

The Dretler Stone Cone® (Boston Scientific, Natick, MA) consists of a 0.43-mm nitinol wire with a 3-F polytetrafluoroethylene (PTFE) sheath and with the distal tip shaped in concentric coils (Fig. 22.5) that, when placed proximal to calculi, prevents proximal migration of stone fragments during lithotripsy [24].

N-Trap

Another tool is the Cook NTrap® (Cook Urological, Spencer, IN). It is a 2.6-F device composed of a tightly interwoven mesh of nitinol wires (Fig. 22.6). The NTrap is capable of blocking smaller fragments (less than 1.5 mm) than the stone cone [25, 26].

Accordion Device

The PercSys Accordion® (Percutaneous System, Palo Alto, CA) is a 2.9-F multifold polyurethane film (Fig. 22.7). It tracks like a guidewire proximal to the stone, secures like a basket during lithotripsy, and clears the fragments easily [23].

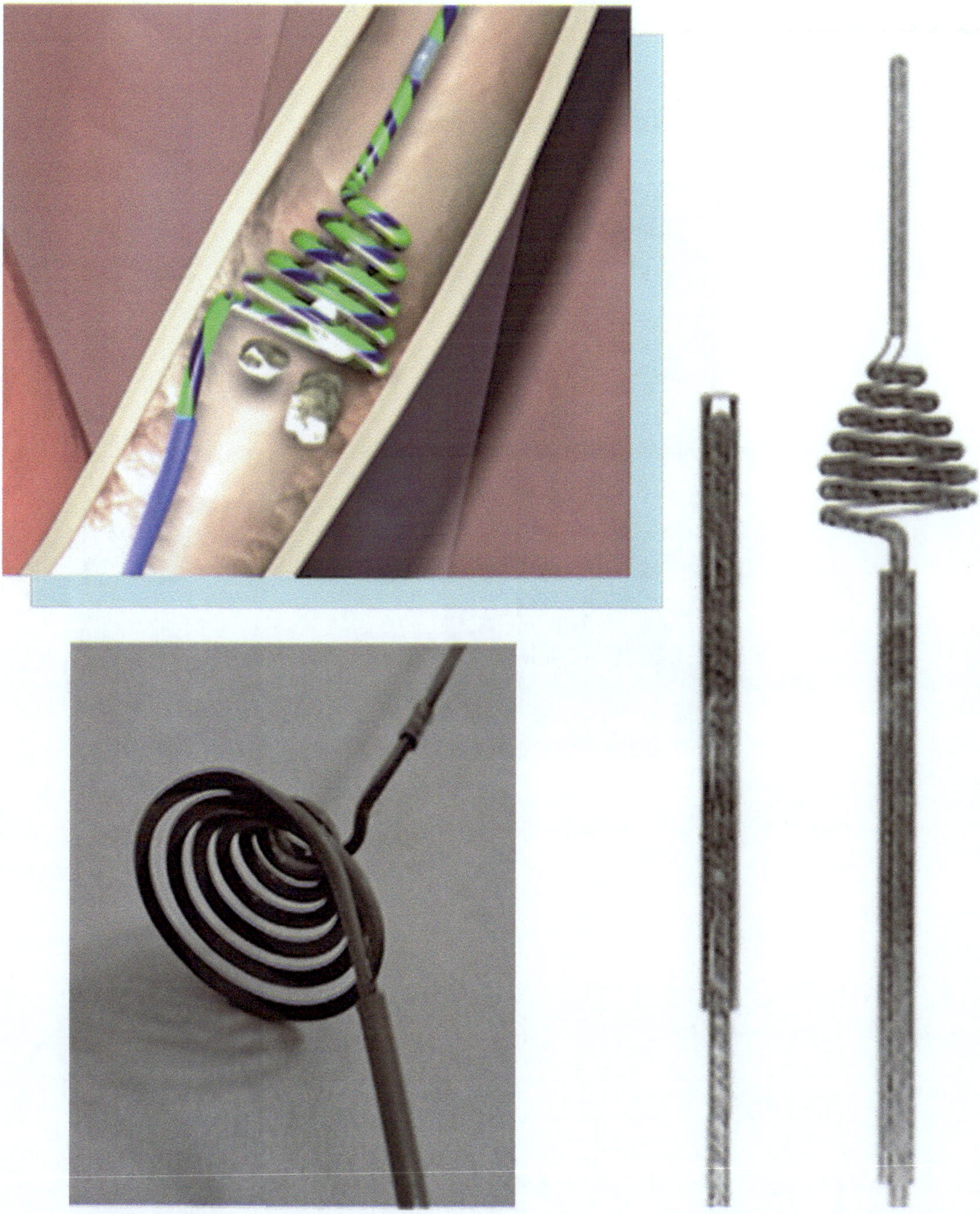

Fig. 22.5 Dretler stone cone® (*Top left image* courtesy of Medsource, Norwell, MA; *Right image* reprinted with permission from Dretler [24])

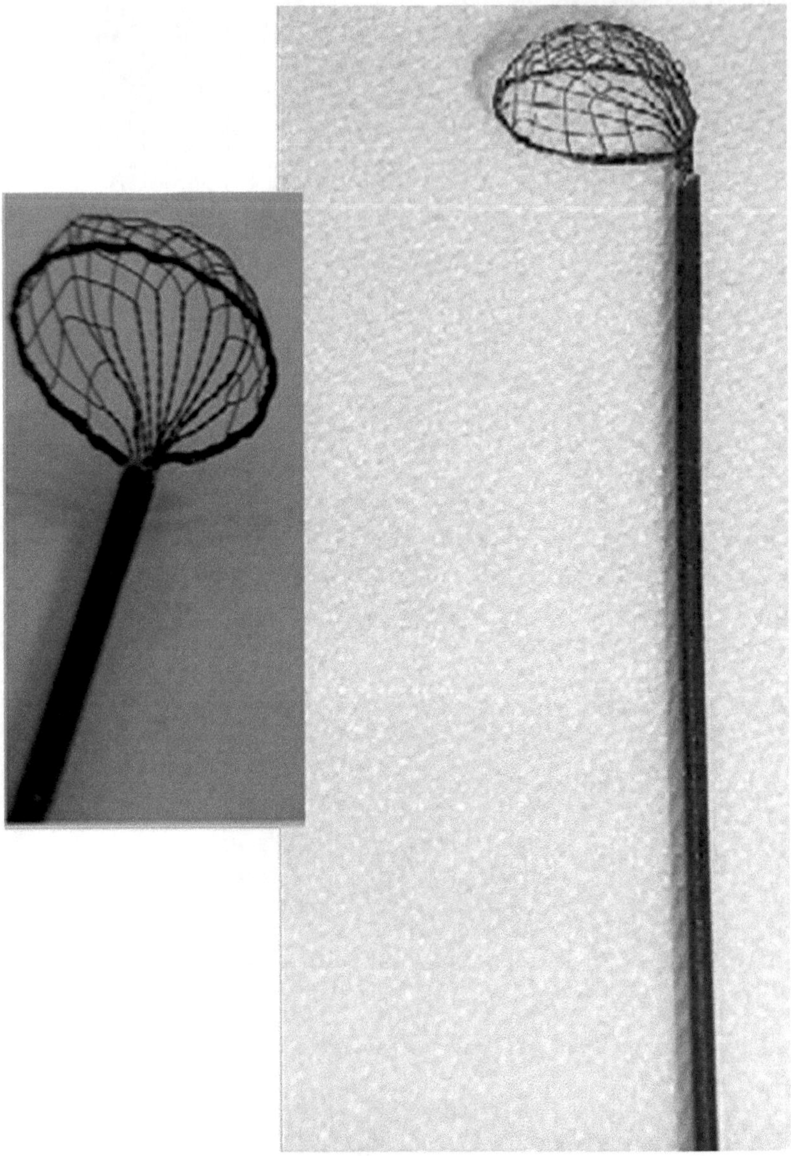

Fig. 22.6 NTrap® device (Cook Urological, Spencer, IN)

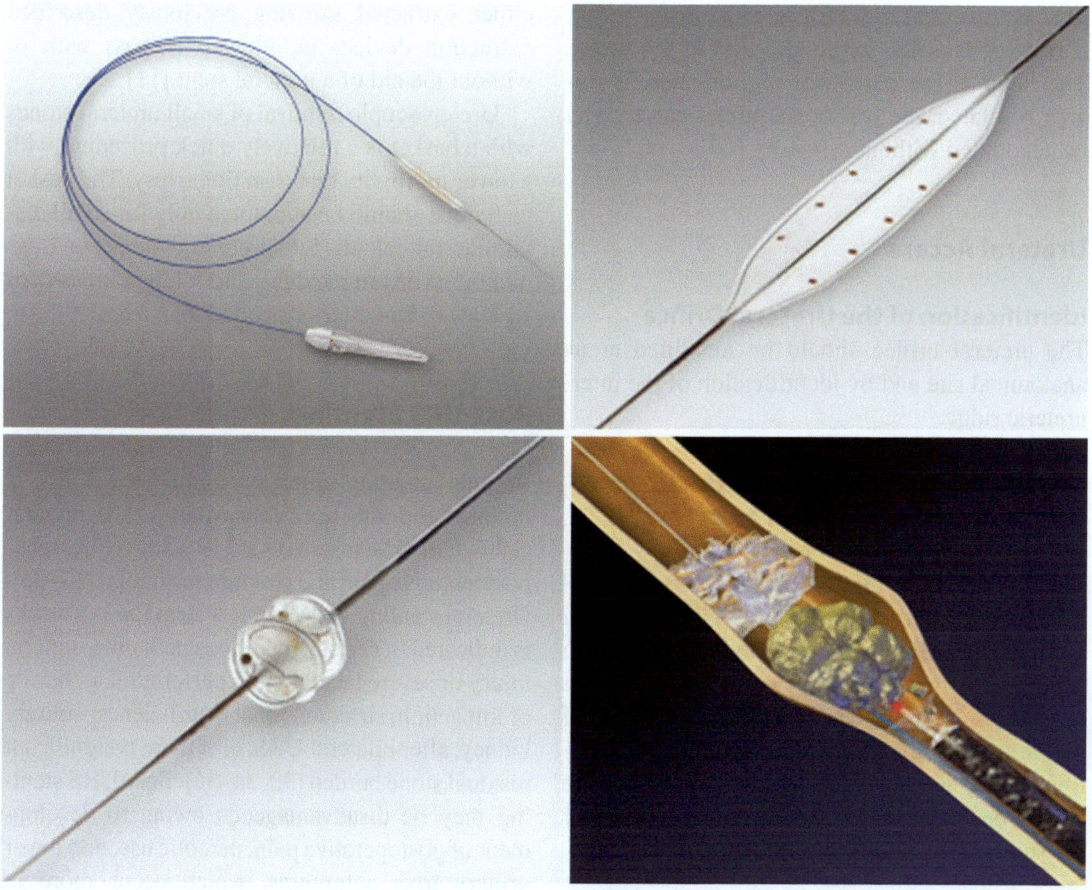

Fig. 22.7 Accordion occlusion device (PercSys Accordion®; Courtesy of Percutaneous System, Palo Alto, CA)

Technical Consideration of Retrograde URS

Patient Preparation

Imaging of both the stone and the upper urinary tract is essential before URS to determine the size, location, and associated anatomy. A noncontrast computed tomography (NCCT) is the most sensitive study for stones and is usually adequate for urolithiasis patients. A urinalysis is performed and if indicated a urine culture.

Urinary tract infections should be treated preoperatively, and obstructed infected pelvicalyceal system due to impacted ureteral calculi must be drained first. Preoperative antibiotic is given routinely. Anticoagulants should be stopped 7–10 days before the procedure with shift to low-molecular-weight heparin which must be stopped at the day of surgery and restarted at first postoperative day. Anticoagulants are restarted 3 days after stoppage of heparin if there is no risk of bleeding [27].

Patient Positioning and Anesthesia

Patient is placed in lithotomy position, under spinal anesthesia which has been demonstrated to be safe and feasible for URS. However, the general anesthesia is preferred for proximal ureteral stones especially with prolonged procedures [28].

Anatomic Consideration of the Ureter

The ureter usually displays three narrow sites at which calculi frequently become impacted. The most proximal is at the ureteropelvic junction, the second is at the crossing of the ureter over the iliac vessels, and the third or most distal site of narrowing is at the intramural part of the ureter. The latter is the narrowest region; thus, if this area is dilated, the rest of the ureter can usually be negotiated without difficulty [29].

Ureteral Access

Identification of the Ureteral Orifice

The ureteral orifice should be identified at its anatomical site and by identification of the inter-ureteric ridge.

Insertion of a Guidewire into the Ureteric Orifice Under Guidance of a Ureteral Catheter and Fluoroscopy

Then, it may be helpful to place a second guidewire to serve as a safety wire after URS insertion. During the procedure, care should be taken to avoid ureteral injury, such as submucosal passage or ureteral perforation, especially with kinked ureter or when the ureter is inflamed and edematous at the level of stone impaction. Also, care should be taken to avoid retrograde migration of the stone during guidewire insertion.

Visualization of the Stone Under Fluoroscopy

When the stone is not visualized, retrograde ureterography may be used [11].

Introduction of the Semirigid URS Along the Safety Wire

The guidewire can be used to open the orifice tent-like when the scope is passed laterally under the wire. After access to the ureter, the scope is passed slowly and carefully until the stone is reached. If primary intubation is not possible with reliable forces, stenting and later URS after 7–14 days offer a safe alternative to mechanical dilation.

Lithotripsy and Stone Extraction

In many cases, the treatment of ureteral calculi will require lithotripsy. Then, fragments can be either extracted utilizing previously described extraction devices or allowed to pass with or without the aid of a ureteral stent [11].

Ureteroscopic removal of small ureteral stones with a basket is a relatively quick procedure with a lower morbidity rate than lithotripsy. The basket technique should be attempted only for small distal ureteral calculi. Small ureteral stones or fragments can be removed fast and safely with forceps which can be better controlled than a basket [30].

Post-URS Stenting

Routine stenting after uncomplicated URS is optional and may not be necessary [2]. A ureteric catheter may be inserted for 2 or 3 days to decrease postoperative pain and stricture formation [31–33]. Ureteral stenting with double-J stent for 2–4 weeks is indicated in certain conditions including ureteral injury or severe laceration or perforation at the site of impaction, stricture, renal insufficiency, solitary kidney, after bilateral URS, or if there is significant residual stone burden [30, 34–36]. Post-URS stenting may be disadvantageous owing to development of postoperative pain, narcotic use, and lower urinary tract symptoms, which occur more in stented than in nonstented patients. Also, additional cost may be added by stenting following uncomplicated URS procedures [31, 34].

Basic Principles During URS

There are certain basic principles that should be considered during URS to make it more safe, easy, and decrease complication rate. These principles can be summarized as follows:

1. Always have a safety guidewire bypassing the ureteral calculus up to the kidney.
2. Never introduce and advance the URS with poor visualization.
3. Never manipulate the stone with poor visualization.
4. When unsure, or when encountering complications, consider stenting over the safety wire and consider scheduling a second session.

Difficulties During URS

Difficulties Reaching the Stone

Next, we cover some of the difficulties that may occur during the trial to reach the ureteral stone during URS.

Failure to Identify the Ureteral Orifice

Indigo carmine may be intravenously injected in case of failure to identify the ureteral orifice at its anatomical site.

Failure to Intubate the Ureteral Orifice

This difficulty can be managed by:

- Use of a second wire which is passed through the working channel
- Emptying the bladder to reduce compression on the intramural ureter
- Rotating the instrument which is not round but oval
- Resectioning of the median prostatic lobe if it causes difficulty for the URS to reach the ureteral orifice

Impacted Stone in the Ureteral Orifice

When the stone is impacted at the ureteral orifice and it is impossible for the guidewire to pass the stone, the easiest option to treat this situation is direct vision ureterotomy at 12 o'clock until the stone is dislodged from the ureter.

If the stone is impacted in the intramural tunnel, ureteroscopy can be carefully placed just inside the ureteral orifice where, under direct vision, a guidewire can be safely placed prior to manipulation of the stone.

If there are ureteral kinks that interfere with advancement of URS, straighten the ureter with a guidewire first or leave a stent for few days.

Difficulty Passing the Guidewire

If a guidewire does not pass beyond the ureteral calculus, special techniques may be necessary to gain access to the renal pelvis. The injection of a small amount of dilute contrast agent from below the calculus may identify the nature of the obstruction and a potential passage around it. The length of the floppy tip of a coaxial guidewire may be increased to provide greater flexibility at the level of the calculus; a J-tipped wire also may permit more ready passage. More commonly, however, the use of hydrophilic guidewires allows the easiest access to the ureter beyond an obstructing stone. Once in place, the hydrophilic wire may be replaced by a standard PTFE-coated wire through a ureteral exchange catheter to permit a straighter ureteral lumen during endoscopic surgery.

In rare instances, it will be impossible to place a wire retrogradely beyond an obstructing ureteral lesion. In such circumstances, the urologist has two options. A percutaneous nephrostomy tube may be placed, and attempts can be made to pass a guidewire down past the obstruction in an antegrade fashion, or, alternatively, ureteroscopy may be undertaken to the level of the lesion and the wire passed beside the calculus under endoscopic vision. This latter technique is associated with a higher rate of ureteral perforation and should never be undertaken unless facilities for percutaneous nephrostomy are available should mural perforation result [37].

Improving Poor Vision Inside the Ureter

To improve vision inside the ureter, we recommend the following:

- Use more irrigation by using manual or automatic devices (Ureteromat™, Karl Storz, Tuttlingen, Germany).
- Inject contrast media through the scope to visualize the ureteral anatomy.
- If the view is poor because of bleeding and cannot be improved by irrigation, stop the procedure and insert a DJ stent over the safety wire.

Minimizing the Risk of Proximal Migration

To minimize the risk of proximal migration, we recommend the following:

- Use of ureteral occlusion devices.
- Decreasing the irrigant force during stone fragmentation if possible.
- Use of Ho:YAG laser lithotripsy is the best choice in disintegration of proximal ureter stones. It has a lower rate of migration than pneumatic and electrohydraulic lithotriptors.
- The lithotriptor probe is better positioned at the anterior aspect of the calculus with some pressure to hold the stone against the posterior ureteral wall during the lithotripsy.
- If retrograde migration is observed during lithotripsy, the stone may be pulled distally in the ureter using URS graspers prior to continuing with lithotripsy.

Entrapped Stone Baskets

Inability to remove the stone basket can result from the manipulation of an excessively large stone, and this occurs mainly at the ureterovesical junction or at the site where the ureter crosses the iliac vessels. This may result in ureteral avulsion or stricture formation [38]. There are many techniques available to remove an entrapped basket containing a stone. First, the handle of the basket can be removed to get the scope out of the body, then URS can be inserted again beside the basket wire enabling endoscopic lithotripsy. Alternatively, insertion of a laser fiber through the second port of the URS allows intracorporeal lithotripsy and simultaneous irrigation, without requiring basket disassembly or removal and reinsertion of the URS [39].

Percutaneous Antegrade URS

Percutaneous antegrade URS is an acceptable first-line treatment in selected cases including patients with large impacted stones in the upper ureter (>15 mm in diameter), either as initial treatment or after failure of ESWL or retrograde ureteric access [40], and when there is combination with renal stones [2] or distal ureteral strictures [41].

Percutaneous antegrade URS may also be indicated in specific conditions such as after urinary diversion [42], after renal transplant [43], and in children with a malformation of the lower urinary tract [44].

Results of URS for Proximal Ureteral Calculi

The current analysis of literature revealed a stone-free rate of 81 % for URS treatment of proximal ureteral stones, with surprisingly little difference in stone-free rates according to stone size (93 % for stones <10 mm and 87 % for stones >10 mm) [2].

The median stone-free rates of URS for proximal ureteric calculi in different series are listed in Table 22.1.

Ureteroscopy Versus SWL

For proximal ureteric calculi, ureteroscopy provides a better success rate compared to SWL, particularly with stones >1 cm (Table 22.2). Retreatment rate, the need of auxiliary procedures, and the average coast were significantly higher with SWL.

Summary

Semirigid URS is a safe and highly effective treatment modality for proximal ureteral stones. URS is generally indicated when less invasive approaches fail to treat those stones and is specifically indicated in certain conditions. Many instruments can be used to make URS more easy and safe including guidewires, dilation devices, lithotripsy devices, stone extraction devices, and ureteral occlusion devices. There are certain basic principles that should be considered during URS which include the following: always have a safety guidewire bypassing the ureteral calculus up to the kidney, and never introduce and advance the URS or manipulate the stone with poor visualization and when unsure. Finally, when encountering difficulties or complications, consider stenting over the safety wire and rescheduling for a second session.

Table 22.1 The median stone-free rate of URS for proximal ureteral calculi

Series	Approach	No. of patients	Stone-free rate%	Complication rate%
Segura et al. [1]	Retrograde	831	86	17
Park et al. [45]	Retrograde	12	75	Not available
Strohamaier et al. [46]	Retrograde	49	94.9	2
Sofer et al. [47]	Retrograde	240	97	4
Lam et al. [6]	Retrograde	17	100 (<1 cm)	0
		14	93 (>1 cm)	0
El-Nahas et al. [42]	Antegrade (In patients with urinary diversion)	4	87.5	0
Preminger et al. [2]	Retrograde	473	80	12
	Antegrade		85	
Basiri et al. [48]	Retrograde	50	76	0
	Antegrade	50	86	0
Youssef et al. [16]	Retrograde	143	88.4 (overall)	14
			87 (<1 cm)	
			90(>1 cm)	

Table 22.2 Comparison between stone-free rates of URS and ESWL for proximal ureteral calculi

Series	Stone free rate	
	URS (%)	ESWL (%)
Grasso et al. [49]	97	62
Park et al. [45]	75	72
Strohamaier et al. [46]	94.4	70
Lam et al. [6]	100 (<1 cm)	80 (<1 cm)
	93 (>1 cm)	50 (>1 cm)
Preminger et al. [2]	81 (overall)	82 (overall)
	80 (<1 cm)	90 (<1 cm)
	79 (>1 cm)	68 (>1 cm)

Percutaneous antegrade URS is an acceptable first-line treatment in selected cases. The median stone-free rate for URS treatment of proximal ureteral stones is 81 and 86 % for retrograde and antegrade approaches, respectively.

References

1. Segura JW, Preminger GM, Glenn M, Assimos DG, Dretler SP, Khan RI, Lingeman JE, et al. Ureteral stones clinical guidelines panel summary report on the management of ureteral calculi. J Urol. 1997; 158:1951.
2. Preminger GM, Tiselius H, Assimos DG, Alken P, Buck C, Gallucci M, et al. Guidelines for the management of ureteral calculi. J Urol. 2007;178:2418.
3. Kijvikai K, Haleblian GE, Preminger GM, de la Rosette J. Shock wave lithotripsy or ureteroscopy for the management of proximal ureteral calculi: an old discussion revisited. J Urol. 2007;178:1157–63.
4. Andreoni C, Afane J, Olweny E, et al. Flexible ureteroscopic lithotripsy: first-line therapy for proximal ureteral and renal calculi in the morbidly obese and super obese patient. J Endourol. 2001;15:493–8.
5. Watterson J, Girvan A, Cook A, et al. Safety and efficacy of holmium:YAG laser lithotripsy in patients with bleeding diatheses. J Urol. 2002;168:442–5.
6. Lam J, Greene T, Gupta M. Treatment of proximal ureteral calculi: holmium:YAG laser lithotripsy versus extracorporeal shock wave lithotripsy. J Urol. 2002;167:1972–6.
7. El-Hefnawy AS, El-Nahas AR, El-Tabey NA, et al. Bilateral same-session ureteroscopy for treatment of ureteral calculi: critical analysis of risk factors. Scand J Urol Nephrol. 2011;45:97–101.
8. Lifshitz D, Lingeman J. Ureteroscopy as a first-line intervention for ureteral calculi in pregnancy. J Endourol. 2002;16:19–22.
9. Watterson J, Girvan A, Beiko D, et al. Ureteroscopy and holmium:YAG laser lithotripsy: an emerging definitive management strategy for symptomatic ureteral calculi in pregnancy. Urology. 2002;60:383–7.
10. Thomas J, DeMarco R, Donohoe J, et al. Pediatric ureteroscopic stone management. J Urol. 2005;174: 1072–4.
11. Rapp D, Gerber G. Ureteroscopy. In: Nakada S, Pearle M, editors. Advanced endourology: the complete

clinical guide. Totowa: Humana Press Inc; 2006. p. 87–104. Chapter 6.
12. Chow G, Patterson D, Blute M, et al. Ureteroscopy: effect of technology and technique on clinical practice. J Urol. 2003;170:99–102.
13. Bagley DH, Kuo RL, Zeltser IS. An update on ureteroscopic instrumentation for the treatment of urolithiasis. Curr Opin Urol. 2004;14:99–106.
14. Abdelrahim AF, Abdelmaguid A, Abuzeid H, et al. Rigid ureteroscopy for ureteral stones: factors associated with intraoperative adverse events. J Endourol. 2008;22:277–80.
15. Yaycioglu O, Guvel S, Kilinc F, et al. Results with 7.5F versus 10F rigid ureteroscopes in treatment of ureteral calculi. Urology. 2004;64:643–7.
16. Youssef R, El-Nahas A, El-Assmy A, et al. Shock wave lithotripsy versus semirigid ureteroscopy for proximal ureteral calculi (<20 mm): a comparative matched-pair study. J Urol. 2009;73:1184–7.
17. Leijte JA, Oddens JR, Lock TM. Holmium laser lithotripsy for ureteric calculi: predictive factors for complications and success. J Endourol. 2008;22:257.
18. Piergiovanni M, Desgrandchamps F, Cochand P, et al. Ureteral and bladder lesions after ballistic, ultrasonic, electrohydraulic, or laser lithotripsy. J Endourol. 1994;8:293–9.
19. Sun Y, Wang L, Liao G, et al. Pneumatic lithotripsy versus laser lithotripsy in the endoscopic treatment of ureteral calculi. J Endourol. 2001;15:587–90.
20. Kupeli B, Biri H, Isen K, et al. Treatment of ureteral stones: comparison of extracorporeal shock wave lithotripsy and endourologic alternatives. Eur Urol. 1998;34:474–9.
21. Chenven ES, Bagley DH. Retrieval and releasing capabilities of stone basket designs in vitro. J Endourol. 2005;19:204.
22. Lee H, Ryan T, Teichman J, et al. Stone retropulsion during holmium:YAG lithotripsy. J Urol. 2003;169:881–5.
23. Ahmed M, Pedro R, Kieley S, et al. Systematic evaluation of ureteral occlusion devices: insertion, deployment, stone migration, and extraction. Urology. 2009; 73:976–80.
24. Dretler S. The stone cone: a new generation of basketry. J Urol. 2001;165:1593–6.
25. Pauletter H, Sameer S, Perry K, et al. Assessment of novel ureteral occlusion device and comparison with stone cone in prevention of stone fragment migration during lithotripsy. J Endourol. 2005;19:200–3.
26. Beiko D, Denstedt J. Advances in ureterorenoscopy. Urol Clin North Am. 2007;34:397–408.
27. Knoll T, Michel M. Ureterorenoscopy. In: Hohenfellner R, Stolzenburg J, editors. Manual endourology. Heidelberg: Springer Medizin Verlag; 2005. p. 105–15. Chapter 12.
28. Cybulski P, Joo H, Honey R. Ureteroscopy: anesthetic considerations. Urol Clin North Am. 2004;11:31–43.
29. Kabalin JN. Anatomy of the retroperitoneum and kidney. In: Walsh PC, Retik AB, Stamey TA, Vaughan Jr E, editors. Campbell's urology. 6th ed. Philadelphia: WB Saunders; 1992. p. 3–39.
30. Harmon W, Sershon P, Blute M, et al. Ureteroscopy: current practice and long-term complications. J Urol. 1997;157:28–32.
31. Denstedt J, Wollin T, Sofer M, et al. A prospective randomized controlled trial comparing non-stented versus stented ureteroscopic lithotripsy. J Urol. 2001; 165:1419–22.
32. Byrne R, Auge B, Kourambas J, et al. Routine ureteral stenting is not necessary after ureteroscopy and ureteropyeloscopy: a randomized trial. J Endourol. 2002; 16:9–13.
33. Cheung M, Lee F, Leung Y, et al. A prospective randomized controlled trial on ureteral stenting after ureteroscopic holmium laser lithotripsy. J Urol. 2003; 169:1257–60.
34. Netto N, Ikonomidis J, Zillo C. Routine ureteral stenting after ureteroscopy for ureteral lithiasis: is it really necessary? J Urol. 2001;166:1252–4.
35. Chen Y, Chen J, Wong W, et al. Is ureteral stenting necessary after uncomplicated ureteroscopic lithotripsy? A prospective, randomized controlled trial. J Urol. 2002;167:1977–80.
36. Hollenbeck B, Schuster T, Seifman B, et al. Identifying patients who are suitable for stentless ureteroscopy following treatment of urolithiasis. J Urol. 2003; 170:103–6.
37. Bolton DM. Chapter 28: Techniques in rigid ureteroscopy. In: Smith AD, editor. Smith's textbook of endourology. St Louis: Quality Medical Publishing; 2006. p. 233–6.
38. O'Connor R, Gerber G. Management of entrapped ureteral stone baskets. Tech Urol. 2000;6:231–3.
39. Low R, George D. Removal of the entrapped basketed ureteral calculus: a novel technique. J Urol. 2000; 163:1863–6.
40. Maheshwari P, Oswal A, Andankar M, et al. Is antegrade ureteroscopy better than retrograde ureteroscopy for impacted large upper ureteral calculi? J Endourol. 1999;13:441–4.
41. Chen C, Wu C, Shee J, et al. Holmium:YAG lasertripsy with semirigid ureterorenoscope for upper-ureteral stones >2 cm. J Endourol. 2005;19:780–4.
42. El-Nahas A, Eraky I, El-Assmy A, et al. Percutaneous treatment of large upper tract stones after urinary diversion. Urology. 2006;68:500–4.
43. Rhee B, Bretan P, Stoller M. Urolithiasis in renal and combined pancreas/renal transplant recipients. J Urol. 1999;161:1458–62.
44. Raza A, Smith G, Moussa S, et al. Ureteroscopy in the management of pediatric urinary tract calculi. J Endourol. 2005;19:151–8.
45. Park H, Park M, Park T. Two-year experience with ureteral stones: extracorporeal shock wave lithotripsy vs. ureteroscopic manipulation. J Endourol. 1998; 12:501–4.
46. Strohmaier W, Schubert G, Rosenkranz T, et al. Comparison of extracorporeal shock wave lithotripsy and ureteroscopy in the treatment of ureteral calculi: a prospective study. Eur Urol. 1999;36: 376–9.

47. Sofer M, Watterson J, Wollin T, et al. Holmium:YAG laser lithotripsy for upper urinary tract calculi in 598 patients. J Urol. 2002;167:31–4.
48. Basiri A, Simforoosh N, Ziaee A, et al. Retrograde, antegrade, and laparoscopic approaches for the management of large, proximal ureteral stones: a randomized clinical trial. J Endourol. 2008;22:2677–80.
49. Grasso M, Beaghler M, Loisides P. The case for primary endoscopic management of upper urinary tract calculi: cost and outcome assessment of 112 primary ureteral calculi. Urology. 1995;45:372–6.

Ureteroscopy for Upper Ureteric and Renal Stones: Overcoming Difficulties with the Flexible Approach

23

Jacob Howard Cohen and Michael Grasso III

Introduction

Advances in flexible endoscope design, miniaturization of accessory equipment, and refinement in ureteroscopic technique have all combined to facilitate upper urinary tract access and treatment of proximal ureteral and renal stones. Smaller caliber endoscopes with improved optics are placed atraumatically throughout the calyceal system, allowing ureteroscopic lithotripsy of calculi of various compositions and sizes. Herein, we will present technical considerations for performing safe and effective flexible ureteroscopy for nephroureterolithiasis as well as reviewing the results and complications of these endoscopic interventions.

Indications

Flexible ureteroscopic lithotripsy is a common alternative to extracorporeal shock wave lithotripsy (ESWL) and percutaneous nephrostolithotomy (PCNL) for proximal ureteral and intrarenal calculi. Ureteroscopy can be employed for stones of all compositions and sizes, including metabolic-based partial staghorn calculi. Ureteroscopic technique may be especially helpful in the morbidly obese patient and in those in whom anticoagulation cannot be stopped. The only relative contraindication to ureteroscopic lithotripsy is in treating infectious, struvite calculi which are best addressed with PCNL.

Instrumentation

The ideal flexible ureteroscope has pristine optics, a small outer caliber, and a capacious working channel which facilitates simultaneous irrigation and placement of an array of accessory instruments and lithotrites. New-generation digital ureteroscopes contain a digital CMOS chip delivering 40,000 pixel image clarity as compared to 3,500 pixels with similar diameter, standard fiber-optic ureteroscopes. Endoscopes maintain two-way, logical tip deflection of 270° and one to one shaft torquability and have shaft diameters less than 8.5 French (Fr). Most contemporary, flexible ureteroscopes have a single 3.6-Fr working channel (Fig. 23.1a, b). When accessory equipment is placed through the working channel, a piston syringe is commonly employed to help facilitate irrigation through the partially occupied lumen.

Necessary accessory equipment to access the upper urinary tract includes ureteral catheters

J.H. Cohen, M.D., MPH (✉)
Department of Urology, Lenox Hill Hospital,
100 E 77th Street, New York, NY, 10075, USA
e-mail: jhcohen4@gmail.com

M. Grasso III, M.D.
Department of Urology, Lenox Hill Hospital,
100 E 77th Street, New York, NY, 10075, USA

Department of Urology, Medical College of New York,
New York, NY, 10075, USA
e-mail: mgrasso3@earthlink.net

A.M. Al-Kandari et al. (eds.), *Difficult Cases in Endourology*,
DOI 10.1007/978-1-84882-083-8_23, © Springer-Verlag London 2013

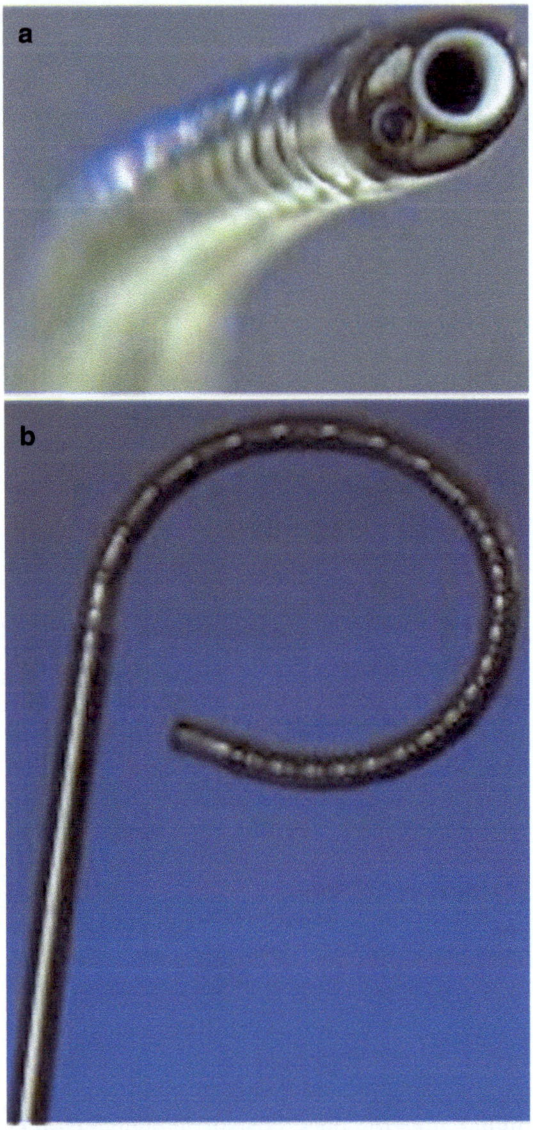

Fig. 23.1 (**a**) Cross-section view of a flexible ureteroscope showing the optical system and 3.6-Fr working channel. (**b**) 270° tip deflection is demonstrated

(typically 5- or 6-French open-ended catheters) for retrograde contrast imaging to define ureteral and calyceal anatomy and an array of access guide wires used to straighten a torturous ureter or to act as a guide facilitating endoscope placement. A variety of guide wires, typically ≤0.038 in. in diameter, may be employed for ureteral access. Angled-tip, lubricious, nitinol-based guide wires (e.g., Terumo Glidewire®, Boston Scientific, Natick, MA) are excellent for gaining access to the obstructed ureter and maintaining kink resistance. Teflon-sheathed nitinol guide wires (Zebra® Wire, Boston Scientific, Natick, MA) and the stainless steel with nitinol core guide wire (Sensor® Wire, Boston Scientific, Natick, MA) facilitate endoscope passage and stent placement.

Twelve- to fourteen-Fr ureteral access sheaths may be used at the surgeon's discretion, facilitating repeated ureteroscope access to the ureter and helping to avoid overdistension of the collecting system. Disadvantages of the ureteral access sheath include overdilation with placement, potentially increased rate of stricture formation from prolonged use, and potential oversight of distal ureteral pathology.

In general, the smallest diameter accessory equipment, such as 1.3- to 2.4-Fr nitinol baskets and 200- or 365-μ laser fibers, is desirable to maximize concurrent irrigation flow through the endoscope. Nitinol-based baskets are typically spherical, conforming to the ureteral lumen, facilitating retrieval of fragments post endoscopic lithotripsy. When stones are relocated or moved from one area of the intrarenal collecting system to facilitate more efficient lithotripsy (e.g., from the lower pole to upper pole to facilitate lithotripsy with a larger 365-μ laser fiber), then small-caliber nitinol extractors (1.9-Fr Graspit®, Boston Scientific, Natick, MA, or 1.7-Fr NGage™, Cook Urology, Spencer, IN) are employed, as they may easily be disengaged from the stone.

Finally, an array of ureteral stents of varied compositions, lengths, and diameters should be available. Smaller-diameter stents and stents without side holes throughout the length of the stent drain inefficiently and are more likely to obstruct with the debris created with laser lithotripsy. Larger-diameter stents not only drain better but also help facilitate greater passive dilation of the ureter over time. With regard to stent compositions, silicone-based stents cause less tissue reaction, but the soft durometer of this material

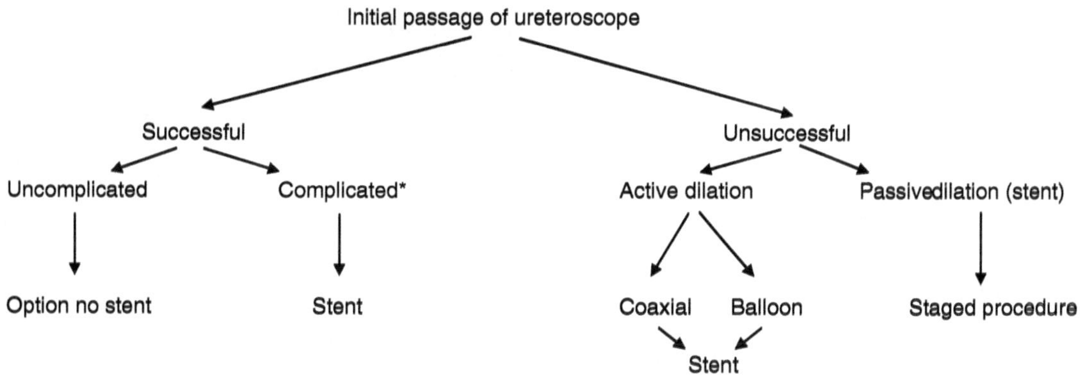

Fig. 23.2 Procedural algorithm

makes placement difficulty in the undilated ureter.

Technique

Ureteroscopic lithotripsy often begins with cystoscopic evaluation of the lower urinary tract and catheter intubation of the ureteral orifice with retrograde instillation of contrast material employed to define the upper urinary tract drainage system (i.e., retrograde ureteropyelography). There are varied techniques employed to obtain endoscopic access to the ureter: endoscope placement under direct vision with or without intramural dilation, endoscope placement over a working guide wire, or placement thru an operating ureteral sheath.

The small-diameter flexible ureteroscopes are commonly placed atraumatically under direct vision into the intramural tunnel without active ureteral dilation (i.e., dilation with a balloon or graduated dilator). This direct placement into the ureter may often be performed without the aid of a "working" guide wire. Termed "no touch" flexible ureteroscopy, this technique minimizes mucosal irritation and trauma and inadvertent stone migration by guide wire passage [1]. If necessary, a guide wire can be placed through the ureteroscope under direct vision to define a narrowed or edematous segment, straighten a kinked portion of the ureter, or increase endoscope tip rigidity during passage. A common pitfall is forgetting to empty the bladder completely prior to passage of the flexible ureteroscope. A full bladder compresses the intramural portion of the ureter, making passage of the flexible ureteroscope more difficult.

If the intramural and distal ureter is narrow (common in young muscular males), active dilation over a guide wire is often required for endoscope access. Active dilation is commonly performed with a small-caliber (5-Fr delivery sheath, 12-Fr outer diameter) balloon dilator. Balloon dilation tends to be less traumatic with only circumferential dilating force, as compared to gradual dilators, which add shearing forces. After dilating, the flexible ureteroscope is often passed over a stiff shaft guide wire into the ureter.

If the flexible ureteroscope fails to traverse the intramural segment after active dilation, a semi-rigid endoscope can be placed to inspect the distal ureter and dilate any narrowing under direct vision. Placement of a ureteral stent and proceeding with flexible ureteroscopy after a period of passive ureteral dilation are frequently employed strategies when endoscope access is challenging (Fig. 23.2).

At the conclusion of ureteroscopic lithotripsy, ureteral stents are commonly placed when passive ureteral dilation is required to help facilitate clearance of stone debris, when significant ureteral edema is encountered from an impacted stone, or to straighten a tortuous segment. Patients are counseled that lower urinary tract voiding symptoms, such as frequency and urgency, are common while the stent is in place and may be managed with anticholinergic agents and/or low-dose benzodiazepines as necessary.

Challenging Cases

Lower Pole Calculi

Lower-pole intrarenal access can be a challenging maneuver with a flexible ureteroscope. Depending on calyceal anatomy, secondary endoscope deflection is often required. Secondary deflection is based on an inherent weakness in the durometer at a predetermined segment of the endoscope which facilitates buckling of the shaft. Advancing the endoscope with the tip maximally deflected (by complete depression of the hand lever), the distal shaft will buckle and thus exaggerate deflection beyond 180° (Fig. 23.3). This is particularly useful when placing an endoscopic accessory into a lower-pole calyx. A thorough inspection of the intrarenal collecting system is essential when a stone-free status is the goal of endoscopic lithotripsy. Stone fragments will often migrate to the lower pole during ureteroscopic lithotripsy of proximal ureteral and renal pelvic stones, for example. Positioning the patient in Trendelenburg (i.e., head down), with the ipsilateral side up, reduces migration of stone fragments into a dependant lower pole, directing them to a more easily accessible cephalad location. Additionally, instillation of contrast material through the ureteroscope will help ensure adequate mapping of the collecting system.

For lower-pole stones, the decision to fragment in situ or move the stone to a more easily accessible location depends on the stone volume, dimensions of the collecting system, and degree of hydronephrosis encountered. Dependent lower-pole stone fragments may not clear over time if the collecting system is markedly dilated and if the infundibulum is particularly elongated. In addition, laser fibers are relatively stiff, inhibiting maximal endoscope deflection and thus efficient in situ lithotripsy. Small-diameter nitinol-based extractors, like the Graspit® or NGage™, do not effect endoscope deflection significantly and can be employed to move lower-pole stones to the upper pole where they may be fragmented more easily with larger-caliber laser fibers. It is important to note that the ability to maintain lower-pole access during endoscopic lithotripsy decreases over time. As the collecting system distends with irrigant, collecting system dimensions change negatively and may ultimately prohibit access. One strategy in the setting of a sizeable lower-pole stone which is too large to engage and move with a basket is to promptly divide the calculus with the laser into sizeable moveable pieces rather than employing a dusting technique. The stone segments are then relocated cephalad and lithotripsy completed, now pulverizing the fragments into fine dust and tiny easily passable debris.

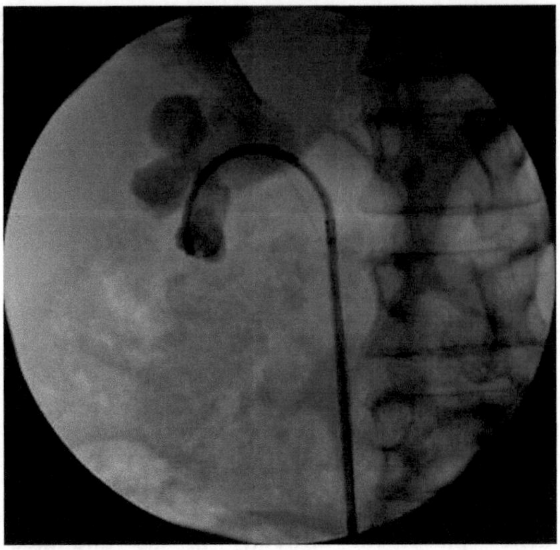

Fig. 23.3 Secondary active deflection is required to achieve access to this right, lower-pole calyx

Obstructing, Proximal Ureteral Calculi

Obstructing, proximal ureteral stones are often impacted and can be associated with significant mucosal edema, engulfing the calculus and limiting endoscopic visualization (Fig. 23.4a–f). In such cases, it may be difficult to fluoroscopically direct a guide wire proximal to the obstructing stone. It is important to remember that disimpacting the calculus with laser energy or irrigant is encouraged,

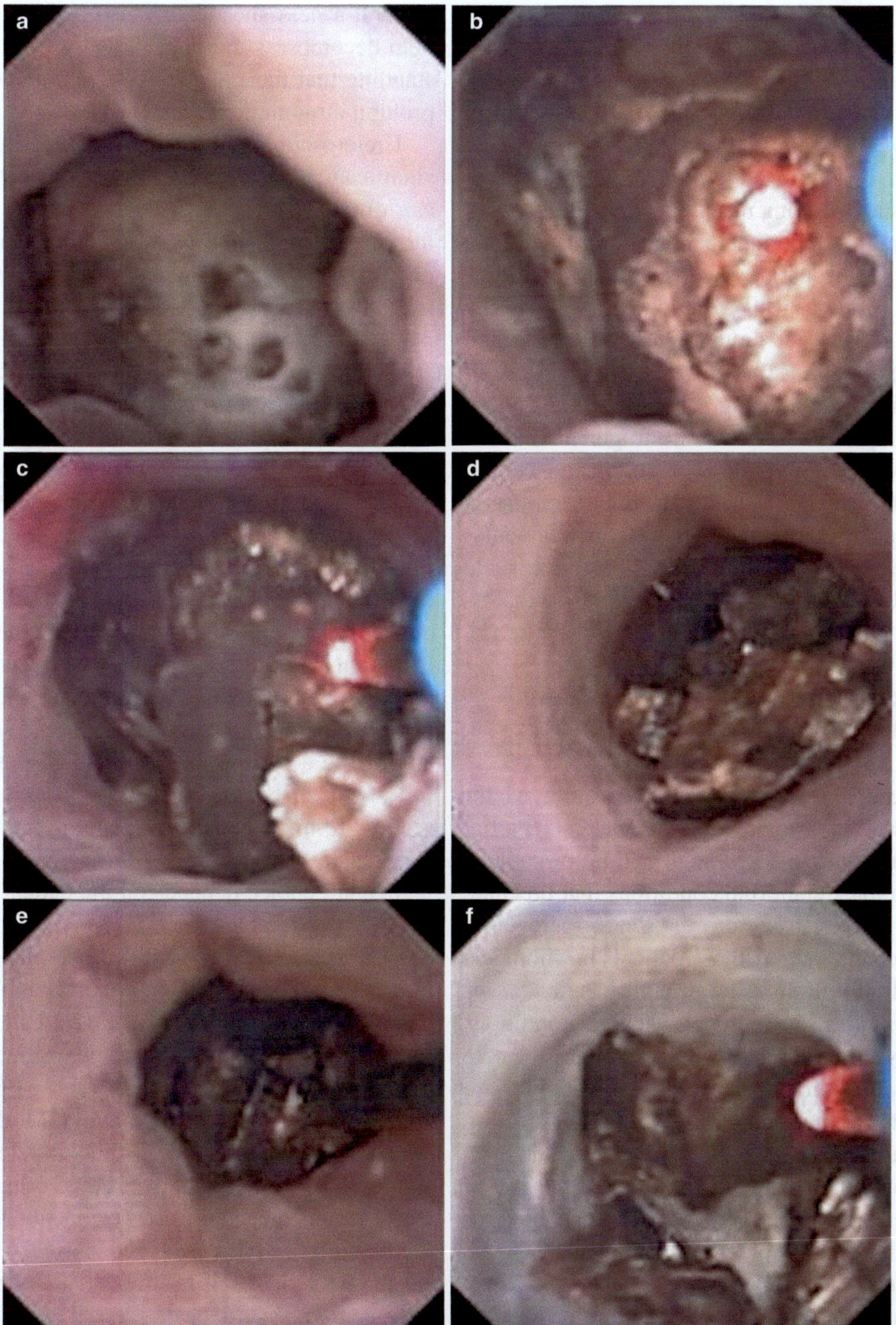

Fig. 23.4 (**a**) A 1.8-cm, impacted proximal ureteral stone with a characteristic appearance of calcium oxalate monohydrate. There is significant ureteral edema. (**b**) Fragmentation begins in the center of the stone. (**c**) Small fragments are pinned, using the main, more proximal stone as a backstop to reduce movement. (**d**) Multiple stone fragments remain in the ureter after disimpacting the stone. (**e**) It is important to basket the most distal fragments first, to avoid engaging multiple fragments which may be too large to pass down the ureter. (**f**) With the patient in Trendelenburg and the ipsilateral side raised, residual fragments wash into an upper-pole calyx, where, using the renal papilla as a backstop, more precise fragmentation may be achieved

with efficient stone therapy now in an intrarenal location. During in situ lithotripsy of an impacted proximal ureteral stone, it is important to maintain the laser fiber tip centrally on the calculus to minimize ureteral wall trauma. Laser energy can, however, be employed to remove central edematous tissue overlying a calculus to facilitate visualization. It is important to move the created stone fragments and debris away from the site of impaction and ureteral wall irritation to minimize the risk of subsequent granulomatous reaction and stricture disease. Relocating the fragments proximally is preferred, using irrigation and the endoscope's tip to direct the stone fragments into an upper-pole calyx where laser lithotripsy can be completed efficiently. Using the renal papilla as a backstop, for example, efficient laser fragmentation creates extractable or more easily passable residual fragments.

Staged Ureteroscopy for Large Pelvic and Partial Staghorn Calculi

Flexible ureteroscopic lithotripsy employed for large (>2 cm), noninfectious renal and partial staghorn stones is a treatment option for patients with complex comorbid conditions that preclude PCNL, those refusing or failing prior percutaneous procedures and in those patients in whom it is desirable to limit renal trauma. Patients, for example, with severe hypermetabolic conditions (e.g., cystinuria, primary hyperoxaluria) where repetitive percutaneous nephrostolithotomies are associated with progressive loss of renal function are ideal candidates for complex retrograde ureteroscopic lithotripsy [2].

When treating a large stone burden ureteroscopically, endoscopic visualization decreases as stone dust created by holmium laser lithotripsy coats the intrarenal urothelium. To improve visibility, it is important to decompress the lower urinary tract, most commonly by simultaneously placing a small-diameter Foley catheter beside the ureteroscope into the bladder. The optical field is cleared with sterile saline irrigant, which will commonly pass around a small-caliber flexible ureteroscope into the bladder. In addition, ureteral access sheaths can also be employed to help decompress the upper urinary tract, understanding that their relatively large diameter may prohibit atraumatic placement.

Ureteroscopic lithotripsy can produce significant quantities of dust and stone debris that can obscure sizeable residual fragments. When the endoscopic field of view is obscured and cannot be cleared with bladder drainage or intrarenal irrigation through the endoscope, it is time to place a stent and plan for a second stage. For stone burdens in excess of 2.5 cm, second-stage ureteroscopic lithotripsy is performed routinely to ensure complete fragmentation. Employing interim intrarenal irrigation between staged endoscopic lithotripsy is an effective strategy to decrease stone dust. Specific metabolic compositions like cystine and uric acid lend themselves to this strategy, but calcium oxalate dust can also be cleared with sterile saline irrigant. The retrograde irrigation is performed with a two catheter system: inflow thru a 5-Fr Cobra catheter with its tip positioned into the lower pole and outflow employing a 6- or 8-Fr single pigtail positioned in an upper-pole/renal pelvis location, both secured to a Foley catheter draining the bladder (Fig. 23.5a–c).

Irrigant choice depends on the patient's stone composition (Table 23.1). In patients with uric acid stones, irrigation with either alkalinizing bicarbonate solution or trometamol tris-hydroxymethyl aminomethane (THAM), serves to both clear and dissolve uric acid residue. When cystine is treated, pH 10 THAM-E with *N*-acetylcysteine (Mucomyst) will clear dust and debris by creating the more soluble cysteine [3]. Inflow rate typically starts at 50 cc/h, increased slowly to tolerance up to 100 cc/h. Clinical signs including fever, flank pain, and nausea with emesis all may reflect rising intrarenal pressure and if encountered should be addressed with manual catheter irrigation and potential termination of the irrigation.

When the second-stage ureteroscopic lithotripsy is performed, endoscopic visualization is commonly improved, and residual fragments are readily identified. Additionally, the ureter has been passively dilated over time, with many

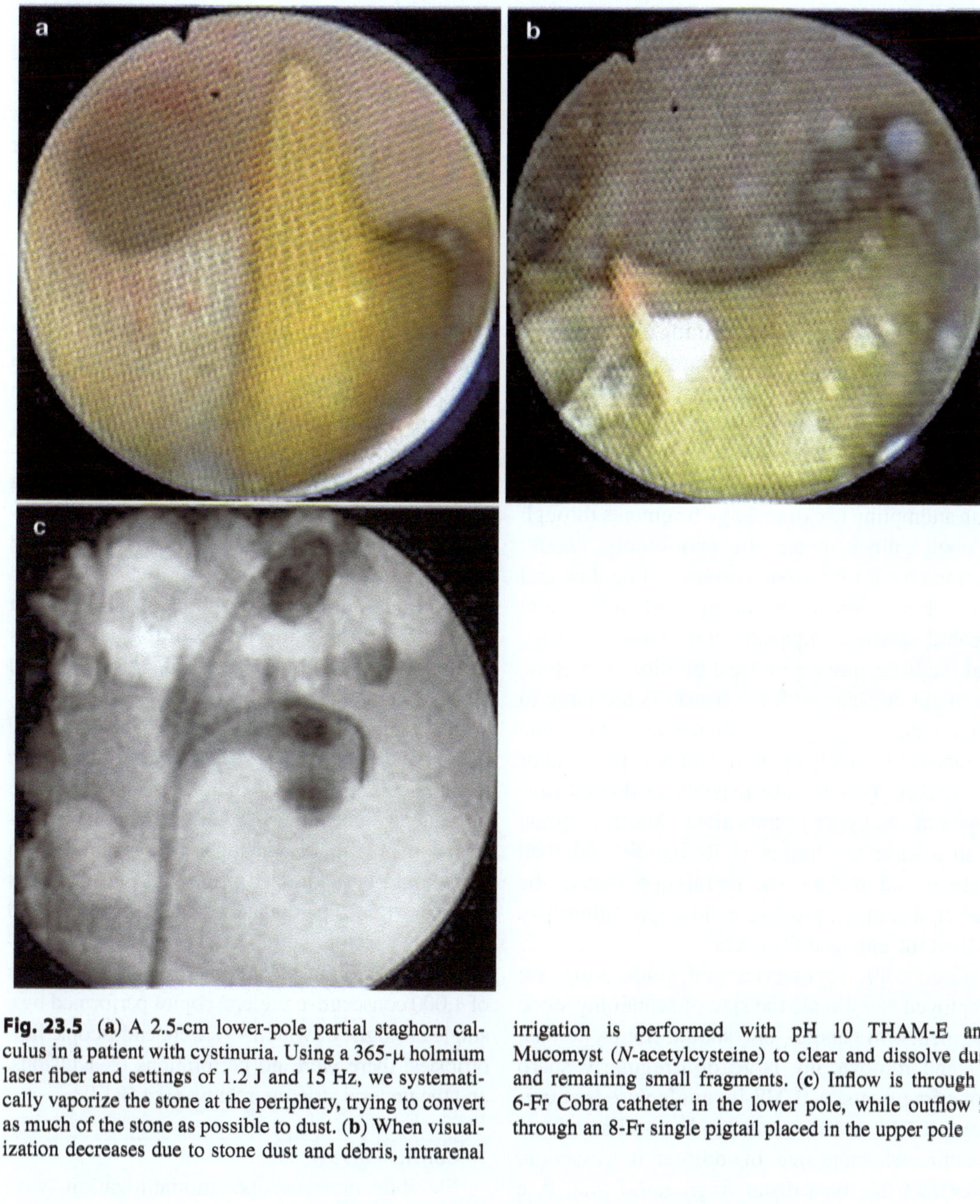

Fig. 23.5 (**a**) A 2.5-cm lower-pole partial staghorn calculus in a patient with cystinuria. Using a 365-μ holmium laser fiber and settings of 1.2 J and 15 Hz, we systematically vaporize the stone at the periphery, trying to convert as much of the stone as possible to dust. (**b**) When visualization decreases due to stone dust and debris, intrarenal irrigation is performed with pH 10 THAM-E and Mucomyst (*N*-acetylcysteine) to clear and dissolve dust and remaining small fragments. (**c**) Inflow is through a 6-Fr Cobra catheter in the lower pole, while outflow is through an 8-Fr single pigtail placed in the upper pole

Table 23.1 Irrigant choice for intrarenal irrigation

Stone type	Irrigant choice	Effect
Cystine	THAM-E and Mucomyst[a]	Clear dust and debris
Uric acid	THAM	Dissolve fragments, clear dust and debris
Calcium-based	Saline and antibiotic[b]	Clear dust and debris

[a]THAM-E is pH 10 trometamol tris-hydroxymethyl aminomethane, with 0.4 M Mucomyst (*N*-acetylcysteine)
[b]Antibiotic is usually 80 mg of gentamicin per liter of normal saline

patients being left stent-free at the conclusion of their second stage. Several series have demonstrated that staged ureteroscopy, with or without intrarenal irrigation, is safe and effective for large (>2 cm) proximal ureteral and renal stones, with stone-free rates of approximately 90 % [4–6].

Stone Basketing with Caution

A common pitfall when performing ureteroscopic lithotripsy is attempting to extract stones or fragments with a basket extractor that are too large to pass down the ureter, with subsequent difficulty disengaging the stone from the basket. Surgeon experience is crucial to avoid this pitfall. Rather than attempting to extract large fragments through a small-caliber ureter, the endoscopist should plan to convert the stone burden to fine dust and small debris with laser energy, with subsequent ureteral stenting employed to maintain drainage and facilitate passive ureteral dilation. If a stone fragment engaged within a basket is too large to extract, disengagement can be performed in some instances by widely opening and past pointing of the basket. This is only feasible in dilated segments of the upper urinary tract. Another option is to release the basket at its handle and then remove and replace the endoscope beside the basket sheath, employing endoscopic lithotripsy to treat the engaged fragment.

Endoscopic accessories and guide wires are employed to estimate the size of remaining stone fragments. In general, one should not try to basket and remove any large or irregularly sharp stone fragments. A 0.038-in. guide wire is equivalent to 3 Fr or 1 mm and can be used as a scale to define fragment size. In addition, it is essential to extract the most distal fragment(s) first, in a sequential stepwise fashion. When treating a ureteral steinstrasse, for example, it is important to extract the most distal fragments first and not engage in a basket a stone fragment in the distance, thus potentially trapping the basket behind distal stone debris.

Disengaging a stone fragment from a basket is most easily facilitated in the intrarenal collecting system. Using a papilla as a backstop, for example, one can try to brush the stone out of the open basket by past pointing and inverting. Nitinol-based baskets are uniquely designed to help facilitate this maneuver. In addition, nitinol graspers can more easily disengage a fragment and are preferred.

Complications

Improvements in instrumentation and refinement in technique have decreased complications from flexible ureteroscopy. Reported complication rates are low, ranging from 1 to 5 %, with major complications (e.g., large perforations with subsequent strictures) at well less than 1 %. Infectious events, such as pyelonephritis, are the most commonly reported complication and are minimized by ensuring a sterile preoperative urine and appropriate antibiotic prophylaxis. Significant gross hematuria with clots is infrequent and is treated with vigorous hydration, Lasix-induced diuresis, and catheter drainage if necessary.

If small-diameter endoscopes and auxiliary instruments are employed and careful atraumatic technique is employed, major complications are infrequently encountered. Large ureteral perforation, with or without avulsion, is a rare complication and should be addressed promptly with proximal drainage (e.g., percutaneous nephrostomy) and subsequent definitive repair with either ileal interposition or autotransplantation. In a published series of 1,000 consecutive ureteroscopies performed by a single urologist of which 491 were endoscopic lithotripsies, there were no perforations or avulsions, and the ureteral stricture rate was 0.4 % [7].

Conclusions

Flexible ureteroscope miniaturization with improved fiber-optic and digital imaging, combined with small, powerful, and precise energy sources, advanced accessories, and refined surgical technique have combined to facilitate safe and effective lithotripsy of proximal ureteral and renal calculi of all sizes and common compositions. Urologists commonly employ retrograde ureteroscopic lithotripsy of proximal upper urinary tract calculi, with large and complex stone burdens addressed with staged therapies, achieving stone-free rates superior to ESWL with minimal morbidity.

References

1. Johnson GB, Portela D, Grasso M. Advanced ureteroscopy: wireless and sheathless. J Endourol. 2006;20(8):552–5.
2. Rudnick DM, Bennett PM, Dretler SP. Retrograde renoscopic fragmentation of moderate-size (1.5–3.0 cm) renal cystine stones. J Endourol. 1999;13(7):483–5.
3. Dretler SP, Pfister RC. Percutaneous dissolution of renal calculi. Annu Rev Med. 1983;34:359–66.
4. Grasso M, Conlin M, Bagley D. Retrograde ureteropyeloscopic treatment of 2 cm or greater upper urinary tract and minor staghorn calculi. J Urol. 1998;160:346–51.
5. Ricchiuti DJ, Smaldone MC, Jacobs BL, Smaldone AM, Jackman SV, Averch TD. Staged retrograde endoscopic lithotripsy as alternative to PCNL in select patients with large renal calculi. J Endourol. 2007;21(12):1421–4.
6. Riley JM, Stearman L, Troxel S. Retrograde ureteroscopy for renal stones larger than 2.5 cm. J Endourol. 2009;23(9):1395–8.
7. Grasso M. Ureteropyeloscopic treatment of ureteral and intrarenal calculi. Urol Clin North Am. 2000;27(4):623–31.

Ureteroscopy for Ureteral Strictures

24

Ahmed M. Harraz, Ahmed M. Shoma, and Ahmed A. Shokeir

Introduction

Ureteral strictures may occur due to intrinsic or extrinsic causes. Intrinsic stricture is usually caused by benign pathologies such as iatrogenic trauma, schistosomiasis [1–3], tuberculosis [4–6], and ureteral endometriosis [7–9]. On the other hand, extrinsic strictures are usually of malignant nature, the ureter is encased by primary or metastatic, or retroperitoneal tumors, and the situation can be aggravated by periureteral fibrosis, a long-term adverse event of previous chemotherapy or radiotherapy [10–12].

Iatrogenic ureteral injury is the most common cause of benign ureteral strictures. Gynecological procedures account for most of the injuries especially after introduction of laparoscopic surgery with hysterectomy accounting for more than half of the cases [13, 14]. Urologic procedures, notably ureteroscopy, were described mainly because of ureteral trauma from instrumentation, calculus impaction, and the use of larger semirigid ureteroscopes [15, 16]. General surgical procedures including vascular surgery then follow [17, 18]. It has been reported also following a variety of surgical procedures including sympathetic nerve bloc and thoracolumbar lateral revision instrumentation and fusion [19, 20]. Penetrating rather than blunt trauma is the most common and may be caused by gunshots or explosive devices shells [21, 22].

Ureteral strictures are commonly associated with ureteral stones and are related to either stone impaction [23] or stone lithotripsy [24]. Impacted stones are associated with edema, inflammation, and fibrosis of the ureteral wall. Furthermore, impacted stones represent an obstacle for good navigation and predispose to subsequent stricture formation. Coupling of impacted stone and stricture add more surgical challenge during management.

Resolutions of obstruction with preservation of renal function are the main management objectives. A wide array of therapeutic modalities ranging from endoscopic, laparoscopic, and open approaches exists within urologist hands. Increasing application and experience of minimally invasive techniques render benign ureteral stricture and or associated ureteral stones amenable for endoscopic treatment [25]. Benign ureteral strictures have been treated with balloon dilation or endoureterotomy. Various endoureterotomy methods have been described and include cold knife incision, electrocautery incision, and Acucise® cutting balloon device (Applied Medical, Rancho Santa Margarita, CA) [26]. Nevertheless, laser endoureterotomy has gained worldwide acceptance currently and has become the preferred option for benign ureteral stricture treatment. In this chapter, we will discuss basic technique and outcome of balloon dilation and

A.M. Harraz, M.D. (✉) • A.M. Shoma, M.D.
A.A. Shokeir, M.D., Ph.D., FEBU
Department of Urology, Urology and Nephrology Center, Mansoura University, El Gomhoria Street, Mansoura 35516, Egypt
e-mail: ahmed.harraz@hotmail.com; ahmedshoma@hotmail.com; ahmed.shokeir@hotmail.com

A.M. Al-Kandari et al. (eds.), *Difficult Cases in Endourology*,
DOI 10.1007/978-1-84882-083-8_24, © Springer-Verlag London 2013

laser endoureterotomy for managing benign ureteral strictures and stones. In addition, we will focus on challenging and troublesome situations and reported methods for optimum treatment.

Indications and Precautions of Endoureterotomy

Endoureterotomy is indicated in cases of short-segment benign ureteral strictures (less than 1 cm). Relative contraindications for endoureterotomy include extensive long ureteral defect, the presence of hydroureter with severe infection, abnormal coagulation, presence of vascular grafts in the retroperitoneum, and finally abnormally positioned ureters [27].

Management Strategy of Benign Ureteral Strictures

Balloon dilation has been advocated as primary therapy for short nonischemic ureteral strictures in patients who have few risk factors for devascularization (previous simple ureteroscopy, retroperitoneal fibrosis, idiopathic causes). In patients with longer strictures, fibrotic bands, or ischemic ureters, different techniques of endoureterotomy are viable options. For patients with more complex and blind-ended ureter, variable techniques have been described to overcome these situations. It is essential to keep in mind the possibility of open, laparoscopic surgeries for management of severe cases not suitable for endoureterotomy [25].

Balloon Dilation

Balloon dilation is one of the least invasive and cost-effective modalities for management of benign ureteral strictures. It has been advocated for dilating very short nonischemic ureteral strictures not associated with devascularizing lesions, e.g., retroperitoneal fibrosis [28]. It can be also used for dilating ureteral orifice before introduction of ureteroscope [16, 25] and for dilation of the ureter after laser incision of the stricture [25].

Instruments

Four- to ten-cm-long balloons are usually used to dilate short benign ureteral strictures. The balloon should be rated to withstand pressure up to 20 Atm. A pressure gauge is placed between the syringe and the balloon; the pressure limit of the balloon should not be exceeded, or else the balloon may rupture within the ureter. The balloon has a proximal and distal marks allowing appropriate positioning under fluoroscopic guidance.

Technique

Under fluoroscopic guidance, the dilating balloon catheter is passed over the guidewire into the ureter. After appropriate positioning at stricture site, the balloon is gradually inflated under fluoroscopic monitoring with a 50:50 mixture of contrast medium and saline solution until the waist in the balloon at stricture site disappears. Hence, the inflated balloon is maintained in position for 4–10 min before it is deflated; the balloon is then reinflated. If the stricture has truly been torn, the balloon should now fill out at a low pressure. In contrast, if the balloon fails to fill out at low pressure, then the stricture has not been treated adequately and an endoincision will be necessary.

Outcome

Promising results have been demonstrated when using balloon dilation for short ureteral strictures with intact blood supply. It showed success rate up to 89.2 % [29]. Byun and associates have demonstrated better outcome in strictures less than 2 cm in length [30]. Overall, balloon dilation of benign ureteral strictures has a lower reported success rates than endoureterotomy, often necessitating multiple procedures to achieve the desired outcome.

Laser Endoureterotomy

The Holmium:YAG (Neodymium:Yttrium-aluminum-garnet) laser provides the finest, most precise incision that provokes minimal peripheral damage with depth of penetration less than 0.5 mm [31]. In addition, it is available as short as 200-μm fiber that can fit into 6.9 F flexible ureteroscopy and can be used for concomitant stone lithotripsy. All of these characteristics make it the preferred option for endoureterotomy [23].

Instruments

The energy is delivered through a low water content flexible quartz fiber. The fibers are available in size of (200, 365, 500, and 1,000 μm) and are reusable. The pulse rate and energy can be varied from 5 to 30 Hz and 0.2–2.0 J, respectively. The peripheral zone of thermal injury is 0.5–1 mm and a helium-neon aiming beam is used for targeting the laser. The preferred settings for laser endoureterotomy are energy of 0.8–1.2 J and frequency of 5–10 Hz to provide a power output of 10 W.

Technique

Gaining access to ureteral stricture is done by a retrograde, antegrade, or combined approaches. An antegrade approach allows for better estimation of stricture length by simultaneous antegrade and retrograde contrast fluoroscopy. In addition, it provides long-term drainage of incision site. It may also used to traverse strictures failed to pass by a retrograde one.

Under spinal or general anesthesia, a 0.035-in. floppy tip safety guidewire is passed across the stenotic segment cystoscopically with the patient in the lithotomy position or percutaneously through a nephroscope with the patient prone. Cystoscopically, the guidewire is used to cannulate the ureteral orifice with the help of an open tip ureteral catheter placed at the ureteral orifice. A semirigid ureteroscope is then advanced through the ureteral orifice and is used to passively dilate the lower end of the ureter and the ureteral orifice and to examine grossly for any associated lesions. If it is difficult to negotiate the ureteral orifice, a second superstiff wire is introduced through the working channel of the ureteroscope and is introduced into the ureteral orifice; then the ureteroscope is rotated to lie in between the two guidewires and then advanced over this "railroad." If there is still difficulty, a balloon can be used to dilate the ureteral orifice. Then the stricture site and length are estimated by combined antegrade or retrograde ureteropyelography.

A red helium-neon targeting beam is used to precisely guide laser application with a reusable 365-μm quartz fiber placed in direct contact. The ureteroscope is advanced through the stricture site guided by a second safety guidewire. If failed to pass, a balloon dilatation may be used to widen the stricture. Then the ureteroscope is further advanced, and cutting is begun proximally and is proceeded down as the ureteroscope is gradually retracted [20, 32]. The Holmium:YAG laser has the advantage of simultaneous cutting and hemostasis; in addition, the availability of fiberoptic delivery system and the accuracy of incision make it the preferred modality for endoureterotomy [33].

A full-thickness incision is performed until paraureteral fat appears. The incision is extended approximately 5 mm to 1 cm above and below the stricture. The location of incision is largely dependent on ureteral portion affected. A thorough knowledge of ureteral anatomy is crucial to avoid any vascular injury during incision. The endoureterotomy is usually done laterally in the lumbar ureter to avoid cutting a possible crossing vessel, whereas over the iliac vessels, it is done anteriorly (toward the abdominal viscera) to avoid iliac vessels injury. Below the iliac vessels, the incision is made directly medial to avoid the branches of the internal iliac artery and vein traveling along the lateral surface of the ureter. For ureteral orifice meatal stenosis and distal stricture, the incision is done at 12 o'clock position.

After making the incision, the adequacy of the incision can be judged by injecting diluted contrast to demonstrate the extravasation or using balloon dilation to confirm disappearance of "balloon wasting" and therefore confirm a complete incision of the stricture. After verification of procedure adequacy, a ureteral stent (either 6 F, or 7 F, or 8 F, or 7/10, or a 8/12 F) is placed fluoroscopically over the guidewire then maintained for 4–6 weeks to allow regeneration of urothelial and muscle layers with an adequate caliber lumen. After placement of the ureteral stent and according to the route employed for access, a Foley catheter and/or a nephrostomy tube is left in place for 24–48 h to minimize ureteral reflux and leak into the retroperitoneum. Figures 24.1, 24.2, and 24.3 represent radiographic findings during laser endoureterotomy for a stricture at right lumbar ureter.

Outcome

Endoureterotomy is relative simple procedure with low complication rate particularly with use of laser. Nevertheless, the success rate varies greatly in literature because of different inclusion criteria (Table 24.1). Most of literature depicted 75 % success rate or less.

Other Modalities for Endoureterotomy

Cold Knife

Cold knife endoureterotomy could be performed with one a cold knife urethrotome. Knife blades are available in variety of configurations, including straight, half-moon, and hook shape. It has a lumen that allows it to move back and forth over a guidewire to ensure that the cold knife at all times remains within the ureteral lumen. Because of the size of endoscopic instrument needed to perform the incision, cold knife incision is generally limited to the distal ureter via a retrograde approach. If the stricture is in the proximal ureter, the incision can be performed through a nephroscope with an antegrade approach [38].

Once the stricture segment is encountered; the best maneuver is to withdraw the scope partially, which will give a wide view of the strictured area. From this position, the cold knife is advanced and one can direct the cold knife into the narrow lumen of the strictured area. The tip of the cutting knife should be seen as soon as it leaves the ureteroscope sheath. Then, it should be directed into the lumen of the stricture along or over the guidewire. After one or two arc-like strokes along the stricture, the ureter slowly widens. This procedure should be continued until the lumen will allow the scope to advance beyond the stricture [36].

Electrosurgical Incision

Electrocautery incision can be performed using 2–3 F electrodes, which are available in straight, pencil point, hook, angled, and loop designs. The electrode is usually set at 50 W of pure cutting current [36]. The only advantage of electroincision over the cold knife is that the reduced caliber probes can be placed through smaller semirigid and flexible endoscopes and therefore permit the incision to be made anywhere along the course of the ureter [38].

Acucise Endoureterotomy

The Acucise cutting balloon was developed by Chandhoke and associates in the early 1990s. They reported on the first clinical use of this device in 21 patients with ureteropelvic junction obstruction [39]. The Acucise cutting balloon catheter is a 5–7 F device incorporating a monopolar electrocautery cutting wire and a low-pressure balloon. It is used for incising obstructions in the proximal and distal ureter and at the ureteropelvic junction. The balloon not only defines the area of stenosis but also carries the cutting wire into the strictured area.

The cutting balloon catheter is positioned in the appropriate orientation considering the blood supply and the ureteral parastructures using two-plane fluoroscopy since it will allow rotational views of the position of the cutting balloon catheter within the ureter. If one is unsure whether the balloon straddles the stricture, the balloon can be gently inflated using 1 cc dilute contrast medium, with demonstration of a waist with inflation of the balloon. The balloon is then deflated before activation of the cutting wire. After ensuring proper grounding of the patient and that the guidewire does not cross or touch the balloon, the balloon is inflated with 2 ml of 50:50 contrast solution and saline mixture, as the cutting wire is simultaneously activated with 75–100 W pure cut electrical current [39–42].

Ureteroscopy for Impacted Stones and Ureteral Stricture

Impacted stones in the ureter are commonly referred to when the stone stays in ureter for more than 2 months and/or failure to pass a guidewire or catheter beyond the stone during first attempt [43]. Impacted ureteral stone represents a surgical challenge during ureteroscopic lithotripsy owing to

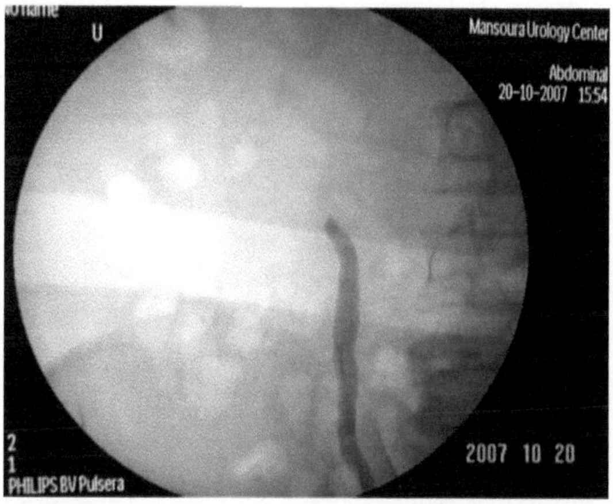

Fig. 24.1 Retrograde ureteropyelography revealed a complete arrest of dye at right lumbar ureter

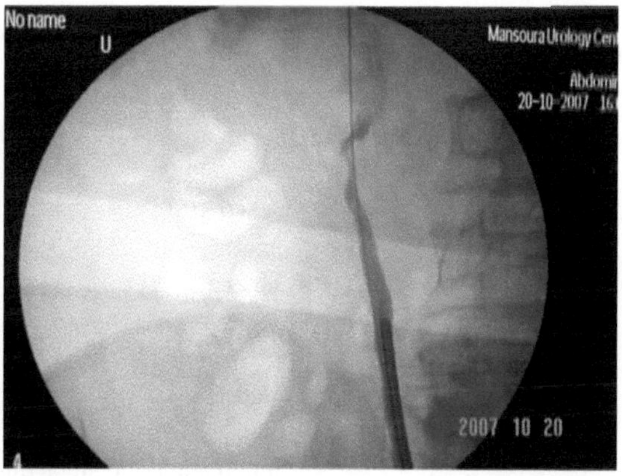

Fig. 24.2 A rigid guidewire has successfully passed through the strictured area

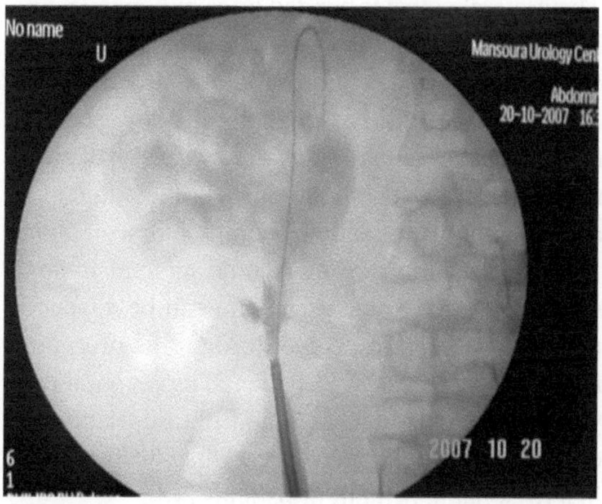

Fig. 24.3 Retrograde ureteropyelography after cutting of the strictured are showing extravasation of dye

pathologic changes in ureteral wall secondary to stone impaction. There might be edema and inflamed ureteral mucosa at stone bed as well as compression induced ischemia facilitating stricture formation. In addition, difficult navigation with iatrogenic injury during lithotripsy predispose for subsequent stricture formation [16, 23, 43, 44].

Instruments

A holmium:yttrium-aluminum-garnet (YAG) laser with 365- and 200-μm laser fiber for semirigid and flexible ureteroscopes, respectively, are the instruments needed. Energy is set at 0.8–1.5 J at a pulse rate of 5–10 Hz. Initial adjustment are 8 Hz and 0.8 J and pulse rate can be increased to achieve adequate stone fragmentation. Continuous irrigation is used to obtain and sustain a clear operative visual field.

Technique

The ureteroscope is introduced over the guidewire after balloon dilatation of the ureteral orifice until the stone is clearly visualized; then lithotripsy is performed using the laser energy. The stones are fragmented to 2- to 3-mm particles, and no effort is needed to extract the stones fragments.

Outcome

Stone impaction has been demonstrated to reduce success rate of endoureterotomy for concomitant ureteral stricture. Gdor and associates reported success rate of 55.5 and 75 % for impacted and nonimpacted stones over mean of 13.7 and 34 months follow-up, respectively [23]. This incidence is in concordance with others; Hibi and coworkers reported success rate of 75 % after 46–74 months of follow-up [33]. Xi et al. reported 26.2 % incidence of iatrogenic stricture after ureteroscopy for impacted stone which was significantly higher than

Table 24.1 Results of Ho:YAG laser endoureterotomy

Group	No. of patients	Average follow-up (months)	Success rate (%)
Lin et al. [34]	19	40.2	52.6
Gnessin et al. [32]	35	27[a]	82 clinically 78 radiologically
Fu et al. [35]	17	17	94
Corcoran et al. [25][b]	34	25.2	85
Gdor et al. [23]	13	21	62
Hong et al. [31]	5	45	75
Razdan et al. [36]	17	–	74
Shoma et al. [37]	43	19.4	60.5

[a]Median
[b]Combination of balloon dilation and laser endoureterotomy

after open procedure [45]. The authors recommended open surgical procedure for impacted stones associated with ureteral strictures. Impacted stone location has been empathized as a predisposing factor for high stricture rate after ureteroscopy with proximal ureteral stone impaction being of highest risk of perforation with subsequent stricture formation [44].

Challenging Situations During Endoureterotomy

It is clear that optimum visualization and the ability of ureteroscope to pass the stricture are considered the corner stone for performing successful endoureterotomy. Nevertheless, the urologist might encounter challenging situations when the ureteroscope could not be advanced through the stricture site or the stricture site is blind-ended. In this context, different endoscopic techniques have been described to get through the stricture and making it passable, and then a standard endoureterotomy could be performed.

Subtotal Ureteral Strictures

In stricture situation where only a guide wire can be passed, a preincision step was described to enable the surgeon to pass an endoureterotomy device. Bach et al. inserted a Foley-type bended ureteral catheter above the level of the stricture, then a laser fiber is passed through the catheter and extended for 2–3 mm beyond the catheter tip. This 2–3 mm limit can be guaranteed by marking the length of ureteral catheter and laser fiber prior to surgery. The ureteral catheter bended tip is radiopaque, giving the surgeon control over the direction of laser energy. Then, under fluoroscopic control, the laser fiber is slowly pulled through the stenotic area until the contrast medium begins to flow freely all along the ureter. This technique enables the surgeon to abstain from using endoscope in the first step procedure and allow for managing subtotal ureteral strictures as long as a guidewire can be advanced through the stricture. Nevertheless, this procedure has a 38.8 % (7 out of 18 patients) reoperation rate; yet taking into consideration the difficulty of encountered cases, open surgery had been avoided in a reasonable percent of patients [46].

When ureteral stricture is so tight that the conventional guidewire cannot be advanced through, a microwire–microcatheter combination may be considered in a trial to traverse the stricture. Microwires and catheters are being used frequently for different vascular interventional techniques. The smaller size of these instruments allows for passing more tight ureteral strictures. In this situation, the microwire is used to pass the stricture; then the microcatheter is advanced on and the guidewire is replaced with a superstiff one followed by dilating the stricture and finally JJ stent insertion [47].

Blind-Ended Short Ureteral Strictures

Inability to pass a guidewire through the stricture area represents a great challenge notably in situations where patients are not candidates for open surgery. When the stricture length has been assessed by combined antegrade and retrograde fluoroscopy, cut to the light or core-through procedures have been advocated as methods of intervention [48, 49]. In such a situation, a combined retrograde and antegrade access is mandatory to assess the length of stricture. In short strictures less than 2 cm, a transluminal puncture technique can be adopted; the stiff end of 0.035-in. guidewire could be advanced through the blind end to the proximal ureter. However, it is necessary to use C-arm in different planes to align the ureteroscope with the proximal end of the ureter. When the guidewire is advanced, an open tip ureteral catheter can be inserted with subsequent placement of the guidewire to its original position with floppy end directed proximally and a standard endoureterotomy can be performed [50].

Another technique have been described by Thomas and associates providing more precise incision of the blind ended ureter "laser uretero-ureterosotomy"; a laser fiber is used to core-through the obliterated segment under direct vision while energy is applied using the Ho:YAG laser light source. Then two endoscopes are used while the light of receiving endoscope is dimmed to allow better visualization of the aiming laser beam. Then the laser fiber is advanced while on hemostatic cutting mode of 0.8 J and 10 pulses/s under antegrade and retrograde visualization. When laser fiber penetrated through the obliterated segment, it will be grasped by the receiving endoscope and brought extracorporeally to provide through and through access. Then the laser fiber is exchanged with an open tip ureteral catheter with subsequent guidewire fixation and a standard endoscopic endoureterotomy is approached.

This procedure allows for assurance of patency during incision, dilation, and stenting of the stricture. Nevertheless, it encounters a few disadvantages, namely, a possible loss of the laser fiber after the procedure has been completed and the risk that the laser fiber could be broken during grasping; in addition, this technique is reserved only for blind-ended strictures less than 2 cm in length as otherwise the light will not be able to penetrate through the fibrosed obliterated segment.

Alternatively, the procedure can be accomplished in an antegrade manner. The reverse end of a stiff Dasher 0.014-in. steerable guidewire with a permaglide hydrophilic coating can be used to "puncture" through the dense inflammatory tissue into the bladder. Then the guidewire is used to introduce a cardiac angioplasty balloon for dilating the ureterovesical junction with subsequent fixation of antegrade JJ stent [51].

For lower end ureteral strictures, an incision could be done through the bladder wall until the opening of the ureteral wall to achieve continuity between bladder and ureter. A stone impacted at the lower end ureter or dye injected from percutaneously fixed tube can be the guide. Under fluoroscopic guidance, the tip of Colling's knife is adjusted to be overlying the stone or dye shadow; then, an incision is made through bladder wall until one reaches the stone or the dye; then, a JJ stent can be fixed for long-term drainage [52]. Alternatively, a rigid ureteroscope can be advanced in antegrade manner down to the ureteral end and is used to adjust the tip of a superstiff guide wire against the obstructed area. Then, an incision can be done cystoscopically to gain access to ureteral lumen and to grasp the guidewire [53].

In another approach, an 18-gauge needle, 35 cm in length, can be introduced into the bladder along the Sachse urethrotome through the bridge generally used for laser fiber; then under fluoroscopic guidance and cystoscopic orientation, the ureteral wall is pierced and the lumen is approached; then a guidewire is fixed with subsequent indwelling stent fixation [54].

Blind-Ended Long Ureteral Strictures

Long ureteral strictures with a gap between the proximal and distal ureter are surgically challenging and present a troublesome situation. The ideal management of these cases is restricted to open surgery. Nevertheless, the need of long-term PCN is crucial to allow for periureteral adhesions and leakage to subside. Consequently, patients are more prone to complications, frequent episodes of PCN dislodgement and refixation in addition to deterioration of renal function, and undoubtedly serious quality of life problems. On the other hand, the situation is so complex that results of open surgery would be questionable.

"Rendezvous" procedure has been advocated for inserting JJ stent into long impassable ureteral strictures in case open surgery is not feasible or long-term internal drainage is required. A proximal access to retroperitoneum is obtained via puncture with guidewire or laser incision using ureteral access sheath. Then the retroperitoneum is approached and a guidewire is passed through. The retroperitoneum is then punctured distally by the rigid end of the wire and grasped from the opposite side. Then bidirectional traction on the wire is applied to allow placement of an indwelling ureteral stent [55]. A modification of the technique has been described; retroperitoneum puncture could be obtained by the rigid ureteroscope or incised by laser through ureteral access sheath. The ureteroscope is advanced in the retroperitoneum under strict fluoroscopic guidance until the guidewire is seen in the retroperitoneum. The guidewire is either grasped to the distal end or followed up till the proximal end of the ureter is approached. Then a JJ stent can be fixed [56].

It is to be noted that these maneuvers could only be done by an experienced endourologist and when all other modalities fail. In addition, the paucity of the patients' number, unfamiliarity with these blind techniques, and the lack of long-term follow-up restrict the widespread use of these techniques.

Summary

The first-step procedure for endourological management of a ureteral stricture is obtaining through and through access with a guidewire through the area in question. Optimum visualization and advancing the endoscopic instrument through the stricture site are crucial for better outcome. A variety of endourological instruments had been described; however, laser endoureterotomy is gaining worldwide acceptance. For difficult situations when the ureter is blind ended or a long segment stricture is encountered, various techniques have been described, including transluminal puncture, laser uretero-ureterostomy and Rendezvous procedure. Nevertheless, these procedures should be adopted with great caution for only select patients as there is a high risk for complication.

References

1. Abou-Elela A, Torky M, Salah E, Morsy A, Elsherbiny M. Inverted ureteral nipple as antireflux technique in surgical management of bilharzial ureteral strictures. Urology. 2010;76:983–7.
2. Badmos KB, Popoola AA, Buhari MO, Abdulkadir AY. Ureteric schistosomiasis with obstructive uropathy. J Coll Physicians Surg Pak. 2009;19:456–8.
3. Hussein A, Rifaat E, Zaki A, Abol-Nasr M. Stenting versus non-stenting after non-complicated ureteroscopic manipulation of stones in bilharzial ureters. Int J Urol. 2006;13:886–90.
4. Goel A, Dalela D. Options in the management of tuberculous ureteric stricture. Indian J Urol. 2008;24: 376–81.
5. Zarrabi AD, Heyns CF. Clinical features of confirmed versus suspected urogenital tuberculosis in region with extremely high prevalence of pulmonary tuberculosis. Urology. 2009;74:41–5.
6. Kamyshan IS. Choice of surgical correction of urodynamics in ureteral tuberculosis. Urologiia. 2008;6:24–8.
7. Khong SY, Lam A, Coombes G, Ford S. Surgical management of recurrent ureteric endometriosis causing recurrent hypertension in a postmenopausal woman. J Minim Invasive Gynecol. 2010;17:100–3.
8. Lee TH, Kim W, Lee S, et al. Hydroureteronephrosis caused by endometriosis around the ureter. Clin Nephrol. 2009;72:418–9.
9. Bosev D, Nicoll LM, Bhagan L, et al. Laparoscopic management of ureteral endometriosis: the Stanford University Hospital experience with 96 consecutive cases. J Urol. 2009;182:2748–52.
10. Sountoulides P, Kaplan A, Kaufmann OG, Sofikitis N. Current status of metal stents for managing malignant ureteric obstruction. BJU Int. 2010;105(8):1066–72.
11. Liatsikos EN, Karnabatidis D, Katsanos K, et al. Ureteral metal stents: 10-year experience with malignant ureteral obstruction treatment. J Urol. 2009;182: 2613–7.
12. Ganatra AM, Loughlin KR. The management of malignant ureteral obstruction treated with ureteral stents. J Urol. 2005;174:2125–8.
13. Parpala-Sparman T, Paananen I, Santala M, Ohtonen P, Hellstrom P. Increasing numbers of ureteric injuries after the introduction of laparoscopic surgery. Scand J Urol Nephrol. 2008;42:422–7.
14. Lim MC, Lee BY, Lee DO, et al. Lower urinary tract injuries diagnosed after hysterectomy: seven-year experience at a cancer hospital. J Obstet Gynaecol Res. 2010;36:318–25.

15. Brandt AS, von Rundstedt FC, Lazica DA, Roth S. Ureteral reconstruction after ureterorenoscopic injuries. Urologe A. 2010;49:812–21.
16. Adiyat KT, Meuleners R, Monga M. Selective postoperative imaging after ureteroscopy. Urology. 2009;73: 490–3, discussion 3.
17. Nakamura LY, Ferrigni RG, Stone WM, Fowl RJ. Urinary bladder injuries during vascular surgery. J Vasc Surg. 2010;52:453–5.
18. Koukouras D, Petsas T, Liatsikos E, et al. Percutaneous minimally invasive management of iatrogenic ureteral injuries. J Endourol. 2010;24:1921–7.
19. Dirim A, Kumsar S. Iatrogenic ureteral injury due to lumbar sympathetic block. Scand J Urol Nephrol. 2008;42:395–6.
20. Bjurlin MA, Rousseau LA, Vidal PP, Hollowell CM. Iatrogenic ureteral injury secondary to a thoracolumbar lateral revision instrumentation and fusion. Spine J. 2009;9:e13–5.
21. Abid AF, Hashem HL. Ureteral injuries from gunshots and shells of explosive devices. Urol Ann. 2010; 2:17–20.
22. Helmy TE, Sarhan OM, Harraz AM, Dawaba M. Complexity of non-iatrogenic ureteral injuries in children: single-center experience. Int Urol Nephrol. 2011;43(1):1–5.
23. Gdor Y, Gabr AH, Faerber GJ, Roberts WW, Wolf Jr JS. Success of laser endoureterotomy of ureteral strictures associated with ureteral stones is related to stone impaction. J Endourol. 2008;22:2507–11.
24. Elashry OM, Elgamasy AK, Sabaa MA, et al. Ureteroscopic management of lower ureteric calculi: a 15-year single-centre experience. BJU Int. 2008; 102:1010–7.
25. Corcoran AT, Smaldone MC, Ricchiuti DD, Averch TD. Management of benign ureteral strictures in the endoscopic era. J Endourol. 2009;23:1909–12.
26. Hafez KS, Wolf Jr JS. Update on minimally invasive management of ureteral strictures. J Endourol. 2003; 17:453–64.
27. Meretyk S, Albala DM, Clayman RV, Denstedt JD, Kavoussi LR. Endoureterotomy for treatment of ureteral strictures. J Urol. 1992;147:1502–6.
28. Lojanapiwat B, Soonthonpun S, Wudhikarn S. Endoscopic treatment of benign ureteral strictures. Asian J Surg. 2002;25:130–3.
29. Richter F, Irwin RJ, Watson RA, Lang EK. Endourologic management of benign ureteral strictures with and without compromised vascular supply. Urology. 2000;55:652–7.
30. Byun SS, Kim JH, Oh SJ, Kim HH. Simple retrograde balloon dilation for treatment of ureteral strictures: etiology-based analysis. Yonsei Med J. 2003;44:273–8.
31. Hong JH, Jeon SS, Lee KS. Result of endoscopic ureteroureterostomy with holmium:YAG laser for complete ureteral obstruction. J Endourol. 2005;19: 979–83.
32. Gnessin E, Yossepowitch O, Holland R, Livne PM, Lifshitz DA. Holmium laser endoureterotomy for benign ureteral stricture: a single center experience. J Urol. 2009;182:2775–9.
33. Hibi H, Ohori T, Taki T, Yamada Y, Honda N. Long-term results of endoureterotomy using a holmium laser. Int J Urol. 2007;14:872–4.
34. Lin CM, Tsai TH, Lin TC, et al. Holmium: yttrium-aluminum-garnet laser endoureterotomy for benign ureteral strictures: a single-centre experience. Acta Chir Belg. 2009;109:746–50.
35. Fu YM, Ni SB, Chen QY, et al. Treatment of ureteral obstruction by holmium: YAG laser endoureterotomy: a report of 18 cases. Zhonghua Yi Xue Za Zhi. 2009;89:335–7.
36. Razdan S, Silberstein IK, Bagley DH. Ureteroscopic endoureterotomy. BJU Int. 2005;95 Suppl 2:94–101.
37. Shoma A, Faisel R, Mansour O, El Kappany H. Laser endoureterotomy: long term results and predection of the outcome. Eur Urol Suppl. 2006;5:72.
38. Conlin MJ, Gomella LG, Bagley DH. Endoscopic ureteroureterostomy for obliterated ureteral segments. J Urol. 1996;156:1394–9.
39. Chandhoke PS, Clayman RV, Stone AM, et al. Endopyelotomy and endoureterotomy with the acucise ureteral cutting balloon device: preliminary experience. J Endourol. 1993;7:45–51.
40. Wolf Jr JS, Elashry OM, Clayman RV. Long-term results of endoureterotomy for benign ureteral and ureteroenteric strictures. J Urol. 1997;158:759–64.
41. Preminger GM, Clayman RV, Nakada SY, et al. A multicenter clinical trial investigating the use of a fluoroscopically controlled cutting balloon catheter for the management of ureteral and ureteropelvic junction obstruction. J Urol. 1997;157:1625–9.
42. El-Nahas AR, Shoma AM, Eraky I, El-Kenawy MR, El-Kappany HA. Prospective, randomized comparison of ureteroscopic endopyelotomy using holmium:YAG laser and balloon catheter. J Urol. 2006;175:614–8.
43. Mugiya S, Ito T, Maruyama S, Hadano S, Nagae H. Endoscopic features of impacted ureteral stones. J Urol. 2004;171:89–91.
44. Brito AH, Mitre AI, Srougi M. Ureteroscopic pneumatic lithotripsy of impacted ureteral calculi. Int Braz J Urol. 2006;32:295–9.
45. Xi Q, Wang S, Ye Z, Liu J. Combined removal of stones with resection of concurrent pathologic ureter may be a preferred treatment for impacted ureteral stones with stricture lesions. J Endourol. 2009;23:243–7.
46. Bach T, Geavlete B, Herrmann TW, Gross AJ. Retrograde blind endoureterotomy for subtotal ureteral strictures: a new technique. J Endourol. 2008;22:2565–70.
47. Keeling AN, Lee MJ. Crossing ureteric strictures: microcatheters to the rescue when conventional methods fail. Cardiovasc Intervent Radiol. 2007;30: 1234–7.
48. Goda K, Kawabata G, Yasufuku T, et al. Cut-to-the-light technique and potassium titanyl phosphate laser ureterotomy for complete ureteral obstruction. Int J Urol. 2004;11:427–8.

49. Thomas MA, Ong AM, Pinto PA, Rha KH, Jarrett TW. Management of obliterated urinary segments using a laser fiber for access. J Urol. 2003;169: 2284–6.
50. Egilmez T, Guvel S, Kilinc F, Yaycioglu O, Ozkardes H. Management of complete ureteral obstructions with a transluminal puncture technique. Int Braz J Urol. 2005;31:264–8.
51. Govender P, Delaney H, Guiney M. Traversing tight ureteric strictures. Cardiovasc Intervent Radiol. 2009;32:199–201.
52. Miskowiak J. Transurethral ureterocystostomy. Scand J Urol Nephrol. 2000;34:123–5.
53. Strup SE, Bagley DH. Endoscopic ureteroneocystostomy for complete obstruction at the ureterovesical junction. J Urol. 1996;156:360–2.
54. Slongo LE, de Fraga R, Mitre AI. Endoscopic stented ureterocystostomy. J Endourol. 2010;24:1817–20.
55. Macri A, Magno C, Certo A, et al. Combined antegrade and retrograde ureteral stenting: the rendezvous technique. Clin Radiol. 2005;60:257–60.
56. Yates DR, Mehta SS, Spencer PA, Parys BT. Combined antegrade and retrograde endoscopic retroperitoneal bypass of ureteric strictures: a modification of the 'rendezvous' procedure. BJU Int. 2010;105:992–7.

Ureteroscopic Management of Ureteral and Renal Pelvic Tumors: Overcoming the Difficulties

25

Demetrius H. Bagley and Kelly A. Healy

Abbreviations

CTU	Computed tomographic urography
F	French
HNPCC	Hereditary nonpolyposis colorectal carcinoma
mL	Milliliter
Nd	Neodymium
RPG	Retrograde ureteropyelogram
UC	Urothelial carcinoma
UTUC	Upper tract urothelial carcinoma
YAG	Yttrium-aluminum-garnet

Introduction

The techniques for endoscopic treatment of urinary tumors have been carried from the bladder into the ureter and intrarenal collecting system with the development of appropriate, small endoscopes and other working devices. Ureteroscopy has been extremely important in both the diagnosis and treatment of upper urinary tract neoplasms. Small rigid and flexible ureteroscopes can provide access to the entire upper tract to deliver devices to not only sample tissue but also to ablate neoplasm. Thus, the minimally invasive diagnosis, treatment, and surveillance of upper tract pathology have become possible.

Upper urinary tract urothelial carcinoma (UTUC) is a relatively rare yet potentially lethal disease, which accounts for approximately 5 % of all urothelial carcinoma (UC) [1]. While the majority of UC occurs in the bladder, UTUC is more common in patients with a previous history of bladder carcinoma [2, 3]. Historically, the gold standard treatment for upper tract tumors was radical nephroureterectomy with bladder cuff excision [4]. Thus, the diagnosis of UTUC resulted in the loss of an entire renal unit. Endoscopic treatment, however, may result in equivalent cancer control and maintenance of the kidney in appropriately selected patients, albeit at the expense of frequent retreatments [5–7]. Nevertheless, not all tumors are amenable to ureteroscopic treatment. Small low-grade tumors are ideal for endoscopic treatment, while more complex lesions require more advanced endoscopic techniques.

Indications for the Ureteroscopic Treatment of Upper Tract Tumors

The two main goals of ureteroscopic treatment for upper tract tumors are oncological control and nephron preservation. Recently, several series have shown that patients undergoing radical nephrectomy for renal cortical tumors are at a greater risk of chronic renal insufficiency than a similar cohort undergoing partial nephrectomy [8–10].

D.H. Bagley, M.D., FACS (✉) • K. A. Healy, M.D.
Department of Urology, Thomas Jefferson University Hospital, 1025 Walnut Street, Suite 1112 College Building, Philadelphia, PA, 19107, USA
e-mail: Demetrius.bagley@jefferson.edu; Kelly.healy@jefferson.edu

A.M. Al-Kandari et al. (eds.), *Difficult Cases in Endourology*,
DOI 10.1007/978-1-84882-083-8_25, © Springer-Verlag London 2013

In turn, chronic kidney disease is associated with adverse cardiovascular and noncardiovascular events, hospitalization, and increased mortality [11, 12]. These findings have served as an impetus for nephron-sparing surgery for localized renal cancer. This same argument can be extended to UTUC, and most cases can be managed ureteroscopically.

The strongest indication for ureteroscopic treatment is in those patients with baseline renal insufficiency who would develop renal failure if the affected renal unit were removed. Therefore, the strongest indication is the patient with a solitary kidney. Patients with a compromised, poorly functioning or nonfunctioning contralateral kidney, which would not maintain adequate renal function, can be considered in the same group. Similarly, patients with bilateral upper tract neoplasms are appropriate candidates for conservative endoscopic treatment. In another group of selected patients, upper tract lesions can be treated ureteroscopically on an elective basis [13, 14]. These include patients with small, low-grade tumors, which are most amenable to endoscopic removal. Any patient being considered for endoscopic treatment should also demonstrate consistent compliance, as a strict surveillance protocol is mandatory [15].

Instruments

Both small, standard rigid and flexible ureteroscopes should be available for the endoscopic management of UTUC. Rigid ureteroscopes of approximately 7 F can be passed directly into the ureter without dilation. These are most useful in the distal ureter and can often be passed to the level of the iliac vessels in both male and female patients. In fact, rigid ureteroscopes may be passed even more proximally to the level of the renal pelvis in elderly female patients.

Actively deflectable, flexible ureteroscopes offer access to the entire upper urinary tract. The smaller diameter, flexible ureteroscopes can often be passed directly into the ureter without prior dilation. However, some larger scopes may require dilation of the ureterovesical junction or even more proximal portions of the ureter. This is particularly true for the newer digital video "chip on the tip" scopes, which offer improved image quality at the expense of a larger overall diameter and limited deflectability compared to fiberoptic scopes. Available flexible ureteroscopes range from 7.4 F to nearly 10 F.

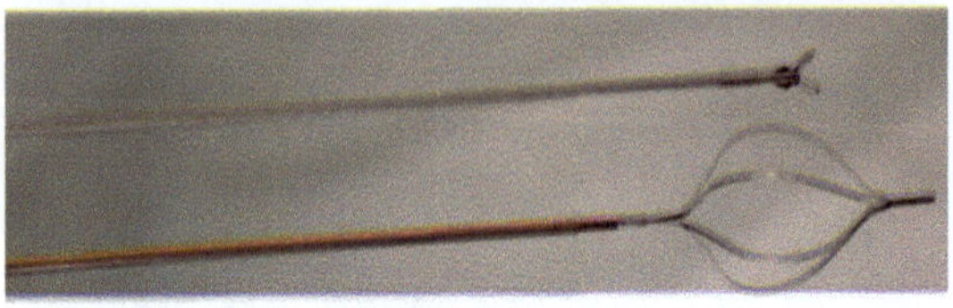

Fig. 25.1 The most commonly used ureteroscopic biopsy devices are the cup forceps and the flat-wire basket

Endoscopic diagnosis of UTUC includes direct visualization and sampling. Visualization alone provides some information on the nature of the tumor, but it is impossible to grade the lesion accurately or confirm its malignancy. In one series, visual inspection alone was only 70 % accurate in determining the malignancy or grade of an upper tract neoplasm [16]. Therefore, it is essential to obtain tissue for pathologic study. Urine, fluid adjacent to the tumor, and a sample of the tumor itself can be aspirated through the channel of the ureteroscope. A large syringe such as 60 mL should be utilized to give the most effective suction. All specimens, including aspirates and biopsies, are sent to the cytopathologist for pathologic diagnosis [17–22]. Samples are examined with both a smear and cytospin preparation. Additionally, a cell block is also prepared if there is any macroscopically visible tissue in the sample. Multiple biopsies of the lesion are taken, as well as aspirates pre- and postbiopsy and posttreatment.

Several different biopsy devices may be employed to obtain a tissue sample, including forceps, baskets, pronged graspers, snares, and brushes [23]. However, the two most commonly used and most effective devices are the cup forceps and basket (Fig. 25.1). Small cup forceps are typically 1-mm diameter and are quite useful for any lesion, including small papillary lesions and more sessile lesions. If the tissue sample is contained within the cup, the forceps can be withdrawn through the working channel and replaced to obtain multiple biopsies in an expeditious manner. However, the forceps shaft is relatively rigid and consequently limits endoscopic deflection beyond approximately 90–110°. In addition to cup forceps, stainless steel flat-wire baskets are also effective for tissue sampling and large tumor debulking. This basket design is most effective as it can trap the tumor between the angles of the wire and remove a large sample even up to 1 cm in diameter. While flat-wire baskets provide a larger tissue sample than cup forceps, the entire unit consisting of tumor sample, basket, and ureteroscope must be removed from the ureter and bladder. Recently, one of the newer biopsy devices incorporates larger cup forceps and thus obtains larger specimen samples. However, this device requires use of a ureteral access sheath and must be back-loaded through the ureteroscope. The search for the ideal biopsy device which maximizes specimen size while maintaining ureteroscope deflectability is ongoing.

Following endoscopic biopsy, treatment requires the use of small caliber instruments to destroy tumor [24]. As aforementioned, the instrument used for biopsy can also be employed to mechanically debulk tumor volume. Small 2–3 F electrodes can be used to coagulate or, in some cases, resect tumor; however, their application is typically avoided in the ureter due to increased risk of stricture formation. The smaller devices are quite flexible and often useful for lesions in difficult intrarenal collecting system locations. In particular, the 2 F electrocautery probe can fulgurate with lateral contact rather than the directly forward approach needed for a laser.

Lasers have gained their place in treatment due to their unique capabilities. The two main lasers currently available for treating upper tract neoplasms include the holmium and neodymium (Nd):yttrium-aluminum-garnet (YAG) lasers. Both lasers can be delivered through small, flexible fibers of either 200 or approximately 400 μm core diameter. The different capabilities of the holmium and Nd:YAG lasers allow for their selective application. The holmium:YAG laser is a solid state pulsed laser with a wavelength (λ) of 2,100 nm. The holmium energy has limited tissue or fluid penetration of <0.5 mm with some coagulative effect but a dominant ablative effect. Longer pulse duration of the holmium laser (350 or 700 μs) causes more coagulation than the shorter duration with the same limited penetration. It is effective for treatment of more extensive tumors within the ureter. In contrast, the Nd:YAG laser (λ 1,064 nm) is a continuous wave device which produces coagulation alone. It gives a deeper effect with up to 1 cm penetration. However, it does not remove tissue as the holmium can with its ablative effect. These two lasers are best used in combination.

Diagnostic Techniques

The most common presentation for upper tract neoplasms is gross or microscopic hematuria, which is seen in approximately 80 % of patients [1, 25, 26]. Less frequently, flank pain or unsuspected hydronephrosis is detected. Upper tract tumors are most common in those patients with a previous history of bladder cancer but are also associated with prior smoking history and the relatively rare syndrome of hereditary nonpolyposis colorectal carcinoma (HNPCC) or Lynch syndrome [27].

Upper tract urothelial neoplasms are commonly defined by radiographic studies. Traditionally, intravenous pyelography (IVP) was used to evaluate upper tract tumors. IVP can demonstrate both the filling defect(s) and indicate the presence of ureteral obstruction. However, it does not define renal parenchymal lesions as well. IVP has been supplanted by computerized tomographic urography (CTU), which is currently the most commonly used imaging study. CTU is now considered the gold standard because it accurately distinguishes calculi from soft tissue masses and identifies hydronephrosis which is suggestive of obstruction. Furthermore, CTU simultaneously evaluates for extraluminal extension, lymphadenopathy, renal parenchymal lesions, and possible metastasis [28, 29]. Multidetector CTU has demonstrated very high diagnostic accuracy, sensitivity, and specificity [28]. Notably, however, smaller lesions

<3 mm may not be detected on some CT urograms. Both IVP and CTU are contraindicated in patients with contrast allergies and renal insufficiency.

Alternatively, magnetic resonance urography (MRU) may be employed in patients with poorly functioning kidneys or severe contrast allergies. Like CTU, MRU is quite useful for parenchymal lesions. However, MRU lacks the resolution to define smaller lesions [30] and, although very rare, is associated nephrogenic systemic fibrosis (NSF) in patients with severe renal insufficiency.

Renal ultrasonography is probably the least useful of the renal imaging studies for UTUC. While ultrasound can indicate possible larger masses in the renal pelvis and the presence of obstruction, it cannot provide information on lesions within the ureter.

At the time of endoscopic evaluation, a cone-tipped retrograde ureteropyelogram (RPG) is quite useful to demonstrate the presence and even the full extent of the ureteral or intrarenal tumor. In addition, RPG also outlines the collecting system and thereby clearly defines the anatomy to ensure a complete endoscopic survey. Nevertheless, several studies have shown that RPG suffers from low accuracy in detecting UTUC [25, 31].

Endoscopic Techniques-Diagnostic

Evaluation and preparation for treatment of any patient with upper tract tumor or suspected lesions includes inspection of the entire urothelium. The procedure starts with cystourethroscopy. Using both a 30- and 70-degree lens, the urethra and bladder are fully inspected to identify concomitant intravesical pathology. At the time of cystoscopy, an RPG may also be performed typically with a cone-tipped catheter to outline the entire ureter. The ureteral orifice is occluded with the cone tip and injected contrast often distends the ureter and intrarenal collecting system sufficiently to demonstrate any filling defects which may be located along the mucosa. Care should be taken not to overfill the collecting system with contrast since it may obscure the filling defect. We prefer to use dilute 50 % iodinated contrast. Both the involved and the contralateral collecting system should be evaluated unless it has been recently cleared by other studies.

A "no-touch" ureteroscopic technique is used, either with rigid and flexible ureteroscopes or with a flexible ureteroscope alone [32]. In doing so, the urothelium may be inspected without prior instrument trauma, which can induce bleeding and impair visualization. Adherence to a "no-touch" technique is critical for a nonconfounded, meticulous endoscopic evaluation. In our practice, we prefer to start with a rigid ureteroscope with a small 6.9 F tip diameter and self-dilating shaft. Under direct vision, the rigid ureteroscope is placed through the urethra and into the ureteral orifice to inspect the ureter. The ureteroscope is advanced as far proximally as possible. If it becomes difficult to pass the rigid instrument, for example, at the level of the iliac vessels, then a wire is left in place to the level that has been inspected and the ureteroscope is removed. Next, a flexible ureteroscope is inserted over this wire. The flexible ureteroscope is advanced under fluoroscopic imaging through the bladder and into the orifice to the level seen by the rigid endoscope. Care must be taken to prevent proximal migration of the wire with flexible ureteroscope insertion. The wire is then removed, and the flexible ureteroscope is advanced under vision through the more proximal portions of the ureter and into the intrarenal collecting system.

Alternatively, a flexible ureteroscope of the smallest diameter can be passed under vision through the urethra and bladder into the ureteral orifice. Irrigation is maintained as the ureteroscope is passed into the ureteral orifice and advanced proximally to inspect the ureter to the level of the renal collecting system. If the flexible instrument fails to pass, then it is possible to return to the rigid scope initially to dilate the ureter. As previously described, inspect as far proximally as possible and then leave a wire for placement of the flexible ureteroscope. Normal-sized ureters may not readily accommodate some of the larger flexible ureteroscopes (9 F). In such cases, it may be inappropriate to attempt to use the larger flexible ureteroscopes in a diagnostic manner alone.

Within the intrarenal collecting system, a renal pelvis aspirate is obtained through the ureteroscope using a 60 milliliter (mL) syringe, which obtains the best suction. The renal pelvis aspirate is sent for cytology. Then, inspection should be carried out systematically. The ureteropelvic junction and the renal pelvis are first inspected. Attention is then turned to the upper infundibuli and calyces, the mid, and then finally the lower. In some cases, it may be more difficult to access the lower calyces and manipulation within the pelvis can cause trauma with resulting mucosal erythema. For this reason, the lower calyces are inspected last.

If a neoplasm is visualized, it should be defined as fully as possible. Is it papillary or sessile and is there is a small base? Are there multiple separately based lesions and are there remote lesions?

The first step for sampling is to aspirate with a 60-mL syringe through the ureteroscope with the channel placed near or on the tumor itself. The aspirate, which is used for cytologic study, can provide a sample of the tumor itself as well as the remainder of the collecting system.

The major portion of the tumor is then biopsied. A flat-wire basket is ideally used on a papillary lesion more than approximately 3–4 mm in diameter. It can remove an entire lesion of that size and a good portion of a lesion up to 1 cm. The basket is placed around the tumor to engage as large a portion as possible. It is then closed snugly but not fully against the lesion. Next, the basket is used to avulse a piece of tumor away as a sample. The entire unit of tumor, basket, and ureteroscope are withdrawn to retrieve the largest fragment of tissue possible. It is usually quite friable and comes away with surprisingly little bleeding. Again, the entire unit of tumor, basket, and ureteroscope are removed since the sample is too large to come through the channel of the ureteroscope. If on inspection, however, only a very small fragment is in the basket, then the basket and tumor can be withdrawn through the channel of the ureteroscope and replaced for repeat biopsy.

Alternatively, a cup forceps is used for smaller papillary lesions which cannot be engaged with a basket and for more sessile or flat lesions. The forceps should be aimed near the base of the tumor parallel to the wall of the ureter or the renal pelvis and perpendicular to the tumor itself. The forceps is closed on the tumor to sample it by excision. Again, if the entire sample is contained within the cup, then it may be removed through the lumen of the ureteroscope. On the other hand, if there is tumor extending beyond the edge of the cups, the specimen would be sheared off as it came through the lumen. Therefore, the entire unit of tumor, forceps, and ureteroscope need to be withdrawn. Multiple biopsies should be taken to obtain sufficient sample for cytopathologic analysis.

There is variable difficulty in sampling tumors at different sites. Within the ureter, most lesions can be approached for biopsy relatively easily. Those in the most distal ureter may be the most difficult, and these are discussed below. In the intrarenal collecting system, the most difficult site is the lower pole. This area can usually be inspected with the flexible ureteroscope. However, it is often not accessible for biopsy forceps and may be relatively difficult to reach even with a basket. The smaller, flat-wire baskets (1.7–2.2 F) may be most useful to minimize the loss of deflection and allow access into the lower infundibulum.

Ureteroscopic Treatment of Upper Tract Neoplasms

The difficulty in treating upper tract tumors ureteroscopically is related to the location and the size of the lesion. The lesions which are easy to treat are those located within the length of the ureter itself or in the renal pelvis. They should be <1 cm in diameter and papillary in configuration. These lesions can be approached directly with a ureteroscope and can be sampled and removed. Other locations and sizes of tumors can present more difficulty in access for visualization, biopsy, and treatment.

Tumor at Ureteral Orifice

Tumor at the ureteral orifice can often be seen initially cystoscopically. It may protrude from the orifice and then withdraw with respiration or urinary flow. These lesions may be biopsied cystoscopically, usually with a basket placed into the ureter. However, this technique suffers from several pitfalls as it fails to visualize the base of the tumor and its distribution as well as the adequacy of removal. Therefore, direct vision with ureteroscopy to inspect the tumor in its entirety is important. The most distal ureter, however, is an area that is difficult to distend or maintain in a stable position for visualization and manipulation.

Maneuvers may be used to promote access to the site of the tumor in the distal ureter. The small rigid ureteroscope is best suited to access tumors in this area. Compared to the flexible ureteroscope, it is easier to maintain position in the distal ureter and prevent withdrawal during respiration and also easier to readvance into the ureteral orifice with the small rigid scope.

Smaller tumors can be removed intact using a flat-wire basket to remove the volume of tumor. This volume varies with the size of the tumor and the position of the basket. However, a 5–8 mm papillary tumor can usually be removed intact. A larger tumor can be sequentially debulked with this technique.

As noted, it may be difficult to distend the most distal portion of the ureter to help to visualize the lumen and the ureteral walls. It also may become difficult to visualize the orifice if there is bleeding from the biopsy or from the instrumentation. Therefore, a safety guidewire can be used to maintain access to the ureter. Although this may make fluid distension of the lumen more difficult, it does provide a guide back into the orifice. A safety wire is also useful to keep the lumen tented open. Its presence can have an advantage or disadvantage depending on the original site of the tumor. If the lesion is located posteriorly or laterally in the ureter, then that area is usually visualized more completely. If the lesion is along the anteromedial segment of the ureter, the wire may be in the way and obscure visualization. The goal of the maneuver is to revisualize the area of the tumor and identify the base so that it can be treated. In the case of the smaller tumor (<1 cm), with a single base, it can usually be identified and treated with the holmium laser or an electrode.

Considerable manipulation of the ureteroscope may be required to place a device, either biopsy forceps or an ablative device. It may be necessary to angle the ureteroscope from the opposite side of the ureter to approach the lesion or place it parallel to the ipsilateral ureteral wall. Furthermore, it may be necessary to work around the wire. Occasionally, it is necessary to advance the wire manually to move it from the medial ureteral wall.

The entire collecting system must be examined endoscopically. This can be done initially if it will make a difference in the treatment. Conversely, it can be done after biopsy and treatment of the distal tumor if there is a risk of damaging the tumor, particularly a very small lesion, during the flexible ureteroscopy.

Large Ureteral Tumor

Large tumors in any location pose additional different problems. In the ureter, tumors that can be considered large may be voluminous or extensive. There are different approaches to each type of lesion. Both biopsy and treatment techniques are different.

Extensive patches of low grade and low volume papillary tumor can be seen coating the walls of the ureter. In our experience, we have seen it ranging from up to 2–3 cm in length. The tumor may be located on one ureteral sidewall or circumferentially. Generally, these lesions are usually of such small volume that they are best biopsied with a cup forceps. Several different areas should be biopsied. The tumor is then treated very carefully. Every effort must be made to avoid circumferential damage to the ureteral wall itself in order to decrease risk of stricture formation. The holmium laser appears to be the safest device for treatment of superficial ureteral lesions [33, 34]. If a holmium laser of variable pulse duration is available, the longer duration (700 vs. 350 μs) should be employed to maximize the coagulative effect and minimize bleeding. The fiber can be placed just off the surface of the lesions to coagulate and ablate the tumor. It is most efficiently applied in an arching movement across the surface of the tumor and parallel to the ureteral wall to remain a safe distance from the wall. It is also usually more effective to start proximally along the lesion and work distally. By approaching it in the opposite direction from distal to proximal, it is easy to lose visualization of the adequacy of treatment and also to inadvertently perforate the ureteral wall.

While it is typically undesirable to treat the ureter circumferentially due to the risk of stricture, it may be necessary for certain extensive tumors in order achieve oncological control. However, the integrity of the ureteral wall can be maintained by a superficial application of the holmium laser. In doing so, structural damage to the muscularis with resultant stricture can be avoided.

A small cautery electrode may be used for these lesions but is much riskier and discouraged. In contrast to the controlled and precise holmium laser which penetrates <0.5 mm, there is a chance of deeper penetration of the electrical energy with damage to the wall of the ureter itself. If it is the only device available, then a very small electrode (2 F) is used to sweep across the papillary tumor very superficially. The desired result is coagulation of the individual papillary lesions.

After resection of such extensive tumors, an indwelling stent should be left in place for several days to 2 weeks to allow drainage through the edema expected in the resected area.

Large ureteral tumors can be considered those that are >1 cm in length. We have been able to resect papillary transitional cell carcinomas up to 3 cm in length. These lesions demand the application of several different techniques for complete tumor removal. Preoperative studies may provide some preliminary information regarding the location, size, and extent of the tumor. Namely, CTU has emerged as the gold standard imaging study and may even suggest extraluminal extension of the lesion. Intraoperatively, the lesion is first defined by radiographic and endoscopic inspection.

During intraoperative inspection of the bladder, a retrograde ureteropyelogram is performed using a cone-tipped catheter and dilute 50 % iodinated contrast (Fig. 25.2). It may demonstrate

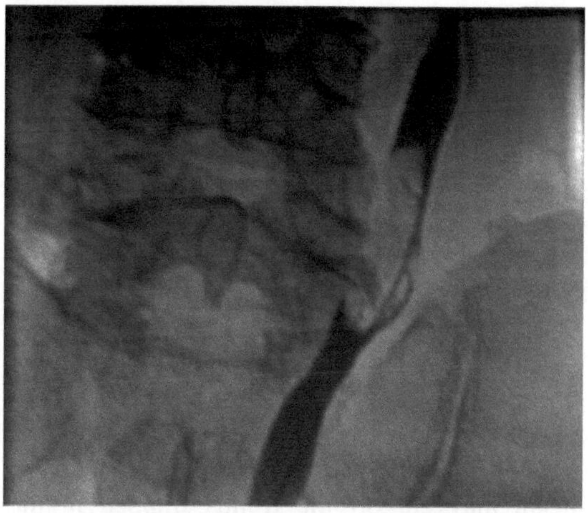

Fig. 25.2 A retrograde ureteropyelogram shows a 3-cm ureteral tumor

obstruction at the site of the large ureteral tumor or may show contrast flowing beyond it to define its extent. The distal portion of the ureter from the orifice to the lower margin of the tumor is then inspected ureteroscopically. Any lesions noted are biopsied and treated prior to defining and treating the dominant ureteral lesion. As the tumor is inspected, the total extent and the ureteral wall should be defined circumferentially. Every attempt should be made to gain access proximal to the tumor either with a guidewire or preferably with the ureteroscope itself. Contrast can be injected directly through the ureteroscope at the level of the tumor and above it, if possible, to give an outline on fluoroscopy of the entire extent of the tumor. If access is gained above the tumor, it is preferable to examine the proximal portions of the ureter and the intrarenal collecting system to define the full extent and any multifocality of the neoplasm. This can help in making a decision regarding treatment.

The ureteral lesion(s) should then be biopsied endoscopically. If it is a large papillary lesion, then it is usually fragile enough to be biopsied with a flat-wire basket. A basket is opened with the largest portion adjacent to the papillary section. Next, it is manipulated to bury the wires into the tumor. The basket is then closed with appropriate advancement of the basket to compensate for the movement expected during closure. In this

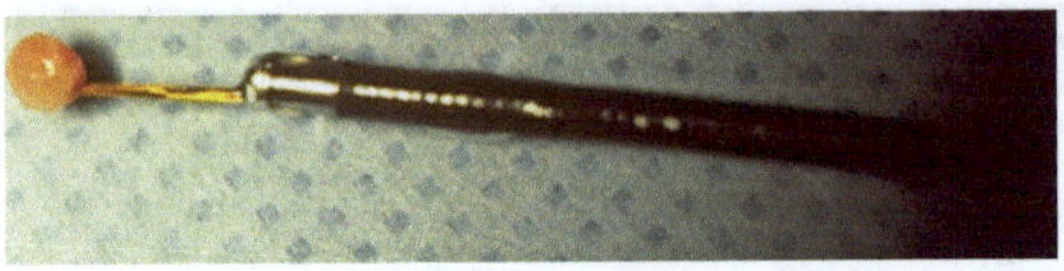

Fig. 25.3 A fragment of tumor, which is too large to pass through the channel of the ureteroscope is trapped within the basket. Therefore, the entire unit of tumor, basket, and ureteroscope are removed

way, the wires of the tumor are maintained in the same position of the tumor to close it onto the captured fronds. The basket should be closed snugly but not tightly. If it is too tight, then the sheath may cut off the fronds trapped in the wires.

If the tumor specimen is too large to pass through the channel of the ureteroscope (approximately 1 mm), then the entire unit of tumor, basket, and ureteroscope should be removed (Fig. 25.3). Otherwise, the tumor would be sheared off and lost. There is always some bleeding with this procedure, but it is usually surprisingly minor. The procedure can be repeated to retrieve additional tissue samples and also to debulk the volume of the tumor. Care should be taken not to entrap a larger fragment of the tumor. The goal in sampling is to avulse a sample of the tumor, not the ureteral wall. If too large a fragment has been entrapped and it cannot be removed easily, then it should be released. The basket is opened and the process reversed to disengage the wires.

Following adequate tumor biopsy and mechanical debulking, treatment of the ureteral tumor is then continued with one of the ablative devices. The holmium laser is the device of choice for all ureteral lesions because of the lower risk of ureteral stricture with this controlled energy source. Again, if a holmium laser with variable pulse duration is available, then the longer duration (700 vs. 350 μs) is preferred to maximize coagulation. The longer duration provides the same energy per pulse yielding less intensity and improved coagulation; the longer pulse retains some ablative properties; the shorter pulse maximizes ablation. We tend to start with settings of 0.6 J and 10–15 Hz. If it is possible to access the proximal portion of the tumor, then it is best to initiate resection proximally and work distally. Any papillary tumor is treated as it is seen against the wall of the ureter. The ureteroscope and fiber should be moved in an arc-like fashion along the ureteral contour at the base of the tumor. As the tumor is ablated, the ureteroscope is moved more distally to treat lower portions of the tumor. It may not be possible to get a good position to treat the tumor proximally and, in such cases, the distal face must be approached initially. The volume of tumor usually within the central portion of the lumen is ablated with the holmium laser. Again, the fiber should be moved across the surface to cut across tumor and to maximize the surface affected by the laser. If a small base of the tumor can be defined by the initial or subsequent inspection along the ureteral wall, then the resection is aimed to resect the base. This is rarely possible and the major volume of the tumor must be resected first before finding and treating the base.

In addition to the holmium:YAG laser, the Nd:YAG laser is also an effective device for treating neoplasms throughout the urinary tract. However, we prefer to avoid the use of the Nd:YAG laser in the ureter because of its deeper penetration and attendant higher risk of ureteral stricture. Instead, the Nd:YAG is used in the renal pelvis and certainly within the bladder. Its major effect is coagulative, and thus, it is very useful for deeper coagulation of larger tumors. However, it does not ablate and coagulated tissue must be removed mechanically or with the holmium laser. Combined use of the holmium and Nd:YAG lasers is very helpful in minimizing bleeding and accomplishing resection, but its use in the upper tract should be restricted to the intrarenal collecting system.

Lower Infundibulum

The lower infundibulum can present the greatest challenge to total treatment of intraluminal neoplasm. Small, flexible ureteroscopes with full deflection can usually examine the lowest infundibulum to detect the presence of a neoplasm. They are also effective to deliver a working instrument, such as a basket to that area for stone retrieval. However, tumor biopsy and treatment requires much greater precision in placing working instruments. The stiff shaft of the cup forceps extremely limits the deflection of the flexible ureteroscope to no more than 90–110°. Obviously, this is inadequate to reach the lower pole. Instead, a flat-wire basket may prove useful to access difficult to biopsy lower pole tumors.

In addition to tissue sampling, treatment of tumors located in the lower infundibulum also presents a challenge. The medial wall of the lower infundibulum is the most difficult to access for adequate treatment. It is usually necessary to use a 200-μ laser fiber or smaller, if it is available. However, even with this instrument, there is some loss of deflection. It also should be noted that the lasers are aimed directly from the fiber with little lateral scatter. The holmium does have some lateral effect which is more an ablative or blast effect when the tip is close to but not pointed directly at tissue. In this situation, when it cannot directly target the tissue, the energy can be increased, for example, to 1 J to maximize this blast effect.

An electrode can be used for electrofulguration. A 2 F electrode allows more deflection of the tip of the flexible ureteroscope than the 200-μ laser fiber. The electrode also has the advantage of coagulation from the side of the tip. As opposed to laser fibers, it is not necessary to point the device directly at the tissue. The major disadvantage is deeper penetration with resultant scarring. Therefore, we reserve use of the electrode only for the most difficult access situations such as the lower infundibulum.

Extensive Renal Pelvic Tumor

Extensive, even low-grade tumors in the renal pelvis can be difficult to encompass. It could appear as a carpeting of papillary lesions throughout the pelvis and possible extending into infundibula. When it is truly limited to the renal pelvis, it is easier to encompass than that extending into the infundibula.

In preparation for treatment, careful retrograde pyelographic studies should be performed to define the extent of tumor. RPG may demonstrate the classic finding of a filling defect. There may be irregularity of the collecting system with diffuse small papillary tumors (Fig. 25.4). Less commonly, RPG may reveal excluded calyces due to calyceal obstruction by tumor. These are not seen directly but must be inferred from the overall pattern of the collecting system when there is a suggestion of an infundibulum or calyx that should be present but fails to opacify. Although initial RPG from the level of the bladder may not demonstrate extensive small papillary lesions, additional studies may be performed by injecting contrast through the ureteroscope itself. The tumor should be sampled extensively by biopsy and washing. The cup forceps is most effective to biopsy small papillary lesions. Several different sites of the involved area should be biopsied. Additionally, the pelvis should be washed with saline introduced through the ureteroscope

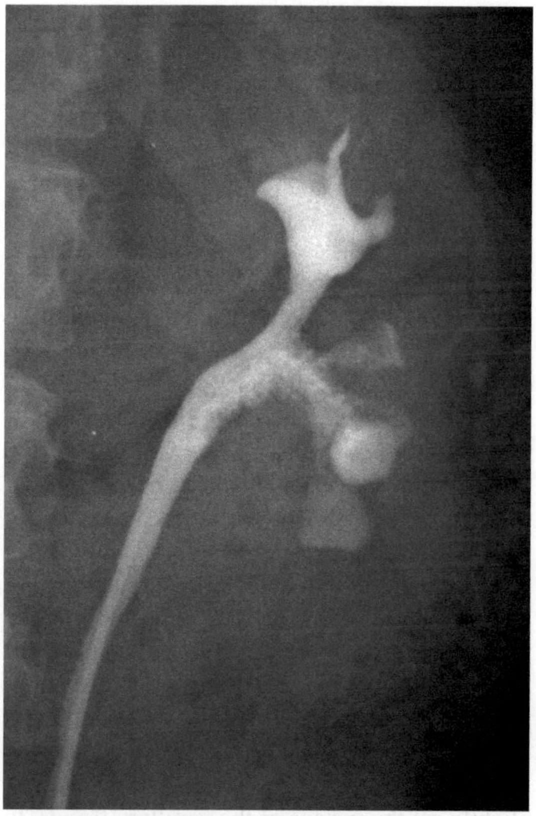

Fig. 25.4 Irregularity of the entire collecting system reflects the presence of papillary tumor

onto the affected area and aspirated directly, both before and after biopsies to improve sample yield. Low-grade papillary lesions can be expected to be low grade, low stage UC, while the presence of high-grade cells in the irrigant raises the suspicion of carcinoma in-situ which may necessitate further treatment [35–41].

After sufficient sampling, tumor in the renal pelvis can be treated most effectively with the holmium laser. A relatively low energy setting (0.5–0.6 J) and a rapid frequency at least 10–15 Hz should be utilized to maximize the coagulation. A longer pulse duration is also beneficial for hemostasis.

In treating the lesion, the laser beam is aimed at the tumor and then moved across the surface in a painting or spraying pattern. Generally, it is more effective to move side to side rather than in and out because of the risks of perforation for the latter pattern. However, if there is renal movement with respiration, it is often possible to maintain the position of the ureteroscope and allow the tumor-bearing renal pelvis to pass through the laser treatment area. The tip should be maintained slightly off the surface of the papillary fronds, to coagulate and ablate, while the renal pelvic wall stays intact. Often, it is not necessary to use the Nd:YAG laser for these lesions. However, since it penetrates more deeply and does not require tissue contact, it can reach tumors that can be seen in the distance and not approached directly. Due to the greater surface area, there is less risk of scarring and stricturing in the renal pelvis than in the ureter.

The treatment becomes even more difficult if the papillary tumor extends into the infundibula and calyces. In such cases, as in the ureter, there is a risk of circumferential damage to the infundibulum with resultant scarring and stricture. Therefore, only holmium:YAG is recommended to decrease the risk of infundibular stenosis. If an infundibulum is seen and essentially obscured by small papillary tumor, the ureteroscope should be advanced into the calyx to determine the extent of the tumor. Here, as in the ureter, it is safest to start the resection proximally and then work distally toward the renal pelvis to maintain orientation and to prevent perforation.

Large-Volume Renal Pelvic Tumors

Adequate biopsies should be taken to obtain sufficient material for an accurate diagnosis. The renal pelvis should be washed with saline for collection of cytologic specimen in a search for unsuspected high-grade cells. In fact, it could suggest the presence of carcinoma in-situ or a focus of high-grade tumor, not adequately sampled and necessitating further diagnosis or treatment.

In the renal pelvis, there is more room to maneuver the ureteroscope than in the ureter. There is also much less risk of stricture from damage to the renal pelvis. Some of the tumor can be debulked with baskets and biopsies. However, this may induce bleeding that will obscure visibility. This seems to be more common within the renal pelvis than in the ureter. If bleeding does occur, it may slow with several minutes without irrigation or aspiration to allow some clot to form on the surface. Treatment can then be started on a visible papillary tumor. In the renal pelvis, the combination holmium and Nd:YAG laser is ideal and their unique capabilities can be exploited. While the Nd:YAG provides excellent coagulation, the holmium:YAG offers some coagulation but better ablation. The Nd:YAG is first applied to the papillary tumor which will blanch and turn white as it is adequately coagulated. Again, a painting motion is used to offer greater exposure of the surface of the tumor. It is important not to allow the laser fiber to penetrate into the papillary mass or tumor beyond the visual field. This tends to cause bleeding and perforation when either laser is being used. With this combined laser technique, the tumor is gradually reduced in volume and removed. As the renal pelvis is approached, the contour of the wall must be taken into consideration. As in the ureter, the ureteroscope should be rotated side to side to paint the tumor as it conforms to the wall of the renal pelvis. However, in the renal pelvis, the cranial-caudal contour is also more prominent. For example, in the upper or cranial portion of the pelvis, it may taper toward the upper infundibula. Large tumors may obscure infundibula which must be defined both radiographically and endoscopically. These areas of the contours also must be considered in planning and carrying out the resection. At the end of the resection, it is then safe to coagulate the base with the Nd:YAG laser. Following laser ablation and resection, additional renal pelvis aspirates should be obtained to increase the biopsy yield.

High-Grade Tumors

High-grade tumors of the ureter and renal pelvis may not be identified by inspection alone [16]. However, some findings are very suggestive of a higher-grade lesion. For example, sessile tumors are more likely to be high grade. It is usually more effective to biopsy sessile lesions with a cup forceps. Multiple samples should be taken to obtain adequate tissue for diagnosis. In the renal pelvis, these lesions can be treated with a combination of the lasers but with preponderance of the Nd:YAG which will provide the deepest coagulation. In the ureter, however, the preference should be for the holmium:YAG laser to minimize the risk of scarring.

Another finding suggestive of a higher grade tumor is loss of pliability of the ureter or renal pelvis. In the ureter, this may be manifest as a narrow or a strictured area at the tumor which does not open easily with the passage of the endoscope. In the renal pelvis, it may appear as an area that does not distend easily or change contour as the surrounding pelvis changes shape or volume.

Grade on endoscopic biopsy has been strongly correlated with grade of the overall tumor with reasonable accuracy [35–37]. Furthermore, grade obtained on ureteroscopic biopsy has been well correlated with pathologic stage on nephroureterectomy specimen and prognosis [35, 38–41]. High grade tumors are more likely to be high stage, and thus, radical nephroureterectomy with bladder cuff excision is advocated in the majority of patients. In patients with previously diagnosed high-grade UTUC, either by biopsy or the presence of high-grade malignant cells localized to the area of the tumor, ureteroscopic treatment may be indicated in certain circumstances. For example, the patient may refuse nephroureterectomy which would render them either anephric or in chronic renal failure. Others may be too ill to tolerate a more extensive, nonendoscopic procedure. These are very extenuating circumstances and the patients should understand the risks, including scarring from treatment, recurrence, and the high probability of progression and even metastases with death. For high-grade tumors in the renal pelvis which must be treated, we tend to maximize the use of the Nd:YAG laser to coagulate the majority of the tumor and to provide deeper penetration. If there is, for example, a 15-mm lesion in the renal pelvis, it can be treated with the combination of lasers. It is first coagulated deeply with the neodymium and then resected with the holmium laser. As the base is approached, the Nd:YAG is used to treat that basal area where the extension is likely. In the ureter, a similar treatment can be employed with a combination of the two lasers. However, there the risk of damage to the ureter with scarring and stricture is very high. If such treatment were planned, then the patient should be informed to expect the placement and maintenance of a stent for drainage. Although it is unusual to treat high-grade tumor endoscopically, many reported series have included some high-grade lesions which have been treated successfully [42].

Irrigation

As with other endoscopic procedures, irrigation is maintained to clear the visual field and distend the lumen. Saline is the preferred irrigant since it is physiologic and is harmless if there is some absorption [43]. In very rare instances, it may be helpful and valuable to irrigate with water to lyse some of the red cells and improve the visualization. However, there is a risk of absorption, which is greater in these difficult and long procedures. Importantly, the irrigation solution should not be switched from saline to water until all cytologic aspirates have been obtained because water is hypoosmotic and thus result in cell lysis.

We use a handheld 50- to 60-mL disposable syringe for irrigation to permit total control over the flow rate and pressure. The outflow travels along the ureter to the bladder. When working within the pelvis, the outflow can be diminished. As the pelvis becomes full by visual inspection, the irrigant should be aspirated from the pelvis mainly through the working channel. The effluent can be used as a cytologic specimen if needed. Similarly, if there is bleeding in the visual field, it can be irrigated and aspirated again as necessary. The bladder should also be emptied intermittently as it fills with irrigant. A Foley catheter may be inserted alongside the flexible ureteroscope and the bladder is then decompressed. Alternatively, the ureteroscope is removed and the bladder is emptied with the cystoscope sheath before ureteroscope reinsertion. At all times, care must be taken to avoid overfilling the collecting system since this may induce submucosal hemorrhage and forniceal rupture.

Ureteral Access Sheath

A ureteral access sheath is not necessary for the vast majority of ureteroscopy in the upper tract for neoplasm. The problems with placement of the sheath, the risks of mucosal trauma, and the difficulty deflecting the ureteroscope after the sheath has been passed are well noted. Additionally, premature placement of a ureteral access sheath may obscure detection of any unexpected ureteral tumors. One advantage of the sheath is to provide a relatively low pressure within the renal pelvis. However, for a tumor procedure, it is helpful to have the pelvis slightly distended to visualize the extent of the pelvis. It is necessary to note the distension and to aspirate the pelvis intermittently to prevent overdistension.

Staged Procedures

For the larger and more extensive tumors, it may be impossible to achieve complete treatment in one procedure, either because of limitation of time or because of difficulty visualizing the field secondary to bleeding. For the extensive low-grade tumors, the procedure can be discontinued. The pelvis is drained with a double pigtail ureteral stent until returning for a second procedure within 2–6 weeks. In the case of larger tumors where the actual bulk of the tumor limits completion, one useful maneuver is to treat the remaining visible tumor extensively with the Nd:YAG laser to get deep coagulation. Repeat inspection should not be less than 4 weeks to allow time for necrosis and resolution of any coagulated tumor.

Conclusions

Ureteroscopic laser resection is an efficacious minimally invasive, nephron-sparing approach for the management of upper tract urothelial carcinoma. Developments in flexible ureteroscopy and use of the holmium and neodymium:YAG lasers have been integral to the success of this approach. Although initially reserved for patients with imperative indications including solitary kidney, compromised contralateral kidney, or preexisting renal insufficiency, ureteroscopic laser resection is being increasingly used on an elective basis to preserve renal function. More challenging cases such as tumors at the ureteral orifice, large ureteral or renal pelvic tumors, and lower infundibulum tumors may be effectively treated with application of more advanced endoscopic techniques. Due to the high risk of bladder and/or upper tract recurrence, all patients must adhere to a strict endoscopic surveillance protocol.

References

1. Batata M, Grabstald H. Upper urinary tract urothelial tumors. Urol Clin North Am. 1976;3:79–86.
2. Shinka T, Uekado Y, Aoshi H, et al. Occurrence of uroepithelial tumors of the upper urinary tract after the initial diagnosis of bladder cancer. J Urol. 1988;140:745–8.
3. Rabbani F, Perrotti M, Russo P, Herr HW. Upper tract tumors after an initial diagnosis of bladder cancer: argument for long term surveillance. J Clin Oncol. 2001;19:94–100.
4. Libertino JA, Bosco PJ, Ying CY, et al. Renal revascularization to preserve and restore renal function. J Urol. 1992;147:1485–7.

5. Rouprêt M, Hupertan V, Traxer O, et al. Comparison of open nephroureterectomy and ureteroscopic and percutaneous management of upper urinary tract transitional cell carcinoma. Urology. 2006;67:1181.
6. Lucas SM, Svatek RS, Olgin G, et al. Conservative management in selected patients with upper tract urothelial carcinoma compares favorably with early radical surgery. BJU Int. 2008;102:172.
7. Gadzinski AJ, Roberts WW, Faerber GJ, et al. Long-term outcomes of nephroureterectomy versus endoscopic management for upper tract urothelial carcinoma. J Urol. 2010;183:2148–53.
8. Lau WK, Blute ML, Weaver AL, et al. Matched comparison of radical nephrectomy vs nephron-sparing surgery in patients with unilateral renal cell carcinoma and a normal contralateral kidney. Mayo Clin Proc. 2000;75:136.
9. McKiernan J, Simmons R, Katz J, et al. Natural history of chronic renal insufficiency after partial and radical nephrectomy. Urology. 2002;59:816–20.
10. Snow DC, Bhayani SB. Rapid communication: chronic renal insufficiency after laparoscopic partial nephrectomy and radical nephrectomy for pathologic T1a lesions. J Endourol. 2008;22:337–41.
11. Go AS, Chertow GM, Fan D, et al. Chronic kidney disease and the risks of death, cardiovascular events, and hospitalization. N Engl J Med. 2004;351:1296.
12. Mathew A, Devereaux PJ, O'Hare A, et al. Chronic kidney disease and postoperative mortality: a systematic review and meta-analysis. Kidney Int. 2008;73: 1069–81.
13. Chen GL, Bagley DH. Ureteroscopic management of upper tract transitional cell carcinoma in patients with normal contralateral kidneys. J Urol. 2000;164:1173–6.
14. Elliott DS, Segura JW, Lightner D, et al. Is nephroureterectomy necessary in all cases of upper tract transitional cell carcinoma? Long-term results of conservative endourologic management of upper tract transitional cell carcinoma in individuals with a normal contralateral kidney. Urology. 2001;58:174–8.
15. Lee D, Trabulsi EJ, McGinnis D, et al. Totally endoscopic management of upper tract transitional cell carcinoma. J Endourol. 2002;16:37–41.
16. El-Hakim A, Weiss GH, Lee BR, et al. Correlation of ureteroscopic appearance with histologic grade of upper tract transitional cell carcinoma. Urology. 2004;63:647–50.
17. Bian Y, Ehya H, Bagley DH. Cytologic diagnosis of upper urinary tract neoplasms by ureteroscopic sampling. Acta Cytol. 1995;39:733–40.
18. Chaubal A, McCue PA, Bagley DH, et al. Multimodal cytologic evaluation of upper urinary tract urothelial lesions. J Surg Pathol. 1995;1:31–5.
19. Zincke H, Aguilo JJ, Farrow GM, et al. Significance of urinary cytology in the early detection of transitional cell cancer of the upper urinary tract. J Urol. 1976;116:781–3.
20. Bagley DH, Kulp DA, Bibbo M. Ureteroscopic biopsy optimized by cytopathologic techniques. J Urol. 1994;151:387A.
21. Low RK, Moran ME, Anderson KR. Ureteroscopic cytologic diagnosis of upper tract lesions. J Endourol. 1993;7:311–4.
22. Tawfiek ER, Bibbo M, Bagley DH. Ureteroscopic biopsy: technique and specimen preparation. Urology. 1997;50:117–9.
23. Abdel-Razzak OM, Ehya H, Cubler-Goodman A, Bagley DH. Ureteroscopic biopsy in the upper urinary tract. Urology. 1994;44:451–7.
24. Conlin MJ, Marberger M, Bagley DH. Ureteroscopy, instrumentation and development. Urol Clin North Am. 1997;24:25–42.
25. Murphy DM, Zincke H, Furlow WL. Management of high grade transitional cell cancer of the upper urinary tract. J Urol. 1981;125:25–9.
26. Bloom NA, Vidone RA, Lytton B. Primary carcinoma of the ureter. A report of 102 cases. J Urol. 1970;103:590–8.
27. Crockett DG, Wagner DG, Holmäng S, et al. Upper urinary tract carcinoma in Lynch syndrome cases. J Urol. 2011;184:1627–30.
28. Wang LJ, Wong YC, Chuang CK, et al. Diagnostic accuracy of transitional cell carcinoma on multidetector computerized tomography urography in patients with gross hematuria. J Urol. 2009;181:524–31.
29. McCoy JG, Honda H, Reznicek M, Williams RD. Computerized tomography for detection and staging of localized and pathologically defined upper tract urothelial tumors. J Urol. 1991;146:1500–3.
30. Milestone B, Friedman AC, Seidmon EJ, et al. Staging of ureteral transitional cell carcinoma by CT and MRI. Urology. 1990;36:346–50.
31. Chen GL, El-Gabry EA, Bagley DH. Surveillance of upper urinary tract transitional cell carcinoma: the role of ureteroscopy, retrograde pyelography, cytology and urinalysis. J Urol. 2000;165:1901–4.
32. Grasso M, Bagley DH. A 7.5/8.2 F actively deflectable, flexible ureteroscope: a new device for both diagnostic and therapeutic upper urinary tract endoscopy. Urology. 1994;43:435–41.
33. Bagley DH. Ureteroscopic laser treatment of upper urinary tract tumors. J Clin Lasers Med Surg. 1998;16:55–9.
34. Bagley DH, Erhard M. Use of the holmium laser in the upper urinary tract. Tech Urol. 1995;1:25–30.
35. Keeley FX, Kulp DA, Bibbo M, et al. Diagnostic accuracy of ureteroscopic biopsy in upper tract transitional cell carcinoma. J Urol. 1997;157:33–7.
36. Daneshmand S, Quek MD, Huffman JL. Endoscopic management of upper urinary tract transitional cell carcinoma: long term experience. Cancer. 2003;98: 55–60.
37. Skolarikos A, Griffiths TRC, Powell PH, et al. Cytologic analysis of ureteral washings is informative in patients with grade 2 upper tract TCC considering endoscopic treatment. Urology. 2003;61:1146–50.
38. Brown GA, Matin S, Buzby JE, et al. Ability of clinical grade to predict final pathologic stage in upper urinary tract transitional cell carcinoma: implications for therapy. Urology. 2007;70:252–6.

39. Charbit L, Gendreau M-C, Mee S, et al. Tumors of the upper urinary tract: 10 years of experience. J Urol. 1991;146:1243–6.
40. Nielsen K, Ostri P. Primary tumors of the renal pelvis: evaluation of clinical and pathological features in a consecutive series of 10 years. J Urol. 1988;140:9–21.
41. Mufti GT, Gove JRW, Badenoch DF, et al. Transitional cell carcinoma of the renal pelvis and ureter. Br J Urol. 1989;63:135–40.
42. Suh RS, Faerber GJ, Wolf JS. Predictive factors for applicability and success with endoscopic treatment of upper tract urothelial carcinoma. J Urol. 2003;170:2209–16.
43. Zeltser I, Pearle MS, Bagley DH. Saline is our friend (commentary). Urology. 2009;74:28–9.

Endourologic Management of Nonmalignant Bilharzial Urinary Complications

26

Hamdy Mohamed Ibrahim, Ahmad Samy Bedair, and Ahmed M. Al-Kandari

Introduction

Urinary schistosomiasis is a chronic parasitic infection of the circulatory system caused by *S. haematobium* which affects the bladder and subsequently the urinary tract system of man. The effect of *S. haematobium* infection is due to deposition of eggs in the bladder and ureter which elicits chronic granulomatous injury. This granulomatous inflammation causes nodules, polypoid lesions, and ulcerations of the lumen of the ureter and bladder, which results clinically in urinary frequency, dysuria, and terminal hematuria. The disease may progress and terminate in renal failure or carcinoma of the bladder. The clinical picture and disease outcomes in persons infected with *S. haematobium* vary dramatically, ranging from mild symptoms to severe damage of the urinary tract including the kidney and bladder [1].

H.M. Ibrahim, M.D. (✉)
Department of Urology, Faculty of Medicine, Fayoum University, 83-Area D, Pyramids Gardens, Giza 63514, Egypt
e-mail: hamdyibrahim4@yahoo.com

A.S. Bedair, M.D.
Department of Urology, Faculty of Medicine, Cairo University, Gamal Salem Street, Mohandeseen, Giza 11559, Egypt
e-mail: asbedair@hotmail.com

A.M. Al-Kandari, M.D., FRCS(C)
Department of Surgery, Kuwait University, Jabriyah, Kuwait City 13110, Kuwait
e-mail: drakandari@hotmail.com

More than 100 million people in the world, especially in rural and agricultural areas, are affected by bilharziasis of the urogenital tract, a parasitic disease caused by *Schistosoma haematobium* [2]. The prevalence of the disease is closely linked to the educational and economic level of the population, absence of adequate sanitation, and unprotected contact with contaminated fresh water. Bathing, swimming, and fishing are the main activities leading to infection. Frequency of contact is more important than duration of exposure. In this chapter, we describe our experience with the evaluation and endourologic treatment of difficult cases of complicated bilharzial lesions.

Pathogenesis and Pathology

Schistosomal disease results directly from the granulomatous host response to schistosome eggs. Furthermore, the spectrum of serious disease ascribed to *S. haematobium* results from the interaction of four factors: intensity, duration, activity, and focality. These variables determine the morbidity, mortality, and treatment of urinary schistosomiasis [3].

Microscopic examination shows that the polypoid patch consists of scattered or massed composite granulomas separated by edematous granulation tissue diffusely infiltrated by eosinophils, lymphocytes, and plasma cells. Grossly, these areas of granulomatous inflammation result in large, bulky, hyperemic, and polypoid masses

A.M. Al-Kandari et al. (eds.), *Difficult Cases in Endourology*,
DOI 10.1007/978-1-84882-083-8_26, © Springer-Verlag London 2013

projecting into the lumen. Schistosomal polyposis of the urinary bladder consists of multiple large inflammatory polyps and is related to heavy localized egg burdens during the active stage of the disease [4]. As egg laying then ceases, entrapped eggs are destroyed or calcified and the inflammation wanes, being supplanted by fibrous tissue to produce the sandy patches characteristic of chronic urinary schistosomiasis.

Inactive urinary schistosomiasis is characterized by the absence of viable eggs in tissues or urine and the presence of "sandy patches" relatively flat, tan mucosal lesions of various depths, often not sharply defined. Patients also develop schistosomal obstructive uropathy as a result of chronic disease. There are two components to schistosomal obstructive uropathy: obstruction and its effect on the proximal ureter. Schistosomal obstructive uropathy is usually bilaterally asymmetrical [5]. It may occur at the ureteral meatus (1 %), interstitial ureter (10–30 %), juxtavesical ureter (20–60 %), lower third (pelvic) of the ureter (15–50 %), or a contiguous combination of these areas (30–60 %) [6, 7]. The results of these obstructions are hydroureter and hydronephrosis. Three types of hydroureter are associated with schistosomal obstruction: segmental (i.e., cylindrical or fusiform), tonic, and atonic [6]. Segmental ureteral dilatations constitute 25 % of schistosomal obstructive uropathy; nearly 80 % of these are in the lower ureter and are accompanied by concentric ureteral muscular obliteration by fibrosis and sandy patches. Segmental lesions are rarely associated with important hydronephrosis. Tonic hydroureter, found in 25–30 % of patients with schistosomal obstructive uropathy, is a dilated, tortuous, thick-walled, and trabeculated ureter with marked ureteral muscle hypertrophy and retarded peristaltic action. It involves the entire ureter proximal to an obstructive lesion, often a functional stenosis, and is often accompanied by significant hydronephrosis, which usually resolves after relief of obstruction. Atonic hydroureter, seen in 35 % of patients with schistosomal obstructive uropathy, is a markedly dilated, very tortuous, thin-walled ureter, without peristalsis and with atrophic fibrotic ureteral muscle [6].

Hydroureter usually precedes hydronephrosis. Schistosomal hydronephrosis passes from progressive renal pelvic dilatation, then medullary atrophy, to nearly total medullary effacement, before cortical atrophy ensues [5, 6].

Clinical Features

The classic clinical presentation of active schistosomiasis is hematuria with terminal dysuria. Patients may also develop polypoid lesions of the bladder during this phase that can present clinically as a urethral or ureteral obstruction or bleed enough to produce clot retention [8].

After some years, active infection enters a more quiescent period, in which egg deposition and excretion continues at a lower rate and symptoms are diminished. Over 30 % of light infections "resolve" spontaneously in some endemic areas [9]. However, although symptoms are absent, silent obstructive uropathy may develop throughout this phase, as fibrosis replaces polypoid lesions, and the bladder and ureters undergo irreversible damage.

Patients finally enter a chronic inactive phase, in which viable eggs are no longer detected in urine or tissues. Signs and symptoms at this stage are caused by sequelae and complications rather than by the schistosomal infection itself. Of patients with schistosomal obstructive uropathy, 40–60 % present to urologists during this stage of their disease [10].

In up to 50 % of patients, chronic or acute bacterial urinary tract infection is superimposed on their schistosomal obstructive uropathy. Bacterial urinary tract infections associated with schistosomal obstructive uropathy are usually ascending infections caused by the same organisms that cause infections in patients without schistosomiasis [11].

Another manifestation of schistosomal disease is the development of bladder ulcers, which occur in two types. Acute schistosomal ulcers will rarely present in the active stage, when a necrotic polyp sloughs into the urine. The more common chronic schistosomal ulcer is a late sequelae of heavy infection. This lesion is associated with a constant "burning" micturition and intense pelvic and suprapubic pain. Gross hematuria and gross pyuria are found in over half of these patients [12].

Diagnosis

The presence of terminally spined eggs in urinary sediment is diagnostic of active *S. haematobium* infection. In moderate to heavy infections, eggs are almost always present in a routine examination of urinary sediment. In lighter infections, routine urinalysis does not always reveal eggs, so the sedimentation or filtration of a 10-mL volume of urine may be necessary [13].

Diagnostic Markers

Serologic tests (Western blot) that are sensitive and specific for *S. haematobium* are available at the Centers for Disease Control and Prevention (CDC). The tests are highly sensitive and about 95 % specific. They may be useful in diagnosing infection when eggs are not present but do not distinguish between acute infection and chronic disease [14]. Although serologic testing is a valuable diagnostic and epidemiologic tool, finding eggs is the gold standard for diagnosis of active infection.

Other Diagnostic Tests for Urinary Tract Sequelae

Radiography is an important diagnostic tool in the evaluation of the sequelae and complications of urinary schistosomiasis. A plain radiograph of the abdomen may reveal calcification within the urinary tract. The classic presentation of a calcified bladder, which looks like a fetal head in the pelvis, is pathognomonic of chronic urinary schistosomiasis (Fig. 26.1). The seminal vesicles, prostate, posterior urethra, distal ureters, and, in rare instances, the colon may also be calcified. The earliest radiographic changes appear to be striations in the ureters and renal pelvis [15]. Ureteral calcification is typically mural, and the ureter is dilated. This differs from the calcification seen in tuberculous disease, which forms a cast of a nondilated ureter.

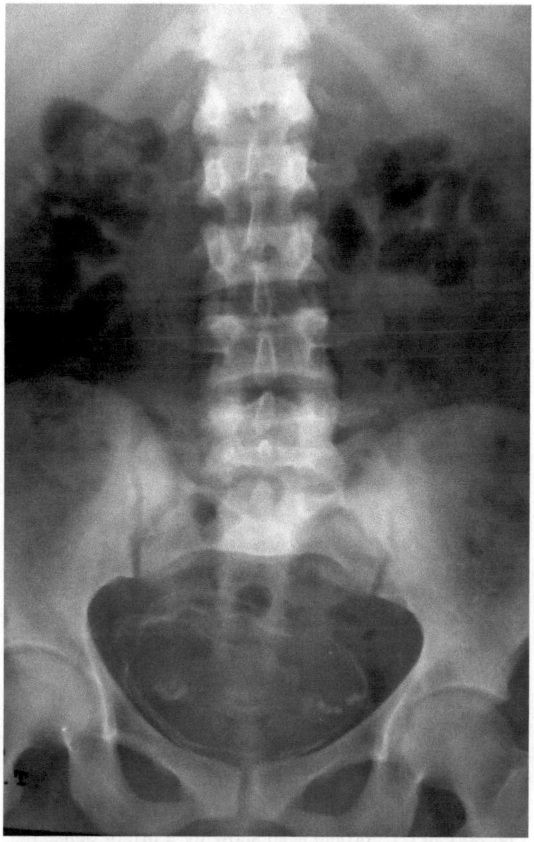

Fig. 26.1 Bladder calcification in a 27-year-old female. Plain x-ray film of the abdomen shows a rim of calcification surrounding the urinary bladder and the lower end of the ureter

Hydroureter, hydronephrosis, nonfunctioning kidney, ureteral stenosis, and bladder and ureteral filling defects such as polypoid lesions are readily observed in a standard intravenous urogram. In the presence of severe obstructive uropathy, delayed films are often needed to discern distended ureters and kidneys. Postvoid films may indicate bladder neck obstruction with retention. Fluoroscopy can differentiate tonic and atonic ureters [16] and identify nonstenotic, immotile ureters. CT, however, can detect both obstructive uropathy and calcified lesions in the urinary tract and the colon and thus complements or substitutes for IVU (Fig. 26.2) [17].

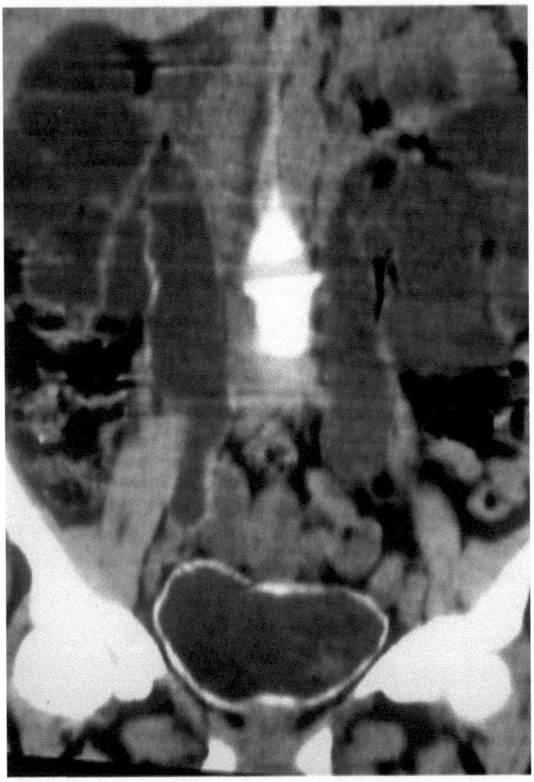

Fig. 26.2 Bladder calcification of the same patient as in Fig. 26.1 in CT coronal scan showing a bright dense line surrounding the bladder

Another useful imaging modality is voiding cystourethrography (VCUG). It indicates the presence of vesicoureteral reflux, which occurs in 25 % of infected ureters. Abdominal ultrasonography is also a useful method to detect focal thickening of the bladder wall and polypoid lesions of the urinary tract, hydroureter, and hydronephrosis in endemic areas, and it detects heavily calcified patches [18].

Preoperative Evaluation

The preoperative evaluation included urinalysis, culture, biochemical profile, and imaging studies (US, CT scan, contrast studies, and radionuclide scan). Antegrade and retrograde ureteropyelography are done when indicated. Renal dynamic scintigraphy is used to determine the split function (split GFR mL/min) of the hydronephrotic units. Kidneys with split GFR of <10 mL/min were considered unsalvageable. Large hydronephrotic kidneys with split GFR of 10–20 mL/min were treated initially by inserting a PCN to predict more accurately the recoverability of function and also to minimize subsequent surgical risks in patients presenting with severe uremia.

Initial percutaneous nephrostomy (PCN) was performed in cases presenting with hugely dilated infected kidney, tense hydronephrosis especially in bilateral obstruction, and in cases with severe azotemia to help improve the general condition and subsequently the operative outcomes.

Surgical Treatments

Endourological options used in this series are covered in the following sections.

Endoscopic Bladder Procedures

Cystoscopic findings are very characteristic. Cystoscopy is generally followed by transurethral resection of the proliferative bladder lesions to provide histologic samples for examination, to reduce bladder irritative symptoms, and to reduce hematuria. Inflammatory polypoid erythematous lesions are mostly found on the dome and lateral walls of the bladder. The "sandy" patches may be seen around the bladder neck and ureteral orifices. Cystoscopy may also be used to evaluate bladder neck stenosis, bladder calcification, and ureteral orifice stenosis.

Chronic bladder ulcers should be biopsied and coagulated or resected.

Bladder neck stenosis often requires incision or a transurethral resection, particularly if an augmentation cystoplasty has to be done, to avoid high-pressure vesicoureteral reflux [19].

Ureteroscopy in Bilharzial Ureter

The wall of bilharzial ureter is thick and may be dilated without obstruction. The ureters may show a generalized or segmental dilatation due to hypotonia or even aperistalsis of the ureter [17, 20]. Thus, it is expected that manipulation of stones in bilharzial ureter is, in particular, less risky due to its natural thick wall and luminal dilatation [21].

Technique of Ureteroscopy

Under either general or spinal anesthesia, all patients undergo initial formal cystoscopy. The ureteric orifices are identified, and a guidewire is passed to the kidney. In most of the cases, the intramural part of the ureter is dilated using 18-Fr balloon dilator. Standard ureteroscopic stone extraction is done using a dormia basket or forceps with or without intracorporeal lithotripsy. A holmium:YAG laser or pneumatic lithotripsy is used through a 7- to 10.5-Fr graduated semirigid ureteroscope. The stent used in the study was 6 Fr in diameter with the appropriate length determined by the surgeon intraoperatively based on patient height. In all patients, the stent was left for 2 weeks.

At the end of the procedure, patients were transferred from the postanesthesia care unit to the same day surgery ward, where they received intravenous narcotics and/or diclofenac sodium and oral pain medication. All patients were given prophylactic antibiotics at the time of anesthesia induction that is a single dose of 1 g ceftriaxone intravenously. Subsequently, 500 mg ciprofloxacin tablets were given twice daily for 5 days.

In our series published in 2008, all patients with distal ureteral calculi and who had clear evidences of bilharzial lesions in the urinary tract (radiologic/cystoscopic) underwent ureteroscopy (Figs. 26.3 and 26.4). In contrary to the non-bilharzial ureter, ureteral dilatation was done for all bilharzial ureters to overcome varying degrees of narrowing or stenotic segments [22].

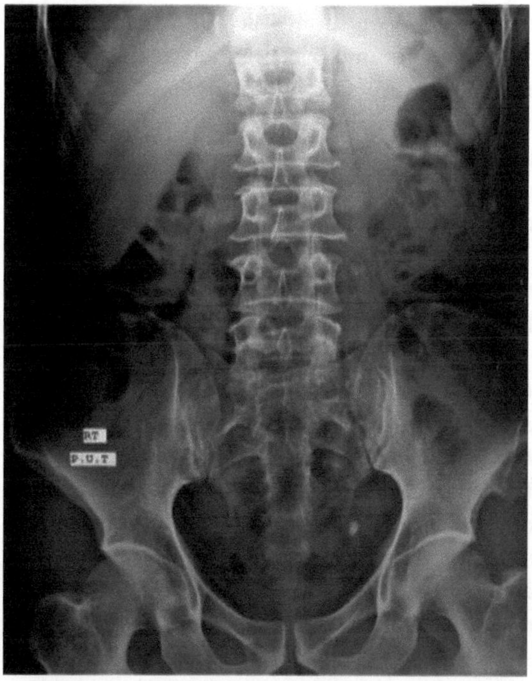

Fig. 26.3 Plain x-ray shows ureteric stone in the lower third of the left ureter

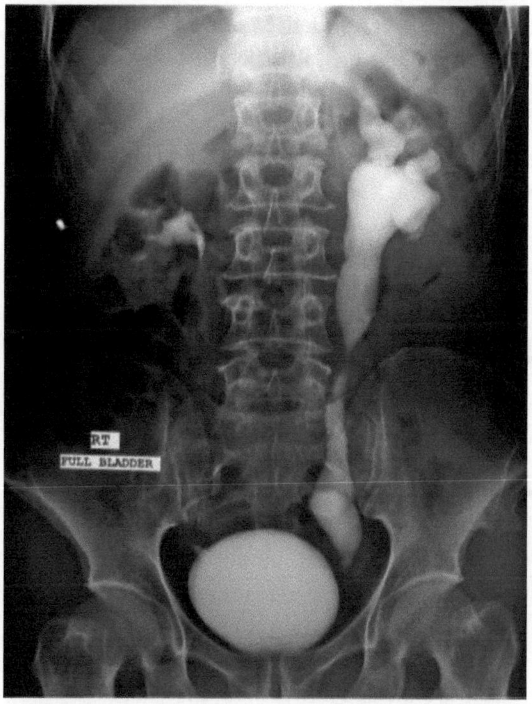

Fig. 26.4 Intravenous urography of the same patient as in Fig. 26.3 showing bilharzial segmental dilatation of the left ureter due to the ureteric stone and bilharziasis

Endoscopic Management of Bilharzial Ureteral Stricture

The advent of endourological techniques and accumulating experience has allowed endoureterotomy to supplant open surgical repair as the treatment of choice for most benign ureteral strictures. Benign ureteral strictures are classified as ischemic and nonischemic or as acute or insidious, but the clinical implications of these distinctions and their impact on the success rate of endoureterotomy remain unclear [23, 24].

Ureteral strictures have traditionally been treated with open operative repair, but success has been achieved with balloon dilation and incision. Davis et al. reported intubated ureterotomy for ureteropelvic junction obstruction and upper ureteral strictures in an animal model and in humans [25, 26]. They noted that the ureteral musculature regenerates around the ureterotomy defect. This simple modification of open reconstructive techniques became the foundation of endoscopic treatment of upper urinary tract obstruction. Cold-knife and electrocautery incisions have been made for endopyelotomy. With the development of retrograde endopyelotomy using a ureteroscopic approach, these principles were easily translated to the management of ureteral stricture. The Acucise® electrosurgical balloon catheter (Applied Medical, Rancho Santa Margarita, CA) has also been used successfully to incise ureteral strictures [27].

There are several important technical considerations in performing endoureterotomy:

- To achieve a successful result, it is essential to make a full-thickness incision through the ureteral wall until fat is visualized and to extend this incision proximally and distally into healthy tissue for 1–2 cm [28].
- In some cases in which this is difficult due to extensive periureteral fibrosis, the use of balloon dilation to open the ureteral incision gently may be helpful [29].
- The incision must be planned carefully to avoid injury to periureteral vessels, which can lead to significant hemorrhage. In general, strictures between the ureteropelvic junction and iliac vessels should be incised in a posterolateral direction, while those below the vessels are incised anteromedially [28, 30].
- Extreme proximal or distal strictures can be marsupialized into the renal pelvis or bladder, respectively [28].
- The greatest potential for bleeding occurs with strictures close to the level of the iliac vessels, which are best treated with a direct anterior incision [30].
- Endoluminal ultrasound and preoperative angiography may be helpful in select cases to avoid vascular injury [31, 32].
- The optimal duration of ureteral splinting and stent size remain controversial. Human and animal studies suggest that placement of a stent following endoscopic incision of the ureter is helpful to avoid urinoma formation, which may increase the risk of recurrent stricture [28, 33].
- Since full regeneration of the muscular wall of the ureter may require up to *6* weeks, this interval of postoperative splinting is most commonly chosen. However, successful results with endopyelotomy have been achieved with stents left as briefly as 4 days postoperatively [25].
- The most appropriate stent size also has not been clearly defined, although tapered (14/7 F) double pigtail catheters are used most commonly [28].
- Finally, cold-knife incision is preferred by some investigators, since it may result in less periureteral fibrosis and scarring [29, 34]. However, others who favor electrocautery believe that use of a small Greenwald electrode (3 F) allows for a more precise incision of the proper depth [28]. Recently. holmium laser endoureterotomy emerged as the leading cutting modality; the holmium laser currently seems to be the preferred modality since it allows efficient cutting through a small-diameter ureteroscope [35].

Techniques of Endoureterotomy

Under either general or spinal anesthesia, all patients underwent initial formal cystoscopy. The ureteric orifices were identified, and a retrograde pyelography was done for initial assessment of the ureteral stricture site and length. A guidewire was then advanced across the strictured area to the kidney. A semirigid 8-Fr ureteroscope was advanced up to the stricture level, and contrast material was injected retrograde to better delineate stenosis length, site, and degree. Pulsations at the stricture area were also evaluated.

After passing a second safety wire, balloon dilation was performed, and ureteroscope advancement was attempted through the strictured segment.

Endoureterotomy was done under direct vision using a 550-μ, end-firing fiber, with energy setting of 1–1.2 J and rate of 10–15 Hz of holmium:YAG laser (Lumenis®, Germany, GmbH), starting at the proximal stricture segment and cutting while retracting the ureteroscope. A full-thickness incision was made into the periureteral fat, extending about 5 mm above and below the strictured segment. To minimize the risk of vascular injury, the incision was tailored to the involved segment that is lateral in the proximal ureter, anterior over the iliac vessels, and medial in the distal ureter.

Appropriate incision depth was confirmed by direct vision and by documenting contrast extravasation. After laser endoureterotomy, the strictured area was further dilated by a 6- to 7-mm (18 Fr to 21 F) ureteral balloon dilator, then an endopyelotomy stent (14/7 Fr or 10/6) was placed with the thick part lying along the previous stricture, or two double-J stents (6/7 Fr) were used instead (Figs. 26.5 and 26.6). Ureteral stents remained in situ for 6 weeks.

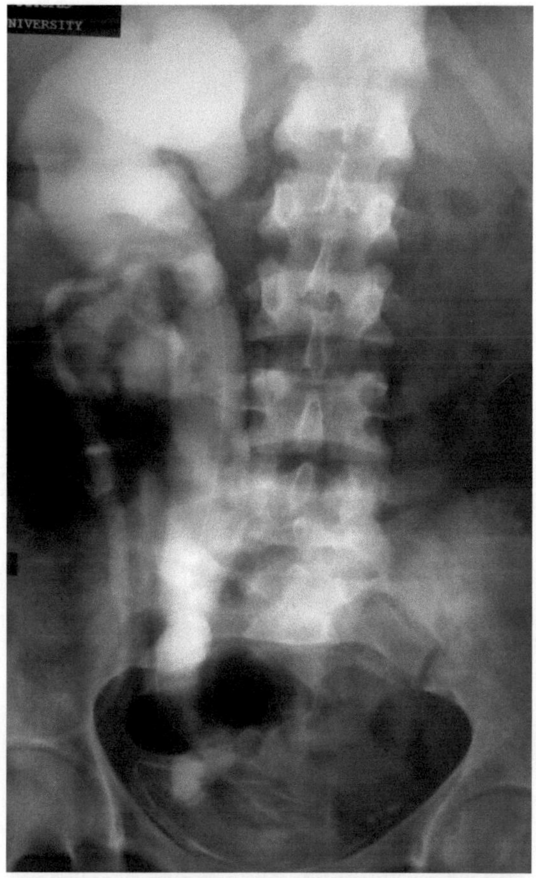

Fig. 26.5 Antegrade study shows markedly dilated kidney and ureter. The contrast is arrested at the distal part of the right ureter (complete obstruction)

Distal Endoureterotomy Technique (for Complete Ureteral Obstruction)

The initial strategy was to bypass the area of the obstruction, which was achieved in various ways depending on individual anatomy. When a ureteral orifice was visible, a 0.038-in. guidewire was passed retrograde with or without a rigid ureteroscope through the stenotic area in an attempt to restore continuity with the upper tract. When it was not possible, percutaneous antegrade access was achieved, and antegrade nephroureteroscopy was performed to the level of obstruction. The stiff end of a 0.038-in. guidewire was then used to puncture through the stricture into the bladder. If the wire did not pass into the bladder from above, it was placed as distal as possible, and a resectoscope with a cautery loop was used retrograde to cut down on the wire under visual guidance when it was visible through the bladder wall or under fluoroscopic guidance at a point nearest the most natural ureteral orifice location. After the guidewire was in place, the procedure was continued or a stent was placed, and definitive treatment was completed later.

During the stage 2 procedure, the endoureterotomy was done using holmium:YAG laser as previously described, or a cutting balloon catheter/ Colin's knife was used to incise the stricture site through the ureter into the bladder under direct vision, marsupializing the dilated ureter proximal to the obstruction into the bladder. An endopyelotomy stent (7/14 Fr) or two 6-Fr double pigtail stents were placed for 6 weeks postoperatively.

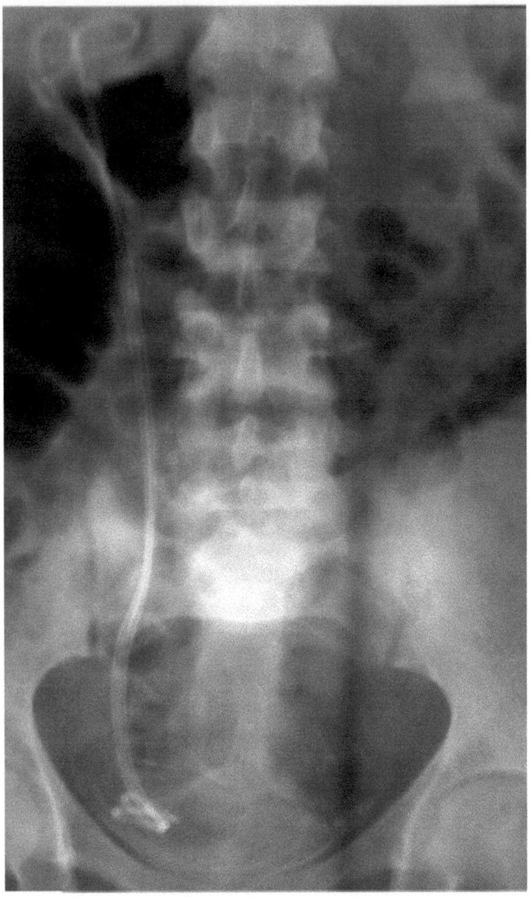

Fig. 26.6 KUB of the same patient shows two double-J stents fixed after endoureterotomy of the right ureter

All patients were followed postoperatively with cystoscopy at 6 weeks to examine the surgical site and remove the ureteral stent. Retrograde pyelography was done at this time to determine ureteral patency. At 6 months, the patients were evaluated by renal ultrasound and/or computerized tomography, and at 1 year, cystoscopy, retrograde pyelography, and furosemide renal scan were performed. Further routine follow-up consisted of history, physical examination, and renal ultrasound every 6 months. When recurrent stricture was suspected, further evaluation by intravenous urogram (IVU) or renal scan was ordered. Success was defined as absence of symptoms and resolution of obstruction on imaging.

References

1. Brouwer KC, Ndhlovu PD, Wagatsuma Y, Munatsi A, Shiff CJ. Epidemiological assessment of *Schistosoma haematobium*-induced kidney and bladder pathology in rural Zimbabwe. Acta Trop. 2003;85:339–47.
2. Savioli L, Renganathan E, Montresor A, Davis A, Behbehani K. Division of Control of Tropical Diseases, Schistosomiasis and Intestinal Parasites Unit, World Health Organization. Control of schistosomiasis – a global picture. Parasitol Today. 1997;13:444–8.
3. Waine GJ, McManus DP. Schistosomiasis vaccine development – the current picture. Bioassays. 1997;19:435.
4. Smith JH, Torky H, Kelada AS, Farid Z. Schistosomal polyposis of the urinary bladder. Am J Trop Med Hyg. 1977;26:85.
5. Smith JH, Torky H, Mansour N, Cheever AW. Studies on egg excretion and tissue egg burden in urinary schistosomiasis. Am J Trop Med Hyg. 1974;23:163.
6. Smith JH, Kelada AS, Khalil A, Torky AH. Surgical pathology of schistosomal obstructive uropathy: a clinicopathologic study. Am J Trop Med Hyg. 1977;26:96.
7. Al-Shukri S, Alwan MH. Bilharzial strictures of the lower third of the ureter: a critical review of 560 strictures. Br J Urol. 1983;55:477.
8. Wilkins HA, Goll PH, Moore PJ. *Schistosoma haematobium* infections and hemoglobin concentrations in a Gambian community. Ann Trop Med Parasitol. 1985; 79:159.
9. Rutasitara WK, Chimbe A. Spontaneous cure in schistosomiasis. East Afr Med J. 1985;62:408.
10. Smith JH, Christie JD. The pathobiology of *Schistosoma haematobium* infection in humans. Hum Pathol. 1986;17:333.
11. King CH. Disease in schistosomiasis haematobia. In: Mahmoud AAF, editor. Schistosomiasis. London: Imperial College Press; 2001. p. 265.
12. Smith JH, Kelada AS, Khalil A. Schistosomal ulceration of the urinary bladder. Am J Trop Med Hyg. 1977;26:89.
13. Mott KE. A reusable polyamide filter for the diagnosis of *Schistosoma haematobium* infection by urine filtration. Bull Soc Pathol Exot. 1983;76:101.
14. Al-Sherbiny MM, Osman AM, Hancock K, et al. Application of immunodiagnostic assays: detection of antibodies and circulating antigens in human schistosomiasis and correlation with clinical findings. Am J Trop Med Hyg. 1999;60:960.
15. Hugosson CO. Striation of the renal pelvis and ureter in bilharziasis. Clin Radiol. 1987;38:407.
16. Abdel-Halim RE, Al-Mashad S, Al-Dabbagh A. Fluoroscopic assessment of bilharzial ureteropathy. Clin Radiol. 1985;36:89.
17. Jorulf H, Linstedt E. Urogenital schistosomiasis: CT evaluation. Radiology. 1985;157:745.
18. Medhat A, Zarzoura A, Nafeh M, et al. Evaluation of an ultrasonographic score for urinary bladder morbidity in *Schistosoma haematobium* infection. Am J Trop Med Hyg. 1997;57:16.

19. Kameh D, Smith A, Brock MS, Ndubisi B, Masood S. Female genital schistosomiasis: case report and review of the literature. South Med J. 2004;97:525–7.
20. Umerah BC. The less familiar manifestations of schistosomiasis of the urinary tract. Br J Radiol. 1977;50:105–9.
21. Hussein A, Rifaat E, Zaki A, et al. Stenting versus non-stenting after non-complicated ureteroscopic manipulation of stones in bilharzial ureters. Int J Urol. 2006;13:886.
22. Ibrahim HM, Al-Kandari AM, Shaaban HS, et al. Role of ureteral stenting after uncomplicated ureteroscopy for distal ureteral stones: a randomized, controlled trial. J Urol. 2008;180:961.
23. Elliot PS, McAninch JW. Ureteral injuries: external and Iatrogenic. Urol Clin North Am. 2006;33:55.
24. Richter F, Irwin RJ, Watson RA, et al. Endourologic management of benign ureteral strictures with and without compromised vascular supply. Urology. 2000;55:652.
25. Abdel-Hakimn AM. Endopyelotomy for ureteropelvic junction obstruction: is long-term stenting mandatory? J Endourol. 1987;1:265.
26. McDonald JH, Calams JA. Experimental ureteral stricture: ureteral regrowth following ureterotomy with and without intubation. J Urol. 1960;84:52.
27. Chandhoke PS, Clayman RV, Stone AM, McDougall EM, Buelna T, Hilal N, Chang M, Stegwell MJ. Endopyelotomy and endoureterotomy with the acucise ureteral cutting balloon device: preliminary experience. J Endourol. 1993;7:45.
28. Meretyk S, Albala DM, Clayman RV, Denstedt JD, Kavoussi LR. Endoureterotomy for treatment of ureteral strictures. J Urol. 1992;147:1502.
29. Conlin MJ, Bagley DH. Incisional treatment of ureteral strictures. In: Smith AD, editor. Smith's textbook of endourology. St. Louis: Quality Medical Publishing; 1996. p. 497–505.
30. Eshghi M. Endoscopic incisions of the urinary tract. Parts I and II. AUA update series. 1989;8:Lessons 37 and 38.
31. Bagley DH, Liu JB, Grasso M, Goldberg BB. Endoluminal sonography in evaluation of the obstructed ureteropelvic junction. J Endourol. 1994;8:287.
32. Bales GT, Jarrard DF, Gerber GS. Ureteroscopic endopyelotomy in an ectopic kidney. Urology. 1995;46:104.
33. Elgammal M, Hassouna M, Li JS, Wang NS, Coolsaet B, Elhilali MM. Effect of balloon catheter dilatation of the ureter on upper tract dynamics and ureteral wall in swine. J Endourol. 1990;4:15.
34. Schneider AW, Conrad S, Busch R, Otto U. The cold-knife technique for endourological management of stenoses in the upper urinary tract. J Urol. 1991;146:961.
35. Lane BR, Desai MM, Hegarty NJ, et al. Long-term efficacy of holmium laser endoureterotomy for benign ureteral strictures. Urology. 2006;67:894.

27 Ureteroscopy During Pregnancy

Hamdy Mohamed Ibrahim
and Ahmed M. Al-Kandari

Introduction

Pregnancy is a physiological state with complex hemodynamic changes. Pain (renal colic) is the most common presentation of urolithiasis, as well as the most common nonobstetric cause of hospitalization during pregnancy. Symptomatic urolithiasis, an uncommon event in pregnancy, is nevertheless of clinical concern because it may adversely affect birth outcome with an increased risk of preterm delivery. In the 9-month duration of pregnancy, the incidence of symptomatic stones appears not to differ from the incidence during a similar interval in women of childbearing age despite increased urinary calcium excretion in pregnancy [1–3].

The gravid uterus causes displacement of intra-abdominal structures whose affliction may mimic renal colic. Misdiagnosis in these cases may have disastrous consequences on the mother and fetus. Consequently, early and accurate detection of urinary lithiasis is of paramount importance. The least invasive radiation-free test is preferred. In patients with refractory ureteral colic, early intervention such as stent placement or ureteroscopic extraction of the stone may be necessary [4].

It is likely that recent improvements in surgical technology may be responsible for the increased use of ureteroscopy (URS) in the treatment of pregnant women. In recent years, there have been great advances in semirigid and flexible ureteroscopes. Consequently, accessing all aspects of the renal collecting system in a safe and expedient manner is now a straightforward endeavor that generally does not require ureteral dilation or another extraordinary maneuver. The widespread use of intracorporeal lithotrites, such as the holmium laser, permits the safe and atraumatic fragmentation of calculi at any location. Improvements in flexible grasping devices have enhanced the efficiency of stone extraction [5].

In this chapter, we describe our experience with the diagnosis and management of difficult conditions in pregnant women. By assessing the clinical data and reviewing the literature, we have tried to set up a diagnostic and management modality for patients with urinary stones during pregnancy.

Anatomical Considerations

Significant anatomic and functional changes occur in the urinary tract during pregnancy. Of these, hydronephrosis has particular relevance in the diagnosis and presentation of urolithiasis. Hydronephrosis occurs in up to 90 % of right

H.M. Ibrahim, M.D. (✉)
Department of Urology, Faculty of Medicine, Fayoum University, 83-Area D, Pyramids Gardens, Giza 63514, Egypt
e-mail: hamdyibrahim4@yahoo.com

A.M. Al-Kandari, M.D., FRCS(C)
Department of Surgery, Kuwait University, Jabriyah, Kuwait City 13110, Kuwait
e-mail: drakandari@hotmail.com

A.M. Al-Kandari et al. (eds.), *Difficult Cases in Endourology*,
DOI 10.1007/978-1-84882-083-8_27, © Springer-Verlag London 2013

kidneys and 67 % of left kidneys in pregnant women [6]. Upper tract dilatation is usually present by 6–10 weeks' gestation and may persist until up to 6 weeks after delivery. Some studies show an increased incidence of hydronephrosis in nulliparous women, which may be secondary to stronger abdominal musculature that is less accommodating to an enlarging uterus [7]. Although physiologic hydronephrosis of pregnancy is typically asymptomatic, it may uncommonly present with renal colic. Regardless, unilateral flank pain associated with hydronephrosis should raise one's suspicion of ureteral stone [8].

Both anatomic and physiologic causes for hydronephrosis of pregnancy have been proposed. One likely factor is extrinsic obstruction of the ureter by the gravid uterus against the fixed pelvic brim. The left ureter may be more protected from this compression by the left colon, accounting for the higher incidence on the right side. Also, the right ureter may be more frequently compressed by the engorged right uterine vein [1]. Ureteral dilatation is generally not present below the level of the uterus at the pelvic brim. Some have attributed this to restriction by Waldeyer's sheath around the distal ureter [9].

Pathophysiology of Urolithiasis

Myriad metabolic conditions affect the risk for urolithiasis. Of these, the three that occur most often in pregnancy are hypercalciuria, hyperuricosuria, and hypercitraturia.

Hypercalciuria

The cause of hypercalciuria of pregnancy is multifactorial. Glomerular filtration rate (GFR) increases in pregnancy. The subsequent increase in tubular flow leads to decreased tubular reabsorption and increased net excretion of calcium. Also, placental formation of 1,25-dihydroxycholecalciferol promotes intestinal reabsorption of calcium and mobilization of calcium from bone [10].

Hyperuricosuria

Hyperuricosuria may also occur during pregnancy [8, 11]. It has been attributed to the increased GFR and subsequent increase in net urinary excretion of uric acid. Even in those who do not have uric acid urolithiasis, hyperuricosuria is of clinical importance because it is a well-recognized risk factor for calcium oxalate nephrolithiasis [12].

Hypercitraturia

Citrate prevents urolithiasis by way of multiple mechanisms. Complexed with calcium, it is more soluble than other calcium salts. Additionally, citrate can act as an inhibitor of crystal growth and aggregation. Citrate depletion is a known cause of urolithiasis in the general population; however, in pregnancy, urine citrate is increased [8, 13].

Clinical Presentations

In many cases, the classic presentation of renal colic because of an obstructing calculus is unmistakable. Symptomatic urolithiasis in the expectant mother may present differently than in the nonpregnant patient, however. Additionally, pregnant women may suffer from abdominal and flank pain, nausea, emesis, and irritative lower urinary tract symptoms unrelated to urolithiasis. The anatomic changes that occur in the gravid abdomen and pelvis can alter the perception, radiation, and localization of pain, making the clinical assessment of abdominal pain difficult [14].

In general, patients present with stone symptoms in the second or third trimesters of pregnancy. At this point in pregnancy, the gravid uterus has enlarged above the pelvic brim and may be impinging on the distal ureter. The most common symptoms of renal or ureteral stones in pregnancy are flank or abdominal pain, microscopic or gross hematuria, and irritative lower urinary tract symptoms. Presenting symptoms may vary depending on the clinical scenario. For example, ureteral stones are more likely to present with classic renal colic. Distal stones may elicit more irritative voiding symptoms [15]. Struvite stones may present with urinary tract infection rather than renal colic [14]. Hydronephrosis of pregnancy may occasionally present with abdominal or flank pain, mimicking stone disease [16, 17].

Diagnostic Imaging

Radiographic imaging is important for treatment planning and diagnosis. Therapy can be planned based on estimation of renal function, stone size, location, configuration, and potential composition, all information gleaned from appropriately selected radiographic studies. Conversely, some of these studies have limited or no use in pregnant women because of concerns regarding fetal risk. The effects of cumulative and threshold doses on fetal risk, the gestational age at which these risks are most pronounced, and the dose delivered by the respective studies are all considered. Some studies can be tailored to reduce fetal risk. Taking all of this into account, one may formulate a plan for using these studies in properly selected patients.

Radiation-Induced Risks

Cell death and teratogenic effects are believed to have a threshold dose below which these effects are unlikely to occur, but above which there may be increasing severity with increasing exposure. Such effects include intrauterine growth retardation and mental retardation. High doses of radiation before implantation and during the first 2 weeks postconception are most likely to result in fetal loss [14]. During the 4- to 10-week gestational period of organogenesis, the fetus is most susceptible to the teratogenic effects of radiation. Doses of less than 5 cGy are not believed to cause intrauterine growth retardation or other fetal anomalies [1, 18]. The delivered dose of radiation varies with the study performed. Most uroradiologic studies can be modified to be performed within the aforementioned 5-cGy limit. This limit can be surpassed, however, with standard computed tomography or excessive fluoroscopy; thus, communication with the radiologist is suggested.

Use of Radiographic Studies

Ultrasound

For most pregnant women who have possible urolithiasis, evaluation may proceed without radiation exposure. Ultrasound shows the renal parenchyma, calyces, and pelvis. Significant renal cortical thinning may suggest chronic obstruction. Dilation of the calyces and renal pelvis is also easily seen. In pregnant patients, the high prevalence of physiologic hydronephrosis further complicates the interpretation. In hydronephrosis of pregnancy, however, ureteral dilation is only above the pelvic brim. If the ureteral dilation extends below the pelvic brim, one should consider distal ureteral obstruction.

Currently, the most promising modification of ultrasonography to better discern obstruction is Doppler ultrasonography, which adds a functional element to the evaluation of the kidney. With Doppler techniques, the velocity of intrarenal blood flow can be quantitated, and the resistive index (RI) can be calculated. Doppler ultrasonography holds significant promise in the evaluation of urolithiasis and in the differentiation of stone obstruction from hydronephrosis of pregnancy (Fig. 27.1a–c).

Excretory Urography

The intravenous pyelogram (IVP) provides anatomic evaluation of radiopaque structures and may reveal radiolucent structures within the urinary tract as filling defects. A proposed protocol includes a scout film followed by a 30-min film. If insufficient information can be gleaned from these, the acquisition of additional films should be based on the 30-min film. A faint nephrogram suggesting a high-grade obstruction may prompt a 2- to 3-h delayed film. Additional measures include judicious collimation, short exposure times, maximal fetal shielding, and prone positioning [14]. With such measures, the exposure may be potentially limited to approximately 1–2 cGy.

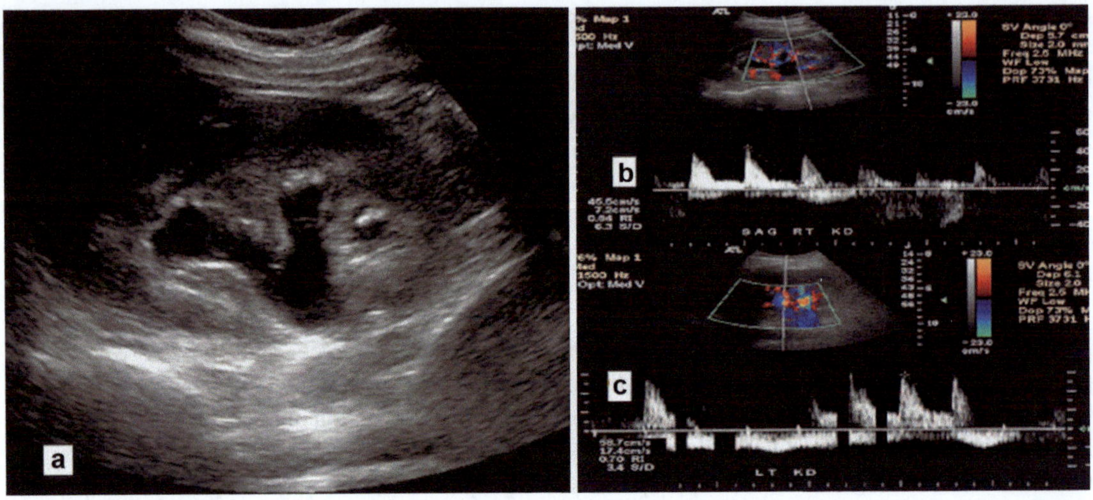

Fig. 27.1 (**a–c**) Thirty-year-old woman with right flank and right lower quadrant pain in the second trimester of pregnancy. (**a**) The right kidney shows moderate hydronephrosis. (**b**, **c**) Doppler US images show RIs of 0.84 in the right kidney (**b**) and 0.70 in the left kidney (**c**). The RI difference between the right and left kidneys (0.14) is consistent with obstruction

CT Scan

Because of its increased speed, elimination of intravenous contrast, and superior sensitivity, the unenhanced helical CT has become the gold standard for diagnosis of a suspected ureteral stone. Renal stone protocol CT on newer multidetector scanners has potential radiation doses of 0.88–1.2 cGy [19]. Low-dose and ultra–low-dose CT protocols have been developed to further limit delivered radiation dose. At present, such techniques remain second-line diagnostic studies, reserved only for those in whom an adequate treatment plan cannot be determined based on clinical examination and ultrasonography. With further evolution of techniques and continued diminishment of dose, CT may become more widely used in this population [20]. The current trend of using low-dose multidetector CT coupled with high accuracy (>95 % sensitivity and >98 % specificity) for detection of calculi in the general population has lowered the threshold for use of abdominal and pelvic nonenhanced CT as a second-line test in pregnancy (Fig. 27.2a, b).

MRI

MRI provides detailed, cross-sectional images without exposure to ionizing radiation. As such, it has been advocated as a nonradiating, noninvasive way to investigate ureteral obstruction in pregnant women. Unfortunately, calculi do not have a distinct appearance on MRI, as they do on CT [21]. High sensitivity has been reported for detection of urinary tract dilatation and identification of the site of obstruction. MR urography was noted to show different appearances in physiologic hydronephrosis and pathologic obstruction. Renal enlargement and perirenal fluid suggestive of obstruction were absent in physiologic dilatation (Fig. 27.3a, b).

Currently, ultrasound remains an appropriate first-line imaging study in the pregnant patient who has possible urolithiasis/obstruction. When second-line studies are necessary, several options are available. A limited excretory urogram, MR urogram, or the emerging ultra–low-dose tailored CT may be considered in these cases. The selection of the best second-line study will depend on the local institution's capabilities and should be performed in consultation with the obstetrician and radiologist.

Indications

The management of a symptomatic stone diagnosed during pregnancy poses multiple challenges to the patient, obstetrician, and urologist. An understanding of the natural history of urolithiasis

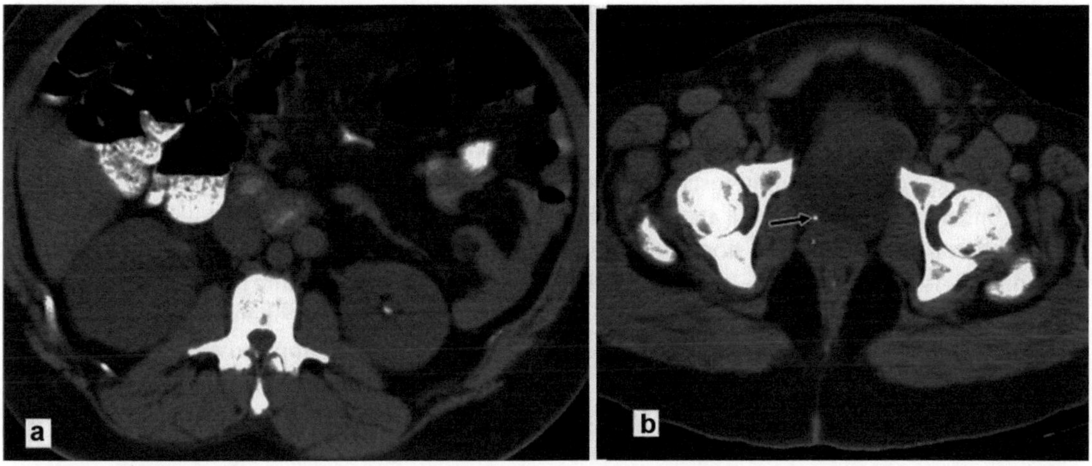

Fig. 27.2 (**a, b**) Same patient in Fig. 27.1 with right flank pain in the second trimester of pregnancy. (**a**) Axial CT image of the abdomen shows moderate right hydronephrosis. (**b**) Axial image of the pelvis shows a small calculus (*arrow*) of the right ureterovesical junction

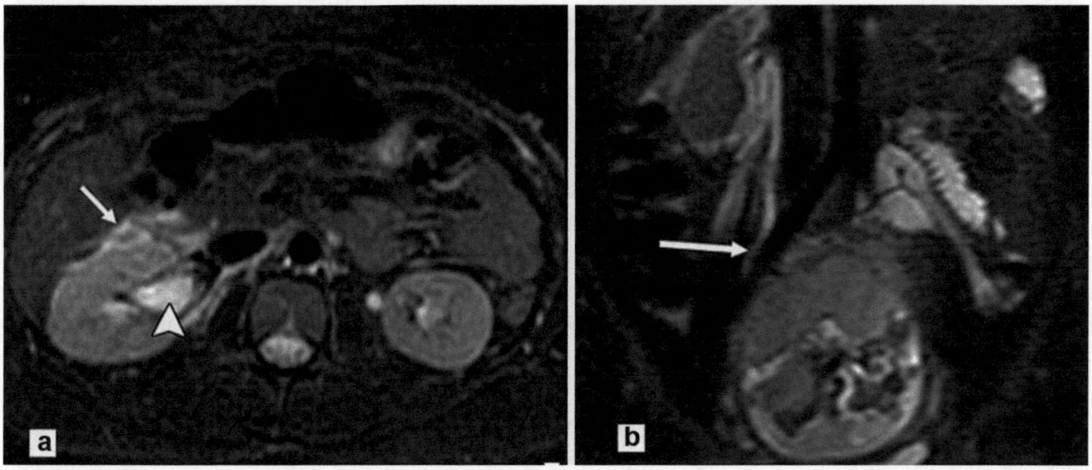

Fig. 27.3 (**a, b**) Twenty-eight-year-old woman with right lower quadrant pain in the second trimester of pregnancy. Axial (**a**) and coronal (**b**) T2-weighted MR images show moderate right hydronephrosis (*arrowhead* in **a**) with perinephric stranding (*arrow* in **a**) and mild right hydroureter (*arrow* in **b**). No calculus was visualized

in pregnancy and the limitations imposed by the pregnancy aids in the formulation of a rational approach to each patient. Despite attempts at conservative management, surgical intervention may ultimately be required. Absolute indications to intervene parallel those in the nonpregnant patient and include febrile urinary tract infection, pyonephrosis, sepsis, obstruction of a solitary kidney, intractable pain, nausea, or vomiting.

Selection of the appropriate intervention must take into consideration the capabilities and limitations of the institution and should respect the wishes of the patient and comfort level and clinical judgment of the urologist, obstetrician, and anesthesiologist [22].

Ureteroscopy

With continued advancement in endoscopic technology and endourologic techniques, ureteroscopy has become less invasive and less traumatic, such that many now consider it a first-line treatment for pregnant patients who have failed expectant management. Several small series have reported stone-free rates ranging from 70 to 100 %, with displacement of proximal ureteral stones into the kidney accounting for most residual calculi [16, 23–29]. As described by Watterson and colleagues, ureteroscopy is performed under general anesthesia in a modified dorsal lithotomy position. The floppy tip guide or glidewire is passed into the ureteral orifice under direct vision, using fluoroscopy only if resistance to wire advancement is encountered. Either semirigid or flexible ureteroscopy can be performed, as dictated by the clinical circumstances. Stones amenable to basket extraction are removed intact. Currently, the holmium laser is the preferred means of lithotripsy for those stones that cannot be removed intact. The versatility of the holmium laser allows efficient lithotripsy of all stone compositions, and its physics allows a large margin of safety, provided the tip is kept at least 1 mm from the ureteral wall [27].

In vitro studies suggest that the peak pressures generated by endoscopic lithotripsy are unlikely to damage fetal hearing, although the data are limited and largely theoretic [30]. The decision to proceed with endoscopic management of a ureteral stone during pregnancy should be determined by the clinical scenario, and the availability and expertise of urologic, obstetric, and anesthetic care.

It is generally agreed that x-ray examinations should be kept to a minimum, although the potential hazard of x-ray exposure to the fetus may be slight. X-ray visualization of a ureteral calculus may be complicated by poor bowel preparation and overlying fetal bony structures [3]. The most accurate detection and location of a suspected stone are probably achieved with retrograde pyelography but our experience is that introducing a ureteral catheter blindly or under fluoroscopic control is not much less invasive than performing ureteroscopy under direct vision. In some cases, it may be possible to reveal calculi in the proximal or most distal portion of the ureter by ultrasound examination [3, 9, 18–20], but visualization of stones in the mid ureter is still the uncommon exception. Improved technology and skill will probably minimize this problem [31, 32].

In our series, if conservative management fails and there is presence of infection, obstructed solitary kidney, or pain refractory to analgesia, then temporary urinary diversion is indicated. The introduction of a double-J stent is a less invasive and efficient method. In most situations, we introduce a ureteral catheter over a wire to the kidney and aspirate urine before insertion of the double-J stent to avoid the exposure to radiation. We placed a double-J stent in 13 patients, and their locations were confirmed postoperatively by US. In one patient, double-J stent insertion was not successful, and we chose percutaneous nephrostomy for urine drainage. The procedure was done under ultrasonic guidance and has the advantage of rapid decompression of the obstructed kidney.

As a result of the innovation through smaller instruments allowing easier access to the ureteral orifice, ureteroscopy has been used as an initial treatment modality for urolithiasis during pregnancy. Using a 6/8 F semirigid ureteroscope in seven pregnant patients (gestation time varied from 10 to 24 weeks), access to the ureteral meatus in pregnant women must be particularly gentle. During the entire procedure, it must be remembered constantly that complications, such as small perforations that would not be serious in a normal patient, could become extremely dangerous in pregnant women [24].

Ureteroscopy was performed with epidural anesthesia in most of the cases. The women were placed on the operating table in a modified dorsal lithotomy position, or some authors recommended an oblique position with the left side down when necessary to decrease the pressure of the pregnant uterus on the inferior vena cava. In our patients, we accessed the ureter without dilation. Ureteral calculi were extracted with a stone basket or forceps under direct vision in four cases; the remaining three stones had to be disintegrated with holmium: YAG laser. In all patients, the ureteroscope was passed through the entire ureter, and in the three patients who underwent laser disintegration, it was advanced into the renal pelvis as well. At the end, a double-J stent was fixed to drain the kidney for 1–2 weeks. In late gestations, the use of flexible ureteroscope will be easier to manipulate in a tortuous ureter, reducing

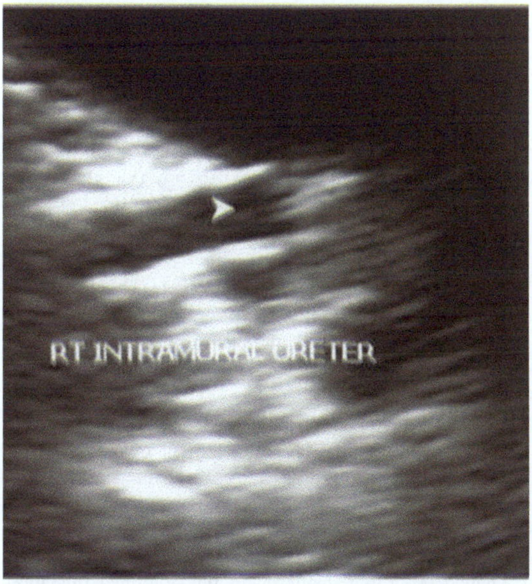

Fig. 27.4 Pelvic ultrasound showing a dilated lower ureter (*arrow*) with a stone in the intramural part in a pregnant patient. This was managed by ureteroscopy

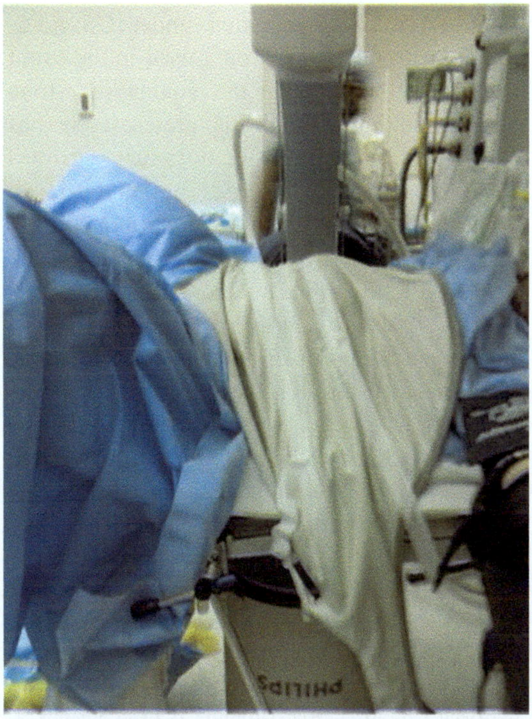

Fig. 27.5 Picture showing inverted C-arm, with lead shield over the abdomen of the patient exposing the right kidney for right ureteroscopy in a 30-week-pregnant patient with stone in right lower ureter

the risk of perforation. Intracorporeal lithotripsy devices, such as the holmium laser, can be used safely and effectively. No complications, such as perforations, bleeding, or sepsis, were reported in any of our series. Convalescence was uneventful without obstetrical complications. After the procedure, the pain, renal dilatation, and fever disappeared. The use of an inverted C-arm, where the radiation tube is on top of the patient and the image intensifier is on the bottom, has been described to cut down radiation exposure during interventions in pregnant patients. This was also combined by shielding the fetus with lead [33]. We have used this approach and found it very practical and helpful. In a 26-year-old pregnant patient at 30 weeks gestation with an obstructing lower ureteric stone, ureteroscopy with holmium laser lithotripsy was done successfully. The inverted C-arm approach was very helpful to confirm the proper position of the proximal wire and double-J stent at the end of the procedure. This is very important especially when the dilated ureter in pregnant patients could be tortuous (Figs. 27.4 and 27.5).

Complications associated with URS in pregnant and nonpregnant patients do not differ significantly. Meta-analysis has been done and demonstrated that URS is a safe and reasonable treatment paradigm in pregnant women with obstructing ureteral calculi refractory to conservative treatment [5].

Conclusion

Numerous small series have demonstrated ureteroscopy to be safe and effective in all stages of pregnancy with stone-free rates between 70 and 100 %. Concerns had previously persisted regarding technical difficulties because of the tortuous nature of the lower ureter from uterine compression, but the physiologic ureterohydronephrosis makes manipulation easier. Ureteral dilatation is therefore avoided [16, 24, 25].

Ureteroscopy (both rigid and flexible) may be performed under a general or spinal anesthesia or even sedation, with the patient in the modified dorsal lithotomy position. The majority of procedures can be performed without ionizing radiation under US guidance, with fluoroscopy only used in the event of failure to advance the guidewire. Stone fragmentation/retrieval via ureteroscopy has been performed using the holmium: yttrium-aluminum-garnet (YAG) or basket retrieval. The holmium: YAG laser has a large safety margin, is effective against all stone types, can be used in the rigid as well as flexible instrument, has very little periureteral thermal effect, and its use does not result in any energy transmission through the patient or fetus [5, 31, 32]. The use of inverted C-arm technique with fetus lead shielding is an attractive and safe way to use limited helpful fluoroscopy during ureteroscopy in pregnant patients [33].

References

1. Biyani CS, Joyce AD. Urolithiasis in pregnancy. I: pathophysiology, fetal considerations and diagnosis. BJU Int. 2002;89:811.
2. Lewis DF, Robichaux 3rd AG, Jaekle RK, et al. Urolithiasis in pregnancy. Diagnosis, management and pregnancy outcome. J Reprod Med. 2003;48:28.
3. Swartz MA, Lydon-Rochelle MT, Simon D, et al. Admission for nephrolithiasis in pregnancy and risk of adverse birth outcomes. Obstet Gynecol. 2007; 109:1099.
4. Parulkar BG, Hopkins TB, Wollin MR, Howard Jr PJ, Lal A. Renal colic during pregnancy: a case for conservative treatment. J Urol. 1998;159:365.
5. Semins MJ, Trock B, Matlaga BR. The safety of ureteroscopy during pregnancy: a systematic review and meta-analysis. J Urol. 2009;181:139.
6. Khoo L, Anson K, Patel U. Success and short-term complication rates of percutaneous nephrostomy during pregnancy. J Vasc Interv Radiol. 2004;15: 1469–73.
7. Faundes A, Bricola-Filho M, Pinto E, Silva JL. Dilation of the urinary tract during pregnancy: proposal of a curve of maximal caliceal diameter by gestational age. Am J Obstet Gynecol. 1998;178:1082–6.
8. Goldfarb R, Neerhut G, Lederer E. Management of acute hydronephrosis of pregnancy by ureteral stenting: risk of stone formation. J Urol. 1989;141:921–2.
9. Waltzer W. The urinary tract in pregnancy. J Urol. 1981;125:271–6.
10. Gertner JM, Coustan DR, Kliger AS, et al. Pregnancy as state of physiologic absorptive hypercalciuria. Am J Med. 1986;81:451–6.
11. Coe FL, Parks JA, Lindheimer MD. Nephrolithiasis during pregnancy. N Engl J Med. 1978;298:324–6.
12. Coe FL, Kavalich AG. Hypercalciuria and hyperuricosuria in patients with calcium nephrolithiasis. N Engl J Med. 1974;291:1344–50.
13. Maikranz P, Coe F, Parks J, et al. Nephrolithiasis in pregnancy. Am J Kidney Dis. 1987;9:354–8.
14. Swanson SK, Heilman RL, Eversman WG. Urinary tract stones in pregnancy. Surg Clin North Am. 1995; 75:123–42.
15. Kroovand RL. Stones in pregnancy. In: Coe FL, Favus MJ, Pak CYC, Parks JH, Preminger GM, editors. Kidney stones: medical and surgical management. Philadelphia: Lippincott-Raven Publishers; 1996. p. 1059–64.
16. Juan YS, Wu WJ, Chuang SM, Wang CJ, Shen JT, Long CY, Huang CH. Management of symptomatic urolithiasis during pregnancy. Kaohsiung J Med Sci. 2007;23:241–6.
17. Spencer JA, Chahal R, Kelly A, et al. Evaluation of painful hydronephrosis in pregnancy: magnetic resonance urographic patterns in physiological dilatation versus calculous obstruction. J Urol. 2004;171:256–60.
18. Bulletins ACOG. ACOG Committee Opinion No 299: Guidelines for diagnostic imaging during pregnancy. Obstet Gynecol. 2004;104:647–51.
19. Hurwitz LM, Yoshizumi T, Reiman RE, et al. Radiation dose to the fetus from body MDCT during early gestation. AJR Am J Roentgenol. 2006; 186:871–6.
20. White WM, Gash J, Hatcher P, et al. Low-dose computed tomography for the evaluation of flank pain in the pregnant population. In: Podium presentation 76, annual meeting of the SES AUA, Puerto Rico, 4 Mar 2006.
21. Birchard KR, Brown MA, Hyslop WB, et al. MRI of acute abdominal and pelvic pain in pregnant patients. AJR Am J Roentgenol. 2005;184:452–8.
22. Pais VM, Payton AL, LaGrange AC. Urolithiasis in pregnancy. Urol Clin North Am. 2007;34:43–52.
23. Jarrard DJ, Gerber GS, Lyon ES. Management of acute ureteral obstruction in pregnancy utilizing ultrasound-guided placement of ureteral stents. Urology. 1993;42:263–8.
24. Scarpa RM, De Lisa A, Usai E. Diagnosis and treatment of ureteral calculi during pregnancy with rigid ureteroscopes. J Urol. 1996;155:875–7.
25. Lifshitz DA, Lingeman JE. Ureteroscopy as a first-line intervention for ureteral calculi in pregnancy. J Endourol. 2002;16:19–22.
26. Evans HJ, Wollin TA. The management of urinary calculi in pregnancy. Curr Opin Urol. 2001; 11:379–84.
27. Watterson JD, Girvan AR, Beiko DT, et al. Ureteroscopy and holmium: YAG laser lithotripsy: an emerging definitive management strategy for symptomatic ureteral calculi in pregnancy. Urology. 2002; 60:383–7.

28. Carringer M, Swartz R, Johansson JE. Management of ureteric calculi in pregnancy by ureteroscopy and laser lithotripsy. Br J Urol. 1996;77:17–20.
29. Shokeir AA, Mutabagani H. Rigid ureteroscopy in pregnant women. Br J Urol. 1998;81:678–81.
30. Karlsen SJ, Bull-Njaa T, Krokstad A. Measurement of sound emission by endoscopic lithotripters: an in vitro study and theoretical estimation of risk of hearing loss in a fetus. J Endourol. 2001;15:821–6.
31. Ulvik NM, Bakke A, Hoisaeter PA. Ureteroscopy in pregnancy. J Urol. 1995;154:1660.
32. Shalom JS, Hickerton B, Van Cleynenbreugel B. Management of urinary calculi in pregnancy: a review. J Endourol. 2008;22:867–76.
33. Cocuzza M, Colombo Jr JR, Lopes RI, Piovesan AC, Borges Mesquita JL, Srougi M. Use of inverted fluoroscope's C-arm during endoscopic treatment of urinary tract obstruction in pregnancy: a practicable solution to cut radiation. Urology. 2010;75(6):1505–8.

Pediatric Percutaneous Nephrolithotomy (PCNL): Overcoming the Difficulties

28

Sinan Zeren and Hakan Çakir

Introduction

The use of the percutaneous route to treat kidney stones was first reported in 1976 and quickly became a routine procedure. Initially, the introduction of shock wave lithotripsy (SWL) therapy dramatically changed the treatment options; however, percutaneous nephrolithotomy (PCNL), with its high success rate, became the procedure of choice, particularly for large stones. Because of the rarity of pediatric cases, instruments were usually produced for adults. Surgeons did not want to operate on children before gaining experience with adult cases; consequently, these techniques were very rarely used in the pediatric population. Approximately 1,000 adult cases had been reported by the 1980s, while only approximately 150 pediatric cases were reported before the year 2000. However, the number of pediatric reports has increased significantly within the last decade.

With increased experience and pediatric-sized instruments, PCNL is a safe and effective procedure. Especially in developing countries, a large number of pediatric kidney stone patients exist, and percutaneous renal surgery is relatively common, with the same indications and techniques as used in the adult population.

S. Zeren, M.D. (✉) • H. Çakir, M.D.
Department of Urology, Acibadem Fulya Hospital, Hakki Yeten Cad. Yesilcimen Sok. No. 23, Besiktas, Istanbul 34349, Turkey
e-mail: snnzeren@gmail.com; drhakancakir@gmail.com

Common Indications for Surgery

The pediatric indications are similar to those for adult patients:

- Stones larger than 2 cm (>1 cm for the lower calyceal calculi)
- Contraindication or failure of SWL or a likelihood of limited SWL success for the following reasons:
  - Ureteropelvic junction obstruction
  - Horseshoe kidney
  - Calyceal diverticulum
  - Stones composed of cystine or calcium oxalate monohydrate

Technique

The technique used for pediatric cases is similar to that used for adult cases. The surgeon must choose appropriate-sized instruments for each case and must know what ancillary equipment may be necessary and have it ready for the operation.

With dilated pelvicalyceal anatomy, the operating technique is similar to that used for adults. Adult-sized instruments have some advantages, such as a wide visual area, more controllable stone disintegration, greater ease of extracting the larger fragments, decreased likelihood of residual fragments, and shorter operation time.

With mildly dilated or nondilated pelvicalyceal anatomy, adult-sized standard instruments may be traumatic to the kidney. Dilating the tract

A.M. Al-Kandari et al. (eds.), *Difficult Cases in Endourology*,
DOI 10.1007/978-1-84882-083-8_28, © Springer-Verlag London 2013

as necessary and using the small caliber sheath and optical devices may improve the safety of the operation.

Fluoroscopy time is kept to a minimum to prevent adverse long-term effects. Because of pediatric patients' small body size, the gonads may not be isolated from the radiated area. It may be necessary to use the collimators on the C-arm device to decrease the radiated area and isolate the operation site. It is also possible to reduce the irradiated area by placing the edges of the X-ray protective lead aprons or thyroid shields under the patient around the work area. The same radiation safety rules are valid for the postoperative antegrade nephrostogram.

The irrigation fluid used in PCNL operations is usually saline. It must be kept close to body temperature. To prevent heat loss during the surgery and maintain a warm, stable body temperature, warm-air blankets may be used. Otherwise, hypothermia complications are common. Expected complications include acidosis, coagulation disorders, cardiac irritability, respiratory depression, delayed awakening, decreases in the enzymatic destruction of drugs, and decreases in tissue oxygenation with increases in vascular resistance.

Preoperative Evaluation

To ensure a safe and accurate treatment plan, it is essential to carefully inspect the radiological images to understand the shape, number, and location of the stones, the intrarenal anatomy, and the perirenal structures. Bleeding disorders and urinary tract infection must be evaluated. Coagulopathy may compromise the feasibility of this procedure. If there is a significant urinary tract infection, appropriate antibiotics must be started before the operation.

Operation

Under general anesthesia, the first step of the operation is retrograde ureteral catheterization. This is necessary for contrast injection or inserting a guidewire, if needed, and to prevent antegrade migration of small stone particles into the ureter

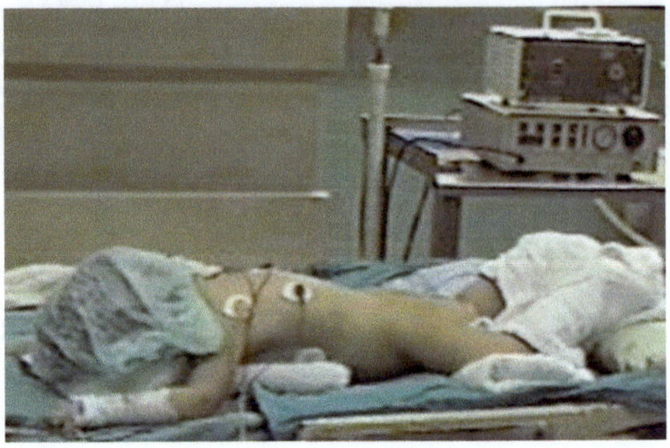

Fig. 28.1 Nine-month-old infant in prone PCNL position

during surgery. After catheterization, the patient is moved into a straight prone position, and the thorax, knees, and ankles are padded with soft materials (Fig. 28.1). Under fluoroscopy, holding the expected size sheath over the back of the patient and superimposing it on the contrast-filled calyceal structures may help to determine the appropriate sheath size. The posterior calix is the preferred initial access site; unfortunately, on fluoroscopy, it is usually superimposed on the lower calyceal infundibulum. The intense contrast filling in that area may help to identify this calix. If there is a stone in the calix that we may puncture, direct access by touching the stone may confirm access without the use of contrast material. Avoiding the use of contrast initially, if possible, may help to prevent confusion between opacified blood clots and contrast-filled small calices that may later appear as suspicious opacities on fluoroscopy. "J" or hydrophilic tip wires are safe to use; however, if their tips are very close to the system wall, careless advancement may also traumatize and easily perforate the system. It is preferable to send them into the ureter or even the bladder; however, this may not always be possible within a reasonable fluoroscopy time. Anatomical structures in kidney or obstruction by a stone may not allow the wire to pass, and a very careful dilation may be needed. Still, at least the flexible part of the guidewire must be inside the kidney during dilatation. Amplatz dilators are usually safe when using over its 8 F stylet, and it may be possible to finalize dilatation at different levels. To work with low pressure, the planned sheath size must be compatible with the scope used inside, leaving enough space for easy irrigation. Low intrarenal pressure during surgery is recommended to decrease the chance of fluid extravasation and antegrade migration of small stone particles into the ureter. It is best to create a new access for the stones behind the nondilated infundibula seen from inside with the flexible scope to avoid touching and traumatizing these areas. By leaving them untouched, there is no need for additional nephrostomy tubes for the additional tracts. A 14 F Malecot reentry catheter is a good choice for a nephrostomy tube at the end of the operation. There is usually no need for the second operation (to reenter the kidney), but the ureteral stent portion of these catheters maintains their stability in children and keeps the ureteropelvic junction open during the early healing of the edematous walls of the renal pelvis. While placing the nephrostomy catheter, the open-end ureteral catheter is removed. In small children, it is necessary to shorten the ureteral stent portion of this catheter before its placement. Before finalizing the operation, a gentle irrigation of the nephrostomy tube with contrast is necessary to remove blood clots, confirm the position of the catheter and its parts, and check the pelvicalyceal structures. While fixing the nephrostomy catheter to the skin and placing the dressings, it is critical to avoid kinking the catheter to ensure safe postoperative drainage (Fig. 28.2).

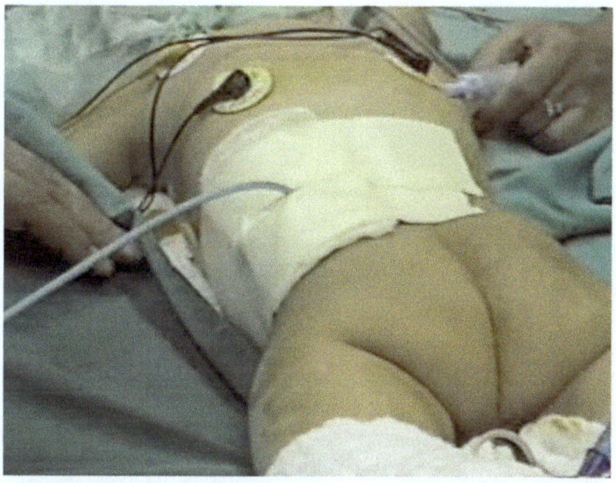

Fig. 28.2 Nine-month-old infant, end of the PCNL operation

Early Postoperative Care

On the day of surgery, patients may eat or drink late in the afternoon, but intravenous fluids must continue until the next morning. The overnight irrigation of the kidney with intravenous hydration helps to keep the nephrostomy tube open and dissolve blood clots. The day after surgery, antegrade nephrostogram is usually necessary to detect residual stones and evaluate the pelvicalyceal structures, extravasations, and the passage of contrast material to the bladder. If everything looks normal and the physicians decide to remove the tube, it can be removed without clamping.

Most renal pelvis extravasations are minor, and there is no need to change the routine care in the early postoperative period. For significant extravasations, a longer nephrostomy drainage period may be necessary. Disintegration of the hard stones and inappropriate manipulations increase the risks to the integrity of the collecting system. Extrarenal collection is mostly retroperitoneal and negligible. Marked collections are rare and may be treated by leaving the nephrostomy catheter for a few more days. Major collections may require drainage. For prolonged urinary leakage from the nephrostomy site, double-J ureteral stent placement may solve the problem.

Instruments and Disposables

Most of the instruments manufactured for adults are also useful in pediatric cases. However, in nondilated systems or when the stone burden is low or the procedure is planned to extract multiple small stone particles, it is better to use instruments specifically designed for pediatric patients.

It is ideal to use appropriate instruments for the procedure:

- Pediatric nephroscope (Fig. 28.3)
- Rigid forceps (note: their mouths are very brittle and must be used with care)
- Small-caliber lithotripsy probes

Alternative instruments:

- Very-small-caliber sheaths
- Ureteroscope
- Pediatric cystoscope and compatible instruments

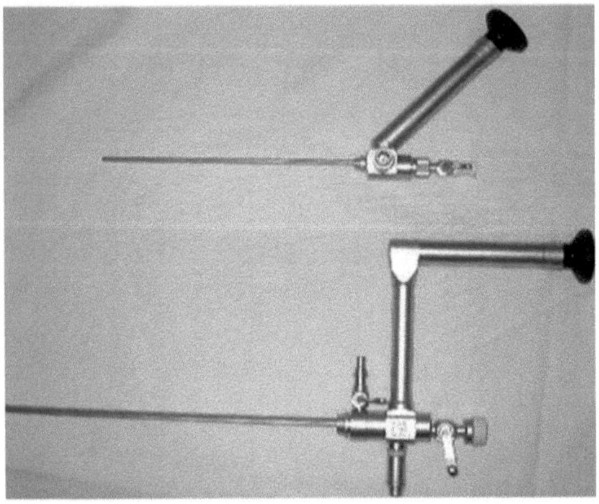

Fig. 28.3 Adult (standard percutaneous nephroscope) and pediatric (miniature nephroscope system) size rigid nephroscopes (Karl Storz Endoskope, Tuttlingen, Germany)

- Flexible extracting devices (i.e., a tipless nitinol basket or other specially designed extractors)

Experienced endourologists usually prefer to have wide range of instruments (i.e., guidewires, catheters, dilation and extraction devices) in different sizes and specifications.

Instruments and disposables used in PCNL surgery:

- Open-end ureteral catheter
- Foley urethral catheter (to maintain bladder drainage and fix the open-end catheter to prevent its accidental dislocation while the patient is positioned)
- Percutaneous needle
- "J" or hydrophilic tip guidewires
- Dilators (Amplatz, balloon, metal coaxial)
- Amplatz sheath
- Rigid and flexible nephroscopes
- Lithotripsy devices
- Stone extractors
- Nephrostomy catheter

Renal balloon catheters may be an alternative for tract dilatation, but their inflated size of 1 cm in diameter may be unnecessarily large and traumatic in some cases. When planning to work with a small sheath, gradual Amplatz dilators offer the best opportunity to stop at any appropriate level. Metal coaxial dilators may be an alternative, but keeping the tip of the unit at a safe point in nondilated kidneys can be difficult, and careless manipulation forced against the unit axis may result in severe kinking of the guidewire due to the unit's nonflexible antenna.

Decreasing the diameter of the sheath results in a remarkable decrease in the cross-sectional area of the tube. As an example, when using a 21 F sheath instead of 28 F (a one-fourth smaller diameter), the cross-sectional area of the working sheath decreases by almost half.

Difficulties Commonly Encountered During the Procedure

Certain uncommon conditions that can cause difficulties during the operation may be resolved with some alternative manipulations.

Retrograde Ureteral Catheterization

Under general anesthesia, ureteral catheterization with an open-end catheter (5 F or 6 F) is the first step of the operation. The size of the ureteral orifice determines the size of the catheter. Larger diameter catheters are best to prevent antegrade migration of the small stone particles during surgery; however, in the pediatric population, two main problems may be encountered during catheterization. The first is the difficulty in placing a Foley catheter while the open-end catheters are inside the urethra, especially in small boys. Sometimes, a thin Nelaton catheter may solve the problem. Rarely, in short cases, the operation may be continued without a catheter in the bladder. The second problem is that pediatric cystoscopes are not wide enough to permit these relatively large-caliber catheters through their working channels, so the catheterization procedure in infants is somewhat different. A guidewire is sent to the kidney through the cystoscope. After the instrument is removed, an open-end catheter is passed over the guidewire into the kidney under fluoroscopy.

Small Sheaths

For the minimally dilated collecting system, the author used a metal coaxial dilator of the desired caliber as a working sheath in early cases. To place one of these dilators into the kidney as a working sheath, Amplatz semirigid dilators that firmly fit into the dilator were used. Metal tubes are the best small-diameter sheaths with a relatively large lumen because their walls are resistant and thin compared with Amplatz sheaths.

Weak Forceps

Because pediatric nephroscopes and their working channels are small in diameter, the bodies of forceps specifically designed for these devices are very thin, and the strength of their mouth joints is low. They must be used with a minimum of squeezing to prevent their breakage while grasping the stones. Nitinol basket-type ureteroscopic extractors are good alternatives to forceps.

Flexible Nephroscopy

It may not be possible to use a flexible nephroscope in nondilated systems or through the small-caliber sheaths. A flexible ureterorenoscope may provide an alternative. When the infundibula of the neighboring calices are very close to the accessed calix, flexible instruments are not useful.

Anecdotal Cases

Figure 28.4a–f illustrates the treatment of an 18-month-old male with PCNL.

Stones in the Calyceal Diverticulum

A 5-year-old female presented with recurrent urinary tract infection. Percutaneous treatment of stones and ablation of the calyceal diverticulum were planned.

After a careful insertion of a percutaneous needle into the calyceal diverticulum, a guidewire was inserted but kept in the diverticular cavity. With careful dilatation with Amplatz dilators, a 21 F metal coaxial dilator was placed as a sheath. After extracting the stone particles from the diverticular cavity with a rigid ureteroscope, the neck of the cavity was found and dilated to 14 F. Before placing a 14 F Malecot nephrostomy tube, the diverticular cavity was fulgurated with a low current. Three days later, the nephrostomy catheter was removed. An intravenous urogram taken 3 months after the operation revealed easy draining of the diverticular cavity (Fig. 28.5a–j).

Pyonephrosis with a Proximal Ureteral Stone

A 3-year-old male with a history of high fever and right flank pain had been hospitalized in another institution for severe urinary tract infection. He was scheduled to receive medical treatment before surgery for a right proximal ureteral stone. After 3 weeks with no improvement in his clinical situation, he was transferred to our hospital with the diagnosis of pyonephrosis (Fig. 28.6a, b). Emergency percutaneous drainage and an antegrade extraction of the stone were completed in the same session. The patient was doing well after the operation, but only 40–50 ml urine drainage was observed daily from the nephrostomy tube. The patient was kept in the hospital for parenteral antibiotic treatment. Contrast material administered via the nephrostomy tube on the third postoperative day showed no extravasation and a slow contrast passage to the bladder (Fig. 28.6c). Four days after surgery, the patient was discharged with the nephrostomy tube to assess his urine output. At home the next day, the urine output increased to 250 ml. On the sixth postoperative day, the patient's nephrostomy tube was removed at an outpatient visit. No leakage was observed from the nephrostomy site.

Bilateral Staghorn Kidney Stones

An 8-year-old female presented with bilateral kidney stones. Open surgery was recommended at another institution. Bilateral PCNL was performed in a single session, and both nephrostomy catheters were removed on the third day postsurgery (Fig. 28.7a–c).

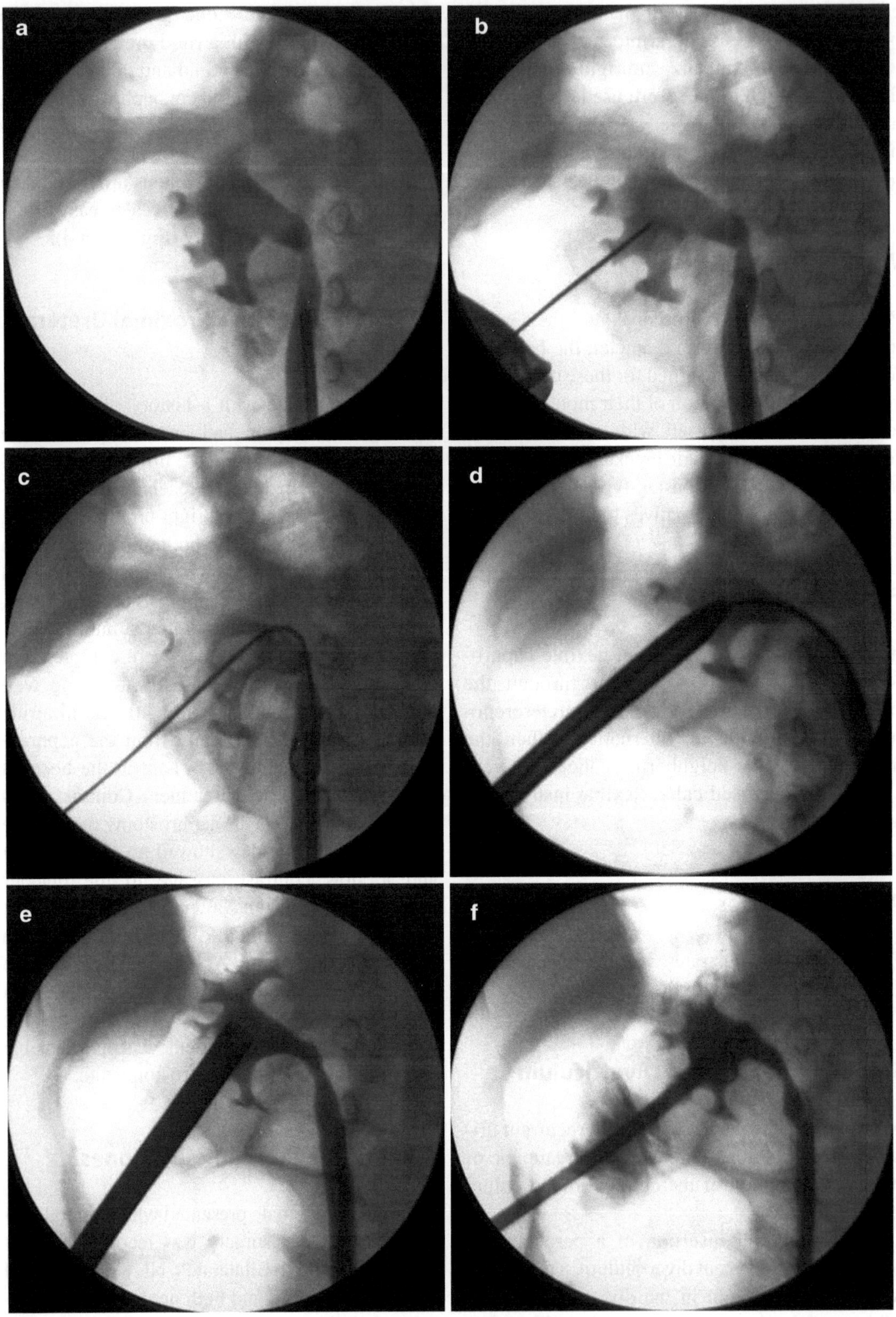

Fig. 28.4 (**a**–**f**) Eighteen-month-old male treated with PCNL. (**a**) Contrast injection. (**b**) Percutaneous needle access. (**c**) Guidewire insertion. (**d**) 18 F dilatation. (**e**) 21 F sheath placement. (**f**) Malecot nephrostomy

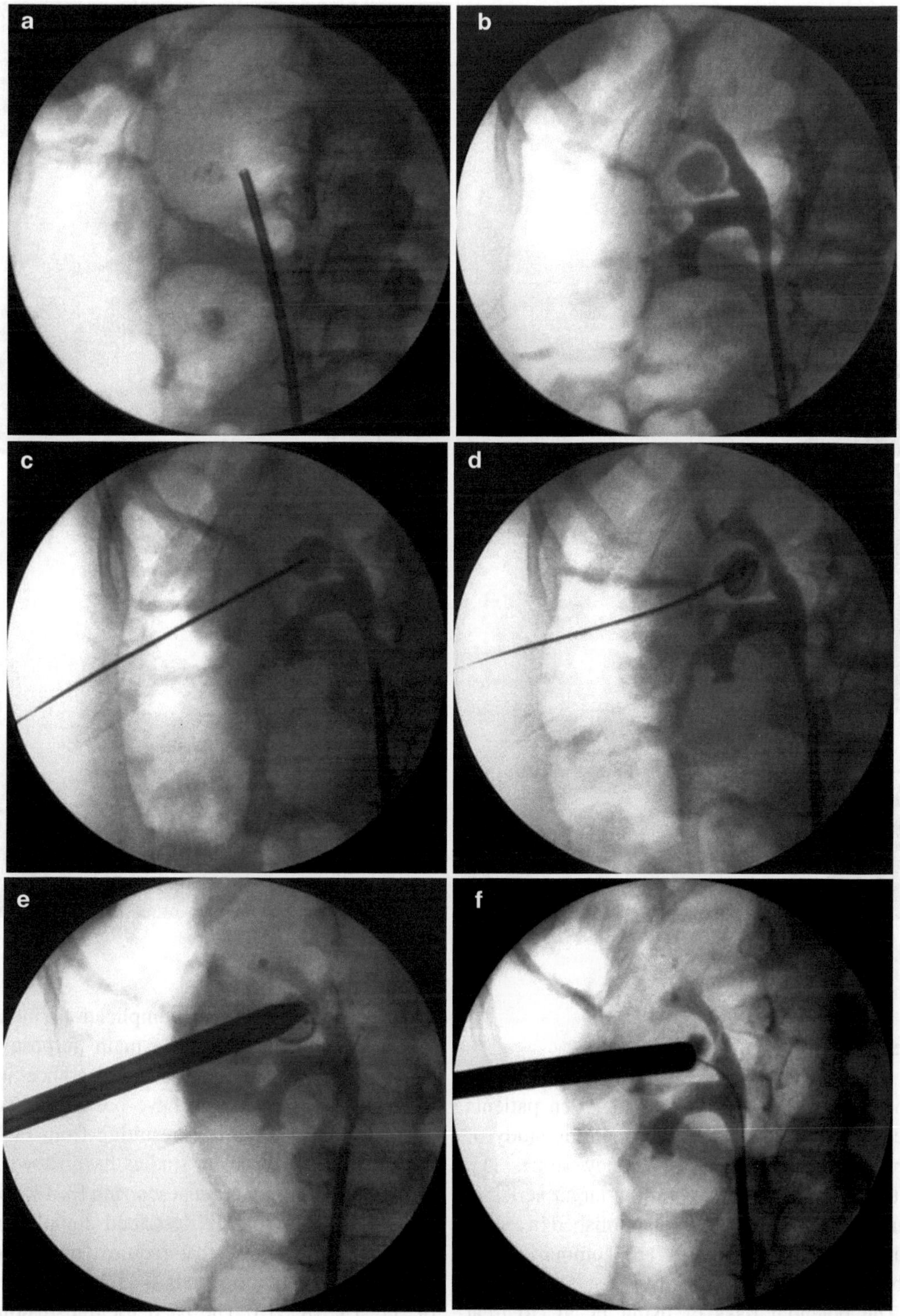

Fig. 28.5 (**a**–**j**) Five-year-old female with calyceal diverticular calculi treated with PCNL. (**a**) Calyceal calculi. (**b**) Calyceal diverticulum. (**c**) Puncture of the diverticulum. (**d**) Guidewire insertion. (**e**) 20 F dilatation. (**f**) 21 F sheath placement. (**g**) 14 F diverticulum neck dilatation. (**h**) Cavity fulguration. (**i**) 14 F Malecot nephrostomy. (**j**) Postop 3 months, IVU

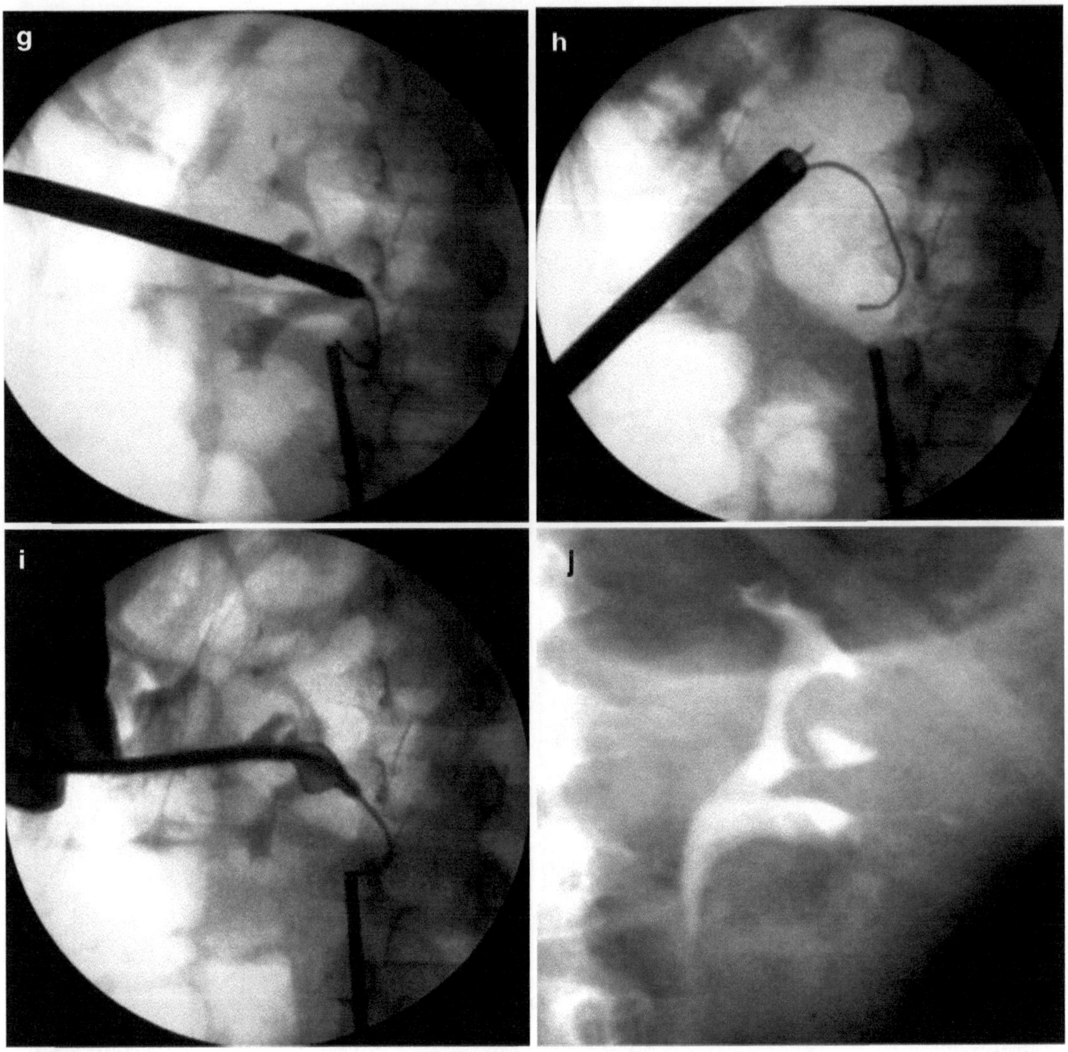

Fig. 28.5 (continued)

Discussion

Woodside et al.'s 1985 report of seven patients aged 5–18 years was the first pediatric study of percutaneous treatment for kidney stones [1]. With wider use of this operation, larger series in younger age groups have been published in recent years. Some recent series are summarized in Table 28.1 [2–18].

The potential risks of using PCNL to treat pediatric kidney stones include parenchymal damage and its associated effects on renal function; radiation exposure resulting from fluoroscopy; and the possibility of major complications, including sepsis and bleeding. The main purpose for using PCNL is achieving stone clearance with minimal morbidity. There have been some concerns about renal damage resulting from PCNL use in children; however, studies have shown no evidence of significant renal scarring [3, 14, 19].

The most commonly described complication of PCNL is bleeding that requires transfusion, which has been reported in 0.7–25.3 % of patients [9, 11, 13, 18, 20]. The need for transfusion is associated with operation time, sheath size, and stone burden [9, 18]. Furthermore, it has been reported that this complication is significant during

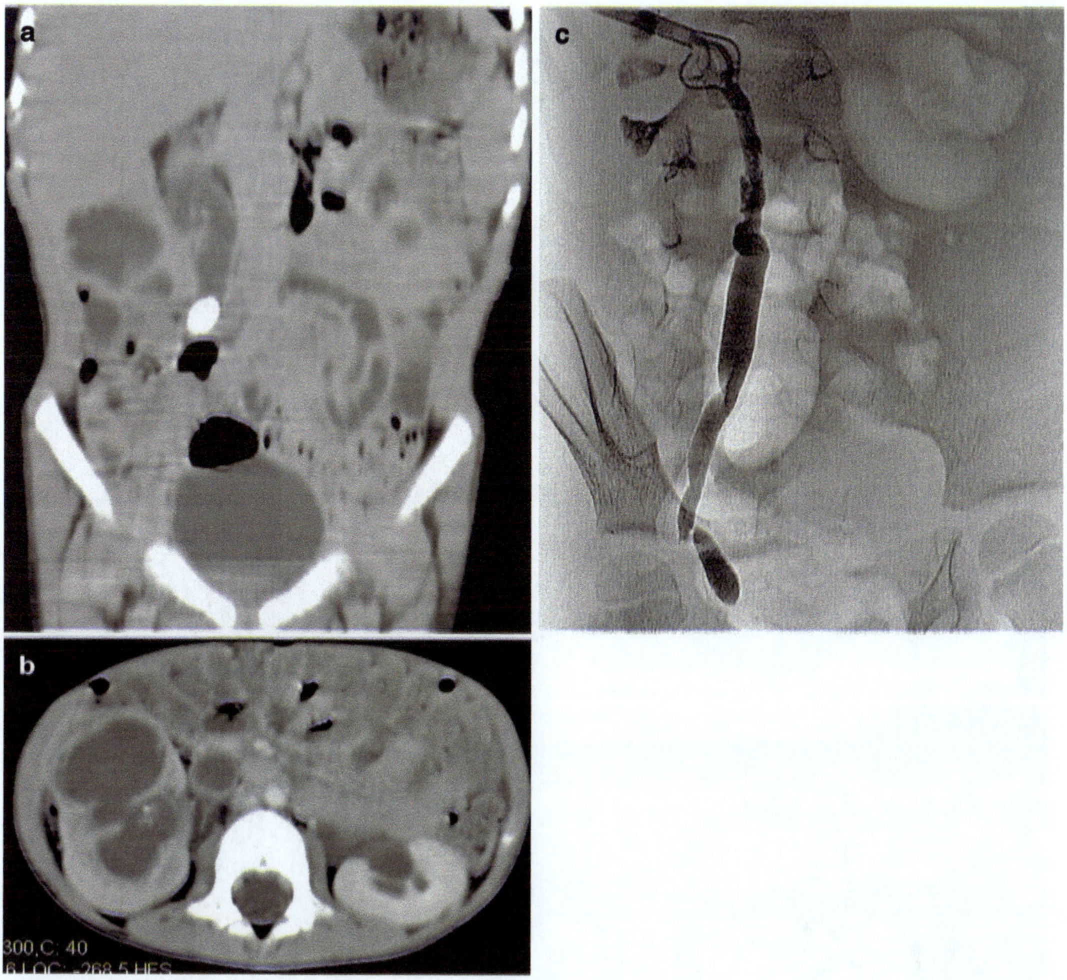

Fig. 28.6 (**a–c**) Three-year-old male, right proximal ureteral stone, pyonephrosis. (**a, b**) CT scans. (**c**) Postoperative antegrade nephrostogram

the initial part of the learning curve but tends to decrease with increasing surgical experience [9]. Some centers prefer to use SWL as a complementary therapy after primary PCNL to treat the residual stone fragments and reduce the renal manipulation-associated morbidity. Studies have reported stone-free rate increases from 60 and 65.5 % with PCNL monotherapy to 100 % and 93.8 % with additional SWL [16, 21]. Nonetheless, we must consider that in children, general anesthesia is usually necessary during SWL. Wollin et al. reported the safety of Holmium:YAG laser use in children [22]. To reduce hemorrhage-related morbidity, flexible instruments and Holmium:YAG lasers play an important role in reaching and breaking stone fragments through the same sheath, without the need for additional access tracts.

Hypothermia is another potential complication of PCNL; it is associated with the length of the operation and insufficient preoperative preparation [7, 23]. Transient fever is a frequent postoperative complication; it has been reported in up to 42.8 % of cases [12].

Thoracic complications are another rare but possible problem, especially after supracostal punctures. Most of the mild hydro/pneumothoraces are asymptomatic, and intervention may not be required; however, some cases indicate fluid aspiration or chest tube insertion. In a recent study, El-Nahas et al. compared subcostal and

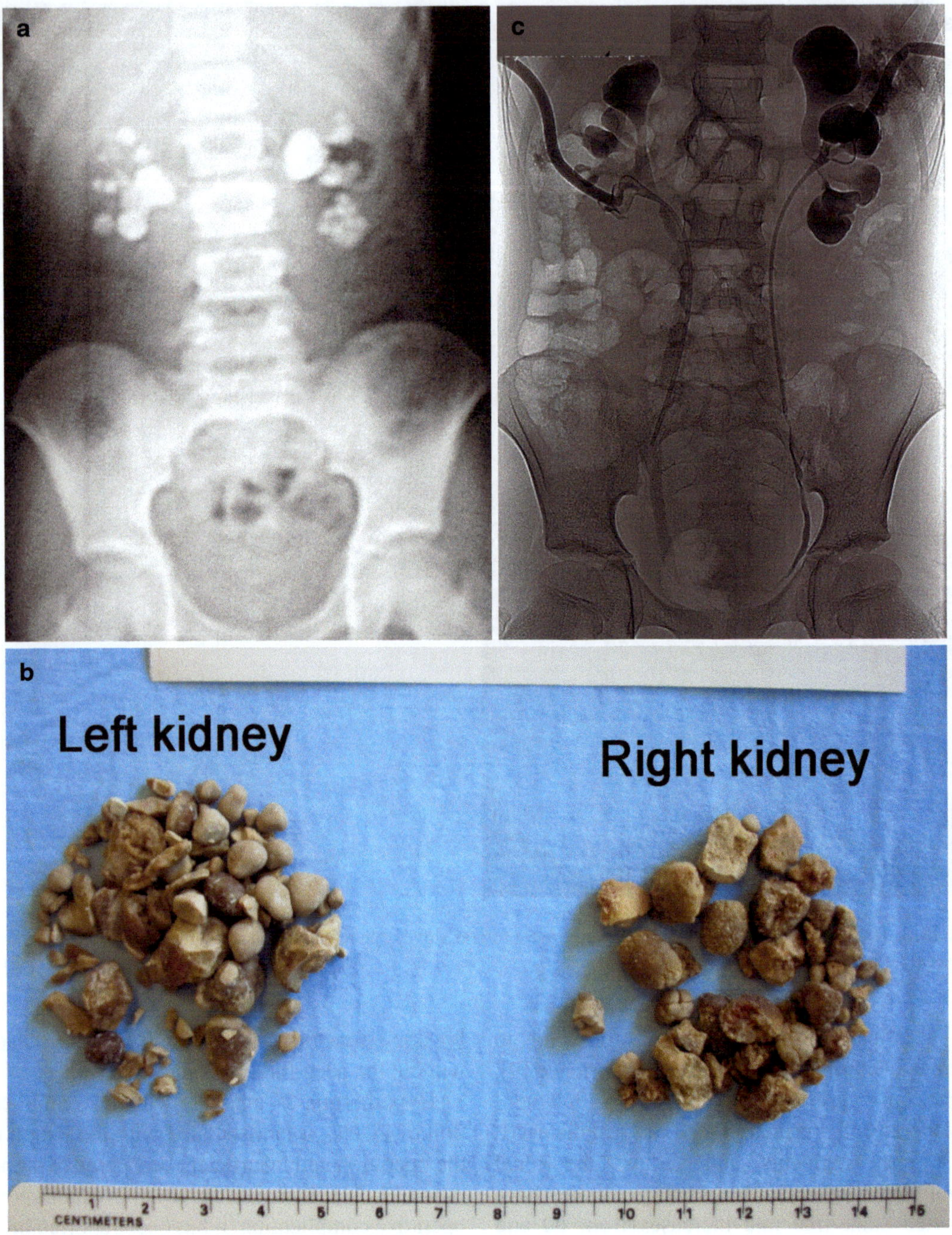

Fig. 28.7 (**a**–**c**) Eight-year-old female with bilateral staghorn kidney stones. (**a**) Preoperative KUB. (**b**) Stones extracted with bilateral PCNL. (**c**) Postoperative antegrade nephrostogram

Table 28.1 Pediatric PCNL series in literature [2–18]

	n	Age	Dilatation	Lithotripsy	Stone-free (%)
Kurzrock et al. [2]	8	3–16	24 F (18 F, one case)	US, EHL	75
Mor et al. [3]	25	3–16	24–26 F	US, EHL	68
Jackman et al. [4]	7 (11 ru)	2–6	11 F "miniperc"	EHL	85
Desai et al. [5]	40 (45 ru)	11 (months)–16	21 F and up	US, Pneum.	91
Badawy et al. [6]	60	3–13	26–28 F	US	83.3
Al-Shammari et al. [7]	8 (9 ru)	4–11	24 F	US, EHL	87.5
Sahin et al. [8]	14 (16 ru)	8–17	24 F and up	US, Laser	69
Zeren et al. [9]	55 (62 ru)	10 (months)–14	18–30	Pneum., US	86.9
Günes et al. [10]	23 (25 ru)	27 (months)–16	24–30	Pneum.	70.8
Rizvi et al. [11]	62	4–14	22	US	67.7
Desai et al. [12]	116 (128)	6 (months)–15	20–24	Pneum.	93.7
Salah et al. [13]	135 (137 ru)	8 (months)–14	19–30	US	98.5
Dawaba et al. [14]	65 (72 ru)	9 (months)–16	≤30	US	86
Raza et al. [15]	37 (43 ru)	1–15	24–30	US	79
Samad et al. [16]	168 (188 ru)	10 (months)–16	28 (max)	NA	59.3
Shokeir et al. [17]	75 (82 ru)	6 (months)–14	22–30	US	95.1
Bilen et al. [18]	46 (48 ru)	2–16	12–26	Pneum., US, Laser	87.8

ru renal unit

supracostal punctures in 40 and 20 patients, respectively. They reported the safety and efficacy of supracostal punctures without major complications, assuming attention to surgical anatomy and avoiding access over the 11th rib [20]. Furthermore, intraoperative thoracic fluoroscopy may help to identify hydro/pneumothorax.

There is also a possibility of adjacent organ injury. Badawy et al. reported colonic injury in 1.7 % of cases [6].

In recent years, it is common to see reports in the literature comparing standard and tubeless PCNLs. In studies with a limited number of pediatric tubeless cases, the reported advantages included a less painful operation with a shorter hospital stay; however, those studies also note that success depends on the surgeon's experience and the patient selection criteria, including whether low-volume and noninfectious stones were removed completely without any bleeding from the tract [24–26].

Small-caliber instruments should be used in nondilated systems, but some authors recommend using them even in dilated systems (i.e., miniperc) to avoid dilating too much renal parenchyma [4]. Small-caliber instruments offer some advantages: they affect less renal tissue, assert less compression on the parenchyma, and are associated with fast healing. However, they also have some drawbacks, including increased operative time in cases of hard and bulky stones. The need to fragment stones into smaller pieces may result in residual stone particles left in situ.

The miniaturization of instruments and tract sizes is ongoing. In a recent study, Desai et al. described the use of microperc, a single-step PCNL method, in a limited number of patients. They used only a 4.85 Fr sheath (a special 1.6-mm needle) placed in a single step without tract dilation and performed the operation with a 0.9-mm flexible telescope and a 200-μm Holmium:YAG laser fiber. Despite the disadvantage of a long stone disintegration duration in some cases, microperc may have a potential role in selected patients, that is, those with a limited stone burden in an anomalous urinary tract, pediatric patients, and those with small stones and lower pole stones. Further clinical studies and a comparison of current modalities are necessary to define microperc's future use in stone treatment [27].

Conclusion

Percutaneous renal surgery is as safe and effective in pediatric patients as in adults. The possibility of retreatment with this procedure when necessary is one of its main advantages in the pediatric population, which has a high risk of recurrence. Experience gained during operations on adults and the use of appropriate instruments (especially in complicated cases) affect the success of this procedure.

References

1. Woodside JR, Stevens GF, Stark GL, et al. Percutaneous stone removal in children. J Urol. 1985;134:1166–7.
2. Kurzrock EA, Huffman JL, Hardy BE, et al. Endoscopic treatment of pediatric urolithiasis. J Pediatr Surg. 1996;31:1413–6.
3. Mor Y, Elmasry YE, Kellet MJ, et al. The role of percutaneous nephrolithotomy in the management of pediatric renal calculi. J Urol. 1997;158:1319–21.
4. Jackman SV, Hedican SP, Peters CA, et al. Percutaneous nephrolithotomy in infants and preschool age children: experience with a new technique. Urology. 1998;52:697–701.
5. Desai M, Ridhorkar V, Patel S, et al. Pediatric percutaneous nephrolithotomy: assessing impact of technical innovations on safety and efficacy. J Endourol. 1999;13:359–64.
6. Badawy H, Salama A, Eissa M, et al. Percutaneous management of renal calculi: experience with percutaneous nephrolithotomy in 60 children. J Urol. 1999; 162:1710–3.
7. Al-Shammari AM, Al Otaibi K, Leonard MP, et al. Percutaneous nephrolithotomy in the pediatric population. J Urol. 1999;162:1721–4.
8. Sahin A, Tekgul S, Erdem E, et al. Percutaneous nephrolithotomy in older children. J Pediatr Surg. 2000;35:1336–8.
9. Zeren S, Satar N, Bayazit Y, et al. Percutaneous nephrolithotomy in the management of pediatric renal calculi. J Endourol. 2002;16:75–8.
10. Gunes A, Ugras MY, Yılmaz U, et al. Percutaneous nephrolithotomy for pediatric stone disease-our experience with adult-sized equipment. Scand J Urol Nephrol. 2003;37:477–81.
11. Rizvi SAH, Naqvi SAA, Hussain Z, et al. Management of pediatric urolithiasis in Pakistan. J Urol. 2003; 169:634–7.
12. Desai MR, Kukreja RA, Patel SH, et al. Percutaneous nephrolithotomy for complex pediatric renal calculus disease. J Endourol. 2004;18:23–7.
13. Salah MA, Toth C, Khan AM, et al. Percutaneous nephrolithotomy in children: experience with 138 cases in a developing country. World J Urol. 2004; 22:277–80.
14. Dawaba MS, Shokeir AA, Hafez AT, et al. Percutaneous nephrolithotomy in children: early and late anatomical and functional results. J Urol. 2004; 172:1078–81.
15. Raza A, Turna B, Smith G, et al. Pediatric urolithiasis: 15 years of local experience with minimally invasive endourological management of pediatric calculi. J Urol. 2005;174:682–5.
16. Samad L, Aquil S, Zaidi Z. Paediatric percutaneous nephrolithotomy: setting new frontiers. BJU Int. 2006; 97:359–63.
17. Shokeir AA, Sheir KZ, El-Nahas AR, et al. Treatment of renal stones in children: a comparison between percutaneous nephrolithotomy and shock wave lithotripsy. J Urol. 2006;176(2):706–10.
18. Bilen CY, Kocak B, Kitirci G, et al. Percutaneous nephrolithotomy in children: lessons learned in 5 years at a single institution. J Urol. 2007;177: 1867–71.
19. Mayo ME, Krieger JN, Rudd TG. Effect of percutaneous nephrolithotomy on renal function. J Urol. 1985; 133:167–9.
20. El-Nahas AR, Shokeir AA, El-Kenawy MR, et al. Safety and efficacy of supracostal percutaneous nephrolithotomy in pediatric patients. J Urol. 2008;180(2): 676–80.
21. Mahmud M, Zaidi Z. Percutaneous nephrolithotomy in children before school age: experience of a Pakistani centre. BJU Int. 2004;94:1352–4.
22. Wollin TA, Teichman JM, Rogenes VJ, et al. Holmium:YAG lithotripsy in children. J Urol. 1999; 152:1714–6.
23. Roberts S, Bolton DM, Stoller ML. Hypothermia associated with percutaneous nephrolithotomy. Urology. 1994;44:832–5.
24. Khairy Salem H, Morsi HA, Omran A, et al. Tubeless percutaneous nephrolithotomy in children. J Pediatr Urol. 2007;3:235–8.
25. Ozturk A, Guven S, Kilinc M, et al. Totally tubeless percutaneous nephrolithotomy: is it safe and effective in preschool children? J Endourol. 2010;24:1935–9.
26. Bilen C, Gunay M, Ozden E, et al. Tubeless mini percutaneous nephrolithotomy in infants and preschool children: a preliminary report. J Urol. 2010;184: 2498–502.
27. Desai MR, Sharma R, Mishra S, et al. Single-step percutaneous nephrolithotomy (microperc): the initial clinical report. J Urol. 2011;186(1):140–5.

Pediatric Ureteroscopy: Overcoming the Difficulties

29

Raguram Ganesamoni, Shashikant Mishra, and Mahesh Desai

Introduction

Pediatric ureteroscopy was first performed in 1929 by Hugh Hampton Young [1]. The procedure was performed on a 2-month-old boy with massively dilated ureters secondary to posterior urethral valves. Young utilized a 9.5-Fr pediatric cystoscope to visualize the ureter as well as the intrarenal collecting system. After many decades, ureteroscopic management of pediatric stone disease was described by Ritchey et al. [2] and Shepherd et al. [3] in 1988. Since then, with the miniaturization of endoscopic instruments, improvement in imaging modalities, improvement in intracorporeal lithotripters and ancillary instruments, ureteroscopy has become a safe and effective endourological treatment in this patient population. But there are some important differences as compared to adult ureteroscopy. In this chapter, we discuss the difficulties which can occur during pediatric ureteroscopy and the tips and tricks to overcome them.

R. Ganesamoni, M.S., MRCS, MCh
S. Mishra, M.S., DNB (✉) • M. Desai, M.S., FRCS
Department of Urology, Muljibhai Patel Urological Hospital, Dr. Virendra Desai Road, Nadiad, Gujarat, 387001, India
e-mail: dr_raguramg@yahoo.co.in; mishra@mpuh.org; mrdesai@mpuh.org

Technique

Choosing the Instrument

Depending on stone location, a semirigid or flexible ureteroscope may be chosen. A semirigid scope (4.5–6 Fr) is preferable in the distal ureter and mid ureter, while a 6 Fr flexible ureteroscope may be required for upper ureteric access. The caliber of ureteroscope has not been shown to affect therapeutic outcomes or complication rates [4]. Sometimes a distal ureteric stone can even be tackled with a 6-Fr pediatric cystoscope (Fig. 29.1).

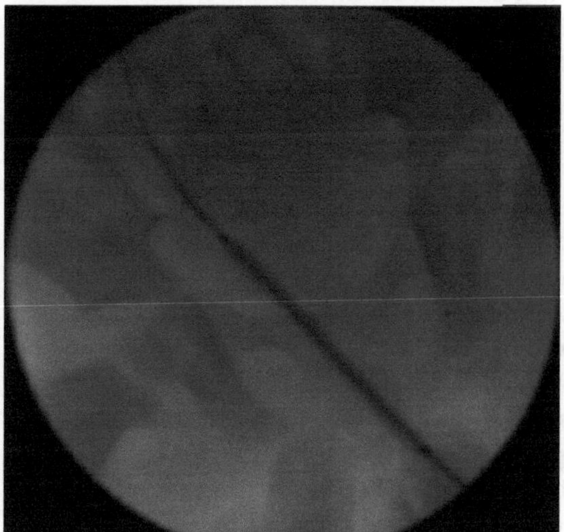

Fig. 29.1 Use of 6-Fr pediatric cystoscope for fragmenting distal ureteric stone

A.M. Al-Kandari et al. (eds.), *Difficult Cases in Endourology*,
DOI 10.1007/978-1-84882-083-8_29, © Springer-Verlag London 2013

Entering the Ureteric Orifice

It is important to enter the bladder with the age-appropriate cystoscope under direct vision with saline irrigation. Once the ureteric orifice is identified, a retrograde study is performed gently using ureteric catheter and contrast to confirm the location of the stone (in case of urolithiasis) and outline the ureteric anatomy. Following this, a safety hydrophilic guidewire (0.025–0.038 in.) should be inserted via the ureteric catheter under fluoroscopic guidance into the ureter and coiled in the renal pelvis.

If the guidewire could not be negotiated easily into the ureter, it is necessary to rule out any false passage. In this situation, a small ureteroscope can be used to directly inspect the intramural part of the ureter and place the guidewire under direct vision. Once the guidewire is placed, the next step is to decide whether the orifice will accommodate the ureteroscope. In the literature, use of active orifice dilation varies widely between 0 and 100 %, reflecting personal and institutional preference rather than evidence-based approach [4–6]. With most modern smaller sized ureteroscopes, active orifice dilation is not routinely required. Just hydrodilation will be sufficient in most of the children. Scarpa and colleagues suggest that dilation is never necessary, and smaller instruments should be chosen if the orifice is small [7]. The options available for active orifice dilation are hydrophilic serial dilators and balloon dilator. Dilation greater than 8 Fr is rarely necessary (i.e., dilatation to 2-Fr sizes greater than the diameter of the endoscope), though it has been shown that dilation up to 12 F in children did not result in vesicoureteral reflux [8]. Care must be taken to avoid dilation at or beyond the level of stone as it can cause ureteric injury. If the orifice is very stenotic or if the caliber of the ureter is too narrow to accommodate the scope, ureteral stent placement for passive dilation is preferred [9]. Ureteroscopy can be safely performed in a few days to a few weeks.

The ureteroscope can be used to displace the guidewire above and laterally, allowing the orifice to be tented open. Knowing the shape and other details of the tip of the ureteroscope before insertion is essential for properly negotiating the orifice. The beveled tip should be allowed to slide in first be rotating the scope accordingly. If required, a second guidewire can be placed through the scope and into the ureteral orifice alongside the safety wire. The scope can then be passed in between the wires by maneuvering such that the wires keep the ureteric orifice open. The second wire should be removed after entry into the ureter to improve the irrigation flow. In small children, an intravenous catheter can be placed suprapubically for bladder drainage (Fig. 29.2a–c).

In case of a cross-trigonal reimplanted ureter, a torquable ureteral catheter and angled wire are useful. Once access has been gained, the initial wire should be replaced with a stiff guidewire, which then straightens the intramural portion of the ureter, allowing access for ureteroscopy. Dilatation of the tunnel is usually not necessary, although the ureteric orifice may require dilation. At the end of the procedure, the ureter will return to its preoperative cross-trigonal position. Percutaneous transvesical ureteroscopy for removal of distal ureteral stone in reimplanted ureter has been described [10]. Sometimes a flexible ureteroscope may be necessary to enter the reimplanted ureter. In case of previously reconstructed bladder neck, care must be taken not to distort the bladder neck excessively while accessing the reimplanted ureter. After successful repair of ureteropelvic junction obstruction, the ureter remains supple at the site of previous surgery and is at no greater risk of injury.

Maneuvering Through the Distal Ureter

Maneuvering the ureteroscope through the distal ureter should be based on keeping the lumen always in the center of the field and following the guidewire. The previous retrograde study and fluoroscopy will further help in knowing the position of the scope. All the maneuvers must be

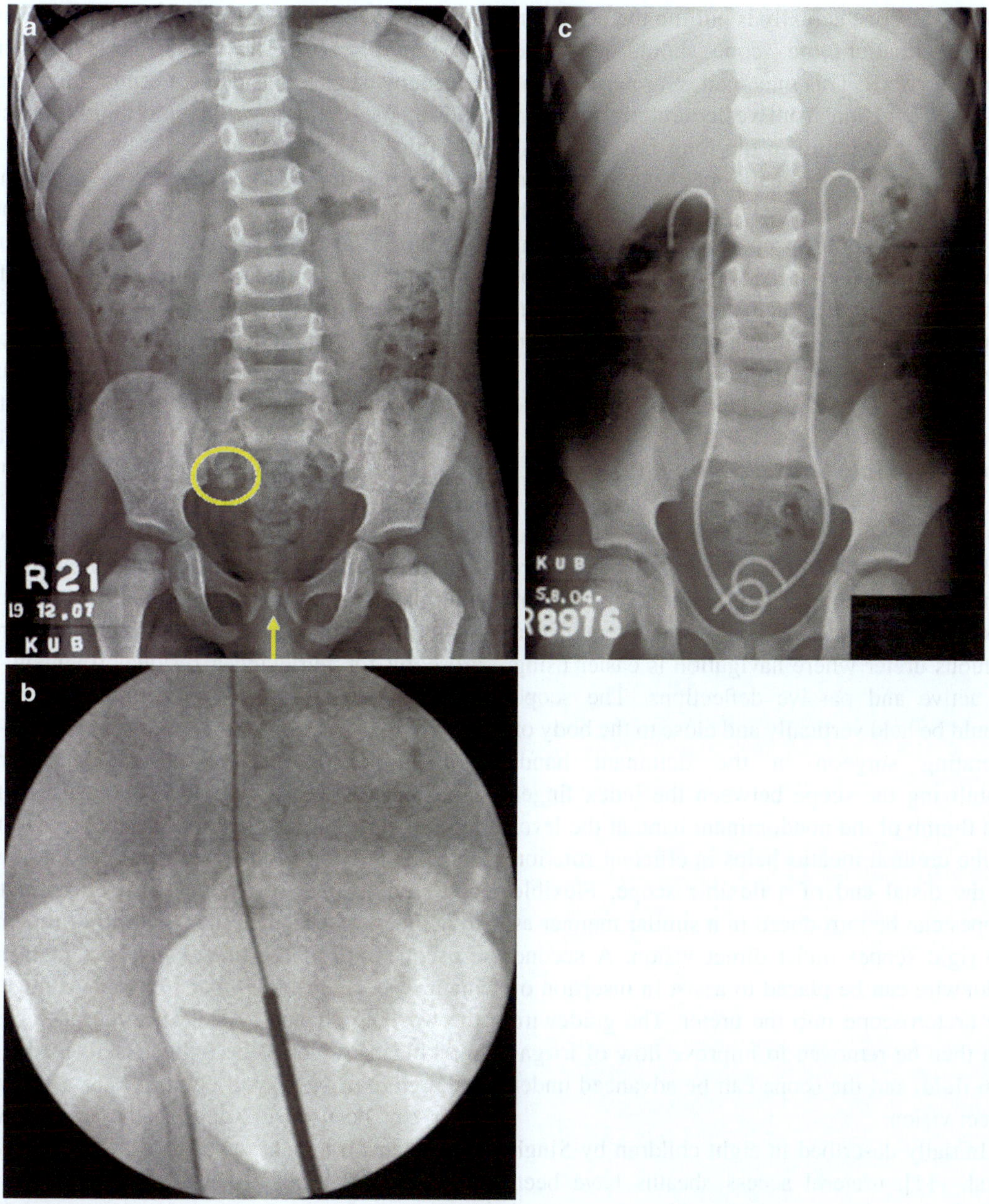

Fig. 29.2 (**a**) Prostatic urethral calculus (*arrow*) and right lower ureteric calculus (*circle*) in a 2-year-old-male child. (**b**) Using 7-Fr ureteroscope, both calculi are fragmented and retrieved in same setting. (**c**) Intravenous catheter used for drainage of bladder

gentle. In case the lumen is collapsing, mild saline irrigation with the help of handheld pump or syringe can be used. In case it is difficult to negotiate a kink in the ureter, a guidewire can be passed through the ureteroscope to straighten the ureter. This can be useful while crossing the pelvic brim.

Care must be taken to note whether the scope is advancing relative to the ureteric mucosa at all times. In case the ureter moves along with the scope, the scope actually is pulling the ureter. In such a situation, the scope should never be forced forward. This may lead to ureteric perforation or avulsion from vesicoureteric junction and ureteric stricture in the long run. The best step is to either do a gentle mechanical dilation over a wire or still safer is passive dilation with a stent. If perforation occurs, a double-J stent should be placed over the safety wire. If it is not possible, a percutaneous nephrostomy tube can be placed. Ureteric avulsion warrants immediate open ureteric reimplantation.

Use of Flexible Ureteroscope

Flexible scopes are useful for proximal ureteric and renal stones or if endoscopy is being performed in a reimplanted ureter. The use of flexible scope is especially advantageous in a tortuous ureter where navigation is easier using its active and passive deflections. The scope should be held vertically and close to the body of operating surgeon in the dominant hand. Stabilizing the scope between the index finger and thumb of the nondominant hand at the level of the urethral meatus helps in efficient rotation of the distal end of a flexible scope. Flexible scopes can be introduced in a similar manner as the rigid scopes under direct vision. A second guidewire can be placed to assist in insertion of the ureteroscope into the ureter. The guidewire can then be removed to improve flow of irrigation fluid, and the scope can be advanced under direct vision.

Initially described in eight children by Singh et al. [11], ureteral access sheaths have been shown to facilitate repetitive upper tract access, reduce intrarenal pressures, decrease operative time, and improve stone-free rates in adults. Use of ureteral access sheaths and a 6 Fr flexible ureteroscope has made possible treatment of lower pole calculi in children that would have previously required shock wave lithotripsy (SWL) or percutaneous nephrolithotomy (PCNL). Cannon et al. reported a 76 % stone-free rate in 21 children with lower pole calculi and a mean stone diameter of 12.2 cm [12]. The success rate for stones <15 mm was 93 % versus 33 % for stones ≥15 mm ($p=0.01$). Thus they suggested that ureteroscopy can be considered a primary treatment option for children with lower pole calculi <15 mm.

Flexible ureteroscopes are more costly and much more prone to damage because of their delicate design. In order to reduce the redundancy of the endoscope outside of the body during the procedure, it is preferable to use the endoscope with the appropriate length according to the age of the child (e.g., 35, 50, and 65 cm). With the use of access sheaths, the difficulty in entering the ureteric orifice is negated. But it must be noted that insertion of access sheath may not be required or possible in every patient and its use increases the cost of the procedure. The use of access sheath can safely be omitted when the need for multiple passages up the ureter is kept to a minimum, as in small-size stone or secondary ureteroscopy for retrieving a residual fragment. In some patients, staged procedures may be required.

In children, secondary passive tip deflection is rarely necessary for complete inspection of the intrarenal pediatric collecting system because the arc of deflection is adequate to access the lower pole in most pediatric kidneys. It is important to remember to straighten the distal tip of the ureteroscope prior to insertion of any working instrument, especially laser fiber to avoid damage to the working channel. Also, after the passage of working instruments, the ability to actively deflect the ureteroscope tip will be decreased. Holmium laser can be used to vaporize the stones. Any significant fragment created can be retrieved using tipless nitinol baskets (2.4–3 Fr).

In some cases of upper ureteric stone, initial stone visualization may require a flexible ureteroscope. But once the ureter is straightened out and a guidewire is passed safely across the stone, a semirigid ureteroscope can be used to rapidly fragment the stone (Fig. 29.3a, b). An antegrade approach to ureter via percutaneous flexible ureteroscopy may be required for large burden upper ureteric stone (Fig. 29.4a–c) or rarely in case of large fibroepithelial polyp which requires complete endoscopic resection.

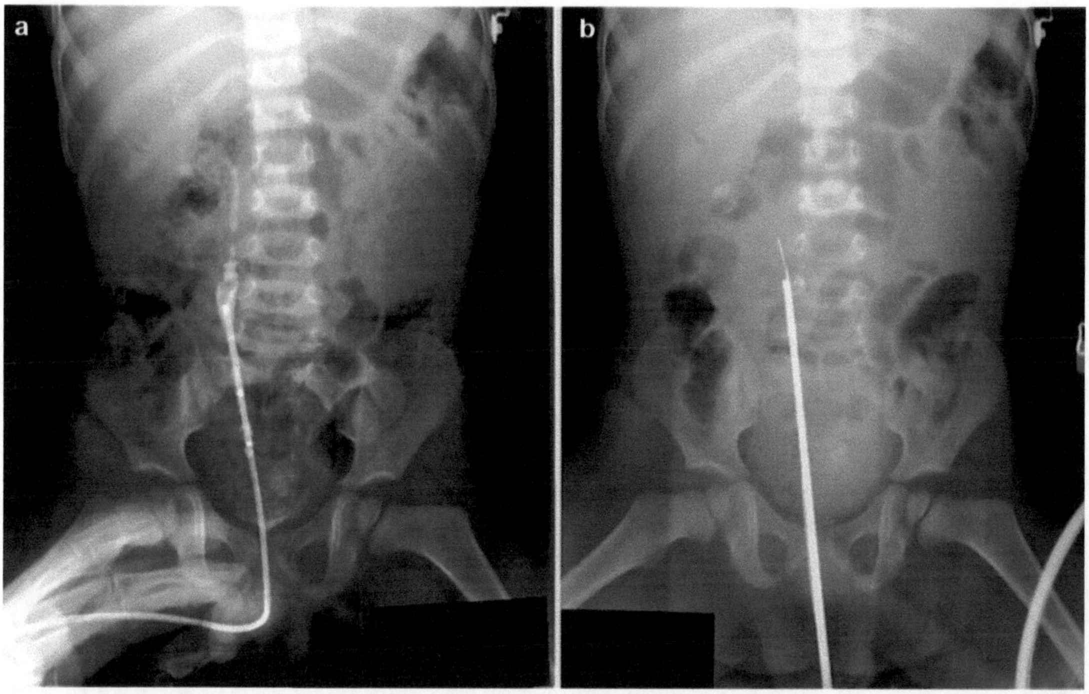

Fig. 29.3 (**a**) Initial use of flexible ureteroscope for difficult to access upper ureteric stone. (**b**) Once stone is reached, guidewire is placed across the stone, and the ureter is straightened out, a semirigid ureteroscope facilitates expedient fragmentation and stone retrieval

Intracorporeal Lithotripsy

Of the four modes of intracorporeal lithotripsy, that is, ultrasonic, ballistic or pneumatic, electrohydraulic, and laser, only pneumatic and laser lithotripsies are commonly used with ureteroscopy. The main disadvantages of pneumatic lithotripsy are retrograde migration of calculus due to pneumatic impaction and reduction in the force of lithotripsy, with significant angulation of the probe. Holmium:yttrium–aluminum–garnet (Ho:YAG) laser lithotripsy is extremely effective at fragmenting all types of urinary calculi [13]. In most centers, Holmium laser has become the preferred modality for stone fragmentation. The tip of the laser fiber should be visualized always to prevent damage to the tip of endoscope. It is necessary to place the tip in direct contact with the stone for efficient stone fragmentation. The preferred technique is "painting" the stone rather than making holes. This makes sure that large fragments are not made and complete stone vaporization occurs.

The small 200–365-μm laser fibers easily pass through the working channel of the flexible ureteroscope, and calculi in all areas of the ureter and kidney have been successfully fragmented in the pediatric population. Because of the high water absorption of the holmium laser with limited tissue penetration of 0.4 mm, there is minimal collateral damage. Thus fibrosis is minimal after incising with holmium laser. So ureterotomy for ureteric strictures and secondary pelviureteric junction obstruction and ablation of urothelial lesions can be performed safely with minimal long-term sequelae.

Postprocedural Stenting

Stenting after ureteroscopy is usually based on the urologist's decision based on the need for ureteric orifice dilation, injury to ureteric wall, and risk of postoperative edema. Other options include leaving a ureteric catheter that is externalized or a

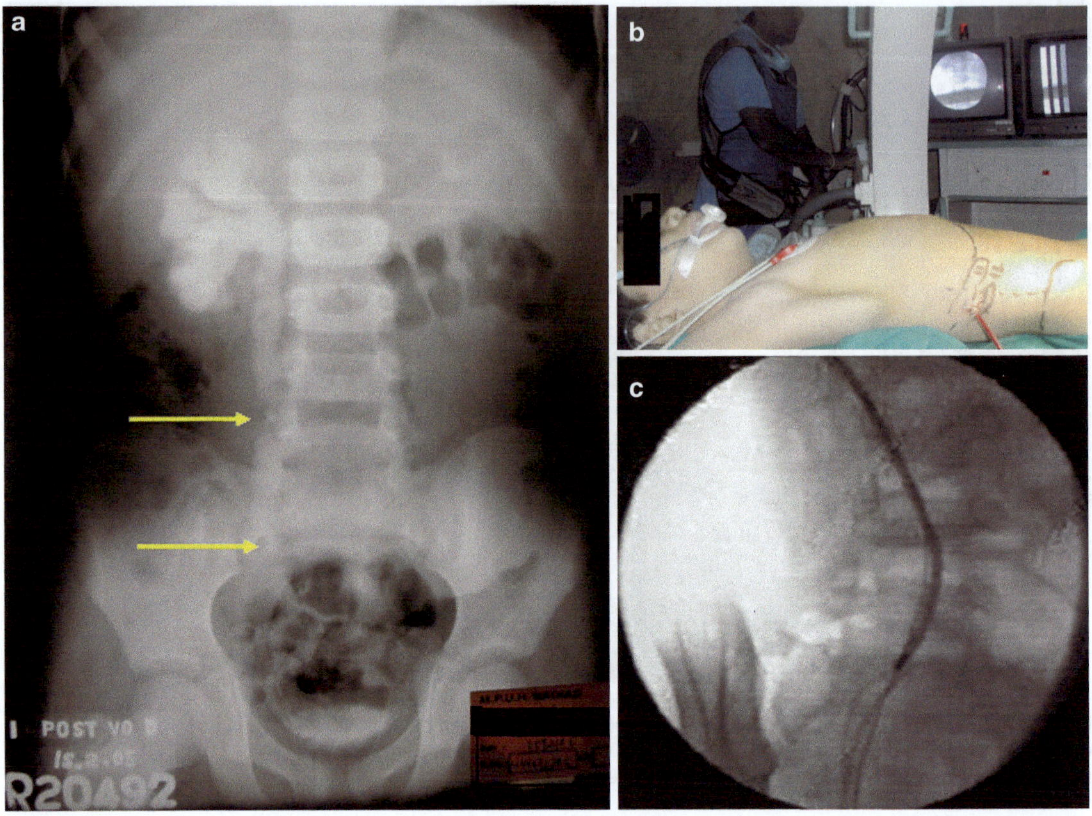

Fig. 29.4 (**a**) Multiple calculi in right upper ureter (shown by *yellow arrows*). (**b**) Supine position avoids the need for change in position and facilitates easy maneuverability of the ureter. Ultrasound-guided puncture is recommended to avoid bowel injury. (**c**) Antegrade flexible ureteroscopy for stone fragmentation and retrieval

double-J stent with a string externalized that can be removed in a few days. Thus the need for another anesthesia is avoided. In selected situations, stent placement can be altogether avoided. Again, the advantages are eliminating the need for another anesthesia and lack of stent-related symptoms.

Conclusion

Although pediatric ureteroscopy has become a safe and effective form of stone management with the help of modern small-sized equipments, care must be taken in proper performance of each procedure. It is important to know your instruments before using and the various small but important tricks in overcoming the difficulties. It is not only important to clear the stones but also monitor the growth of the kidney and prevent further stone formation by identifying and correcting any underlying metabolic abnormality.

References

1. Young HH, McKay RW. Congenital valvular obstruction of the prostatic urethra. Surg Gynecol Obstet. 1929;48:509–11.
2. Ritchey M, Patterson DE, Kelalis PP, Segura JW. A case of pediatric ureteroscopic lasertripsy. J Urol. 1988;139:1272.
3. Shepherd P, Thomas R, Harmon EP. Urolithiasis in children: innovations in management. J Urol. 1988; 140:790–3.
4. Tanriverdi O, Silay MS, Kendirci M, et al. Comparison of ureteroscopic procedures with rigid and semirigid ureteroscopes in pediatric population: does the caliber of instrument matter? Pediatr Surg Int. 2010;26:733.

5. De Dominicis M, Matarazzo E, Capozza N, et al. Retrograde ureteroscopy for distal ureteric stone removal in children. BJU Int. 2005;95:1049.
6. Minevich E, Defoor W, Reddy P, et al. Ureteroscopy is safe and effective in prepubertal children. J Urol. 2005;174:276.
7. Scarpa RM, De Lisa A, Porru D, Canetto A, Usai E. Ureterolithotripsy in children. Urology. 1995;46: 859–62.
8. Thomas R, Ortenberg J, Harmon EP. Safety and efficacy of pediatric ureteroscopy for management of calculous disease. J Urol. 1993;149:1082.
9. Hubert KC, Palmer JS. Passive dilation by ureteral stenting before ureteroscopy: eliminating the need for active dilation. J Urol. 2005;174:1079.
10. Santarosa RP, Hensle TW, Shabsigh R. Percutaneous transvesical ureteroscopy for removal of distal ureteral stone in reimplanted ureter. Urology. 1993;42:313–6.
11. Singh A, Shah G, Young J, Sheridan M, Haas G, Upadhyay J. Ureteral access sheath for the management of pediatric renal and ureteral stones: a single center experience. J Urol. 2006;175:1080.
12. Cannon GM, Smaldone MC, Wu HY, Bassett JC, Bellinger MF, Docimo SG, et al. Ureteroscopic management of lower-pole stones in a pediatric population. J Endourol. 2007;21:1179.
13. Grasso M. Experience with the holmium laser as an endoscopic lithotrite. Urology. 1996;48:199–206.

Difficulties with Ureteral Stents

30

Brandon K. Isariyawongse and Manoj Monga

Introduction

Urinary tract obstruction – whether due to calculus disease, malignancy, or other benign cause – is one of the most common problems encountered by urologists. And while the use of catheters to improve the drainage of the lower urinary tract dates back as far as the ancient Egyptians, it was only in the twentieth century that endourologists and engineers were able to develop devices that achieved upper urinary tract drainage [1]. These tools, initially referred to as "splints" or "stints," have now become most commonly referred to as ureteral stents and are among the most ubiquitous in the urologic armamentarium [2]. However, despite their common use in urology, difficulties may arise with ureteral stents and can be related to insertion or removal of the devices.

B.K. Isariyawongse, M.D.
Department of Urology, Glickman Urological and Kidney Institute, Cleveland Clinic Foundation, 9500 Euclid Avenue, Q10, Cleveland, OH 44195, USA
e-mail: isariyb@ccf.org

M. Monga, M.D., FACS (✉)
Departments of Urology, Glickman Urological and Kidney Institute, Cleveland Clinic Foundation, 9500 Euclid Avenue, Q10, Cleveland, OH 44195, USA

Stevan B. Streem Center for Endourology and Stone Disease, Cleveland, OH, USA
e-mail: mongam@ccf.org

Indications

The most common indication for ureteral stent placement occurs in the setting of upper urinary tract obstruction. Obstruction may be related to a process intrinsic to the ureter – such as ureteral stricture, or extrinsic to the ureter – such as retroperitoneal fibrosis or malignancy. Furthermore, intraluminal processes leading to obstruction such as urothelial tumors or, more commonly, urolithiasis may require ureteral stenting as well. But regardless of the cause of the ureteral obstruction, the indications for relief in general remain the same.

Evidence of pyelonephritis or infection proximal to a ureteral obstruction is an absolute indication for urgent decompression. Failure to do so may result in pyonephrosis with pyelovenous backflow and subsequent urosepsis. As such, many patients will present with evidence of infection, including fever, tachycardia, and/or leukocytosis. A urinalysis along with urine culture should also be obtained to examine the urine directly for evidence of urinary infection, with the caveat that either or both may be negative despite frank pyonephrosis in the setting of complete ureteral obstruction.

Certainly, obstruction of the urinary tract resulting in azotemia or other evidence of renal damage that may result in the permanent loss of nephrons is another absolute indication for intervention. This may occur as a result of obstruction in a patient with a solitary functioning kidney but is also possible in the setting of bilateral ureteral

A.M. Al-Kandari et al. (eds.), *Difficult Cases in Endourology*,
DOI 10.1007/978-1-84882-083-8_30, © Springer-Verlag London 2013

obstruction. Timely decompression in these instances is paramount in preserving the patient's remaining renal function.

Other relative indications for ureteral stenting include significant symptoms of urinary tract obstruction, including intractable pain or inability to tolerate oral intake. This frequently arises in the acute setting in patients with ureteral stones, and while many patients may be managed with symptomatic relief alone – namely, nonsteroidal anti-inflammatory drugs (NSAIDs) or narcotics for pain and antiemetics for nausea – some patients will require endourologic intervention to alleviate these symptoms. The etiology of renal colic-related pain is thought to be a result of increased pressure within the renal pelvis and subsequent stretch of the renal capsule. Thus, bypass of the blockage will reduce intrapelvic pressure and relieve the patient's symptoms.

Stents do have uses outside the realm of upper urinary tract obstruction. Injuries to the ureter can occur in the trauma setting or as a result of iatrogenic misadventure. In these instances, retrograde passage of a ureteral stent can be therapeutic if successful by allowing the ureter to heal over the stent via the principle of the Davis intubated ureterotomy [3]. Stents may also be employed at the time of open repair of ureteral injury in a similar fashion. Pyeloplasties and other urologic procedures requiring violation of the upper urinary tract will often utilize stents to facilitate anastomotic healing as well. Preoperative placement of ureteral stents has been employed to aid colorectal and gynecologic surgeons with intraoperative identification of the ureters, although there is not any conclusive data that this practice does indeed reduce iatrogenic ureteric injury [4].

Ureteral stents are also employed as an adjunct to endourologic procedures such as ureteroscopy and extracorporeal shockwave lithotripsy (ESWL). Chandhoke et al. demonstrated that the placement of a ureteral stent prior to ESWL does not improve stone-free rates; rather, it increases irritative voiding symptoms reported by patients [5]. Following ureteroscopy – particularly when employing a ureteral access sheath – ureteral stents are routinely placed as a measure to prevent transient ureteral obstruction as a result of postoperative edema [6]. Several studies support the theory that placement of a ureteral stent is unnecessary after uncomplicated ureteroscopy, but the decision to leave a stent in place is ultimately left with the surgeon and his or her own clinical judgment [7–9].

The primary alternative to ureteral stenting is placement of a percutaneous nephrostomy tube. Percutaneous nephrostomy tubes are most often placed by an interventional radiologist and function to decompress the upper urinary tract in an antegrade fashion. Under ultrasound or fluoroscopic guidance, a needle is used to gain access into the renal collecting system. Once access is achieved, a nephrostomy tube may be placed over a wire allowing drainage of the renal unit. Surgical diversion of the upper urinary tracts remains a long-term alternative to ureteral stenting, although endourologic and urinary reconstructive options have made this a much less common management approach.

The primary advantages of ureteral stenting are its low cost, relative ease of placement, and the low morbidity associated with its use, relative to the alternative procedures. Stents can be placed in the outpatient setting and can sometimes be performed without the need for general anesthesia. The procedure itself is comparatively straightforward in relation to other urologic procedures, and the morbidity is very low and primarily associated with the irritative voiding symptoms that the stent produces. On the other hand, a percutaneous nephrostomy requires an external appliance to collect urine and can be associated with flank pain. However, in the setting of malignant obstruction, a percutaneous nephrostomy bears the advantage of bypassing the distal drainage, as a ureteral stent may itself be compressed by a growing external malignancy.

Technique

The patient is placed in the dorsal lithotomy position. Care is taken to position the patient such that the fluoroscopy C-arm has appropriate access both above and below the bed between the patient's pubis and the nipple line. Access is gained into the bladder using a standard rigid or flexible cystoscope. Through the working channel of the cystoscope, we employ a 0.035 hybrid guidewire with a hydrophilic tip and a stiffer shaft (Boston Scientific Sensor™, Natick, MA) to cannulate the ureteral orifice. The wire is then advanced under fluoroscopic guidance until coiling is noted in the renal pelvis. In the event that the wire cannot be advanced past a point of obstruction, a 5-French (Fr) open-ended ureteral catheter is advanced over the wire to that point, and the guidewire is removed. A gentle retrograde pyelogram is performed through the open-ended catheter to delineate the ureteral anatomy, and then a Boston Scientific (Natick, MA) Glidewire® is inserted through the catheter. The Glidewire itself is hydrophilic, and so, care must be taken to ensure that it is kept moist for optimal maneuverability; the open-ended catheter may also be flushed with irrigant for this reason as well. Typically, the Glidewire will traverse the level of obstruction, following which the open ended is advanced to the kidney and wire exchanged for the Sensor wire.

The ureteral stent may be placed under a combination of direct cystoscopic vision and fluoroscopic guidance, or it may be placed under fluoroscopy alone. Typically, we will utilize a cystoscopic approach for women with pelvic organ prolapse and men with intravesical extension of BPH. In these situations, the ureteral stent is advanced over the wire utilizing the positioning catheter (pusher) to the level of the renal pelvis. Ideally, if the appropriate stent length was chosen, the thick marking line on the ureteral stent will be visualized at the ureteral orifice. The cystoscope is withdrawn to the bladder neck, and the ureteral stent is visualized as it slides into the ureter. The guidewire is removed. Coils are noted in the kidney (fluoroscopically) and in the bladder (visually), and the bladder is drained.

For many patients after ureteroscopy, the stent is placed under fluoroscopic guidance alone. In this situation, the pusher is advanced until the radiopaque marker on the pusher reaches the mid-pubis in men or the lower edge of the pubic bone in women.

Ureteral stents come in a variety of sizes, lengths, and materials [10, 11]. Stent size is measured in Fr (3 Fr = 1 mm), and stent length is measured along the straight portion of the stent in centimeters (cm). Generally, we generally employ 6- or 7-Fr stents in the adult patient, although stents as small as 4 Fr or as large as 8 Fr may be used. For adults, stent length may be approximated in cm by subtracting 42 from the patient's height in inches. For example, for a 5′10 adult male, an appropriate stent length would be 28 cm [70 – 42] [12]. Intraoperatively, one can also measure the ureter using a calibrated ureteral catheter to choose appropriate length of stent.

Traditional ureteral stents are currently constructed of silicone, polyurethane, and other synthetic polymers with varying degrees of treatments to resist encrustation and infection. It is difficult to draw direct comparisons between stent compositions, and there appear to be disparities in performance even among stents of the same composition. Born out of the need for a device that was less compressible than the standard variety, stents composed of metal or reinforced with a metal coil have become popularized in treating cases of extrinsic ureteral compression, and evidence has shown that they are superior to traditional ureteral stents in relieving malignant obstruction [13, 14]. Tolerability tends to vary from patient to patient, as is the case with traditional stents, but it should be noted that the cost is significantly greater with metal stents.

Complicated Cases

In general, ureteral stent placement is uncomplicated and considered to be one of the most basic of endourologic procedures, but as with any surgical procedure, one may encounter pitfalls and complications along the way.

A common complication occurs when attempting to place a ureteral stent to bypass an obstructing stone in the acute state. If the stone is truly impacted within the ureteral lumen, retrograde passage of a Glidewire, let alone a ureteral stent, may prove extremely challenging. This may occur similarly in cases of tight ureteral strictures.

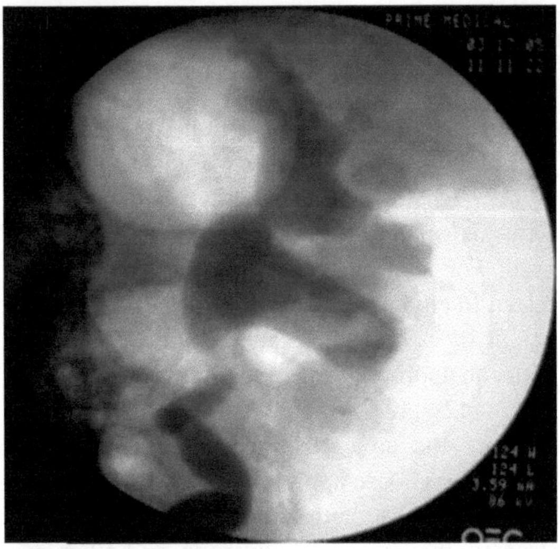

Fig. 30.1 A Kumpe angled catheter was used to manipulate the guidewire through the tortuous ureter and into the renal pelvis

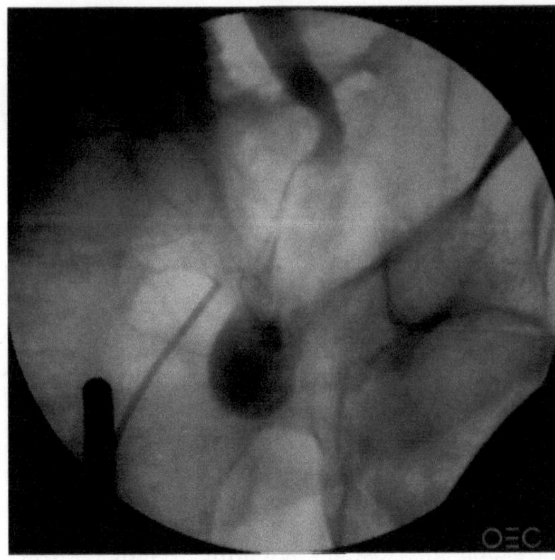

Fig. 30.2 Attempts at retrograde passage of a guidewire led to coiling of a wire within a Hutch diverticulum. A guidewire was successfully advanced into the ureter under direct vision using a 6-Fr semirigid ureteroscope

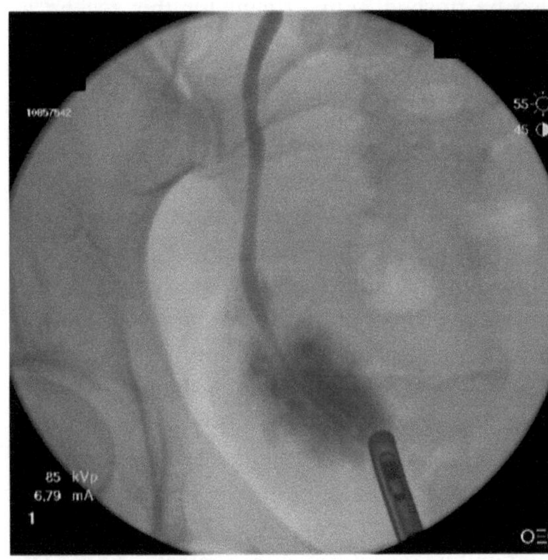

Fig. 30.3 Initial attempts at guidewire placement resulted in a false passage in the distal ureter and extravasation of contrast. A guidewire was subsequently placed under direct vision using a 4.5-Fr semirigid ureteroscope

In these instances, it is useful to utilize an angled hydrophilic guidewire with the assistance of a torque device, which allows controlled manipulation of the wire direction, through an open-ended ureteral catheter with continuous fluoroscopic guidance. Typically, by using this method, it is possible to find a luminal gap through which the wire may be passed into the collecting system. Alternatively, one may employ an angled catheter, such as a Kumpe "hockey stick" catheter or a Cobra "C-shaped" catheter, to facilitate steering of the wire, in particular, if significant tortuosity is noted on retrograde pyelogram (Fig. 30.1).

Should this fail, consideration should be given to performing ureteroscopy utilizing either a semirigid or flexible ureteroscope, which will facilitate passage of a guidewire under direct vision (Fig. 30.2). This technique may be of benefit if a minor ureteral perforation has occurred with prior guidewire placement, resulting in extravasation (Fig. 30.3); in this situation, placement of a wire under direct vision may be of benefit with the semirigid ureteroscope.

Any attempts at manipulation of an obstructing stone must be taken with great care as the ureter is a delicate organ and prone to perforation or avulsion. If needed, one may fragment an obstructing stone with holmium laser lithotripsy until the ureteral lumen opens sufficiently to allow passage of the guidewire, but no attempts at basket extraction should be made unless a safety wire is in place (Fig. 30.4). Once the guidewire is in the collecting system, passage of the stent typically is successful.

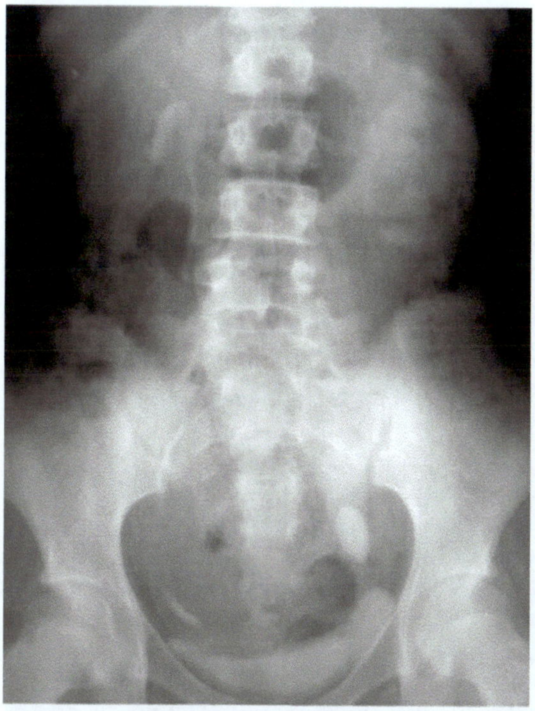

Fig. 30.4 A large distal ureteral stone prevented access to the renal pelvis. Semirigid ureteroscopy and holmium laser lithotripsy were utilized to fragment the stone, after which a guidewire was placed under direct vision through the ureteroscope

However, if difficulty is encountered, which may be the case in instances of considerable extrinsic compression, one may utilize a dual-lumen catheter to exchange the existing guidewire for a superstiff guidewire. The added rigidity will reduce buckling of the wire and facilitate retrograde stent passage. Similarly, by placing the stent under direct vision using a rigid cystoscope, it is possible to utilize rigidity of the scope itself to minimize the risk of buckling in the bladder.

Ureteral obstruction in pregnancy presents a unique problem because of altered anatomy and renal physiology in addition to considerations related to the developing fetus. Ureteral stenting may be accomplished under local anesthesia, as previously mentioned, and with the assistance of ultrasound in place of fluoroscopy to minimize radiation exposure to the fetus. The choice of appropriate stent length is more challenging given the presence of the gravid uterus and generally will require several extra centimeters to account for the distorted anatomy. The ureteral orifice itself may be difficult to localize for similar reasons, and one may need to employ a flexible cystoscope to successfully cannulate the orifice with a guidewire. Finally, as a result of increased urinary calcium excretion during pregnancy, rapid stent encrustation may occur, which must be taken into account in relation to the frequency of stent changes required prior to childbirth. In view of this, it is now recognized the primary ureteroscopy to avoid prolonged ureteral stenting is a good alternative for ureteral calculi during pregnancy [15].

Calcified ureteral stents deserve special mention because of their resultant morbidity and cost. Despite the best efforts of medical device manufacturers to produce stents that resist calcification, stent encrustation remains a very real problem. Stent encrustation is a result of ureteral stents serving as a nidus for crystallization for normal urinary solutes and is directly related to stent dwell time. For stents that have been indwelling for more than 6 months, it is reasonable to check an abdominal X-ray to evaluate for stent encrustation. However, recent studies suggest that computerized tomography is superior to evaluate the degree of proximal coil encrustation – which is prognostic of the need for multiple-staged procedures [16]. Consideration should be given to removal in the operating room under fluoroscopy where one can observe the unfurling of the proximal coil of the stent. If the coil does not unfurl easily, passage of a stiff-shaft guidewire retrograde may straighten the stent and allow uncomplicated removal. However, if significant calcification of the stent is noted preoperatively, adjunctive measures such as ESWL, ureteroscopy, or percutaneous approaches should be employed to free the stent from stone to facilitate removal (Figs. 30.5 and 30.6) [17]. Failure to do so may result in ureteral avulsion.

Advances in reconstructive techniques of the urinary tract in conjunction with early and aggressive oncologic principles for urologic malignancies present a unique problem for the endourologist. Many now consider continent urinary diversion to be the standard of care in the

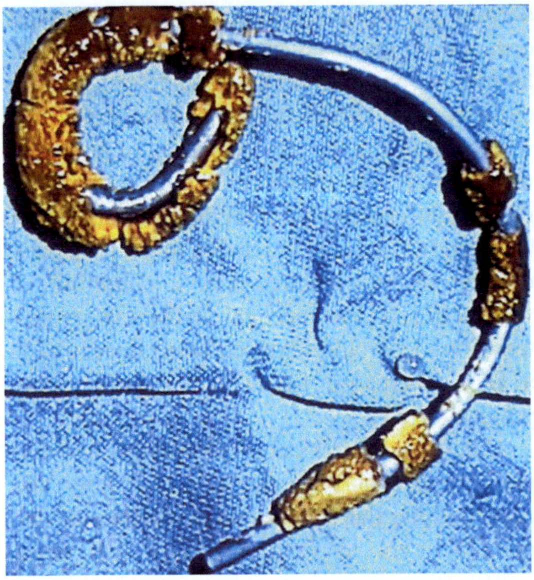

Fig. 30.5 A very large stone burden encrusted on this ureteral stent required percutaneous nephrolithotomy for successful fragmentation and extraction

treatment of urothelial cell carcinoma of the bladder, and patients undergoing neobladder construction following radical cystectomy with subsequent endourologic complications – including strictures and stones – are being seen with increasing frequency. Furthermore, the patients who choose to undergo continent neobladder construction do so primarily with a goal of improved quality of life and, as such, commonly desire to avoid the morbidity associated with the percutaneous approaches used to access the upper urinary tract. With this goal in mind, it is requisite that the treating urologist has a reasonable comfort level utilizing retrograde endoscopic techniques in these bladders with often very unpredictable anatomy. The overriding principles in these situations include prompt identification of the ureteral orifices with successful cannulation using a combination of flexible and rigid endoscopy depending on the situation encountered.

Identifying and locating the ureteral orifices in cases of urinary diversion, and also ureteral reimplantation, are commonly quite trying. Certainly, as with any urologic case involving distorted anatomy, review of preoperative imaging will help to

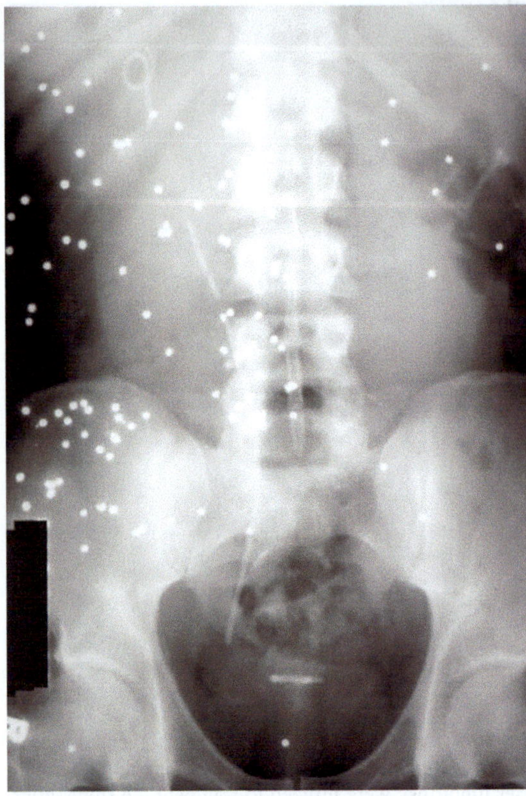

Fig. 30.6 Ureteral stent placed at the time of penetrating trauma (shotgun blast). The patient returned 2 years later with a fragmented stent and a stone in the bladder, requiring open cystolithalopaxy, ureteroscopy, and percutaneous nephroscopy

guide the intraoperative plan. We highly recommend employing intravenous agents that are excreted into the urine – namely, indigo carmine or methylene blue – which can greatly aid in identification of the orifices. In the patient with renal insufficiency, excretion of these agents may be delayed, and consideration should be given to administration at the time of induction.

Oftentimes, the ureteral orifices are not readily identifiable but rather recessed from the mucosa, and the excretion of the dye allows for general localization of the orifice as a starting point for access. We recommend the use of hydrophilic wires with a floppy tip advanced through an open-ended ureteral catheter to gently probe the area of interest, which may be successful if the ureteral orifice is widely patent. If the area of dye excretion is in an unusual location that is not amenable to rigid cystoscopy, a standard flexible cystoscope may be employed which may permit passage of a wire more easily. Consideration can also be given to using a flexible ureteroscope to attempt to localize the orifice; this instrumentation affords the flexibility of the flexible cystoscope but also adds quite a bit of length for distant ureteral orifices. This technique can be particularly useful in cases of Studer neobladder diversion, where the ureters are sewn into a "chimney" located proximal to the bulk of the neobladder. This places the ureteral orifices quite a distance from the urethra and makes it particularly amenable to the use of the flexible ureteroscope. The unusual anatomy of the neobladder also raises the issue of appropriate ureteral stent choice in terms of length. In our experience, the use of a single-J ureteral stent allows for a long distal segment that is amenable to outpatient endoscopic retrieval. The following case will highlight some of the aforementioned techniques.

Ureteral Access with Ureteroscopy and Stenting in a Studer Neobladder

We present a case of a 68-year-old male with a prior history of carcinoma in situ (CIS) of the urinary bladder who had undergone radical cystoprostatectomy with Studer ileal neobladder continent urinary diversion 8 years prior to presentation. Final pathology was significant for CIS at the bilateral ureteral margins. The patient had been followed expectantly by his primary urologist for several years, and he had recently developed positive urine cytologies. Furthermore, CT imaging of the abdomen and pelvis demonstrated bilateral dilation of the renal pelvises and ureters, with some increase on the left-hand side relative to prior imaging. Metastatic evaluation was negative, and the patient was asymptomatic. A cystogram was performed which showed no reflux into either ureter. The patient was counseled regarding the possible etiologies of the radiologic findings, including tumor recurrence and ureteroileal stricture, and he was offered either antegrade or retrograde ureteroscopy for further evaluation and possible management. He elected to undergo retrograde ureteroscopy with ureteral stent placement.

The patient was brought into the operating room and induced under general anesthesia, placed in the dorsal lithotomy position, and prepped and draped in the usual fashion for standard retrograde endoscopy. Access was gained into the urinary bladder using a 20-Fr rigid cystoscope using a 30° lens. Indigo carmine was administered intravenously to help to localize the ureteral orifices; efflux was noted from the right anterior surface of the neobladder, which identified the opening of the neobladder chimney. Attempts were made to cannulate the chimney using a flexible cystoscope, a semirigid ureteroscope, and a flexible ureteroscope. The chimney was successfully cannulated with a Sensor Guidewire via the rigid cystoscope while utilizing compression of the anterior abdomen to adjust the anatomy into a more favorable configuration. A 5-Fr open-ended ureteral catheter was advanced over the Sensor Guidewire, which was then exchanged for an Amplatz Superstiff Guidewire. A dual-lumen catheter was then advanced over the superstiff guidewire to facilitate placement of a second superstiff wire into the ileal chimney. The first superstiff wire was secured as a safety wire, and a 12/14 Fr × 45 cm ureteral access sheath was then placed over the working wire, which was thereafter removed. A Wolf Viper flexible ureteroscope (Richard Wolf Medical, Vernon Hills, IL) was then advanced through the sheath, and endoscopy of the chimney was performed. Indigo carmine was again administered to facilitate localization of the left ureteral orifice. Once the orifice was identified, access was gained into the left ureter under direct vision, and flexible ureteroscopy was performed. After ureteral washings were obtained and a retrograde pyelogram was performed, a superstiff wire was placed through the ureteroscope with good coiling within the renal pelvis. The ureteroscope was then removed, and a 6 Fr × 65 cm Angiocath with a single coil

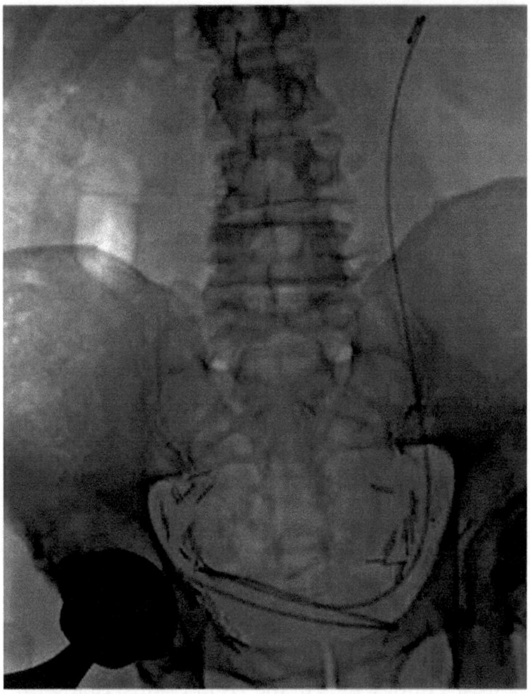

Fig. 30.7 Postoperative image following left ureteral stent placement in Studer neobladder

was advanced under fluoroscopic guidance until a good coil was noted in the renal pelvis. The residual catheter was advanced into the bladder for endoscopic retrieval (Fig. 30.7).

Conclusion

Ureteral stenting is a common urologic procedure with many indications, including urinary tract obstruction and trauma. And though one of its advantages is its ease relative to other urologic procedures, it is not without propensity for complications and pitfalls. Knowledge of basic endourologic principles and comfort with the full armamentarium of available endoscopic equipment will prepare one well for handling difficult cases of ureteral stenting.

References

1. Bitschay J, Brodny M. A history of urology in Egypt. New York: Riverside Press; 1956.
2. Goodwin W. Splint, stent, stint. Urol Dig. 1972;11:13.
3. Davis DM. Intubated ureterotomy: a new operation for ureteral and ureteropelvic strictures. Surg Gynaecol Obstet. 1943;76:513–4.
4. Kuno K, Menzin A, Kauder HH, et al. Prophylactic ureteral catheterization in gynecologic surgery. Urology. 1998;52(6):1004–8.
5. Chandhoke PS, Barqawi AZ, Wernecke C, et al. A randomized outcomes trial of ureteral stents for extracorporeal shock wave lithotripsy of solitary kidney or proximal ureteral stones. J Urol. 2002;167:1981.
6. Rapoport D, Perks AE, Teichman JM. Ureteral access sheath use and stenting in ureteroscopy: effect on unplanned emergency room visits and cost. J Endourol. 2007;21:993.
7. Chen YT, Chen J, Wong WY, et al. Is ureteral stenting necessary after uncomplicated ureteroscopic lithotripsy? A prospective, randomized controlled trial. J Urol. 2002;167:1977.
8. Srivastava A, Gupta R, Kumar A, et al. Routine stenting after ureteroscopy for distal ureteral calculi is unnecessary: results of a randomized controlled trial. J Endourol. 2003;17:871.
9. Preminger GM, Tiselius HG, Assimos DG, et al. Guideline for the management of ureteral calculi. J Urol. 2007;178:2418.
10. Chew BH, Duvdevani M, Denstedt JD. New developments in ureteral stent design, materials and coatings. Expert Rev Med Devices. 2006;3:395.
11. Denstedt JD, Reid G, Sofer M. Advances in ureteral stent technology. World J Urol. 2000;18:237.
12. Wieder JA. Ureteral stents. In: Wieder JA, editor. Pocket guide to urology. 2nd ed. Boise: Griffith Publishing; 2005. p. 151.
13. Borin JF, Melamud O, Clayman RV. Initial experience with full-length metal stent to relieve malignant ureteral obstruction. J Endourol. 2006;20:300.
14. Blaschko SD, Deane LA, Krebs A, et al. In-vivo evaluation of flow characteristics of novel metal ureteral stent. J Endourol. 2007;21:780.
15. Semins MJ, Trock BJ, Matlaga BR, et al. The safety of ureteroscopy during pregnancy: a systematic review and meta-analysis. J Urol. 2009;181:139–43.
16. Weedin JW, Coburn M, Link RE. The impact of proximal stone burden on the management of encrusted and retained ureteral stents. J Urol. 2011;185:542–7.
17. Monga M, Klein E, Castaneda-Zuniga WR, et al. The forgotten indwelling ureteral stent: a urological dilemma. J Urol. 1995;153:1817.

Overcoming the Cost Difficulties in Endourology

31

Ravindra B. Sabnis

Introduction

The fascination with performing surgery through a small incision is as old as the history of surgery itself. Over a period of years, this fascination has led to the development of minimally invasive or keyhole surgery as a separate subspecialty. Rapid advances and all-round developments, especially in last two to three decades, have led endourology to be the most attractive and sought-after branch of urology all over the world. Most procedures now can be performed by minimally invasive methods, thanks to the massive research conducted by biomedical engineers, clinicians, and researchers. Today, we have different types of scopes (rigid, flexible), lithotripsy machines, laser units, high-definition cameras, chip-on-tip technology, and not to forget the emergence of robot. All these have resulted in reducing morbidity, less hospital stay, and early resumption of work. However, looking at the other side of the coin, cost of treatment has escalated to a great extent. Therefore, cost in endourological treatment has become a major concern. Efforts are now being made to overcome cost difficulties irrespective of whether a patient pays for himself or is covered by insurance. This chapter deals with various measures that can be employed to reduce the overall cost of the endourology procedure without affecting safety.

Where the Cost Is Involved

The cost of any endourological procedure (when operative and theater charges – since they vary from country to country – are excluded) largely depends on the cost of investigations, equipments, disposables, and hospital stay. Quite often, several procedures are available to treat particular problems; for example, for 10-mm middle calyx stone, the options could be shock wave lithotripsy (SWL), retrograde interventional renal surgery (RIRS), mini-perc, and others. It is worth considering choosing the most economical method, provided that the success and complications of each method are not significantly different [1]. So, selection of procedure is also important in the discussion of cost-cutting measures. Thus, any cost-cutting measures in endourology will revolve around cost of investigations, cost of equipment, cost of disposables, hospital stay, and selection of procedures.

Cost of Investigations

Imaging has become an integral part of the diagnostic workup for any disease. Newer methods have changed the choice of investigations in several centers across the globe. CT IVU is now

R.B. Sabnis, M.S., MCH
Department of Urology,
Muljibhai Patel Urological Hospital,
Dr. Virendra Desai Road, Nadiad 387001, India
e-mail: rbsabnis@gmail.com

A.M. Al-Kandari et al. (eds.), *Difficult Cases in Endourology*,
DOI 10.1007/978-1-84882-083-8_31, © Springer-Verlag London 2013

preferred over conventional IVU. There is no doubt that CT IVU obtains much more information and is more specific and sensitive than conventional IVU [2–5], but the cost difference is also significant. Many centers in the USA and Europe have stopped doing conventional IVU for renal function evaluation. Is this blanket shift justifiable from a cost point of view? For example, before doing interventions such as URS for a small stone in ureter, one has to do a functional study. In such situations, low-cost conventional IVU will yield equal information as CT IVU and thus the cost burden can be reduced. In the Western world, several investigations are done sometimes in anticipation of avoiding possible lawsuits and to be safe legally. This not only puts a burden on the system but also escalates the cost to a considerable extent. Judicious investigations tailor-made to specific situations will reduce the cost without compromising the outcome. This can be a first step in overcoming cost difficulties.

Cost of Equipment

The state of endourology today is due to the development of newer sophisticated equipment. Progress in last four decades has taken us from conventional cystoscope with bulb at the tip to flexible digital slender cystoscope with camera at the tip. Endourology equipment can be divided according to the usage, for example, equipment required for PCNL, URS, RIRS, transurethral resection of the prostate (TURP), optical urethrotomy, laparoscopy, etc. Or it can be classified as high-end, intermediate-end, and low-end equipment. There are many accessories along with the main equipment. The modern endourology suite cannot be complete unless one has the full armamentarium.

High-End Equipment

High-end equipment such as nephroscopes, semirigid or flexible URS, telescopes, high-definition (HD) camera with monitor, laser units, and SWL are researched over years. A few companies across the globe manufacture them. Their production involves several complexities, precision, and sophistication. The cost of such equipment is usually very high. Since there are few manufacturers globally, this equipment usually must be imported by most countries. For any country, if any item is to be imported, the additional costs of import duties, transportation, and currency differences play a major role. Thus, when such equipment arrives in the hands of the end user, the cost has already increased considerably. If a urologist in a developing country in Asia has to import a laser machine manufactured in the USA or a flexible URS made in Germany, then he has to spend a huge amount of funds available to him in his currency. The return on the investment will be as per the local cost of living and local capacity of expenditure. This imbalance may make investment economically nonviable to many individuals. To overcome these cost difficulties, it is advisable to purchase equipment in groups. If many urologists combine their costs, then they will have to contribute much less as a group than they would have otherwise paid individually. The equipment will also be better utilized. Sharing the equipment not only cuts down the capital cost of purchasing but proves economically attractive in terms of maintenance as many of these high-end instruments have high annual maintenance costs.

Intermediate-End Equipment

Intermediate-end equipment (such as light source and cables, CO_2 insufflators, TUR working element, etc.) is not that expensive and is far less sophisticated than their high-end counterparts. Many companies manufacture them, and the endourologists in different countries have options to choose from. One has to select the cheaper yet better model. Usually, this equipment experiences more usage and more wear and tear, and therefore, it is not a good idea to share it. Overcoming cost is achieved by judicious selection of the make and model of the instrument.

Low-End Equipment

Low-end equipment (such as cystoscope sheaths, PCNL/URS forceps, stone-crushing forceps/stone punch, forceps used in laparoscopy, internal urethrotomy sheath, pneumatic lithotripter, etc.) does not involve high sophistication in manufacturing. In many countries, local companies manufacture them. Whatever is produced locally is always cheaper. However, one has to select which is best among the lot.

Conclusion

A combination of high-end equipment purchased as a group along with accessories manufactured locally and purchased locally will overcome the cost to a considerable extent. For example:

1. Purchase a nephroscope from an international company but purchase forceps and a pneumatic lithotripter from the local market.
2. Purchase a telescope and camera from a high-end manufacturer but purchase the cystoscope sheath, stone crusher, biopsy forceps, light source, and cable from the local market.
3. Purchase a laparoscope telescope and CO_2 insufflator from a high-end manufacturer but all accessories such as suction, forceps, and needle drivers from local manufacturers.
4. Form a group to purchase a lithotripter and laser unit.

Cost of Disposables

A major chunk of budgetary allocation in most hospitals is eaten up by the ever-increasing disposables' cost. Disposables can be classified as major (nephrostomy tract balloon (NephroMax™, Boston Scientific, Natick, MA) or ureteric balloon catheters, nitinol baskets, laparoscopic scissors, forceps, different types of guide wires, etc.) and minor (different catheters, drainage tubes, dilators, etc.). Different countries have different laws which everyone must follow, but from a scientific point of view, whatever items used during procedures have to be sterile and should not transmit any disease from one individual to other. Single-use policy prevents transmission of disease from one person to another but puts a tremendous burden on the budget. Most major disposable items can be resterilized and brought into use again. A set methodology and protocol have to be developed and implemented toward this goal. Items such as guidewires, Amplatz sheath, nitinol baskets, balloon catheters, dilators, and laparoscopic instruments can be thoroughly cleaned by mechanical and enzymatic cleansers. All hollow tubes are cleaned from the inside by pressure flow, resulting in a thorough washing inside the hollow tubes. These are then dried properly, packed, sealed, and sent for sterilization either by gamma radiation, ETO, or plasma sterilization. Such items can then be equivalent to new items with regard to sterility. Implementing such a policy can reduce cost considerably without compromising quality. The situation in the developed world is different. When sterilizing, manpower is required to clean, wash, pack, seal, etc. In many developed countries, manpower is expensive. Each country has to look into their prevailing situation to decide whether pursue the reusable model or stay with a use and throw policy. Several developing countries have adopted the reusage model and are happy to continue with it. Items that are considered as minor disposable items are not worth reusing. They are typically kept indwelling in a patient's body or have very long hollow tubes (ureteric catheter) that are difficult to clean and sterilize. Thus, a balance has to be stuck between single use models, reuse policy, cost of manpower, and safety. Whatever method is adopted, sterility cannot be compromised.

In many countries, disposable gowns and drapes are used. Disposable gowns add to the cost; however, reusing gowns also needs manpower to send the gowns through the sterilization process. Many procedures have dedicated drapes, for example, laparoscopy, TURP, PCNL, etc.

Usage of these can be restricted, and permanent linen drapes can be used which can be autoclaved and reused.

Plasma sterilization has become a method of choice for sterilization of various endourological equipment. This method is quick and therefore can be used so that equipment can be shared by two surgeries. It makes sense to have this unit near the operating theater so that whatever instruments are reusable, disposables can be sterilized. This avoids duplication of instruments and is aided by the fact that many procedures are planned in 1 day thereby further reducing the capital cost of inventory.

Thus, judicious reuse as per the prevailing laws in the country will go a long way in overcoming cost difficulties.

Hospital Stay

Hospital stay costs differ considerably from country to country, and even within a given country, they will vary from region to region. As a general rule, reduced hospital stay would result in quick recovery and early resumption of work. This in turn will prove to be cost beneficial to the patient. Therefore, all endourological procedures are aimed to reduce hospital stay. Tubeless PCNL [6], inserting double J stent after PCNL, or URS are some of the techniques that result in quick catheter removals and reduced hospital stay. Typically in developing countries, hospital stay is far less expensive; therefore, even if you select a procedure that results in a longer hospital stay, this will not add much to the financial burden. For example, if the cost of JJ stent is more than a day or two in terms of hospital stay, then it is better to avoid the stent, thereby reducing cost. But, by and large, a reduced hospital stay will help in decreasing the overall cost of treatment.

Selecting the Procedure

Endourology is a rapidly advancing area. Newer and newer methods are being developed, each with various advantages and disadvantages. It is up to the urologist to decide which modality to adopt depending upon the success rate, safety, and morbidity. If all modalities have almost similar safety and efficacy, then the urologist should select a method that is cost effective. For example, 1-cm stone in the renal pelvis can be treated by SWL, RIRS, or mini-perc. The choice of treatment will largely depend on the surgeon's preference. But cost also should be borne in mind. These implications will vary from country to country and from region to region. Some countries may find SWL cheaper as compared to RIRS or mini-perc, while in some centers, mini-perc may be cheaper than SWL or RIRS. A large burden stone can be treated by RIRS, but it takes a long time, has increased chance of infection, and may result in early damage of flexible URS. Thus, it is not appropriate to do large burden stone by RIRS as PCNL becomes much cheaper. Ureteric strictures of benign etiology that are not candidates for definitive reconstructive surgery are managed by DJ stent and repeatedly changing the stent. Metallic stents are expensive, but using them avoids repeated changes and therefore in turn may prove to be more cost effective in the long run [7].

Thus, all such factors should be carefully considered before selecting a procedure so as to overcome cost difficulties.

Selecting the Energy Source

Like equipment, advances have been made in the development of newer and better energy sources for breaking a stone. Ultrasound, pneumatic, and laser are the most common energy sources. They are not competitive but instead are complementary to each other. Understanding the appropriate choice will make the procedure not only cost effective but safe as well. In PCNL, pneumatic is better than laser; in upper ureteric stone, laser is better; however, in lower ureter, pneumatic energy can take care of stone fragmentation. Pneumatic energy source is cheaper while laser is more expensive. So whenever laser is not required, use alternate energy sources to overcome cost difficulties. Even when holmium laser energy is used, reusable fiber is cost beneficial than the single-use variant [8].

Methods for Overcoming Cost Difficulties in Some Common Endourological Procedures

PCNL

1. In case of simple stone: Limited plates conventional IVU can be done.
2. Drapes can be of linen: reusable.
3. Puncture needle can be reused many times after thorough cleaning and then plasma sterilization.
4. Dilatation of tract up to the desired size by Alken telescopic dilators and then putting Amplatz sheath.
5. Stone breaking by pneumatic energy source, which is cheaper in terms of both purchasing and maintenance.
6. Reuse of Amplatz dilator and Amplatz sheath.
7. Use of locally made instruments such as forceps.
8. Careful planning of punctures, which helps achieve clearance in one or a minimum of stages.
9. Avoiding any complications: Any complications such as bleeding and infection add considerably to the cost. All efforts should be taken in planning the procedure to make sure that complete clearance is achieved in minimal stages and without any complications.

URS

1. Avoid two stages: Inability to dilate ureter up to adequate size results in a staged procedure. Any staged procedure involves additional cost. This can be avoided by the use of ultrathin URS such as 6 or 4.8 Fr.
2. Slender URS does not need dilatation, thus reducing the cost burden further by avoiding use of ureteric dilators.
3. In ureteroscopy especially for upper ureteric stone, there is a chance of migration of stone into the kidney. If this migration occurs, it involves another procedure such as SWL or RIRS. This is an additional cost. Use of laser energy rather than pneumatic reduces the chance of migration, thereby controlling the cost.

Thus, thin (6 or 4.8 Fr) URS and laser disintegration are cost-overcoming tools in this situation.

Flexible URS

1. Flexible URS is a very delicate instrument. It is likely to be damaged if not used properly. A novice should practice on a model in a dry lab for a sufficient length of time. Once accustomed, he should use the instrument under the supervision of an experienced surgeon. This will avoid damage to the instrument.
2. Access sheath can be reused by plasma sterilization.
3. All methods described to prolong the life of flexible URS should be adopted:
   (a) Avoiding repeated extreme bending, which will damage flexion mechanism.
   (b) Lower calyceal stones should be repositioned in other calyx or else they will add to wear and tear.
   (c) Access sheath will prevent damage if repeated in and outs are done.
   (d) Laser fiber should be properly covered, and insulation should be checked before every surgery.
   (e) Laser tip fiber should protrude adequately outside the tip of the scope or else the lens will get damaged by the laser.
4. Judicious use of nitinol baskets: Do not catch fragments that are too big, which may result in damaging the basket. Thus, baskets can be reused.
5. Use of hand-held pump/syringe irrigation instead of expensive pressure irrigation systems.

TURP

1. Standard TURP does not have many cost issues; however, when it comes to other modalities such as laser prostatectomies, bipolar

TURP cost can be a significant factor. TURP still remains the gold standard for treatment of most BPH. Barring certain situations (very large prostates, patient on anticoagulation therapy, patient with pacemaker, patient with bleeding disorders, etc.), the newer modalities may not have added advantages. Thus, these methods can be reserved for special circumstances to overcome cost difficulties.

Laparoscopy

1. Cost of disposable, plastic ports is a great burden. Reusable metal ports serve more or less the same purpose. Thus, use of metal ports should be encouraged, and one should become familiar with these ports and this methodology in order to reduce overall costs.
2. Reusable instruments: Most instruments can be properly sterilized. Even instruments such as scissors can be reused.
3. Judicial use of energy sources such as Harmonic® (Ethicon Endo-Surgery, Somerville, NJ) scalpel, LigaSure™ (Covidien, Boulder, CO), Enseal® (Ethicon Endo-Surgery, Somerville, NJ) bipolar/monopolar cautery, etc.: Every operation does not need all these energies. Use should depend upon the type of surgery. A surgeon should be familiar with all modalities.
4. Use of staplers is recommended for ligating large vessels (renal vein in right-side donor nephrectomy). However, this adds to the cost of the procedure. If a surgeon becomes familiar with alternate methods of ligating the renal vein in such a situation, it will reduce the cost without affecting the safety [8].
5. Bags for specimen retrieval also create additional economic burden. In developing countries, many surgeons innovate some modality to overcome this cost difficulty. Nadiad bag is one such example that reduces the cost but still serves the purpose very well [9].
6. Technique of surgery is of key importance. Any complications will add to the cost. If a dissection is rash, this may result in more bleeding and therefore more surgery; if certain vessels are not properly cauterized, this may result in bleeding, control of which may need too many Hem-o-Lok clips or metal clips, which in turn will add to the cost.
7. Use of locally made instruments.

Summary

Endourological procedures are minimally invasive procedures, resulting in low morbidity, reduced hospital stay, early ambulation, and early resumption to work, thereby becoming cost effective. However, if success is not achieved or if any complications occur, then these procedures may instead turn out to be extremely expensive with high morbidity and occasional mortality as well. All precautions should be taken to prevent complications. For example, in PCNL, if bleeding occurs, it will not only prolong the hospital stay but may also end up in angioembolization. In laparoscopy, if the bowel is damaged or if a vessel is damaged, the procedure will end up as a conversion to open surgery and may prove to be very expensive. This is true for almost all endourological procedures. Thus, taking the utmost care to avoid complications is very cost beneficial. It is also important to ensure that procedures end in total success. For example, achieving complete clearance after treatment for stone disease is important, as residual stones will necessitate vigorous follow-up and possibly yet another procedure. This, in the long term, will be expensive. So achieving complete clearance at any cost is cost beneficial in the long run. Similarly, preventive measures in stone disease are also part and parcel of treatment. All measures taken to prevent stone disease are cost effective [10] for obvious reasons.

With these guidelines, endourological procedures can be performed with the same benefits and the same success rates and additionally be successful in overcoming cost difficulties to a considerable extent.

References

1. Dharaskar A, Mandhani A. Should flexible ureteroscope be added to our armamentarium to treat stone disease? Indian J Urol. 2008;24(4):513–6.
2. Homer JA, Davies Payne DL, Peddinti BS. Randomised prospective comparison of non contrast enhanced

helical CT & IVU in diagnosis of acute ureteric colic. Australas Radiol. 2001;45:285–90.
3. Mendelson RM, Arnold-Reed DE, Kuan M, et al. Renal colic: a prospective evaluation of non-enhanced spiral CT versus IVU. Australas Radiol. 2003;47:22–8.
4. Pfister SA, Deckart A, Laschke S, et al. Unenhanced helical CT vs intravenous urography in patients acute flank pain: accuracy and economic impact. Eur Radiol. 2003;13:2513–20.
5. Wang J-H, Sha S-H, Huang S-S, et al. Prospective comparison of unenhanced spiral CT and IVU in the evaluation of acute renal colic. J Chin Med Assoc. 2008;71:30–6.
6. Yuan H, Zeheng S, Liu L, Han P, Wel Q. The efficacy and safety of tubeless percutaneous nephrolithotomy: a systematic review and meta-analysis. Urol Res. 2011; 39:401–10.
7. Hector LL, Anthony JP, Alex AM, Thomas MT. Metallic ureteral stents: a cost effective method of managing benign upper tract obstruction. J Endourol. 2010;24(3):483–5.
8. Chris HC, Steve YC, Christopher SN, Gerhard JF. Looped silk tie: surgical technique for management of renal vein during laparoscopic live donor nephrectomy. J Endourol. 2005;19(3):401.
9. Ganpule AP, Gotov E, Mishra S, Muthu V, Sabnis R, Desai M. Novel cost effective specimen retrieval bag in laparoscopy: Nadiad Bag. Urology. 2010;75: 1213–6.
10. Knoll T, Wendt NG, Trojan L, Wenke N, Alken P. Current aspects of stone therapy. Aktuelle Urol. 2005;36(1):47–54.

Difficulties in Endourologic Training

32

Ahmed M. Al-Kandari

Introduction

Endourology has evolved tremendously over the years in all aspects. This was mainly possible due to great improvements of technique, technology, and instrumentation. Learning and training in endourology has progressed more than standard surgical training. We will focus mostly in this chapter on the issues related to training in percutaneous renal surgery and ureteroscopy.

Given that urinary stone disease is a common recurrent condition in urology, endourologic interventions, especially percutaneous nephrolithotomy (PCNL) and ureteroscopy (URS), are the commonest surgical modalities in the treatment of urolithiasis.

Methods to learn these important endourologic skills include:

1. Residency training program
2. Endourology fellowship program
3. Endourology workshops and courses
4. Visiting and inviting experts
5. Use of simulators
6. Use of animal models
7. Observing operative videos.

We will discuss the important issues to utilize these methods effectively, and then we will outline some of the difficulties that are encountered with discussion of possible solutions.

A.M. Al-Kandari, M.D., FRCS(C)
Department of Surgery, Kuwait University,
Jabriyah, Kuwait City 13110, Kuwait
e-mail: drakandari@hotmail.com

Residency Training Programs

Nowadays, since more trained endourologic staff are available worldwide and since endourologic procedures, namely, PCNL and URS, are becoming more common, residency training programs are including more of these procedures as a learning task. Studies from one residency program have shown that access for PCNL surgery can be safely and successfully obtained by genitourinary residents under the supervision of trained staff at the time of surgery. We think that access for PCNL is a valuable tool that should be in the armamentarium of all urologic surgeons upon leaving an accredited urology training program [1]. This observation confirms that PCNL access, which is the most important and technically demanding step, can be effectively taught to residents.

An interesting study suggested a relationship between training in percutaneous renal access and subsequent use of percutaneous renal procedures in the urologist's practice. Subsequently, emphasis should be placed on providing continuing education opportunities to maintain competency in this important technique [2]. PCNL is currently the most complicated stone surgery technique to teach. The steep learning curve is mainly related to obtaining renal access. The traditional method of acquiring surgical skills is by apprenticeship in the absence of validated virtual simulators. Given the complexity of the treatment of renal stones, one may consider a centralized renal stone treatment in dedicated stone centers [3].

A.M. Al-Kandari et al. (eds.), *Difficult Cases in Endourology*,
DOI 10.1007/978-1-84882-083-8_32, © Springer-Verlag London 2013

As a suggestion for residency training in PCNL learning, the following steps are given:

1. Teaching residents in each year of residency and especially junior resident indications, preoperative preparations, important investigations, operative steps, and recovery and postoperative care and management.
2. Allowing the junior residents to be involved in PCNL cases and letting them do the first step of cystoscopy and ureteral catheterization. They also need to learn and do the actual patient positioning with all the important details.
3. The junior residents can easily learn and perform some sequential tract dilatation and stone removal after fragmentation using nephroscope and forceps.
4. The senior residents should be taught the full procedure including percutaneous renal access, tract dilatation, lithotripsy, stone removal, and nephrostomy tube insertion.

With regard to ureteroscopy, the following learning issues should be emphasized:

1. The ureter is an important delicate structure, and absolute care is required during its manipulation.
2. Knowledge of important disposables including guidewires, balloon dilator, catheters, and stents with sizes and diameters is essential.
3. Knowledge of important instruments including semirigid ureteroscope, flexible ureteroscope, and lithotripsy machines including pneumatic and laser are important.
4. Knowledge of all possible intraoperative difficulties and complications and methods to deal with them is essential.
5. Emphasis must be placed on the fact that force is not a method of URS and that when the ureter does not allow safe ureteroscopy, then postponing the procedure with stenting is the safest exit.

Ureteroscopy is commonly done by senior residents, but it can be taught and performed safely by junior residents especially in high-volume centers and under supervision. Obviously, the more the residents do during the URS, the better his or her performance will be. Careful curriculum design in high-volume stone centers may be the key to optimizing URS training [3].

Endourology Fellowships

The field of endourology, which encompasses genitourinary endoscopy and percutaneous, laparoscopic, and robotic surgery, has advanced rapidly over the past quarter century, causing endourology to be considered a subspecialty of urology. The Endourological Society, which is recognized by the American Urological Association, offers numerous clinical and research fellowship opportunities throughout the world [4].

Subsequently, more fellowship programs are being recognized by the Endourological Society, which helps more candidates worldwide gain competence in endourology. In an abstract that we presented during the World Congress of Endourology in 2008, we have shown that the endourology fellowship has changed significantly the urological practice of a major institution [5].

We strongly recommend pursuing fellowships in endourology for the residents who are interested in this area, as this will give them superior knowledge, skills, and competence in endourology. This also makes them more attractive to large academic centers and institutions.

Problems and Difficulties with Endourology Training During Residency and Fellowship

1. Non-committed staff: It is a real problem when the staff does most or all the operative procedure themselves without giving the trainees the appropriate opportunity to learn or train. This can even happen in recognized programs. The solution we propose includes the following:
   (a) Logbook: The presence of a logbook for all the endourologic procedures for residents and fellows is helpful in order to

document the minimum number of cases that each has to do or assist on.

(b) Periodic staff evaluation and feedback: This is also an essential tool that can help evaluate the staff in training centers and ensure that the staff is committed to actual training of residents and fellows. If complaints from residents and fellows document non-commitment of a staff member to assigning cases according to the situation and level of the trainee, then this staff member should be confronted and warned. If the staff member does not alter his or her behavior, then actions should be taken against this person to ensure that he or she participate in the training or he or she could be denied the privilege of the assistance of residents and fellows.

2. Conflict between a senior resident and a fellow: This issue can happen in certain programs and can manifest itself as one taking advantage of the other or one taking cases away from another. The solution we propose:
   (a) The distribution of the types and numbers of cases should be clear and illustrated in the program goalbook and logbook of both the resident and the fellow.
   (b) The program director should be responsible for all team members getting their training according to the program guidelines and policy and according to the level of the team member.

Endourology Workshops and Courses

Various endourology workshops and courses are available worldwide nowadays. These courses are excellent chances for learning different endourologic techniques. More urological associations are including different endourologic courses during their annual meetings. Examples of this can be seen during the meetings of the American Urological Association, the Endourological Society, and other associations.

How to Learn Optimally During These Workshops and Courses

1. Look for the useful courses of interest in endourology and pre-register to ensure seating.
2. A thorough knowledge of all the essential disposables and instruments is required to benefit from the courses.
3. Visit the exhibition booths of the manufacturers to see the equipment and make contact with the agents in your country for the different manufacturers. This will help in keeping your interest in learning these procedures active.
4. Make contact with the experts, which is essential for you in order to learn more, exchange knowledge through e-mail, and arrange for future visits or invitations.
5. Obtain operative videos, which is essential, as these can help you in continuing your learning experience after the courses that you attend are over.

Visiting and Inviting Experts

Visiting and inviting experts in order to observe them operate and even asking them to assist you at your center are valuable ways in which to learn and master different endourologic methods.

How to Maximize the Benefit of Visiting Experts

1. Visiting experts at their centers:
   (a) Proper time arrangement especially before or after conferences.
   (b) Inform experts ahead of time and ask them to schedule cases so the visit will be beneficial.
   (c) Take notes of the full setup, instruments, and disposables.
   (d) Record the videos of endoscopic cases since they show real case scenarios.
   (e) Maintain contact with the team that helps *the* expert in case you need further advice regarding instruments, e.g., operating room head nurse, fellow, etc.

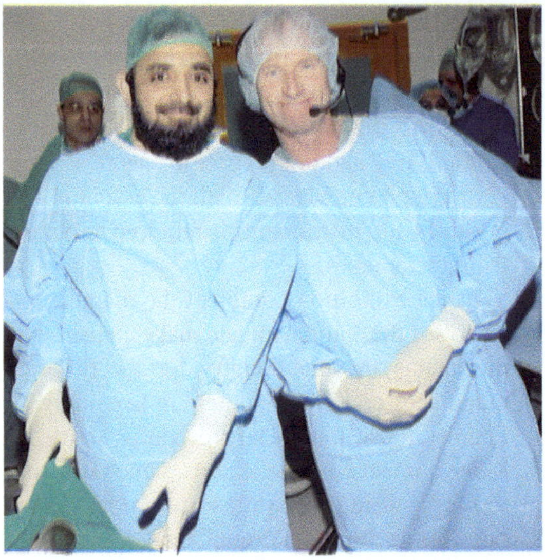

Fig. 32.1 Dr. Al-Kandari and Dr. Gilling during a holmium laser enucleation case (HOLEP) workshop in Kuwait in 2006

2. Inviting experts to your center:
    (a) Prepare all the important instruments and disposables that the expert uses.
    (b) Arrange for a good case selection, with cases that have the least medical risk and are the most ideal.
    (c) Prepare standby cases in to allow for cancelations.
    (d) Involve the best operating team especially with regard to the anesthetist, assistant, and scrubbing and circulating nurses.
    (e) Involve the medical equipment representative and supplies representative; have him or her be available in the operating room to assist in case technical or instrument problems occur.
    (f) Have the medical supply company prepare standby items especially with regard to the disposables.
    (g) If you are personally keen to improve your endourologic skills, then it is best for you to assist the expert, since you will have the maximum time with him or her (Figs. 32.1, 32.2, and 32.3).

Use of Simulators

The use of simulators in endourology is one of the helpful tools for training. Different models have been developed to help gain experience in percutaneous renal access as well as in ureteroscopy. Virtual reality (VR) simulators are now commercially available for various surgical skills training. The URO Mentor™ VR Ureteroscopy Simulator by Simbionix™ (Cleveland, OH) (Fig. 32.4) is one system that may revolutionize the way we assess and teach surgical residents. Surgical educators may no longer have to depend on the operating room as the sole venue for teaching residents technical skills [6] (Figs. 32.5, 32.6, 32.7, and 32.8).
Simbionix's URO Mentor medical simulator provides the most comprehensive endourology hands-on training and practice opportunities for diagnostic and therapeutic procedures. The URO Mentor provides a unique opportunity to work with a variety of scopes, tools, and visual images on a true-to-life system providing a look and feel so close to reality that at times it may be hard to distinguish the difference.

Safe practice of endourology procedures on the URO Mentor includes:

- Simulation of rigid and flexible cystoscopes and ureteroscopes.
- Practice of essential skills, stone extraction, stone lithotripsy, cutting strictures, or taking biopsies.
- Real-time simulation of fluoroscopy and C-arm control.
- An ergonomic platform that provides use of actual scope with a real tool handle and enables actual tool insertion into working channels.
- The Simbionix™ PERC Mentor™ (Cleveland, OH) is a medical simulator for training percutaneous access procedures performed under real-time fluoroscopy.

The PERC Mentor simulator provides healthcare specialists with opportunities for training and practicing basic tasks and skills on a variety

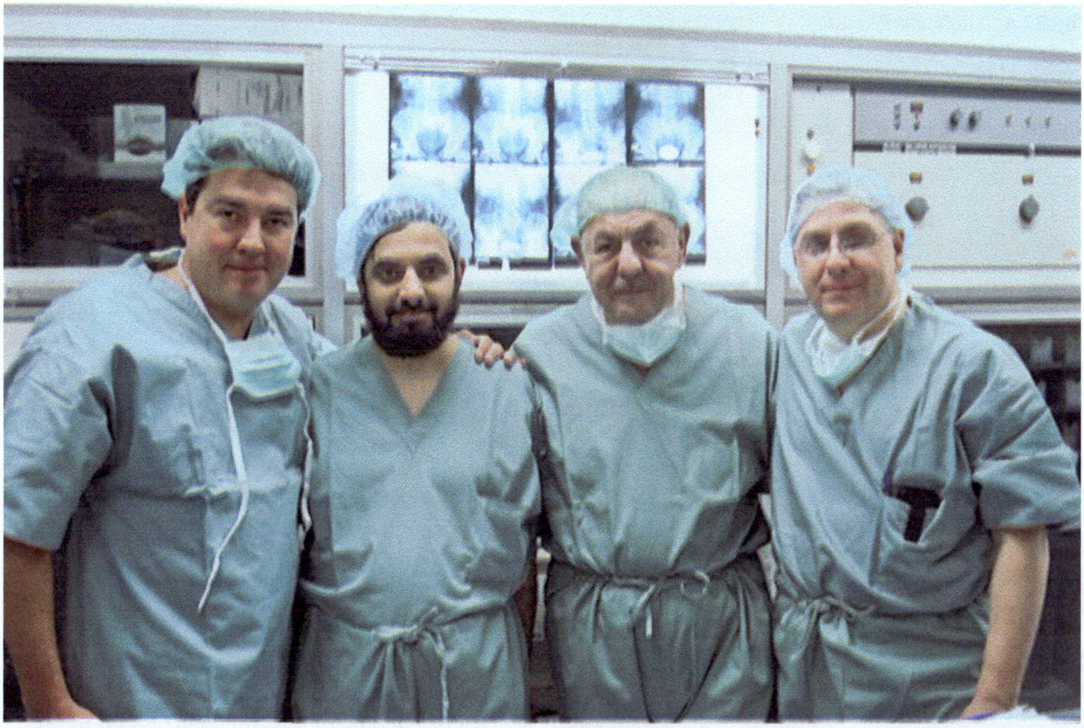

Fig. 32.2 Dr. Smith, Dr. Al-Kandari, Dr. Grasso, and Dr. Sotelo during an endourology and laparoscopy workshop in Kuwait in 2008

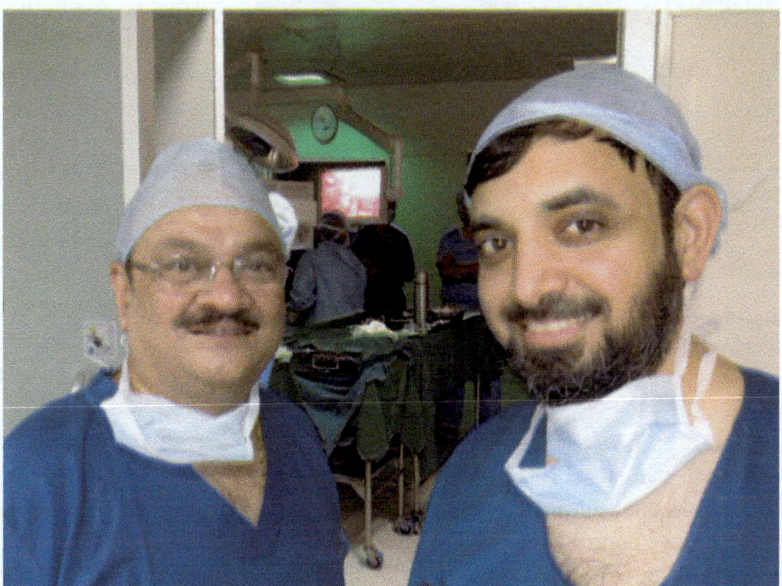

Fig. 32.3 Dr. Desai and Dr. Al-Kandari at Dr. Desai's center in India during a workshop

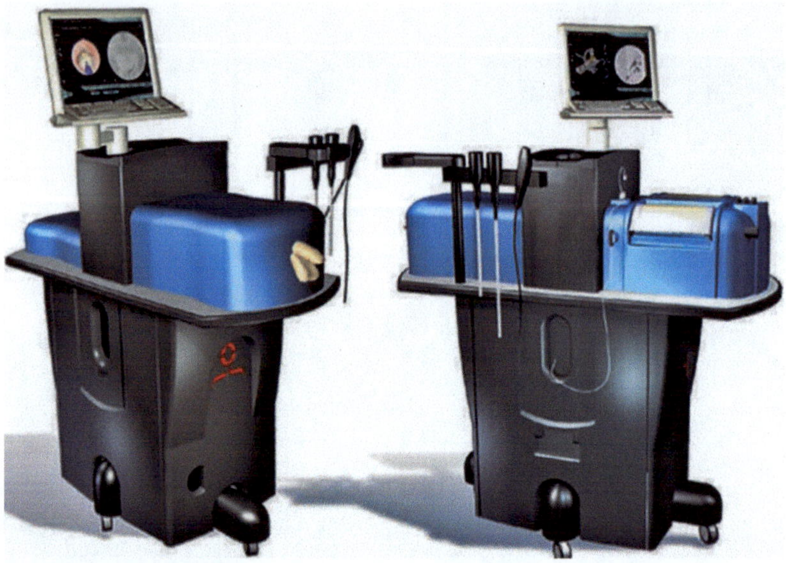

Fig. 32.4 Simbionix™ URO Mentor™ (*left*), Simbionix™ combined PERC Mentor™ and URO Mentor™ (*right*) (Courtesy of Simbionix™, Cleveland, OH)

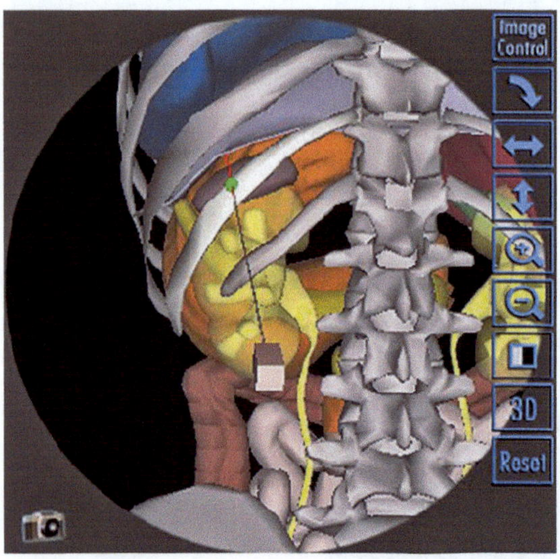

Fig. 32.5 Basic task images from monitor of PERC Mentor™ (Courtesy of Simbionix™, Cleveland, OH)

of virtual patients. PERC Mentor helps specialists acquire the following skills:

- Hand-eye coordination
- Processing of 2D fluoroscopic radiographic imaging into 3D "mind's eye" visualization of anatomies
- Fluoroscopy image manipulation
- Tools and guidewire manipulation
- C-arm manipulation for obtaining ideal access
- Use of needles of varying sizes and lengths

The module offers training on a variety of virtual normal weight patients with different renal anatomies and pathologies. The module provides an ideal opportunity to practice, identifying the correct access to the proper calyx through a variety of access sites. Realistic hands-on training is enhanced by the tactile sensations felt when maneuvering through the various layers and ribs.

The module offers training on a variety of obese virtual patients with different renal anatomies and pathologies. Using a designated cartridge representing the virtual patient's back and an authentic needle, the trainee may practice performing the procedure on this type of patient before encountering the situation live in the operating room.[1]

Some studies have shown that training models may be useful for training in URS and stone disintegration [3]. Others found that virtual reality simulators may have a potential for training for PCNL. To maintain one's expertise, participation in continuing educational programs is recommended [7].

[1] simbionix.com

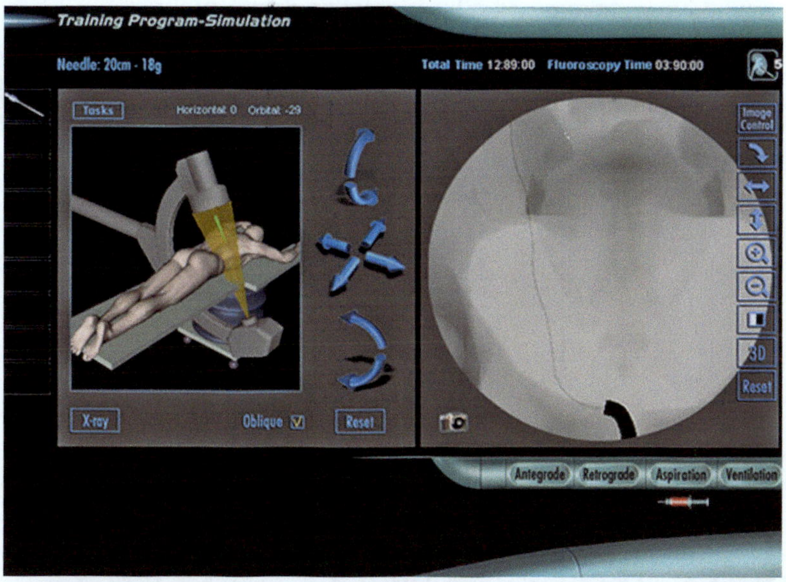

Fig. 32.6 Image from PERC Mentor™ monitor showing fluoroscopic image with a simulator guidewire in ureter (Courtesy of Simbionix™, Cleveland, OH)

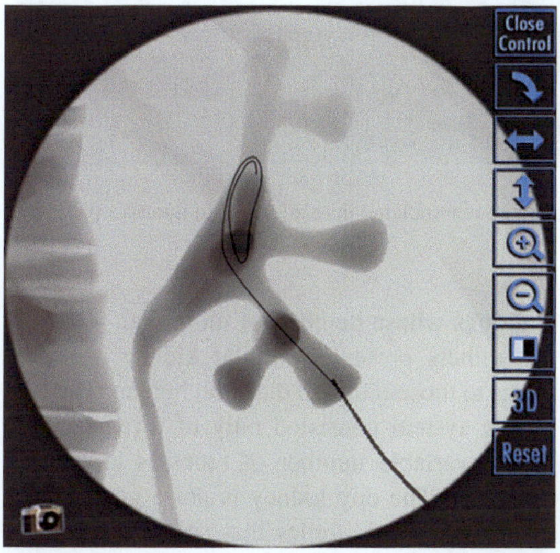

Fig. 32.7 Image from monitor of PERC Mentor™ showing a fluoroscopic image with opacification of collecting system (Courtesy of Simbionix™, Cleveland, OH)

Use of a computer-based ureteroscopy simulator resulted in rapid acquisition of ureteroscopic skills in trainees who had no prior surgical training. Results of this study demonstrate the use of a virtual reality ureteroscopy simulator in endourological training. Correlation of simulator-based measurements with a previously validated endourological global rating scale provides initial validation of the ureteroscopy simulator for the assessment of ureteroscopic skills [8].

The largest number of models has been described for ureterorenoscopy (nine types). Due to growing interest in training models in urology, it is increasingly urgent to determine which of these models are most valuable for postgraduate training. Because the validation studies published so far are few in number, have low evidence levels, and are composed of only a few RCTs, it is important that more randomized controlled validation studies including larger numbers of participants are performed [9]. Simulators are typically more useful and practical in academic and big institutions where there are residency and or fellowship programs focusing on endourology.

Problems and issues related to simulators are as follows:

1. The high cost, especially for virtual reality simulators, is an inherent problem that limits use to most centers interested in training for endourology.
2. The need for dedicated trainers that must be part of a training center to help the trainee gain the most benefit from working with this equipment.
3. The different perception of reality with simulators especially considering the breathing

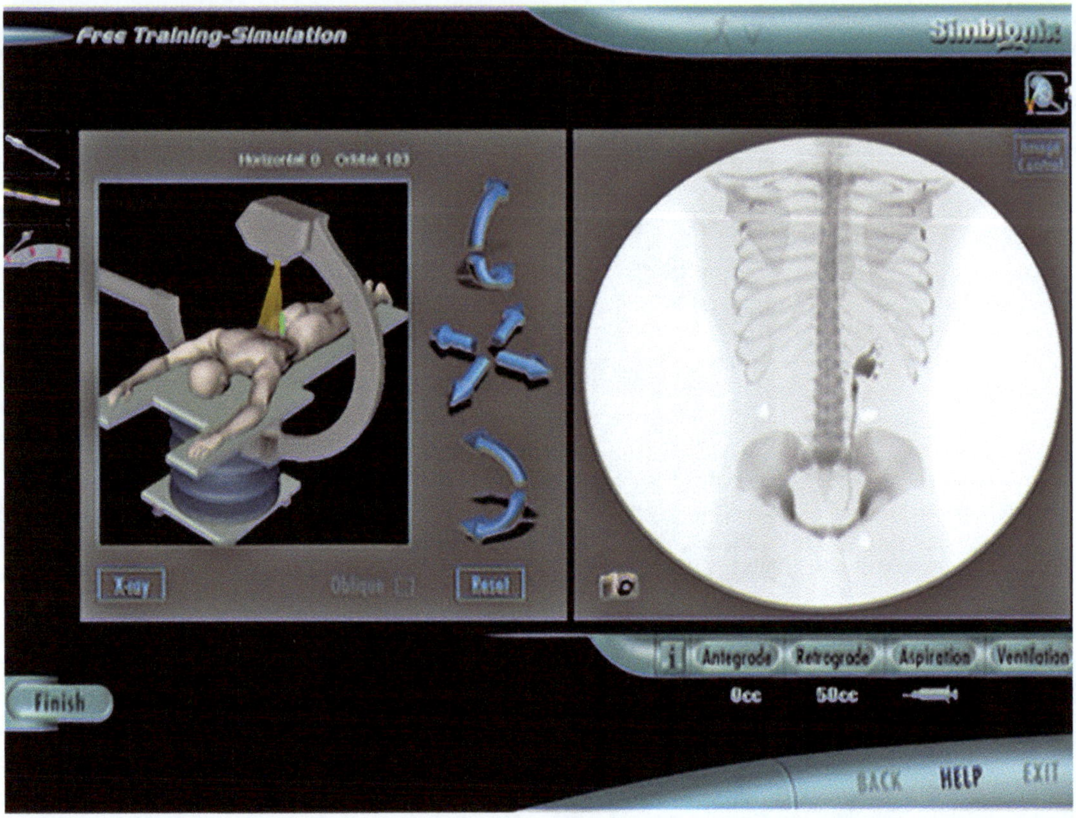

Fig. 32.8 Image from PERC Mentor™ monitor showing guidewire manipulated in renal pelvis in fluoroscopic image (Courtesy of Simbionix™, Cleveland, OH)

issue in patients with the moving target, e.g., renal calyx in PCNL access unlike simulator target.

4. Deficiency in covering most endourological operations. This challenges the manufacturing and simulator developing companies to develop a full menu of simulations in relation to common endourologic surgeries.

In the centers that have the facility for a simulator, we do recommend that trainees go through a structured program of training that includes the simulator.

Use of Animal Models

Animal models are an important method for operative learning and mastering new surgical skills before doing them on patients. Pereira-Sampaio et al. examined dog kidneys and found that dogs whose height was more than 70 cm at the withers presented similar kidney measurements to those found in the adult human. The collecting system consisted only of a renal pelvis with a variable number of recesses around its perimeter. The dog kidney is not a good model for experimental studies that consider the morphology of the collecting system. Kidneys from dogs taller than 70 cm, however, might be useful as a model in experimental studies in which renal volume is an important aspect, such as shockwave lithotripsy and endourology [10].

We have used pigs to study the effects of renal trauma in different methods of tract dilation during percutaneous renal surgery [11]. We believe that pigs are useful animals for percutaneous renal surgery experiments and for training, especially in learning the renal access as well as tract dilatation.

Problems and issues related to animal usage during endourologic training are as follows:

1. The issue of cost of the animal as well as equipment and disposables used during endourologic animal surgery. This equipment is typically dedicated to animals, and this includes a significant cost burden, especially when including such equipment as the X-ray C-arm. The use of some expensive machines such as laser machines does not require full dedication for animals since the fibers are changed.
2. The importance of an experienced technician who can give anesthesia to animals and care for animals after the surgery, especially when survival studies are planned.
3. Although, as mentioned earlier, some animals have some similarities to human kidneys, there are still important differences that the trainee has to master when operating on patients.

Observing Operative Videos

The educational material that many operative videos contain is significant, especially when a urologist has the basic skills but needs to learn certain approaches. A good example is laser endopyelotomy through the outside pelvis. Different authors used this technique, and it can be nicely illustrated by an educational video. This shows the steps for incising the renal pelvis before the ureteropelvic junction (UPJ) and then the steps for incising the UPJ from the outside in an easy way.

Points and issues related to endourologic operative videos are as follows:

1. We do not recommend doing a full complete technique via a video, e.g., PCNL cannot be mastered by just watching a video without going through the more comprehensive learning experience.
2. Operative videos are useful for illustrating a new technique or a modification or a new device through a generally mastered technique. Some examples of this are the following: use of ureteral access sheath during ureteroscopy, use of holmium laser for large renal pelvic stones, and PCNL in certain congenital or acquired renal anomalies, e.g., horseshoe kidney, polycystic kidney.

Learning Curve and Competence

The learning curve is an important aspect of training in any new surgical skill. This is especially important in percutaneous renal surgery. This is specifically obvious in gaining renal access, especially in non-dilated kidneys. It is always better to start PCNL in a dilated system with non-complex cases (e.g., 2-cm renal pelvic stone). Studies have looked into the number of cases needed to gain competence in PCNL. In one study, an improvement in operation duration was observed and an absence of complications was achieved after 45 cases of PCNL. The improvement in stone clearance was observed up to the last subjects. Competence and excellence were achieved after 45 and 105 operations, respectively [12]. In my view, study should not discourage a urologist from doing PCNL or training unless he or she has reached those numbers. The most important thing is knowledge of the technique and safety of the procedure. Whenever there is difficulty in a case, one can insert a nephrostomy tube and return at a later time to complete the procedure. The same applies but probably to a lesser degree for URS. Obviously, the more you do, the better you become.

Summary

Endourologic training is an important aspect of safe and efficient surgery. Thorough knowledge about all instruments and disposables is an essential prerequisite of training. There are variable means for acquiring the training skills including residency training. Since the development of the Endourologic Society and recognition of more endourology fellowship programs worldwide (Table 32.1), the opportunities for trainees have increased significantly. Residents and fellows may have better privileges than others in opportunities to use different training simulators. Nonetheless, more urologists worldwide are in need of training in endourology, which is the fastest evolving subspecialty. Subsequently, different societies and organizations prepare different endourologic workshops and courses. These take

Table 32.1 Recognized endourology fellowships

North America
Albert Einstein College of Medicine/Montefiore Medical Center Department of Urology
Brown University, Department of Urology
Cedars Sinai Medical Center – Minimally Invasive Urology Institute
Cleveland Clinic – Glickman Urologic and Kidney Institute
Columbia University, Department of Urology
Duke University Medical Center – Division of Urology
Eastern Virginia Medical School
Hackensack University Medical Center, Department of Urology
Indiana University Medical Center, Department of Urology
Institute of Endourology, Hospital del Carmen, Mexico
Johns Hopkins University, School of Medicine
Kaiser Foundation Hospital, Department of Urology
Lenox Hill Medical Center
Loma Linda University Medical Center, Department of Urology
Methodist/Clarian Hospital and Indiana University School of Medicine
New York Medical College, Department of Urology
Northwestern University Medical School, Department of Urologic Surgery
The Arthur Smith Institute of Urology
The University of Western Ontario, Division of Urology
Thomas Jefferson University, Department of Urology
Tulane University Medical Center, Department Of Urology
University of California Irvine
University of Cincinnati, Department of Urology
University of Kentucky
University of Miami School of Medicine, Department Of Urology
University of Michigan, Urologic Surgery
University of Minnesota, Department of Urology
University of North Carolina, Chapel Hill, Department of Urology
University of Pittsburgh, Department of Urology
University of Pennsylvania
University of Rochester Medical Center, Department of Urology
University of Texas Southwestern, Department Of Urology
University of Toronto, Department Of Urology
University of Wisconsin Madison Medical School, Department of Urology
Vanderbilt University Medical Center, Department Of Urology
Wake Forest School of Medicine, Department of Urology
Washington University School of Medicine, Department of Urologic Surgery
South America
Instituto Medico La Floresta
Federal University in Sao Paulo, Division of Urology
School of Medicine Universidade Estadual Paulista, Department of Urology
Clinica Indisa Faculty of Medicine, Universidad Andres Bello, Department of Urology
Europe
Asklepios Hospital Barmbeck
L'Instiut Mutualiste Montsouris
University of Patras University Hospital
Klinikum Heilbronn, Department Of Urology

Table 32.1 (continued)

St. Bartholomew's Hospital, Department of Urology
University of Amsterdam, Department of Urology
Middle East/Africa
Hadassah Hebrew University Hospital
Rabin Medical Center Tel Aviv University School of Medicine
Asia
All India Institute of Medicine Sciences, Department of Urology
Muljibhai Patel Urological Hospital, Department of Urology
Yonsei University College of Medicine, Department of Urology

place during most annual meeting to facilitate the participation of more candidates. Finally, using animal models and observing variable operative videos are important helpful tools for training in endourology.

References

1. Spann A, Poteet J, Hyatt D, Chiles L, Desouza R, Venable D. Safe and effective obtainment of access for percutaneous nephrolithotomy by urologists: the Louisiana State University experience. J Endourol. 2011;25(9):1421–5.
2. Lee CL, Anderson JK, Monga M. Residency training in percutaneous renal access: does it affect urological practice? J Urol. 2004;171(2 Pt 1):592–5.
3. Skolarikos A, Gravas S, Laguna MP, Traxer O, Preminger GM, de la Rosette J. Training in ureteroscopy: a critical appraisal of the literature. BJU Int. 2011;108(6):798–805.
4. Chung BI, Matin SF, Ost MC, Winfield HN. Fellowship in endourology, the job search, and setting up a successful practice: an insider's view. J Endourol. 2008; 22(3):551–7.
5. Al-Kandari AM, Ibrahim H, Shaaban H, El-shebiny Y. The effect of Endourology fellowship on the change of urology practice in a general hospital in Kuwait. J Endourol. 2006;20(Suppl 1):52.
6. Matsumoto ED, Pace KT, D'A Honey RJ. Virtual reality ureteroscopy simulator as a valid tool for assessing endourological skills. Int J Urol. 2006;13(7): 896–901.
7. Chou DS, Abdelshehid C, Clayman RV, McDougall EM. Comparison of results of virtual-reality simulator and training model for basic ureteroscopy training. J Endourol. 2006;20(4):266–71.
8. Watterson JD, Beiko DT, Kuan JK, Denstedt JD. Randomized prospective blinded study validating acquisition of ureteroscopy skills using computer based virtual reality endourological simulator. J Urol. 2002;168(5):1928–32.
9. Schout BM, Hendrikx AJ, Scherpbier AJ, Bemelmans BL. Update on training models in endourology: a qualitative systematic review of the literature between January 1980 and April 2008. Eur Urol. 2008; 54(6):1247–61.
10. Pereira-Sampaio MA, Marques-Sampaio BP, Henry RW, Favorito LA, Sampaio FJ. The dog kidney as experimental model in endourology: anatomic contribution. J Endourol. 2009;23(6):989–93.
11. Al-Kandari AM, Jabbour M, Anderson A, Shokeir AA, Smith AD. Comparative study of degree of renal trauma between Amplatz sequential fascial dilation and balloon dilation during percutaneous renal surgery in an animal model. Urology. 2007;69(3): 586–9.
12. Ziaee SA, Sichani MM, Kashi AH, Samzadeh M. Evaluation of the learning curve for percutaneous nephrolithotomy. Urol J. 2010;7(4):226–31.

Avoiding and Overcoming Medicolegal Difficulties in Endourology

33

Donnaline Richman and James H. Robb

Introduction

Physicians commonly fear being sued in a medical malpractice case. Society expects perfect results from physicians, including urologists who perform endourological procedures. The question is not *whether* a urologist will be sued but *when*. In order to understand the rationale behind the risk management best practices discussed in this chapter, the urologist must understand the four legal elements of medical malpractice.

Portions of the risk management advice contained in this chapter have been reprinted with permission from Medical Liability Mutual Insurance Company, 2 Park Avenue, New York, NY 10016.

D. Richman, MN, JD (✉)
Department of Urology, Counsel for Healthcare Law & Risk management, Fager & Amsler, LLP, 2 Clinton Square, Suite 212, Syracuse, NY, 13202, USA
e-mail: drichman@fagerandamsler.com

J.H. Robb, M.B.A.
Department of Urology, Donald J Fager & Associates, Inc., Medical Liability Mutual Insurance Company, 2 Park Avenue, 25th Floor, New York, NY, 10016, USA
e-mail: jrobb@mlmic.com

The first element is the duty of care assumed by the urologist when he/she agrees to see or consult with another physician about a patient. The second element is a breach of that duty. A breach is a deviation from the standard of care applicable to urologists, generally proven by expert witnesses who testify based upon the urologist's documentation of the patient's care and the applicable professional standards in existence at the time the urologist treated the patient. The third element is proximate cause, which means that the deviation from the standard of care was a substantial factor in causing the untoward result experienced by the patient. The fourth element of medical malpractice is damages due to a physical, emotional, and/or financial injury. All four elements *must* be present to have a viable medical malpractice case.

One of the easiest ways to illustrate all of the variables in a medical malpractice case is to review an actual lawsuit. The following case study contains all four of the legal elements of medical malpractice and highlights the importance of implementing risk management best practices in the field of endourology.

In September 2001, a 45-year-old female was seen by her urologist with complaints of pain in her left lower abdomen. She had a history of renal calculi since approximately age 20 and had been followed regularly by her urologist due to her history. Previous urologic treatment included lithotripsy and extracorporeal shock wave lithotripsy (ESWL). On September 26, 2001, a CT scan revealed bilateral renal calculi, calculus in the proximal left ureter, and mild hydronephrosis.

A.M. Al-Kandari et al. (eds.), *Difficult Cases in Endourology*,
DOI 10.1007/978-1-84882-083-8_33, © Springer-Verlag London 2013

The urologist referred the patient to a specialist with expertise in basket extractions. The specialist saw the patient on October 16, 2001, and discussed the results of the CT scan with her. He also very briefly discussed the proposed basket extraction procedure. However, the consent form signed by the patient did not describe the potential risks of the procedure, and no consent discussion was documented in the patient's medical record.

On October 31, 2001, the patient was admitted to the hospital for a basket extraction procedure to remove the left ureteral calculus. The procedure was unsuccessful because the ureteroscope could not be advanced to the area of the ureteral calculus. However, a piece of tissue found when the basket was removed indicated a possible ureteral perforation. The specialist immediately consulted an interventional radiologist. He performed a left nephrostomy and placed a double J stent in the left ureter. The patient subsequently underwent ESLW to break up the ureteral calculus, but the stent became blocked and had to be changed. Persistent flank pain and multiple infections required several hospital admissions. Eventually, a ureteral stricture was diagnosed. The patient underwent surgery to remove a 1.5-cm piece of damaged ureter. After this surgery, the patient did fairly well.

The patient commenced a lawsuit, alleging that the urologist was negligent in his performance of left ureterovesical balloon dilation and left ureteroscopy and also perforated her left ureter during the ureteroscopy. She also alleged a lack of informed consent. Analysis of this case revealed several concerns that made defense of the specialist's care extremely difficult. First, the specialist's dictated operative note described cystoscopy, placement of two wires beyond the ureteral calculus, dilation of the intramural ureter, and passage of a ureteroscope, which failed to reach the calculus at the L3 level. The ureteroscopy was then halted. One of the wires was removed, but the second wire migrated distal to the calculus. No mention of basket extraction was made in the operative report. Further, the tissue discovered at the end of the procedure was not mentioned. However, a pathology report indicated that a specimen determined to be fibroadipose tissue was received. Second, at deposition, the operating room nurses testified that a basket was used and was opened and closed during the procedure. In contrast, the specialist testified that he never opened the basket and thus did not include this in his operative note. He further testified that the tissue sample sent to pathology was found on the patient's drape. Third, while the patient's medical records document that the September 2001 CT scan also revealed the presence of bilateral renal calculi, there is no evidence that a treatment plan for those was proposed by either the urologist or the specialist or that the renal calculi passed spontaneously. Further, there was no evidence that the urologist and the specialist ever discussed this finding.

Expert urologists who reviewed this case felt that perforation was a known complication of a ureteroscopic procedure, which was a recognized and suitable method to treat a ureteral calculus. However, there was no evidence that the patient was informed of this risk *prior* to the procedure. Finally, the discrepancy between the operative report and the testimony of the operating room nurses, the pathology report which identified fibroadipose tissue, and the development of a ureteral stricture requiring major surgery, resulting in references to "iatrogenic injury to the proximal ureter with UPJ obstruction" in the patient's hospital record made this case impossible to defend. Thus, this lawsuit was settled before trial for $375,000.

The specter of patient injuries which might occur during an endourologic procedure and result in legal proceedings may potentially lead to an adversarial element in the urologist/patient relationship. To minimize the possibility of patient injury and decrease the risk of liability, a body of risk management best practices has evolved. These best practices can be adopted by all urologists with little effort.

Competency Assessments

Assessment of physician and staff competency is a crucial element in avoiding the occurrence of untoward events. When a physician joins a practice or the medical staff of a facility, it is incumbent upon the employer to thoroughly review and verify the individual's training and experience in endourology. The urologist's training and experience must be appropriate to perform endourologic procedures. The physician's malpractice experience must also be carefully explored. A physician may appear to have excellent credentials on paper, yet his/her actual skill level may not match those credentials. Therefore, due care must be taken when confirming and checking references. Speaking with a reference provided by the physician may yield more accurate and reliable information than depending solely upon written comments.

The competency, licensure, and credentials of other personnel who are assisting with procedures must be assessed and verified. Physicians may only delegate duties considered to be the practice of nursing or medicine to individuals who are licensed and trained to perform those duties.[1] This is critical because inappropriate delegation exposes the urologist to license restriction, suspension, or revocation. In addition, a lawsuit may be commenced against the urologist and other individuals to whom duties were improperly delegated. If the person to whom medical or nursing duties are delegated is unlicensed, criminal charges may be brought against all parties.

Patient Selection

Well-accepted criteria must be used to select patients who are suitable candidates for endourologic procedures. Failure to adhere to such criteria may be considered evidence of a deviation from the standard of care. Thus, urologists must be knowledgeable of the criteria and apply them appropriately to each patient. The risk of inappropriate patient selection is significant in endourology, thus enhancing the risk of patient injury.

History and Physical Examination

A comprehensive history and physical examination performed at the patient's initial visit helps to obtain pertinent information and determine the best course of treatment for the patient. The following patient examination data must be well documented:

What complaints and symptoms caused the patient to seek treatment? How long has the patient had symptoms? Have those symptoms occurred previously? How do the symptoms impact the patient's daily activities? Does the patient experience pain when urinating? Is there blood in the urine? Pertinent symptoms and the chief complaint must clearly have been addressed.

Further, it is important to document the presence of chronic illnesses such as diabetes, tuberculosis, multiple sclerosis, sickle-cell anemia, or hypertension, as well as other significant conditions revealed by the patient's medical history. A thorough family history may provide critical information about the type of stone a patient may have, since urolithiasis is frequently genetically or family related. If surgery is contemplated, cigarette smoking and consumption of alcohol increase the likelihood of postoperative pulmonary and cardiac complications. Thus, a history of cigarette smoking and alcohol consumption, along with any counseling the patient receives about the risks of such activities, must be documented.

Since certain medications contribute to urinary tract symptoms, *all* medications the patient currently takes must be elicited and documented, including prescriptions, over-the-counter medications, and herbal supplements. Further, allergies to food and medications must be noted prominently in the medical record. All prior surgical procedures must be discussed and documented, particularly if they were in the same anatomical area as the contemplated procedure. To confirm the accuracy of the patient's surgical history, copies of the previous operative report(s) should be obtained and reviewed prior to surgery.[2]

Informed Consent

The informed consent discussion, or lack thereof, often dictates whether a patient or family chooses to seek legal counsel for an unanticipated or

[1]New York Education Law § (Section) 6530 (11) and (25).

[2]Gerber GS, Brendler CB. Chapter 3: Evaluation of the Urologic Patient: History, Physical Examination and Urinalysis. 1–9. Wein: Campbell-Walsh Urology (9th ed. 2007). www.mdconsult.com/das/book/body/224870721-3/1076918018/1445/6.html#4-u1.0. Accessed on 11/1/2010.

untoward result. Informed consent is much more than a signed consent form. It is the discussion between the physician and the patient of all of the pertinent information necessary for the patient to make an informed decision about undergoing a proposed procedure, treatment, or surgery. This critical discussion is the physician's responsibility. Generally, this duty cannot be delegated.

To be valid, the patient's informed consent must be voluntary, the patient must have the capacity to understand the nature and consequences of the decision to give consent, and sufficient information must be provided to make a reasonable decision. If the patient lacks capacity, the physician must discuss the procedure with the individual legally permitted to give consent for the patient's medical treatment and obtain consent.

The required elements of the informed consent discussion may vary, depending upon the legal rules governing a specific geographic area. For example, some jurisdictions require the disclosure of the identity of active participants in a procedure, such as physicians, residents, and mid-level providers.[3] Further, in some areas, if a second physician is expected to perform any portion of a procedure, the physician's identity and the duties he/she is expected to perform must also be disclosed to the patient prior to surgery.[4] In almost all situations, however, the nature, purpose, risks, and benefits of and alternatives to the proposed treatment (including no treatment) and the risks of the alternatives to the proposed treatment must be thoroughly discussed with the patient. The proposed procedure must be discussed using plain language, without medical jargon, and the communication must be at an educational level and in the language that the patient understands. The patient must fully comprehend what is discussed, have the opportunity to ask questions, and have all questions answered to the patient's satisfaction.

The signed consent form merely serves as evidence that the physician had the consent discussion with the patient or the patient's legal representative. The patient's signature may be obtained by a nurse or other staff member. The patient/representative must then sign, date, and time the document. The nurse or staff member serves only as a witness to the patient's signature, *not* to the content of the conversation between patient and physician. A consent document is not always considered conclusive proof that an informed consent discussion has taken place. Thus, physician documentation of the discussion in the patient's record is critical.

A patient's ability to give informed consent may be affected by other circumstances. The patient may be a minor; have a limited capacity to speak and/or understand the language that is customarily used; lack capacity due to developmental disabilities, dementia, or other conditions; or have a disability such as a hearing or visual impairment. Such patients require special attention. Interpreters, guardians, surrogates, or parents must be present to both participate in the discussion and to provide consent, if appropriate. The use of family members, especially children, as interpreters is inappropriate, ineffective, and can enhance the physician's liability.

When discussing risks with a patient, the urologist should disclose several of the most frequent and most severe risks. Although it may not be feasible to disclose every possible risk (even those which are reasonably foreseeable), the risks disclosed must be sufficient for the patient to make a decision about whether or not to proceed. When documenting the discussion in a patient's medical record, any statement of risks should be prefaced by the phrase "including but not limited to...." In endourology, the risks discussed should include, but may not be limited to, known potential injury to surrounding organs, blood vessels, and nerves, risks specific to the patient's general health and urological condition(s), the possibility that multiple procedures may be required to resolve the

[3] New York Education Law § (Section) 6530 (25-a), Interpretive Guidelines, 42 C.F.R. § (Section) 482.24 (c) (2) (v). www.cms.gov/manuals/downloads/som107ap_a_hospitals.pdf. Accessed on December 13, 2010.

[4] Interpretive Guidelines, 42 C.F.R. § (Section) 482.24 (c) (2) (v) www.cms.gov/manuals/downloads/som107ap_a_hospitals.pdf. Accessed on December 13, 2010.

patient's problem, the possibility that an open procedure may be required, and when performing extracorporeal shock wave lithotripsy, the increased risk of hypertension and/or diabetes.[5]

The individuals who are permitted to consent for medical treatment and the type of treatment for which they may give effective consent vary by location. In some areas, pregnant females and married individuals who are under the legal age of majority can consent for treatment for both themselves and their children.[6] In the United States, pursuant to various laws governing advance directives, surrogates may consent for medical care and treatment for patients who lack capacity.[7] On very rare occasions, a urologist may believe that in his/her professional judgment, full disclosure of the risks and alternatives of the proposed procedure would directly, substantially, and adversely affect the patient's condition. In such situations, he/she may use reasonable discretion and not fully disclose the harmful information to the patient. However, a reasonable attempt must be made to contact a close relative or a legal representative of the patient to discuss the proposed procedure and obtain his/her consent as the patient's surrogate. In an emergency, where a delay in obtaining consent would cause risk to a patient's life or medical condition, consent can and should be waived. However, the physician must then document the fact(s) of the emergency in the medical record and the necessity of dispensing with informed consent.

Finally, patients have the right to refuse to consent to treatment. Although this often may place the urologist in an uncomfortable position because the procedure is both indicated and necessary to the patient's future health and safety, careful documentation of the refusal in the patient's medical record should prevent legal repercussions. Documentation must include the fact that the patient had capacity and refused consent for the proposed procedure or treatment after a detailed conversation of the risks of refusing treatment and any available alternatives.

Drugs and devices approved by a government agency, such as the United States Food and Drug Administration (FDA), are often used by physicians for a nonapproved purpose. The drug or device may also be experimental in nature. In such situations, the patient must be fully advised that the drug or device is either experimental or has been approved *only* for a different purpose. The urologist must also disclose his/her prior experience in such use and how it affected prior patients. After full and fair disclosure, the patient can then give informed consent. The urologist should refrain from making any guarantees about successful use of the drug or device in this situation.

Pre-procedure Testing

Once the patient has consented to a procedure, appropriate pre-procedure testing must be performed. Testing provides an opportunity to identify any health concerns, including unrecognized abnormalities of the urinary tract, blood, and other body organs. The results of the testing may affect the choice of procedure and help the physician determine the best course of treatment before, during, and after surgery. The urologist must communicate the results of laboratory and other test results to the patient, referring physician, or any physician retained to provide medical clearance prior to surgery, so that potential abnormalities can be explored. The urologist must also communicate pertinent laboratory test results to anesthesia providers, since not only the choice of anesthesia but also surveillance and nursing care during and after the procedure can be affected by such results.

[5]Grasso M et al. Percutaneous Endourology: Treatment. http://emedicine.medscape.com/article/446934-treatment. Accessed on 10/28/2010. Lingeman J E et al. Current Perspective on Adverse Effects in Shock Wave Lithotripsy. © 2009 American Urological Association Education and Research, Inc. http://www.auanet.org/content/media/whitepaper.pdf. Accessed on 11/1/2010.

[6]New York State Public Health Law § (Section) 2504 (2).

[7]United States Code of Federal Regulations, 42 C.F.R. § (Section) 482.13 (b) (3).

Time-Out

Wrong site/wrong patient procedures are a focal point of government scrutiny and a potential source of legal action.[8] While efforts to reduce wrong side/site procedures have increased, such errors continue to occur. Hospitals have incorporated a system of checks and balances, including multiple "time-outs" into hospital policies and procedures. However, this has not stopped such errors.

Proper patient identification is the first step. This requires speaking to the patient *prior* to sedation. The patient should state his/her name to the physician rather than be asked if he is "Mr. Jones." Patients may not hear or see well or be nervous. Surprisingly, they frequently respond to another person's name. Pertinent x-rays, records, and signed consent form must accompany a patient to surgery. The urologist must confirm that consent was obtained for the procedure that is to be performed for the patient. The proper site and side must also be verified by asking the patient the location, including site and side, where the surgery is to be performed. At any time, if the answers do not match, the procedure must *not* begin. The verified site/side must then be marked by the physician with an indelible marker. Once the procedure, patient identity, site, and side have been confirmed, sedation can be initiated and the procedure commenced.

Documentation

Documentation can be both a sword and a shield. There is an old saying, "if it has not been documented, it was not done." Poor, sparse, late, or inaccurate documentation can subject a urologist, who has actually provided reasonable and appropriate patient care, to significant liability. Accurate, timely, and factual documentation can protect the urologist and may even prevent a medical malpractice lawsuit. Documentation must also reflect all of the information which justifies the diagnosis and the proposed procedure. Any communication with or from the patient, including written correspondence, e-mail, voice mail, text messages, and telephone calls must be incorporated into the patient's medical record. Documentation of such communication must include the date, time, name of the caller or patient, complaint, and gist of the advice or response. Test and procedure results, prior treating physicians' records, consultation reports, consent forms, and progress notes are also important parts of the patient's medical record.

Documentation must be contemporaneous and must *never* be altered after the fact. Alteration of medical records may result in charges of professional misconduct and criminal or civil charges since medical records are considered business records in many areas. If a change or correction is required, it should be done via an addendum. However, an addendum should only be placed in the record when the information is relevant to the patient's future care and is written within 24–48 hours after the care was rendered. After that, addenda often appear self-serving or are not credible. Addenda must be placed after the most recent note, labeled as an addition to the record, dated with the date the addition is actually written, and reference the note which the new information is intended to clarify. Finally, documentation must not include humor or derogatory remarks about the patient, a staff member, or another health care professional. The patient or his/her legal representative is generally entitled to obtain a complete copy of the medical record. Humorous or derogatory comments can be an embarrassment to the physician when the records are viewed by the patient. They are also unprofessional and can provoke the anger of a jury. Use of personal abbreviations is also discouraged, since it may be difficult to remember the meaning of the abbreviation(s) months or years later when a lawsuit is commenced or goes to trial. A patient's medical record must be retained for the appropriate time period required by law. If either the entire record or any portion of it is lost, the physician's defense of a lawsuit may be compromised.

[8]Novello MD, Antonia C et al. New York State Surgical and Invasive Procedure Protocol for Hospitals, Diagnostic and Treatment Centers, Ambulatory Surgery Centers and Individual Practitioners, New York State Department of Health, Office of Health Systems Management, Division of Primary and Acute Care Services, September 2006. Joint Commission on Accreditation of Healthcare Organizations: 2009 Hospital, Accreditation Standards, pp. 245 – 249.

Communication

The physician/patient relationship is based upon effective communication as much as surgical skills. However, the need for complete, accurate, and timely communication is not limited to the physician/patient relationship. It is equally important to have effective communication with covering physicians, consultants, and referring physicians. Documentation of these communications is essential. The transfer of care to a covering physician is an area of high risk since patients frequently develop problems when the treating urologist is not on call or out of town. Thus, a formal hand-off/referral mechanism between the treating and covering urologists is important. The covering urologist should receive the same type and depth of information he/she would provide to others. Appropriate "hand-offs" help decrease errors and improve patient care.

When a patient is referred to a consultant, or for a diagnostic test, the referring urologist must communicate all relevant information so that the consultations and/or tests are appropriate for the patient's condition. However, it is not sufficient to simply refer the patient. A tickler system must be in place in the urologist's office to confirm that the patient has been compliant with the referral, that a report was received, and that the results were communicated to the patient. If a patient's results are abnormal, the consultant, radiologist, or laboratory should contact the urologist, to prevent delays in the patient's future care. When test and/or consultation results are received, the urologist should initial and date the report, indicating that the results have been reviewed. The urologist must then contact the patient, either by telephone or mail, to advise the patient of the results, discuss necessary treatment, and schedule a follow-up appointment with the patient.

Another important aspect of communication occurs both before and after a procedure is performed. The nursing staff, at the direction of the urologist, must provide appropriate pre-procedure education to the patient and confirm that the patient understands the instructions. For instance, if the patient requires someone to drive him/her home after a procedure involving the use of sedation or anesthesia, this must be made clear prior to the day of the procedure. Patients who insist upon driving home, despite offers of alternative transportation, face serious risks. The patient's failure to comply with these instructions and any offer of alternative transportation must be documented in the medical record. Pre-procedure instructions must also be documented. After the procedure, nursing staff, in conjunction with the urologist, must again review the discharge instructions with the patient and/or family members who have accompanied the patient to the procedure, to promote proper care of the patient after discharge. Discharge instructions must provide the patient with information about what to expect in the next few days or weeks, highlight signs and symptoms of complications, and describe required follow-up care, including dates and times of appointments scheduled with the urologist. Contact information for emergency care must be provided. The patient should be told to seek care promptly at the Emergency Department if serious symptoms such as excessive pain or bleeding develop. All discharge instructions must be documented in the medical record.

The Noncompliant Patient

The noncompliant patient presents serious legal jeopardy for urologists. Noncompliance includes failure to keep appointments with both the urologist and specialists to whom the patient is referred and failure to undergo ordered tests. Noncompliant patients may be very nice people but can be very dangerous legally since they do not accept responsibility for their own care. If a patient misses a scheduled appointment, it is very important to document both the missed appointment and any attempts to contact the patient to reschedule the appointment. Sometimes, the patient's reason for noncompliance is readily resolvable (e.g., fear, cultural, emotional, or language obstacles), and the physician can work with the patient to achieve the desired result. However, if a pattern of missed appointments and failure to comply with the proposed treatment plan becomes apparent, the patient should be discharged from the practice, as long as the patient's condition is not urgent, emergent, or does not require continuous care without interruption. All efforts to follow up with these patients must be carefully documented in the patient's medical record.

The Difficult Patient

Every physician deals with difficult patients. Some patients seek narcotics or are actually impaired by drugs or otherwise intoxicated. Patients and/or family members may be rude, hostile, abusive, or threatening to physicians or staff. If the threat appears serious, and realistic, a call to the police might be necessary. Incredibly, some patients wish to continue to see the urologist while simultaneously lodging complaints about their care to the urologist, his/her staff, hospitals, insurers, or government agencies or after commencing malpractice litigation. Patients may threaten to sue the urologist, fail to pay their bills, or even act in a seductive manner toward the physician or staff. Whatever the reason, any one of these difficulties may make the urologist uncomfortable in continuing to treat the patient. When the physician has exhausted reasonable methods to stop this behavior (e.g., pain contracts, warning letters, speaking to the patient/family members, using chaperones), he/she should strongly consider discharging the patient from care after considering several important factors.

If the patient has an urgent or emergent condition or a condition that requires continuous care without interruption, discharge may not be possible, unless another urologist is available immediately and willing to provide care to the patient. The transition must be seamless for patients who require continuous care. Thus, if other providers refuse to assume care or a provider is not available to treat the patient within a reasonable geographic distance, discharge may not be possible. When this occurs, the best course is continuous documentation of the patient's behavior, condition, and failure to comply with the treatment plan as well as written warnings to the patient of the risks associated with failure to comply.

When discharging a patient, a letter should be sent to the patient stating that the patient has been discharged as of the date of the letter, but that the urologist will provide emergency care *only* for 30 days (or longer, if appropriate). The patient should be referred to generic resources such as hospitals or local medical or urological societies to obtain the names of other competent urologists. The reason for discharge should be stated, e.g., there has been a serious disruption of the doctor/patient relationship, failure to keep scheduled appointments and comply with recommendations for treatment, or failure to pay for professional services provided. These reasons, although general, are specific enough for the patient to understand why he/she has been discharged. The letter should be nonconfrontational and not contain a litany of the patient's bad behavior. Finally, an authorization for release of medical records should be sent with the letter to facilitate transfer of records to the new urology practice. The letter should either be hand delivered or mailed, using a method which provides proof of mailing and confirms that the patient has received the letter. When a patient is discharged from care, all future appointments must be canceled and the office staff advised NOT to give the patient another appointment. Computer alerts can be helpful to remind the staff. However, if the urologist is on call for a hospital's Emergency Department and is called to attend the patient in the Emergency Department, the urologist MUST respond to the Emergency Department even if the patient has been discharged by his/her office. In the United States, failure to respond to the Emergency Department under these circumstances could result in an EMTALA violation.[9]

Use of Chaperones

Allegations of inappropriate sexual misconduct against physicians appear to be increasing. The best way to prevent unwanted negative consequences (i.e., publicity, potential criminal and/or civil liability, and licensure actions) is to use chaperones at all times. The chaperone should be a nurse or medical assistant rather than a relative

[9] 42 C.F.R. § (Section) 489.20(r)(2) and 489.24(j).

of the patient. The chaperone's initials, date, time, and the phrase "present during the entire examination" must be documented. If a patient is sexually inappropriate at or outside the office, or writes suggestive letters, the patient should be promptly discharged. A chaperone must then be present at any future visits, until the patient has received the discharge letter.

Confidentiality

Breaches of confidentiality and privacy are regularly in the news. Stories abound about unauthorized access to the medical records of famous people, discussions about patients in public areas with other professionals or friends, and inappropriate use of social media to discuss confidential issues. Yet the overriding reality is that the health information provided to a physician in the course of assessment, care, and treatment is and must remain confidential, unless the patient authorizes release to a third party. Many countries regulate the release and retention of medical records and protected health information. In the United States, compliance with these laws and rules is mandatory. When a breach of confidentiality occurs, a patient may commence a lawsuit or file a complaint with a government agency. The complaint may trigger an investigation and potential financial penalties, in addition to a potential malpractice verdict.

Disclosure of an Unanticipated Result or Adverse Event

When an unanticipated result, complication, or adverse medical error occurs during or as a result of a procedure, transparent communication with the patient is critical. An assessment must be made both of the patient's condition and the level of understanding of the patient and/or family. The patient may lack capacity, or the family may be in shock or grieving. The patient and/or family may also have educational or literacy deficits or cultural differences. Only information which can initially be absorbed should be presented, using professional interpreters, if necessary. The use of layman's terms to explain the occurrence is strongly recommended.

Rather than avoiding the patient/family, the urologist should meet with them as soon as possible. The conversation should be brief, but caring and sincere, since patients and families need time to absorb information. The urologist should sit down at the patient's eye level. The initial statement should be: "We performed this procedure after we gave you complete information about the procedure and obtained your permission. We anticipated X. The result was Y." It is appropriate to apologize for the occurrence of this outcome, but the urologist should NOT say that he/she is sorry he/she *caused* this to happen. Such admissions may later be used in a legal proceeding and be evidence of an admission against the physician's interests. Blame is also inappropriate and can be legally dangerous. When speaking with the patient and/or family, the urologist should only state that the situation will be investigated to determine how and why it occurred and answer questions based only on the facts known at the time. This includes information about the current diagnosis, prognosis, and further treatment needed, if known. The urologist should also indicate that when more definitive information is available, it will be provided. Speculation about the cause or facts of an event before an investigation or review has been completed can be inaccurate and thus unnecessarily damaging. What may appear to be a particular individual's fault may actually be due to a faulty process, a result occurring in the absence of negligence, or a known complication disclosed to the patient prior to the procedure. Communication with the patient and/or family should be continued, if the patient's condition permits. However, no guarantees or promises should be made regarding the patient's prognosis. Finally, all conversations with the patient and/or family after an unanticipated or adverse outcome must be well documented in the patient's record. If the patient has died, flowers or a sympathy card may be sent. The physician may also decide to attend the patient's funeral. This depends on the urologist's comfort level, the attitude of the family, and whether there has been a long-term relationship with the patient and family.

How to Respond to Written Complaints from the Patient or Other Individuals

When a physician receives a written complaint from a patient about the quality of care provided, it should never be ignored. Rather, the physician should send a carefully worded response. The response should acknowledge receipt of the complaint and state that the physician will investigate the matter and that he/she will contact the patient after the review is completed. The letter must be in plain English, factual without being defensive or argumentative, and use no medical or technical jargon.

The investigation should consist of staff interviews, if relevant, and a thorough review of the entire medical record. When the investigation is concluded, a letter should be sent to the patient addressing each complaint or allegation (if more than one) in a factual manner from the information documented in the medical record. The letter should also state whether miscommunication was involved or if office policy and procedure changes or staff counseling and education were indicated as a result of the review. However, admissions or speculation about liability are not recommended. A statement such as, "I am sorry you were so unhappy with your care" is appropriate. This acknowledges the patient's anger without admitting liability. The physician should also thank the patient for bringing these concern(s) to his/her attention, in order to improve the quality of care the practice provides to patients. Be mindful that complaints by someone *other* than the patient (e.g., family members or the Better Business Bureau) should be answered *only* if the patient has previously authorized release of confidential medical information to that third party in writing. The complaint letter and a copy of the response should be included in the patient's medical record. If the doctor/patient relationship has been seriously disrupted by the complaints, this may be a reasonable basis for discharging the patient from care.

If the complaint was verbal rather than written, the person best equipped to handle the complaint should call the patient after the complaint has been investigated. The timing of this call is also important. If the complaint is about the quality of care, the physician should respond and do so at a time when he/she will not be interrupted. Should the patient become angry or abusive during the conversation, the urologist can politely advise the patient that the conversation will be continued at a later date, when the patient is able to calmly resume the discussion. When the conversation has been satisfactorily completed, the urologist must document the date, time, and contents of the discussion. If the patient appeared satisfied with the response, or the conversation was prematurely discontinued due to the nature of the patient's response, this should also be recorded.

There are many potential medical and legal pitfalls in the practice of endourology. However, when faced with liability and/or legal risks, or an adverse action against one's medical license, the implementation of the risk management principles reviewed here may make a substantial positive difference in the outcome of such actions.

Index

A.M. Al-Kandari et al. (eds.), *Difficult Cases in Endourology*,
DOI 10.1007/978-1-84882-083-8, © Springer-Verlag London 2013

MIX
Papier aus verantwortungsvollen Quellen
Paper from responsible sources
FSC® C105338

If you have any concerns about our products,
you can contact us on
ProductSafety@springernature.com

In case Publisher is established outside the EU,
the EU authorized representative is:
Springer Nature Customer Service Center GmbH
Europaplatz 3, 69115 Heidelberg, Germany

Printed by Libri Plureos GmbH
in Hamburg, Germany